中医临床护理学

（双语版）

主　编　周　洁　涂宇明

副主编　谌志远　刘永芬

主　审　陈　骥　刘建军

上海大学出版社

·上海·

图书在版编目（CIP）数据

中医临床护理学：汉文、英文／周洁，涂宇明主编.
上海：上海大学出版社，2024. 12. -- ISBN 978-7
-5671-5098-0

Ⅰ. R248

中国国家版本馆 CIP 数据核字第 2024BW6936 号

责任编辑　高亚雪
封面设计　缪炎栩
技术编辑　金　鑫　钱宇坤

中医临床护理学（双语版）
周　洁　涂宇明　主编
上海大学出版社出版发行
（上海市上大路 99 号　邮政编码 200444）
（https://www.shupress.cn　发行热线 021 - 66135112）
出版人　余　洋

*

南京展望文化发展有限公司排版
江苏凤凰数码印务有限公司印刷　各地新华书店经销
开本 889mm×1194mm　1/16　印张 25.5　字数 630 千
2024 年 12 月第 1 版　2024 年 12 月第 1 次印刷
ISBN 978 - 7 - 5671 - 5098 - 0/R · 83　定价　85.00 元

《中医临床护理学》（双语版）编委会

主　编

周　洁（江西中医药大学）

涂宇明（江西中医药大学）

副主编

谌志远（江西中医药大学）

刘永芬（江西中医药大学）

主　审

陈　骥（成都中医药大学）

刘建军（江西中医药大学）

编　委

（以姓氏笔画为序）

万　琦（江西中医药大学）

皮冬平（江西中医药大学）

刘佳鑫（江西中医药大学）

钟　琴（江西中医药大学）

涂　延（江西中医药大学）

黄依琴（江西中医药大学）

康林之（江西中医药大学）

章　晓（江西中医药大学）

熊　展（江西中医药大学）

编 写 说 明

  本教材是在"健康中国"新形势下,为满足人民群众健康需求,培养适应行业发展要求的高素质应用型护理专业人才,更好地满足从事临床护理工作的需要,以护理专业培养目标为导向,以"三基""五性"为原则而编写的特色教材。为促进中医临床护理学独特的学术理论和丰富的护理方法走向世界,我们在参阅大量文献资料的基础上,编成此书。

  本教材不仅可以作为医学院校护理专业师生的教学及学习用书,还可以作为护士在临床进行中医护理的参考书。

  中医临床护理学是高等医学院校护理专业的一门临床必修课。本教材共有四章,内容包括内科、外科、妇科、儿科25种常见疾病的、具有中医特色的护理。每种疾病包括病因病机、常见证型和护理措施三部分。在护理措施中,对于病情观察、生活起居护理、饮食护理、情志护理、用药护理、中医护理操作技术和健康教育进行了详细的论述。

  本教材的中文编写组成员是周洁、刘永芬、康林之、黄依琴、万琦、钟琴、刘佳鑫、章晓,英文编写组成员是涂宇明、谌志远、涂延、熊展、周洁、皮冬平。本书在编写过程中得到上海大学出版社和江西中医药大学教务处的大力支持和热情帮助。诚挚感谢江西中医药大学刘建军教授和成都中医药大学陈骥教授对教材内容的审定。诚挚感谢在本书编写过程中给予悉心指导的专家学者:上海师范大学李照国教授、浙江中医药大学扈李娟老师、中南大学湘雅三医院主管护师肖静,以及江西中医药大学聂晶教授、丁成华教授、钟凌云教授、程绍民教授。

  编写中医汉英双语教材是一项繁重的工作,全体编者都以高度认真、负责的态度参与了工作,但不当之处在所难免,恳请读者提出宝贵意见,我们将在今后的教学和临床实践中不断总结经验,以祈纠偏正误。

《中医临床护理学》(双语版)编委会

2024 年 8 月

Note for Compilation

This textbook is intended for training high-caliber nursing professionals capable of providing clinical care, adapting to the evolving demands of the industry, meeting the public's healthcare needs under the Healthy China Initiative. It is aimed at cultivating nursing majors and highlighting the basic theories, essential knowledge and fundamental skills of TCM that is ideologically correct, scientific, advanced, inspiring and practical. To internationalize the unique academic theories of clinical nursing of traditional Chinese medicine (CNTCM) and its rich variety of nursing techniques, we have compiled this book after referring to extensive literature.

This book can be used as a coursebook for nursing students and teachers in medical colleges or serves as a reference for TCM clinical care.

Clinical nursing of traditional Chinese medicine (CNTCM) is a compulsory clinical course for nursing majors. This textbook consists of four chapters, elaborating on 25 diseases in internal medicine, external medicine, gynecology and pediatrics, for which TCM provides unique and advantageous clinical care. The description of each disease comprises three sections: etiology and pathogenesis, common syndrome types and nursing measures. In nursing measures, observation of the condition, daily nursing, diet nursing, emotion nursing, medication nursing, manipulation techniques, and patient education are elaborated.

The Chinese sections of the book are compiled by Zhou Jie, Liu Yongfen, Kang Linzhi, Huang Yiqin, Wan Qi, Zhong Qin, Liu Jiaxin and Zhang Xiao and the English sections by Tu Yuming, Chen Zhiyuan, Tu Yan, Xiong Zhan, Zhou Jie and Pi Dongping. Special thanks go to Shanghai University Press and the office of academic affairs of Jiangxi University of Chinese Medicine for their support and assistance. We fare deeply

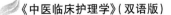

indebted to Professor Liu Jianjun and Professor Chen Ji for their review of the book. Sincere gratitude goes to the experts and scholars who provided invaluable insight and guidance during the writing process of this book: Professor Li Zhaoguo, Shanghai Normal University; Lecturer Hu Lijuan, Zhejiang Chinese Medical University; Head Nurse Xiao Jing, the Third Xiangya Hospital of Central South University; Professor Nie Jing, Professor Ding Chenghua, Professor Zhong lingyun and Professor Cheng Shaomin, Jiangxi University of Chinese Medicine.

Compiling a TCM textbook in both Chinese and English is strenuous work. Despite all the authors' devotion and diligence, mistakes are inevitable. We look forward to the valuable suggestions from readers as we continually learn from classroom instruction and clinical practice in an effort to further improve the book in the future.

Editorial Board of *Clinical Nursing in Traditional Chinese Medicine*

（Chinese-English Version）

August, 2024

目　　录

绪　论 ……………………………………………………………………………… 1

第一章　内科病证的中医护理　　　　　　　　　　　　　　　　　6

第一节　感冒 …………………………………………………………………… 9
　　一、病因病机 …………………………………………………………… 9
　　二、常见证型 …………………………………………………………… 9
　　三、护理措施 …………………………………………………………… 10

第二节　咳嗽病 ………………………………………………………………… 23
　　一、病因病机 …………………………………………………………… 23
　　二、常见证型 …………………………………………………………… 23
　　三、护理措施 …………………………………………………………… 25

第三节　哮病 …………………………………………………………………… 42
　　一、病因病机 …………………………………………………………… 42
　　二、常见证型 …………………………………………………………… 42
　　三、护理措施 …………………………………………………………… 44

第四节　喘病 …………………………………………………………………… 56
　　一、病因病机 …………………………………………………………… 56
　　二、常见证型 …………………………………………………………… 56
　　三、护理措施 …………………………………………………………… 59

第五节　心悸 …………………………………………………………………… 76
　　一、病因病机 …………………………………………………………… 76
　　二、常见证型 …………………………………………………………… 76
　　三、护理措施 …………………………………………………………… 78

第六节　胸痹 …………………………………………………………………… 93
　　一、病因病机 …………………………………………………………… 93

二、常见证型 …………………………………………………………………… 93
三、护理措施 …………………………………………………………………… 95

第七节　中风 ……………………………………………………………………… 109
一、病因病机 …………………………………………………………………… 109
二、常见证型 …………………………………………………………………… 109
三、护理措施 …………………………………………………………………… 111

第八节　呕吐 ……………………………………………………………………… 131
一、病因病机 …………………………………………………………………… 131
二、常见证型 …………………………………………………………………… 131
三、护理措施 …………………………………………………………………… 133

第九节　胃脘痛 …………………………………………………………………… 145
一、病因病机 …………………………………………………………………… 145
二、常见证型 …………………………………………………………………… 145
三、护理措施 …………………………………………………………………… 147

第十节　泄泻病 …………………………………………………………………… 164
一、病因病机 …………………………………………………………………… 164
二、常见证型 …………………………………………………………………… 164
三、护理措施 …………………………………………………………………… 166

第十一节　黄疸 …………………………………………………………………… 180
一、病因病机 …………………………………………………………………… 180
二、常见证型 …………………………………………………………………… 180
三、护理措施 …………………………………………………………………… 182

第十二节　水肿 …………………………………………………………………… 196
一、病因病机 …………………………………………………………………… 196
二、常见证型 …………………………………………………………………… 196
三、护理措施 …………………………………………………………………… 198

第十三节　消渴 …………………………………………………………………… 216
一、病因病机 …………………………………………………………………… 216
二、常见证型 …………………………………………………………………… 216
三、护理措施 …………………………………………………………………… 218

第二章　外科病证的中医护理　　　　　　　　　　　230

第一节　丹毒 ……………………………………………………………………… 235
一、病因病机 …………………………………………………………………… 235
二、常见证型 …………………………………………………………………… 235
三、护理措施 …………………………………………………………………… 236

第二节　湿疮 ……………………………………………………… 246

一、病因病机 ……………………………………………………… 246

二、常见证型 ……………………………………………………… 246

三、护理措施 ……………………………………………………… 247

第三节　蛇串疮 …………………………………………………… 256

一、病因病机 ……………………………………………………… 256

二、常见证型 ……………………………………………………… 256

三、护理措施 ……………………………………………………… 257

第四节　痔疮 ……………………………………………………… 266

一、病因病机 ……………………………………………………… 266

二、常见证型 ……………………………………………………… 266

三、护理措施 ……………………………………………………… 267

第三章　妇科病证的中医护理　　　　　　　　　278

第一节　月经先期、月经后期、月经先后不定期 ………………… 282

一、病因病机 ……………………………………………………… 282

二、常见证型 ……………………………………………………… 282

三、护理措施 ……………………………………………………… 284

第二节　痛经 ……………………………………………………… 298

一、病因病机 ……………………………………………………… 298

二、常见证型 ……………………………………………………… 298

三、护理措施 ……………………………………………………… 300

第三节　胎动不安 ………………………………………………… 311

一、病因病机 ……………………………………………………… 311

二、常见证型 ……………………………………………………… 311

三、护理措施 ……………………………………………………… 312

第四节　产后恶露不绝 …………………………………………… 322

一、病因病机 ……………………………………………………… 322

二、常见证型 ……………………………………………………… 322

三、护理措施 ……………………………………………………… 323

第四章　儿科病证的中医护理　　　　　　　　　330

第一节　肺炎喘嗽 ………………………………………………… 334

一、病因病机 ……………………………………………………… 334

二、常见证型 ……………………………………………………… 334

三、护理措施 ……………………………………………………… 336

第二节　积滞 ……………………………………………………… 354
　　一、病因病机 ………………………………………………… 354
　　二、常见证型 ………………………………………………… 354
　　三、护理措施 ………………………………………………… 355

第三节　水痘 ……………………………………………………… 365
　　一、病因病机 ………………………………………………… 365
　　二、常见证型 ………………………………………………… 365
　　三、护理措施 ………………………………………………… 366

第四节　手足口病 ………………………………………………… 378
　　一、病因病机 ………………………………………………… 378
　　二、常见证型 ………………………………………………… 378
　　三、护理措施 ………………………………………………… 379

参考文献 　　　　　　　　　　　　　　　　　　　　　　389

Contents

Introduction   **3**

Chapter 1   Nursing of Internal Diseases   **7**

Section 1   Common Cold ·· 14
   ETIOLOGY AND PATHOGENESIS ··································· 14
   COMMON SYNDROMES ··· 14
   NURSING MEASURES ·· 17

Section 2   Cough ·· 30
   ETIOLOGY AND PATHOGENESIS ··································· 30
   COMMON SYNDROMES ··· 31
   NURSING MEASURES ·· 35

Section 3   Wheezing ··· 47
   ETIOLOGY AND PATHOGENESIS ··································· 47
   COMMON SYNDROMES ··· 47
   NURSING MEASURES ·· 50

Section 4   Dyspnea ·· 63
   ETIOLOGY AND PATHOGENESIS ··································· 63
   COMMON SYNDROMES ··· 64
   NURSING MEASURES ·· 68

Section 5   Palpitation ··· 82
   ETIOLOGY AND PATHOGENESIS ··································· 82
   COMMON SYNDROMES ··· 83
   NURSING MEASURES ·· 86

Section 6   Chest Impediment ··· 99
   ETIOLOGY AND PATHOGENESIS ··································· 99

COMMON SYNDROMES ·· 100

NURSING MEASURES ·· 103

Section 7　Wind Stroke ·· 117

ETIOLOGY AND PATHOGENESIS ···································· 117

COMMON SYNDROMES ·· 118

NURSING MEASURES ·· 121

Section 8　Vomiting ·· 136

ETIOLOGY AND PATHOGENESIS ···································· 136

COMMON SYNDROMES ·· 136

NURSING MEASURES ·· 139

Section 9　Epigastric Pain ·· 152

ETIOLOGY AND PATHOGENESIS ···································· 152

COMMON SYNDROMES ·· 153

NURSING MEASURES ·· 156

Section 10　Diarrhea ··· 170

ETIOLOGY AND PATHOGENESIS ···································· 170

COMMON SYNDROMES ·· 171

NURSING MEASURES ·· 174

Section 11　Jaundice ··· 186

ETIOLOGY AND PATHOGENESIS ···································· 186

COMMON SYNDROMES ·· 187

NURSING MEASURES ·· 189

Section 12　Edema ·· 203

ETIOLOGY AND PATHOGENESIS ···································· 203

COMMON SYNDROMES ·· 204

NURSING MEASURES ·· 207

Section 13　Wasting-Thirst ·· 221

ETIOLOGY AND PATHOGENESIS ···································· 221

COMMON SYNDROMES ·· 221

NURSING MEASURES ·· 224

Chapter 2　Nursing of External Diseases　232

Section 1　Erysipelas ··· 239

ETIOLOGY AND PATHOGENESIS ···································· 239

COMMON SYNDROMES ·· 239

NURSING MEASURES ·· 241

Section 2   Eczema ·· 250

ETIOLOGY AND PATHOGENESIS ······················· 250

COMMON SYNDROMES ······························· 250

NURSING MEASURES ································· 252

Section 3   Herpes Zoster ···································· 260

ETIOLOGY AND PATHOGENESIS ······················· 260

COMMON SYNDROMES ······························· 260

NURSING MEASURES ································· 262

Section 4   Hemorrhoids ····································· 270

ETIOLOGY AND PATHOGENESIS ······················· 270

COMMON SYNDROMES ······························· 270

NURSING MEASURES ································· 272

Chapter 3   Nursing of Gynecological Diseases   280

Section 1   Early Menstruation, Delayed Menstruation, and Irregular

Menstrual Cycle ································· 288

ETIOLOGY AND PATHOGENESIS ······················· 288

COMMON SYNDROMES ······························· 289

NURSING MEASURES ································· 293

Section 2   Dysmenorrhea ···································· 303

ETIOLOGY AND PATHOGENESIS ······················· 303

COMMON SYNDROMES ······························· 304

NURSING MEASURES ································· 306

Section 3   Threatened Abortion ······························ 315

ETIOLOGY AND PATHOGENESIS ······················· 315

COMMON SYNDROMES ······························· 316

NURSING MEASURES ································· 318

Section 4   Postpartum Lochiorrhea ··························· 325

ETIOLOGY AND PATHOGENESIS ······················· 325

COMMON SYNDROMES ······························· 326

NURSING MEASURES ································· 327

Chapter 4   Nursing of Pediatric Diseases   332

Section 1   Pneumonia with Dyspnea and Cough ················· 341

ETIOLOGY AND PATHOGENESIS ······················· 341

COMMON SYNDROMES 341

NURSING MEASURES 345

Section 2　Food Accumulation 358

ETIOLOGY AND PATHOGENESIS 358

COMMON SYNDROMES 358

NURSING MEASURES 360

Section 3　Chickenpox 370

ETIOLOGY AND PATHOGENESIS 370

COMMON SYNDROMES 371

NURSING MEASURES 373

Section 4　Hand-Foot-Mouth Disease 382

ETIOLOGY AND PATHOGENESIS 382

COMMON SYNDROMES 382

NURSING MEASURES 385

绪　　论

　　中医临床护理学，是指在中医理论体系指导下，基于整体观念，应用辨证施护的方法、传统的护理技术，系统阐述各专科病证的预防、保健、康复和护理的一门学科。中医临床护理学是中医学的重要组成部分，是中医护理知识与技能在临床各科中的具体实践。

　　中医临床护理学以辨证施护为核心，研究内、外、妇、儿各科常见病证的概念、临床特征、病因、病机、诊断、辨证要点、证候分型、护治原则、护理措施和健康教育等内容。其中护理措施包括病情观察、生活起居护理、饮食护理、情志护理、用药护理和中医护理操作技术等内容。

　　古代的中医身兼医生、药师、护士等数职。中医护理知识通常被记载为调理、调养、调慎、侍疾、扶持等内容，分布于历代医学文献中。

　　早在3 000多年前，商代（约公元前1600年至公元前1046年）的甲骨文中就有关于疾病和医药卫生的记载。在周代（公元前1046年至公元前256年），医学有了分科。当时，人们用除虫、灭鼠等方法改善环境卫生，进行防病调护。春秋时期（公元前770年至公元前476年），人们认识到顺应四时气候能预防疾病。

　　《黄帝内经》约成书于战国时期（公元前475年至公元前221年），该书以整体观念为特点，奠定了中医临床护理学的理论基础。书中记载了病情观察、生活起居护理、饮食护理、情志护理、用药护理等内容，包括艾灸、推拿、砭石等中医护理操作技术。华佗（约公元145年至208年）创编了"五禽戏"，首次提出用体育锻炼进行防病调护。《神农本草经》成书于东汉末年（约公元200年），记述了四气五味等中药学理论，对饮食护理和用药护理产生了重要影响。张仲景的《伤寒杂病论》与之成书年代相近（公元200年至210年）。《伤寒杂病论》提出了辨证论治理论，创立了六经辨证、脏腑辨证，提出了中医护理"八法"，即汗、吐、下、和、温、清、消、补。该书涉及用药护理、饮食护理等内容，列举了汤、丸、散、酒、洗、浴、熏、滴、灌、吹等剂型。

　　王叔和的《脉经》成书于西晋初期（约公元3世纪）。《脉经》规范了脉学理论，把脉象归纳为24种，将脉象、症状、护理相结合，为病情观察提供了理论依据。隋大业六年（公元610年），巢元方编著《诸病源候论》。书中描述了各种疾病的病因、病机、症状、诊断、预后和护理等内容，论及小儿的喂养和调护。在公元7世纪的唐代，孙思邈在《备急千金要方》与《千金翼方》中强调了医德的重要性，提出医治应以预防为主。书中首创葱管导尿术，详细描述了换药术等操作技术，记载了水井消毒、空气消毒的方法，提到了饮食疗法和情志护理的重要性。

　　北宋宣和元年（公元1119年），钱乙所著的《小儿药证直诀》开创性地论述了小儿的生理病理特点和小儿常见病的辨证论治。南宋嘉熙元年(公元 1237 年),陈自明所著的《妇人大全良方》详细记载了妇科的常见病和孕产期的护理。金元时期(公元 1115 年至 1368 年),"金元四大家"对于内科疾病诊治的贡献格外突出:李东垣在《脾胃论》中详细论述了脾胃内伤疾病的生活起居护理、饮食护理和情志护理;朱丹溪倡导"养生""节欲",为生活起居护理提供了理论依据;张子和的攻下学说和刘河间的清热学说,至今仍在中医临床护理中广泛使用。

明万历十八年(公元 1590 年),李时珍在《本草纲目》中提出传染病病人的衣被可用蒸汽进行消毒。公元 17 世纪的明末清初,王肯堂所著的《女科证治准绳》和傅青主所著的《傅青主女科》详尽论述了妇产科疾病,对后世影响深远。明万历四十五年(公元 1617 年),陈实功的《外科正宗》记载了外科疾病的调护方法。清乾隆十五年(公元 1750 年),陈复正的《幼幼集成》提出了对小儿保育、儿科杂病调治护理的独到见解。公元 17 至 18 世纪,明代张景岳的《景岳全书》和清代吴谦的《医宗金鉴》等书中都包含丰富的中医临床护理学内容。

1956 年,南京中医学院附属卫校开设了中医护理专业。1984 年,中华护理学会中医、中西医结合护理学术委员会成立,中医护理学正式成为独立学科。2013 年,世界中医药学会联合会护理专业委员会成立,中医护理的国际交流与合作日益加深。时至今日,很多中医医院都开设了中医护理专科门诊,取得了良好的社会效益和经济效益。

Introduction

Clinical nursing of traditional Chinese medicine (CNTCM) is a discipline under the guidance of traditional Chinese medicine (TCM) that utilizes a holistic approach and traditional nursing techniques to provide syndrome-based nursing. It systematically describes the prevention, treatment, rehabilitation and nursing of various diseases. It is an integral component of TCM and applies nursing theories and skills of TCM in clinical practice.

CNTCM focuses on overall analysis of the illness and the patient's condition, and studies the concepts, clinical features, etiology, pathogenesis, diagnoses, syndrome differentiation, common syndromes, nursing principles, nursing measures and patient education of common diseases in internal medicine of TCM, external medicine of TCM, gynecology of TCM, and pediatrics of TCM. Nursing measures include observation of conditions, daily life nursing, diet nursing, emotion nursing, medication nursing and manipulation techniques.

Ancient doctors played multiple roles as a doctor, a pharmacist and a nurse, so that knowledge about CNTCM was interpreted in medical literature down the ages with different names such as *tiao li*, *tiao yang*, *tiao shen*, *shi ji*, *fu chi*, etc. Although the names are different, their essence of nursing and recuperation is the same.

As early as three thousand years ago, records on diseases, medicine and health were found on oracle scripts from the Shang Dynasty (around 1600 B.C. to 1046 B.C.). During the Zhou Dynasty (from 1046 B.C. to 256 B.C.), medicine became divided into various branches. People killed insects and rats to prevent diseases and enhance nursing while improving environmental hygiene. In the Spring and Autumn Period (from 770 B.C. to 476 B.C.), the fact that compliance with the seasonal climate helped prevent illness was generally appreciated.

In the Warring States Period (475 B.C. to 221 B.C.), *Huangdi's Internal Classic* was completed. This book laid the theoretical foundation for CNTCM, characterized with holism. It recorded observation of disease conditions, daily life nursing, diet nursing, emotion nursing, medication nursing and manipulation techniques such as moxibustion, tuina, and bian stone used in acupuncture. Hua Tuo (from 145 A.D. to 208 A.D.) created *five mimic-animal exercise* and was the first to propose the idea of preventing diseases and enhancing nursing through physical exercise. *Shennong's Classic of Materia*

Medica, written in the late Eastern Han Dynasty (about 200 A.D.) summarized the theories in Chinese Materia Medica, such as four properties and five flavors, exerting far-reaching impact on later generations. Zhang Zhongjing's *Treatise on Cold Damage and Miscellaneous Diseases*, finished between 200 A.D. and 210 A.D., proposed the theory of syndrome differentiation, including six-meridian syndrome differentiation and visceral syndrome differentiation, and eight nursing methods, i.e., diaphoresis, emesis, purging, harmonizing, warming, heat-clearing, tonifying and dispersing. It focused on medication and diet nursing approaches and listed dosage forms such as decoction, pills (boluses), powder, lotion, drop, fumigation, insufflation, filling agent, wine preparation, bath preparation, etc.

Pulse Classic was written by Wang Shuhe in the early Western Jin Dynasty (about the third century A.D.). This book standardized theories of sphygmology by dividing pulse conditions into 24 categories and integrating pulse manifestations and symptoms with nursing, thereby providing the basis for observation of disease conditions in CNTCM. *Treatise on Causes and Manifestations of Various Diseases*, completed by Chao Yuanfang in the sixth year of the Daye reign of the Sui Dynasty (610 A.D.), described the etiology, pathogenesis, symptoms, diagnosis, prognosis, and nursing of various diseases, and discussed the feeding and nursing of children. In the Tang Dynasty in the seventh century, Sun Simiao articulated the importance of medical ethics and nursing for the prevention of diseases in *Essential Prescriptions Worth a Thousand Gold for Emergencies* and *Supplement to Prescriptions Worth a Thousand Gold Pieces*. In these two books he also recorded formulas and medicines for sterilizing wells and the air, creatively used scallion tubes for urinary catheterization, elaborated on nursing manipulation techniques like changing dressings, and pointed out the significance of diet and emotion nursing.

In 1119, the first year of the Xuanhe reign in the Northern Song Dynasty, Qian Yi pioneered the description of pediatric physiological features and syndrome-based nursing of common diseases in his book *Key to Medicines and Patterns of Children's Diseases*. In 1237, the first year of the Jiaxi reign in the Southern Song Dynasty, Chen Ziming elaborated on the nursing of patients with common gynecological diseases and maternity nursing in his book, *Complete Collection of Effective Prescriptions for Women's Diseases*. In the Jin and Yuan Dynasties between 1115 and 1368, four medical experts in the Jin and Yuan Dynasties contributed enormously to diagnosis and treatment of diseases in internal medicine. Li Dongyuan elaborated on daily, diet and emotion nursing for spleen and stomach internal injury diseases. Zhu Danxi promoted "health preservation" and "restraining desires", laying theoretical foundation for daily life nursing. The theories of the "School of Purgation" represented by Zhang Zihe and those of the "School of Cold and Cool" represented by Liu Hejian are still widely applied in today's CNTCM.

In 1590, the 18th year of the Wanli reign in the Ming Dynasty, Li Shizhen developed the approach of sterilizing patients' clothes and bedding with steam in his book, *Compendium of Materia Medica*. In the late Ming and early Qing Dynasties in the 17th century, *Standards for Diagnosis and Treatment of Women's Diseases* by Wang Kentang and *Fu Qingzhu's Obstetrics and Gynecology* by Fu Qingzhu elaborated on gynecological diseases, exerting lasting impact on later generations. In 1617, the 45th year of the Wanli reign in the Ming Dynasty, Chen Shigong's *Orthodox Manual of External Medicine* developed nursing techniques for surgical diseases. In 1750, the 15th year of the Qian long reign in the Qing Dynasty, Chen Fuzheng gave an original insight into childcare and nursing for miscellaneous pediatric diseases in his book, *Complete Work on Children's Diseases.* Between the 17th century and 18th century, rich content on CNTCM was delivered in *Jing Yue's Collected Works* by Zhang Jingyue of the Ming Dynasty, and *Golden Mirror of the Medical Ancestors* by Wu Qian of the Qing Dynasty.

In 1956, the nursing school affiliated with Nanjing College of Chinese Medicine (now Nanjing University of Chinese Medicine) launched the major of CNTCM. In 1984, CNTCM became an independent discipline after the establishment of Academic Committee of Traditional Chinese Nursing as well as Academic Committee of Integrated Chinese and Western Medicine Nursing, both of which are under Chinese Nursing Association. In 2013, World Federation of Chinese Medicine Societies set up its nursing committee, facilitating international exchange and cooperation in CNTCM. Nowadays, many TCM hospitals run specialized nursing clinics for outpatients, yielding substantial social and economic benefits.

第一章
内科病证的中医护理

在殷商时期的甲骨文中已有一些关于内科疾病的记载。周朝时,出现了内科医生:疾医。《黄帝内经》奠定了中医学理论基础,书中强调整体观念,记载了200多种内科病证。在汉代,张仲景著成《伤寒杂病论》,开创辨证论治先河,将基础理论与临床实践紧密结合。隋代,巢元方的《诸病源候论》对中医内科的病因学和症状学内容进行了充实。其后,晋代的《肘后备急方》、唐代的《备急千金要方》、北宋的《太平圣惠方》等著作都促进了内科治疗学的发展。金元时期,"金元四大家"对中医内科学的理论和实践进行了创新。中医内科学保持了独特的理论体系,为中华民族的繁衍昌盛做出了巨大的贡献。

中医内科学研究的疾病分为外感病与内伤病两大类。外感病多由外感六淫或疫疠之气所致,主要按六经、卫气营血和三焦理论进行辨证论治。内伤病由七情、饮食、劳倦所致,主要按脏腑、经络、气血津液理论进行辨证论治。中医内科病证的命名多以病因、病机、病理产物、相关脏腑、病位、主症、体征等为依据,有些病名与西医不完全相同。

中医内科学的病因包括外感、内伤等。外感病因包括六淫、疫毒、虫毒。六淫为风、寒、暑、湿、燥、火。风为百病之长;风为阳邪,其性开泄;风性善行数变,动摇不定。寒为阴邪,易伤阳气;寒主收引拘急;寒邪凝滞主痛;寒性清澈。暑为阳邪,其性炎热;暑性升散,易伤津耗气;暑多夹湿。湿为阴邪,易阻遏气机,损伤阳气;湿性黏滞,重浊;湿性趋下。燥邪干涩;燥易伤肺。火为阳邪,其性炎上;火易销烁阴津,生风动血。疫毒致病,发病急骤,病情危笃;具有传染性和流行性;致病呈多样性。内伤病因包括情志失常、饮食失宜、劳逸不当等。情志致病必有明显的精神刺激,直接引起气机紊乱;情志致病是否会伤及五脏,取决于心。过怒伤肝,过喜伤心,过思伤脾,过忧伤肺,过恐伤肾。饮食失宜可致脾胃受损、聚湿生痰或气血化生不足。劳则气耗,逸则气滞,皆伤脾胃。五劳所伤,久视伤血,久卧伤气,久坐伤肉,久立伤骨,久行伤筋。房劳伤肾。内生五邪:内风、内寒、内湿、内燥、内火,皆是脏腑功能失调的病理产物,同时也可成为致病因素。瘀血和痰饮是病理产物,也可成为继发病因。

内科疾病的病势、病性、演变、转归等与病人的体质、情志状态、行为习惯,发病的季节、地域,病邪的性质,就医用药等关系密切。内科病证的基本病机包括邪正斗争、阴阳失调、升降失常。

内科疾病的治疗原则包括整体论治、治病求本、随证施治和医护结合。治疗方法包括汗、吐、下、和、温、清、消、补。其内治剂型有汤、散、丸、膏、丹、酒、注射液等。外治方法包括贴、涂、敷、熨、熏、浸、洗、擦、蒸、扑、吹、塞、填、导等。

Chapter 1
Nursing of Internal Diseases

Records about internal diseases were found in inscriptions on bones or tortoise shells of the Shang Dynasty. In the Zhou Dynasty, internists appeared: Ji doctor. *Huangdi's Internal Classic* laid the theoretical foundations for traditional Chinese medicine. The book emphasized the concept of holism, and recorded more than 200 kinds of internal diseases. In the Han Dynasty, Zhang Zhongjing wrote *Treatise on Cold Damage and Miscellaneous Diseases*, in which syndrome differentiation and treatment was first recorded and basic theories were tightly integrated with clinical practice. In the Sui Dynasty, Chao Yuanfang added supplements on etiology and symptomatology in *Treatise on the Pathogenesis and Manifestations of All Diseases*. After that, the *Handbook of Prescriptions for Emergencies* in the Jin Dynasty, *Essential Prescriptions Worth A Thousand Gold for Emergencies* in the Tang Dynasty, and *Peaceful Holy Benevolent Prescriptions* in the Northern Song Dynasty had all made contribution to the development of therapeutics of internal diseases. During the Jin and Yuan Dynasties, the four famous physicians had innovated the theories and clinical practice of internal medicine of TCM. Internal medicine of TCM has been maintaining its unique theoretical system, and made great contribution to the prosperity of the Chinese nation.

The diseases in internal medicine of TCM fall into two categories: diseases caused by external pathogens and those by internal damage. The former are often caused by six external pathogenic factors and pestilential qi, and the treatments are based on six meridian syndrome differentiation, defense-qi-nutrient-blood syndrome differentiation, and triple energizer syndrome differentiation. Meanwhile, the internal damage diseases are often caused by seven emotions, diet, and overstrain, and the treatments are based on visceral syndrome differentiation, meridian syndrome differentiation, and qi-blood-body fluid syndrome differentiation. Internal diseases are often named on the basis of etiology, pathogenesis, pathological products, related zang-fu organs, locations, main symptoms and signs of the diseases. Some of the disease names are different from those in Western medicine.

The causes of disease in internal medicine of TCM mainly include external pathogens and internal damage. The former include six excesses, pestilential qi and animal toxin. Six excesses are pathogenic wind, cold, summer-heat, dampness, dryness and fire. Wind is the primary pathogen of diseases. As one of the yang pathogens with the nature of opening and discharging, it tends to be mobile, changeable, shaking and shivering. Cold as one of the yin pathogens is characterized by tendency of damaging yang qi, coagulation and stagnation with pain, contracture and tension, clear nasal discharge and watery feces. Summer-heat pathogen as one of the yang pathogens is hot, ascending, dispersive, and likely to consume body fluids and qi, and it often causes diseases together with dampness. Dampness pathogen is one of the yin pathogens, characterized by stickiness and stagnation, downward movement, heaviness and turbidity, and the tendency of obstructing qi movement and damaging yang qi. Dryness pathogen has the dry and astringent nature, which can easily damage the lung. Fire pathogen is one of the yang pathogens with the tendency of flaring upward, consuming yin fluid, generating inner-wind, and causing bleeding. When pestilential qi is the pathogen, the disease is contagious and epidemic with sudden onset, severe condition and various clinical manifestations. For internal damage, there are emotional disorders, improper diet, and imbalance between activity and rest. Emotion-induced diseases usually relate to obvious psychological stimulation, which disturbs the movement of qi. Whether the disease damages zang-organs depends on the heart. Over-anger damages the liver; over-joy damages the heart; over-thought damages the spleen; over-anxiety damages the lung; over-fear damages the kidney. Improper diet may damage the spleen and stomach, generate dampness and accumulate phlegm, or cause deficiency of qi and blood. Overexertion consumes qi, while exessive rest causes stagnated qi, both of which can damage the spleen and stomach. The harms caused by the five overstrains are as follows: to observe over a long time harms the blood; to lie down for a long time harms the qi; to sit for a long time harms the flesh; to stand for a long time harms the bones; to walk for a long time harms the sinews. Overindulgence in sexual intercourse harms the kidney. There are five kinds of internally generated pathogens: internal wind, internal cold, internal dampness, internal dryness and internal fire. They are all pathological products due to disorder of zang-fu organs. In turn, they can all become the causes of diseases. Likewise, static blood and retained phlegm-fluid are pathological products, and they can become the secondary causes of diseases.

The condition, nature, evolution, and prognosis of internal diseases are closely related with body constitution, emotional status and behavioral habits of the patient, as well as the onset season and geographic region of the disease, the nature of pathogen, and the medical treatment. The basic pathogenesis of internal diseases involves battles between pathogenic qi and healthy qi, the disharmony between yin and yang, and the abnormal ascending and descending of qi.

The treatment principles of internal diseases include holistic treatment, treatment aiming at root causes, treatment based on syndrome differentiation, and combination of treatment and nursing. The treatment methods include diaphoresis, emesis, purgation, harmonization, warming, heat-clearing, tonifying, and dispersing. The internal treatment preparations include decoction, powder, bolus (pills), ointment, pellets, wine and injection. The external treatments include preparations for applying, coating, compressing, ironing, fumigating, steeping, washing, rubbing, steaming, puffing, insufflating, inserting, packing and discharging.

第一节　感　冒

感冒,是指因时令外邪侵袭肺表而引起的,以发热、恶寒、头身疼痛、鼻塞、喷嚏、咽喉痛痒。咳嗽为临床特征的外感时病。轻者称伤风,具有一定流行性者为时行感冒。西医的急性上呼吸道感染、流行性感冒可参照本节进行护理。

一、病因病机

感冒的病因包括六淫之邪、时行病毒等。因天气突变,六淫肆虐,冷热失调,人体卫外之气未能及时应变,以致虚邪贼风伤人,可发为感冒。在六淫中,导致感冒的主因是风邪。随季节的不同,风邪常与其他当令之时气相合为患,尤以风寒多见。或因时令不正,天时暴厉之气流行人间,直袭肺卫。病人生活起居不当,寒温失调,如贪凉露宿、冒雨涉水、更衣脱帽,导致外邪乘袭肺卫。或因正气不足,或平素体虚,或过劳,或肺有宿疾,卫外不固,易感外邪,均可发为感冒。

感冒的病机为外邪侵袭肺卫,以致卫表不和,肺失宣肃。病位在肺卫。感冒一般以实证居多。若因体虚感邪,则为本虚标实之证。

二、常见证型

（一）辨证要点

1. 辨伤风与时行感冒　根据发病季节、病情轻重、传变程度等来辨别。若发生于冬春时节,呈散发性,首犯皮毛,病情轻,多不传变,则多为伤风。若发病季节不限,有传染性,易广泛流行,直入经络,病及脏腑,病情重,常继发他病,则多为时行感冒。

2. 辨风寒与风热　根据恶寒发热孰轻孰重、有无口渴、是否咽痛、鼻涕清浊等来辨别。若恶寒重,发热轻,颈背强痛,流清涕,口不渴,无咽痛,舌苔薄白,脉浮紧,多为风寒。若发热重,恶寒轻,流浊涕,口渴,咽肿痛,舌红,苔薄黄,脉浮数,则多为风热。

（二）证候分型

1. 风寒束表证

[主要证候]恶寒重,发热轻,无汗,头痛,肢体酸楚,甚则疼痛,鼻塞声重,打喷嚏,时流清涕,咽痒,咳嗽,痰白稀薄;舌苔薄白,脉浮紧。

[证候分析]风寒外束,卫阳被郁,故恶寒;正邪相争,故发热;足太阳膀胱经主一身之表,寒邪犯表,太阳经气不舒,故头痛身疼;肺开窍于鼻,肺主皮毛,风寒束表,肺气不宣,故鼻塞,流清涕,打喷嚏;舌苔薄白,脉浮紧,均为风寒束表之象。

[护治原则]辛温解表,宣肺散寒。

［常用方剂］荆防败毒散。

2. 风热犯表证

［主要证候］发热较重，微恶风，汗出不畅，咽干甚则咽痛，鼻塞，流黄稠涕，头胀痛，咳嗽，痰黏或黄，口干欲饮；舌尖红，舌苔薄白干或薄黄，脉浮数。

［证候分析］风热外袭，卫表失和，风热为阳邪，易化热生火，故发热较重，微恶风，汗出不畅；风热上受，肺窍为风热所壅，肺失清肃，故鼻塞，流黄稠涕，咳嗽；风热上犯于头则头痛，熏蒸清道则咽痛；舌尖红，舌苔薄白干或薄黄，脉浮数，均为风热犯表之象。

［护治原则］辛凉解表，疏风清热。

［常用方剂］银翘散。

3. 暑湿伤表证

［主要证候］夏令感邪，发热，或身热不扬，微恶风，汗出不畅，肢体困重或酸痛，头重如裹，胸闷脘痞，纳呆，鼻塞，流浊涕，心烦口渴，大便稀溏，小便短赤；舌苔黄腻，脉濡数。

［证候分析］暑湿之邪侵袭，卫气被遏，故发热，或身热不扬，微恶风，汗出不畅；风暑夹湿上犯清空，故头重如裹；湿困中焦，气机不展，故胸闷脘痞；表卫不和，肺气不宣，故鼻塞流涕；舌苔黄腻，脉濡数，均为暑湿侵袭之象。

［护治原则］清暑祛湿解表。

［常用方剂］新加香薷饮。

4. 气虚感冒证

［主要证候］恶寒较甚，或并发热，但觉时时形寒恶风，自汗，鼻塞，流涕，咳嗽，痰白，咳痰无力，气短，乏力，平素神疲体弱，语声低怯，或易感冒；舌淡苔薄白，脉浮无力。

［证候分析］风寒外袭，肺气失宣，故恶寒发热，头痛鼻塞，咳嗽痰白；素体气虚，表卫不固，腠理疏松，故反复易感；气虚失于温煦，故热势不盛，但觉时时形寒恶风；自汗，咳痰无力，气短，乏力，神疲，舌淡苔薄白，脉浮无力，均为气虚、邪在卫表之象。

［护治原则］益气解表，调和营卫。

［常用方剂］参苏饮。

5. 阴虚感冒证

［主要证候］身热，微恶风寒，无汗或微汗，或寐中盗汗，干咳少痰，头痛，心烦，口干，甚则口渴；舌红少苔，脉细数。

［证候分析］外感风热或感邪后邪从热化，卫表失和，故身热，微恶风寒，头痛，口干；阴虚之体，内有燥热，热郁伤津，感邪之后，发热汗出，更伤阴液，故无汗或微汗，盗汗，干咳少痰，心烦；舌红少苔，脉细数，均为阴虚内热之象。

［护治原则］滋阴解表。

［常用方剂］加减葳蕤汤。

三、护理措施

对于感冒的病人，应观察恶寒、发热的轻重程度，咳嗽的发作时间、持续时长、声音，痰的量、色、质、鼻涕的量、色、质、头痛的部位。观察病人有无汗出、口渴、咽痛。对于体虚感冒者,应观察感冒的诱因、发病次数、病程长短和病人的体质特点。若有高热,每4小时测1次体温、心率、心律、呼吸。若病人出现头痛项强、高热、抽搐,应立即报告医生。

（一）辨证施护

1. 风寒束表证

（1）生活起居护理　居室温暖避风,空气新鲜,阳光充足,不可有强风、对流风。注意保暖,衣被宜厚,随天气变化及时增减衣物,外出时戴口罩。若恶寒较重,可用热水袋保暖,服热汤以散寒。若鼻塞,可用热毛巾敷鼻、额部。

（2）饮食护理　饮食宜温热,多喝热稀粥和热水。可用连须葱白3茎,生姜9 g,陈皮6 g,红糖30 g,用水快煎后代茶饮。宜食解表散寒的食物,如白胡椒、紫苏叶。食疗方:芥菜牛肉汤。不宜食生冷、油腻的食物。

（3）情志护理　病人恶寒较重,头痛身疼,可能会心烦、焦虑,护士可运用语言开导疗法,做好解释和安慰工作,讲解疾病的发展过程,使病人积极配合治疗。

（4）用药护理　中药汤剂应武火快煎,热服。服后避风,覆被取汗,或食热稀饭、热米汤以助药力,以微微出汗为佳。中病即止,不可过汗,以防伤阴。忌服补敛之品。

（5）操作技术　① 灸法:取大椎、风门、肺俞,用温和灸,艾条燃着端悬于施灸部位上,距离皮肤2~3厘米,灸至病人有温热舒适无灼痛的感觉,皮肤稍有红晕,每日1次。② 拔罐疗法:取风门、大椎、肺俞,留罐10分钟,隔日1次。③ 推拿疗法:在背部循足太阳膀胱经,用掌平推法、拇指揉法,按摩至周身微微汗出,适用于头痛身疼者;或取迎香,用拇指揉法,按摩至局部发热或有酸麻重胀感,每日1次,适用于鼻塞者;孕妇禁用。④ 膏药疗法:取大椎、肺俞、定喘,将麝香壮骨膏剪成1厘米见方,贴在腧穴上,每日1次。⑤ 敷贴疗法:取劳宫,用白胡椒、丁香各7粒碾碎,与葱白泥调匀后外敷,合掌握定,夹于大腿内侧,加盖衣被,微微汗出。

2. 风热犯表证

（1）生活起居护理　居室凉爽避风,光线柔和,空气新鲜。衣被宜薄,清洁干燥。保持口腔清洁,饭后用金银花甘草液漱口。若汗多,应及时擦干,并换掉湿衣被。若高热,应卧床休息,用温水擦浴,不可使用冷敷法。若咳嗽,可取半仰卧位,由护士告诉病人有效的咳嗽及咳痰方法,或协助翻身、拍背。

（2）饮食护理　多饮水,可饮薄荷茶、菊花茶、淡竹叶茶。多吃高纤维的水果和蔬菜,以保持大便通畅。若咳嗽伴喘,可食枇杷、白萝卜。若高热,以素流食为宜,热退第1天食素半流食,3天后改为荤半流食,如瘦肉丝、鲜鱼汤,恢复期予普食。宜食疏风清热的食物,如薄荷、葛根。食疗方:银花山楂汤、绿豆茶叶冰糖汤。戒烟限酒,不宜食油腻、辛辣的食物,如大蒜、大葱、韭菜。

（3）情志护理　病人可能出现烦躁,护士可运用移情易性疗法,转移其注意力。

（4）用药护理　薄荷后下。中药汤剂宜武火快煎,饭后温服。服药后观察出汗和体温的变化。中病即止,忌服补敛之品。

（5）操作技术　① 刺血疗法:取大椎,皮肤消毒后揉按局部使其充血,用三棱针的3毫米针尖,快速刺入并出针,放出1.0 mL以下的血液,用无菌干棉球擦拭或按压,适用于高热者;或取少商,适用于咽痛者。② 雾化吸入疗法:用桂枝、薄荷各10 g煎汤,以43℃中药蒸汽吸入呼吸道,每次10分钟,每日1~2次;适用于鼻塞者。③吹喉疗法:用双料喉风散或西瓜霜吹喉,需在病人屏息时吹药;适用于咽痛者。

3. 暑湿伤表证

(1) 生活起居护理　居室凉爽避风,光线柔和,空气新鲜。衣被宜薄,清洁干燥。保持口腔清洁,饭后用金银花甘草液漱口。若高热,应卧床休息,用温水擦浴,不可使用冷敷法。

(2) 饮食护理　饮食宜清淡、素净、稀软。多饮水,可饮鲜芦根茶、金银花茶、薄荷茶、荷叶茶。可食香蕉,以保持大便通畅。二豆羹:豆腐250 g,淡豆豉、葱白各15 g,糖适量;豆腐略煮,加入淡豆豉,放水一大碗,煎取小半碗,再放葱白,水开后趁热服用,服后盖被取微汗,每日1次。宜食清暑祛湿的食物,如荸荠、西瓜皮、丝瓜皮、番茄、薏苡仁、绿豆、赤小豆。不宜食油腻、过甜、生冷、油炸的食物。

(3) 情志护理　病人头昏胀重,胸闷泛恶,可能会心烦、焦虑,护士可运用顺意疗法,倾听病人的诉说,满足其合理要求。

(4) 用药护理　中药汤剂宜武火快煎,饭后温服。服药后,可食薏苡仁粥。中病即止,忌服补敛之品。

(5) 操作技术　① 刮痧疗法:自大杼开始,经风门,到肺俞,每侧刮拭20~30次,以皮肤出现潮红或起痧为度,不可太过用力,两次刮痧之间宜间隔3~6日;女性月经期或妊娠期禁用。② 灸法:取大椎,用温和灸,艾条燃着端悬于施灸部位上,距离皮肤2~3厘米,灸至病人有温热舒适无灼痛的感觉,皮肤稍有红晕,每日1次;适用于头昏胀重者。③ 热敷疗法:用热毛巾敷鼻、额部;或用薄荷、紫苏叶各10 g煎汤,毛巾浸药,热敷鼻、额部10分钟;适用于鼻塞者。

4. 气虚感冒证

(1) 生活起居护理　居室温暖安静,光线柔和,空气新鲜,不可有强风、对流风。衣被宜厚,床单干燥舒适。卧床休息,减少外出,外出时戴口罩,注意保暖,不可过劳。若病情稳定,可进行轻缓的运动,如太极拳、八段锦。若汗多,应及时擦干,并换掉湿衣被。若头痛恶风,可戴帽子或用棉布包扎头部。若发生面色苍白、烦躁不安、气喘、心跳加快,应取半仰卧位,吸氧,并立即报告医生。

(2) 饮食护理　宜食健脾补气的食物,如荔枝、山药、大枣、茯苓。食疗方:葱白鸡肉粥。不宜食生冷、油腻、辛辣的食物。

(3) 情志护理　病人气虚且病情反复,容易悲观、消沉,护士可运用语言开导疗法和移情易性疗法,多与病人沟通,向病人介绍预防感冒的措施和重要性,安慰和鼓励病人,帮助其树立战胜疾病的信心。

(4) 用药护理　中药汤剂宜饭前温服。服药后卧床休息。

(5) 操作技术　① 膏摩疗法:取劳宫、涌泉、足三里、气海,用玉屏风膏(取玉屏风散,在75%酒精中浸泡24小时,再与凡士林调成膏状,微火加热至微黄,冷却后使用)按揉各个腧穴,每处2分钟,手法宜轻缓,每日早晚各1次;孕妇禁用。② 敷贴疗法:取大椎、肺俞、膻中、中府、肾俞,用白芥子、细辛、延胡索、甘遂、肉桂打粉,与生姜汁调成糊状,在三伏(头伏、中伏、末伏的第1天或第2天)、三九(一九、二九、三九的第1天或第2天)敷贴,共6次,每次4~6小时;此法发泡,可能会留疤,治疗前应征得病人同意;孕妇禁用。③ 灸法:取足三里、悬钟,在春夏季节进行瘢痕灸,每处1壮,每年1~2次;或取外关,用麦粒灸,灸至皮肤潮红,最后一壮保留艾灰,用创可贴覆盖;孕妇忌用。

5. 阴虚感冒证

（1）生活起居护理　居室凉爽湿润,安静避风,光线柔和,空气新鲜。衣被宜薄。起居有常,多卧床休息,减少外出,不可熬夜及过劳。若病情稳定,鼓励病人进行轻缓的运动,以增强体质。若盗汗,应及时擦干,并换掉湿衣被。

（2）饮食护理　可饮玉竹茶、黄精茶。若干咳少痰,可食白蜜炖雪梨。宜食养阴生津的食物,如银耳、百合、海参、鳖肉、鸭肉。不宜食燥热伤阴的食物,如羊肉、狗肉。

（3）情志护理　病人阴虚且病程较长,容易产生烦躁情绪,护士可运用语言开导疗法,多和病人沟通,讲解体质与情绪的关联,帮助病人保持情绪稳定。

（4）用药护理　薄荷后下。中药汤剂宜温服。服药后卧床休息。

（5）操作技术　① 膏摩疗法:取劳宫、涌泉、足三里、照海、太溪,用玉屏风膏按揉各个腧穴,手法宜轻缓,每处 2 分钟,每日早晚各 1 次;孕妇禁用。② 耳压疗法:取肺、气管、肾等耳穴,用耳穴压丸贴片贴压,每日按揉 4~5 次,以局部发热泛红为度,留置 2~4 日;孕妇禁用。

（二）健康教育

居室宜避风,空气新鲜。起居有常,注意休息。防寒保暖,避免淋雨,盛夏时不可贪凉露宿。

擤鼻涕时,按住一侧鼻孔,轻轻擤出,不可同时按住两侧鼻孔或用力过猛,以防止发生耳咽管、鼻窦的并发症。

多饮水。宜食高热量的流食、半流食或软食,如鱼汤、肉末菜粥、蒸鸡蛋。忌烟酒、浓茶,不宜食滋腻、生冷的食物,如肥肉、糕点、冷饮。

对于老年人、婴幼儿、体弱或时感重症者,必须予以重视。早发现、早治疗,以防止疾病发生传变。

对于时行感冒,按照呼吸道传染病进行隔离。时行感冒流行期间,可服药预防。冬春季节,可遵医嘱用紫苏叶、荆芥各 10 g,甘草 3 g,水煎服,连用 3 日。夏季,可遵医嘱用广藿香、佩兰各 5 g,薄荷 2 g,煎汤代茶饮。或遵医嘱用贯众 9~15 g,煎汤代茶饮,连用 2~3 日。

Section 1　Common Cold

Common cold is an externally contracted disease clinically characterized by fever, aversion to cold, headache and body pain, nasal congestion, sneezing, sore or itching throat and cough. It is caused by the invasion of seasonal external pathogens into the lung defense. Its mild condition is called wind damage and it is called seasonal influenza when epidemic. This section may be referred to for the nursing of acute upper respiratory tract infection and influenza in Western medicine.

ETIOLOGY AND PATHOGENESIS

The etiology includes six pathogenic excesses and seasonal epidemic toxin. Sudden weather change, six pathogenic excesses, and cold-heat disharmony make the body's defense qi fail to stay alert and result in common cold. Among the six pathogenic excesses, the main pathogen responsible for common cold is pathogenic wind that usually combines with other seasonal pathogens to attack the human body, of which wind-cold is the one mostly seen in clinic. Other causes include epidemic toxin attacking the lung defense; unhealthy lifestyle as well as cold-heat disharmony, such as sleeping in the open to keep cool, braving in rain and wading in water, changing clothes and taking off hat; insufficient healthy qi, weak constitution, overstrain, chronic illness in the lung, and insecurity of defense qi.

The pathogenesis is external pathogens attacking the lung defense that causes disharmony of defensive exterior and failure of lung qi to disperse and descend. The location of disease is lung defense. Common cold mostly belongs to excess syndrome. If the case is caused by body deficiency, it is the syndrome of root deficiency and branch excess.

COMMON SYNDROMES

Key Points in Syndrome Differentiation

1. Differentiation of Wind Damage from Seasonal Influenza

The differentiation is based on the onset of season, severity, and degree of development and transmission of disease. Wind damage usually occurs in winter and spring, which invades the skin and hair firstly with sporadic onset, mild condition, and no transmission. Seasonal influenza may occur all around the year, with pathogens directly entering into meridians and zang-fu organs, it is infectious and severe, and often leads to other diseases.

2. Differentiation of Wind-Cold from Wind-Heat Syndrome

The differentiation is based on the predominance of aversion to cold or fever, presence of thirst and sore throat, and nature of nasal discharge. Severe aversion to cold, mild fever, stiffness and pain of the nape and back, thin nasal discharge, no thirst or sore throat, thin white tongue coating, and floating tight pulse indicate wind-cold syndrome. Severe fever, mild aversion to cold, thick nasal discharge, thirst, sore throat, red tongue with thin yellow coating, and floating rapid pulse signify wind-heat syndrome.

Syndrome Differentiation

1. Wind-Cold Fettering Exterior Syndrome

[Clinical Manifestations] Severe aversion to cold, mild fever, no sweating, headache, aching limbs, nasal congestion with a heavy voice, sneezing, frequent thin nasal discharge, itching throat, cough, white clear and thin phlegm, thin white tongue coating, and floating tight pulse.

[Manifestations Analysis] Wind-cold that fetters the exterior obstructs defensive yang, so aversion to cold is felt. Healthy qi struggles with pathogenic qi, so fever occurs. The bladder meridian of foot-taiyang governs the exterior of the body, therefore, when pathogenic cold invades the exterior and obstructs its meridian qi, headache and generalized pain present. Lung opens into the nose and governs the skin and hair, therefore, when wind-cold fetters the exterior and causes failure of lung qi to disperse, symptoms of nasal congestion, sneezing, and thin nasal discharge appear. Thin white tongue coating and floating tight pulse are signs of wind-cold fettering the exterior.

[Nursing Principle] Releasing exterior with pungent-warm medicinals; ventilating lung and dissipating cold.

[Suggested Formula] Jingfang Baidu Powder.

2. Wind-Heat Invading Exterior Syndrome

[Clinical Manifestations] Severe fever, mild aversion to cold, inhibited sweating, dry or even sore throat, nasal congestion, yellow thick nasal discharge, distending headache, cough, sticky or yellow phlegm, dry mouth with desire for drinking, red tongue tip, thin white and dry tongue coating or thin yellow coating, and floating rapid pulse.

[Manifestations Analysis] Wind-heat invading the exterior leads to disharmony of defensive exterior. And wind-heat belongs to yang pathogen that is likely to transform into heat and generate fire. So the patients have severe fever, mild aversion to cold, and inhibited sweating. Wind-heat obstructing the nose leads to failure of lung qi to disperse and descend, so nasal congestion, yellow thick nasal discharge, and cough happens. Wind-heat upward attacks the head and dries the upper respiratory tract, so headache and sore throat occurs. Red tongue tip, thin white and dry tongue coating or thin yellow coating, and floating rapid pulse are signs of wind-heat invading the exterior.

[Nursing Principle] Releasing exterior with pungent-cool medicinals; dispersing wind and clearing heat.

[Suggested Formula] Yinqiao Powder.

3. Summerheat-Dampness Damaging Exterior Syndrome

〔Clinical Manifestations〕Invasion of pathogenic qi in summer, fever or hiding fever, slightly aversion to wind, inhibited sweating, heavy or aching limbs, head heavy as if swathed, chest oppression, gastric stuffiness, anorexia, nasal congestion, thick nasal discharge, heart vexation, thirst, loose stool, scanty dark urine, yellow slimy tongue coating, and soggy rapid pulse.

〔Manifestations Analysis〕Summerheat-dampness obstructs defense qi and leads to fever or hiding fever, slight aversion to wind, and inhibited sweating. Wind-summerheat with dampness upward invades the head, so the head is heavy as if swathed. Dampness encumbering the middle energizer inhibits qi movement, resulting in chest oppression and gastric stuffiness. Disharmony of defensive exterior and failure of lung qi to ventilate are responsible for nasal congestion with thick nasal discharge. Yellow slimy tongue coating and soggy rapid pulse are signs of summerheat-dampness damaging the exterior.

〔Nursing Principle〕Clearing summerheat, removing dampness, and releasing exterior.

〔Suggested Formula〕Xinjia Xiangru Drink.

4. Syndrome of Common Cold due to Qi Deficiency

〔Clinical Manifestations〕Severe aversion to cold, or accompanied with fever, constant physical cold and aversion to wind, spontaneous sweating, nasal congestion, cough, white phlegm, weakness in expectoration, shortness of breath, lassitude, mental fatigue and weak constitution, timorous low voice, susceptibility to cold, pale tongue with thin white coating, and floating weak pulse.

〔Manifestations Analysis〕External invasion of wind-cold causes failure of lung qi to disperse and descend, leading to symptoms such as aversion to cold, fever, headache, nasal congestion, cough and white phlegm. Qi deficiency constitution and insecurity of defensive exterior explain frequent susceptibility to cold. Deficient qi cannot to warm the body, resulting in mild fever, constant physical cold and aversion to wind. Spontaneous sweating, weakness in expectoration, shortness of breath, lassitude, mental fatigue, pale tongue with thin white coating, and floating weak pulse all are signs of qi deficiency with pathogens in defensive exterior.

〔Nursing Principle〕Replenishing qi and releasing exterior; harmonizing nutrient and defensive aspects.

〔Suggested Formula〕Shensu Drink.

5. Syndrome of Common Cold due to Yin Deficiency

〔Clinical Manifestations〕Fever, slight aversion to wind-cold, no or scanty sweating, or night sweat, dry cough with scanty phlegm, headache, heart vexation, dry mouth or even thirst, red tongue with scanty coating, and thready rapid pulse.

〔Manifestations Analysis〕External invasion of wind-heat or pathogenic qi transforming into heat, and disharmony of defensive exterior are responsible for fever, slight aversion to wind-cold, headache, and dry mouth. Yin deficiency constitution with internal dryness-heat further consumes body fluids after invasion of pathogens, thus leading to no or scanty sweating, night sweat, dry cough with scanty phlegm, and heart vexation. Red tongue with scanty coating and thready rapid pulse are signs of yin deficiency with internal dryness.

[Nursing Principle] Nourishing yin and releasing exterior.

[Suggested Formula] Jiajian Weirui Decoction.

NURSING MEASURES

For patients with common cold, nurses should observe the degree of aversion to cold and fever; the onset time, duration and sound of cough; the amount, color and texture of phlegm and nasal discharge, and the location of headache. They should check the presence of sweat, thirst and sore throat. Moreover, for patients with weak constitution, the inducing factors, onset frequency and course of disease as well as the constitution should also be observed; for those with high fever, the body temperature, heart rate, heart rhythm and breathing should be checked once every four hours. If the patient experiences headache with a stiff neck, high fever and seizure, report to the doctor immediately.

Syndrome-Based Nursing Measures

1. Wind-Cold Fettering Exterior Syndrome

(1) Daily life nursing. The ward should be warm, full of fresh air and plenty of sun light, and avoid strong and convective wind. The coverings should be thick. The patients should keep warm, and increase or decrease clothing according to weather changes. A mask is required when the patient is outdoors. For patients with severe aversion to cold, place a hot water bag on the body, or drink hot soup to dispel the cold pathogen. For patients with nasal congestion, a hot towel covering the nose and forehead could help.

(2) Diet nursing. The patients may eat warm foods and drink more hot porridge and hot water. Herbal tea is recommended: three stalks of congbai (scallion white) with root, shengjiang (fresh ginger) 9 g, chenpi (aged tangerine peel) 6 g and brown sugar 30 g, which are decocted fast with strong fire. It is advisable to eat foods that relieve the exterior and dispel cold, such as baihujiao (white pepper) and zisuye (perilla leaf). Food therapy: leaf mustard beef soup. Raw, cold and greasy foods should be avoided.

(3) Emotion nursing. The patients have been suffering from severe aversion to cold, headache and generalized pain, which may lead to dysphoria and anxiety, so nurses may use verbal enlightenment therapy to comfort the patients and impart the knowledge about the disease to make them confident and cooperative.

(4) Medication nursing. Decoction should be prepared fast with strong fire and taken hot. To boost the efficacy of medicine, the patients should stay away from wind, and tuck themselves in at night, or eat hot porridge or rice soup to perspire slightly after taking the decoction. Stop taking the medicine immediately after the disease is cured. Profuse sweating should be avoided to prevent yin damage. Tonic and astringent products should be avoided.

(5) Manipulation techniques. ① Moxibustion therapy: select Dazhui (GV 14), Fengmen (BL 12)

and Feishu（BL 13）; place the moxa stick 2～3 centimeters away from the skin to perform mild moxibustion on each of the acupoints until the area turns red and the patient feels warm and comfortable without the sensation of burning pain, once per day. ② Cupping therapy: select Fengmen（BL 12）, Dazhui（GV 14）, and Feishu（BL 13）; retain the cup on the acupoints for 10 minutes, once every other day. ③ Tuina therapy: select the bladder meridian of foot-taiyang on the back of the trunk for patients with headache and generalized aching, and apply palm flat pushing and thumb kneading manipulations until mild generalized sweating starts; or select Yingxiang（LI 20）for patients with nasal congestion, and apply thumb kneading manipulation on the acupoint until the area turns hot or the patient has the feelings of soreness, numbness, heaviness and distension in the area. And it is contraindicated in pregnancy. ④ Plaster application therapy: select Dazhui（GV 14）, Feishu（BL 13）and Dingchuan（EX－B1）; apply on them Shexiang Zhuanggu Plaster（Musk Plaster for Strengthening tendons and bones）in the size of one square centimeter, once per day. ⑤ Paste application therapy: select Laogong（PC 8）; grind into powder seven grains of baihujiao（white pepper）and seven grains of dingxiang（clover flower）, blend the powder with mashed scallion white to make pastes, and apply them on the acupoint. Hold both hands together tightly, clamp them between the thighs, and put on more clothes to perspire slightly.

2. Wind-Heat Invading Exterior Syndrome

（1）Daily life nursing. The ward should be cool, full of fresh air and gentle light, and away from wind. The coverings should be thin, clean and dry. The patients should pay attention to oral hygiene and rinse the mouth with jinyinhua gancao（honeysuckle flower and licorice root）liquid after meals. For patients with profuse sweating, wipe the sweat away and change the wet clothes and bedding timely. For patients with high fever, stay in bed and apply warm sponge bath rather than cold application therapy. For patients with cough, take a semi-supine position; nurses should instruct the patients about the right method of effective cough and expectoration, or assist with turning-over and back-patting.

（2）Diet nursing. The patients should drink more water. They may drink bohe（field mint）tea, juhua（chrysanthemum flower）tea, or danzhuye（lophatherum herb）tea, and eat more vegetables and fruit rich in fiber to guarantee a normal defecation. For patients with cough and panting, eat loquats and white radishes. For patients with high fever, eat vegetarian liquid foods, then semi-liquid foods once the body temperature is normal, and semi-liquid foods with meat three days after the body temperature returns to normal, such as shredded lean meat and fish soup, and finally, general diet during remission stage. They may eat foods that dispel wind and clear heat, such as bohe（field mint）and gegen（kudzuvine root）. Food therapy: yinhua shanzha（honeysuckle flower and Chinese hawthorn fruit）soup, and lüdou（mung bean）tea leaf crystal sugar soup. The patients should refrain from smoking, drinking, and eating foods that are greasy, pungent and spicy, such as garlic, scallions, and Chinese chives.

（3）Emotion nursing. The patients may have dysphoria, so nurses may use emotional transference and dispositional change therapy to distract the patients' attention.

（4）Medication nursing. Bohe（field mint）should be decocted later. Decoction should be prepared fast with strong fire and taken warm after meals. After taking medicine, observe the change of sweating and body temperature. Stop taking the medicine immediately after the disease is cured. Tonic and astringent products should be avoided.

（5）Manipulation techniques. ① Blood-letting therapy: after the skin is disinfected, rub the local area to make it hyperemic, use a three-edged needle to quickly pierce the skin at a depth of 3 millimeters and remove the needle to release blood less than 1.0 mL, and wipe or press the pierced point with a sterile dry cotton ball. Select Dazhui（GV 14）for patients with high fever; or select Shaoshang（LU 11）for patients with sore throat. ② Spray inhalation therapy: boil guizhi（cinnamon twig）10 g and bohe（field mint）10 g together; inhale the steam of the decoction at a temperature of 43℃ into the respiratory tract, 10 minutes each time, once or twice per day. It is suitable for patients with nasal congestion. ③ Laryngeal insufflation therapy: insufflate Shuangliao Houfeng Powder or Xiguashuang（watermelon frost）into the throat while the patient is holding breath. It is suitable for patients with sore throat.

3. Summerheat-Dampness Damaging Exterior Syndrome

（1）Daily life nursing. The ward should be cool, full of fresh air and gentle light, and away from wind. The coverings should be thin, clean and dry. The patients should pay attention to oral hygiene and rinse the mouth with jinyinhua gancao（honeysuckle flower and licorice root）liquid after meals. For patients with high fever, apply warm sponge bath rather than cold application therapy.

（2）Diet nursing. The patient should eat light, vegetarian, thin and soft food, and drink more water. They may drink xianlugen（fresh reed root）tea, jinyinhua（honeysuckle flower）tea, bohe（field mint）tea, or heye（lotus leaf）tea, and eat bananas to keep a normal bowel movement. Erdou broth: take 250 g of tofu, 15 g of dandouchi（prepared soybean）, 15 g of congbai（scallion white）, and some sugar; cook tofu for a short time with a large bowl of water, add in dandouchi（prepared soybean）and continue to cook untill most of the water is evaporated, then add in congbai（scallion white）for further boiling, and eat the hot broth after the water is boiling again, then tuck themselves in to perspire slightly; once per day. The patients may eat foods that clear summerheat and resolve dampness, such as biqi（waternut）, xiguapi（watermelon peel）, luffa peel, tomato, yiyiren（coix seed）, lüdou（mung bean）and chixiaodou（adzuki bean）. Greasy, too-sweet, raw, cold, and fried foods should be avoided.

（3）Emotion nursing. Because the patients are suffering from vertigo, head distention with heavy sensation, chest oppression and nausea, they may have dysphoria and anxiety, so nurses may use submission therapy to listen to them and meet their reasonable requirements.

（4）Medication nursing. Decoction should be prepared fast with strong fire and taken warm after meals. Eat yiyiren（coix seed）porridge after taking the decoction. Stop taking the medicine immediately after the disease is cured. Tonic and astringent products should be avoided.

（5）Manipulation techniques. ① Scraping therapy: select the areas starting from Dazhu（BL 11）to Fengmen（BL 12）and Feishu（BL 13）use scraping plate to gently scrape from top to bottom, and repeat the manipulation for 20~30 times on each side till the area turns red or *qi sha* (rashes occur). An interval of 3~6 days is preferred between two sessions. And it should be avoided for women during menstruation or pregnancy. ② Moxibustion therapy: select Dazhui (GV 14); place the moxa stick 2~3 centimeters away from the skin to perform mild moxibustion on the acupoint until the area turns red and the patient feels warm and comfortable without the sensation of burning pain, once per day. ③ Hot compress therapy: apply a hot towel on the nose and forehead; or use bohe (field mint) 10 g and zisuye (leaf of purple perilla) 10 g to make a decoction, and apply a towel steeped in the hot decoction on the nose and forehead; 10 minutes each time; it is suitable for patients with nasal congestion.

4. Syndrome of Common Cold due to Qi Deficiency

(1) Daily life nursing. The ward should be warm, quiet, full of fresh air and gentle light, and avoid strong and convective wind. The coverings should be thick, and the sheets should be dry and comfortable. The patients should stay in bed, reduce going outside, wear a mask when going outside, keep themselves warm and avoid overstrain. When the condition is stabilized, they may do gentle exercise, such as Taiji and Baduanjin. For patients with profuse sweating, wipe the sweat away and change the wet clothes and bedding timely. For patients with headache and aversion to wind, wear a hat or wrap the head with a piece of cotton cloth. If the patient has pale complexion, dysphoria, panting and rapid heartbeat, take a semi-supine position with oxygen inhalation, and nurses should report to the doctor immediately.

(2) Diet nursing. The patients may eat foods that invigorate spleen and replenish qi, such as lychee, shanyao (common yam rhizome), dazao (Chinese date) and fuling (poria). Food therapy: congbai jirou (scallion white and chicken) porridge. Avoid raw, cold, greasy, pungent or spicy foods.

(3) Emotion nursing. Because the patients have qi deficiency that causes the disease to occur repeatedly, they may easily be pessimistic and depressed. To help patients be confident in winning the battle against disease, nurses may use verbal enlightenment therapy as well as emotional transference and dispositional change therapy to communicate with them, and explain the methods and importance of preventing common cold to comfort and encourage them.

(4) Medication nursing. Decoction should be taken warm before meals. After taking medicine, the patients should take a rest in the bed.

(5) Manipulation techniques. ① Therapy of massage with paste: select Laogong (PC 8), Yongquan (KI 1), Zusanli (ST 36) and Qihai (CV 6); prepare Yupingfeng Paste: immerse Yupingfeng Powder in 75% alcohol for 24 hours, blend it with vaseline to make a paste, then heat it at low temperature until it turns yellowish, and cool it for later use; smear the paste on the skin of the acupoints and gently press and knead each acupoint for 2 minutes; once in the morning and once in the evening. And it is contraindicated in pregnancy. ② Paste application therapy: select Dazhui (GV 14), Feishu (BL 13), Danzhong (CV 17), Zhongfu (LU 1) and Shenshu (BL 23); grind into powder baijiezi (white mustard seed), xixin (Manchurian wild ginger), yanhusuo (corydalis rhizome), gansui (gansui root) and rougui (cinnamon bark), blend the powder with shengjiang (fresh ginger) juice to

make paste, and apply the paste on the acupoints during the dog days (on the first or second day of the three ten-day periods after the summer solstice) and cold days (on the first or second day of the three nine-day periods after the winter solstice), 6 times in total, 4~6 hours each time; this therapy may cause blisters and scars on the skin, so an informed consent is demanded. And it is contraindicated in pregnancy. ③ Moxibustion therapy: select Zusanli (ST 36) and Xuanzhong (GB 39), apply scarring moxibustion on each of the acupoints in spring and summer, one moxa cone on every acupoint, once or twice every year; or select Waiguan (TE 5), apply grain-sized moxa cone moxibustion on the acupoint until the area turns red, keep the ashes of the last moxa cone on the skin, and cover it with woundplast; it is contraindicated in pregnancy.

5. Syndrome of Common Cold due to Yin Deficiency

(1) Daily life nursing. The ward should be cool, moist, quiet, full of gentle light and fresh air, and away from wind. The coverings should be thin. The patients should live a regular life, stay in bed, reduce going outside, and avoid staying up late and overstrain. When the condition is stabilized, the patients should do gentle and slow exercise to improve their health. For patients with night sweat, wipe the sweat away and change the wet clothes and bedding timely.

(2) Diet nursing. Yuzhu (fragrant solomonseal rhizome) tea and huangjing (rhizoma polygonati) tea are advisable. For patients with dry cough and little phlegm, white honey stewed with snow pear is recommended. The patients may eat foods that nourish yin and engender liquid, such as yin'er (tremella), baihe (lily bulb), sea cucumber, meat of soft-shelled turtles and duck meat. Avoid foods that are dry and hot in nature and damage yin, such as mutton and dog meat.

(3) Emotion nursing. Because the patients have yin deficiency with a long disease course, they may have dysphoria. Nurses may use verbal enlightenment therapy to communicate with them as much as possible and explain the relationship between constitution and the state of mind so as to calm them.

(4) Medication nursing. Bohe (field mint) should be decocted later. Decoction should be taken warm. After taking medicine, the patients should take a rest in the bed.

(5) Manipulation techniques. ① Therapy of massage with paste: select Laogong (PC 8), Yongquan (KI 1), Zusanli (ST 36), Zhaohai (KI 6) and Taixi (KI 3); smear Yupingfeng Paste on the skin of the acupoints and gently press and knead each acupoint for 2 minutes; once in the morning and once in the evening. And it is contraindicated in pregnancy. ② Auricular pressure therapy: select the auricular points of lung (CO14), trachea (CO16) and kidney (CO10); apply specialized pasters on the points, knead each of them till the area turns hot and red, 4~5 times per day, and keep the pasters for 2~4 days. And it is contraindicated in pregnancy.

Patient Education

The room should have fresh air, away from wind. The patients should live a regular life, have sufficient rest, and keep themselves warm. Avoid braving rain and sleeping outdoors in summer.

When blowing the nose, press one nostril and gently blow, instead of pressing two nostrils simultaneously or blowing forcefully, in order to prevent complications of eustachian tube and paranasal sinus.

The patients should drink more water, and eat calorie-rich liquid, semi-liquid or soft foods, such as fish soup, minced meat vegetable porridge, and steamed egg. The patients should refrain from smoking and drinking alcohol and strong tea. Greasy, cold and raw foods should be avoided, such as fatty meat, cakes, and cold drinks.

For the elderly, infants, and those with weak constitution or severe common cold, extra attention should be paid to make early diagnosis and treatment to prevent development and transmission of the disease.

For influenza, the patients should be put into quarantine as those with respiratory infectious diseases. During the influenza epidemic, preventive medicine is recommended based on the doctor's advice. In winter and spring, boil zisuye (leaf of purple perilla) 10 g, jingjie (schizonepeta) 10 g, and gancao (licorice root) 3 g to make medicated tea for drinking 3 days in a row. In summer, boil guanghuoxiang (cablin patchouli) 5 g, peilan (eupatorium) 5 g, and bohe (field mint) 2 g to make medicated tea; or drink medicated tea made of guanzhong (cyrtomium rhizome) 9~15 g, for 2~3 days in a row.

第二节　咳　嗽　病

咳嗽病,泛指因六淫外邪袭肺,有害气体刺激,或因脏腑内伤,肺脾气虚,痰饮停肺,肝火犯肺,或因久病气阴两亏,导致肺失清肃宣降,肺气上逆,以咳嗽、咯痰为临床特征的一类肺系病。咳嗽病包括外感咳嗽和内伤咳嗽。西医的急性气管-支气管炎、慢性支气管炎、咳嗽变异型哮喘,以咳嗽为主要表现的,可参照本节进行护理。

一、病因病机

咳嗽病的病因有外感与内伤两大类。外感六淫,从口鼻或皮毛而入,使肺气被束,肺失肃降,上逆作声,可发为咳嗽病。风为六淫之首,外感咳嗽多以风为先导,以风寒者居多。内伤脏腑,多由肺脏自病或他脏之病累及肺脏所致。或可因肺系本有多种疾病,迁延不愈,耗损肺气,灼伤肺阴,而致肺失宣降;或过度劳倦,损伤脾胃,脾失健运,痰湿内生,上渍于肺;或饮食不节,嗜食烟酒,助火熏灼肺胃;或情志刺激,肝失条达,日久化火,肝火上逆犯肺,致肺失宣降,肺气上逆,均可发为咳嗽病。

咳嗽病的病机为邪犯于肺,肺失宣肃,肺气上逆。病位在肺,与肝、脾、肾有关。外感咳嗽,属于实证。内伤咳嗽,为虚实夹杂之证,或以邪实为主,或以正虚为主。

二、常见证型

（一）辨证要点

1. 辨外感与内伤　根据病程长短、病情轻重、病位等来辨别。若起病急,病程短,病情轻,病变局限于肺,没有涉及其他脏腑,易于治疗,多为外感咳嗽。若病程长,反复发作,病情重,病变主要在肺,但涉及肝、脾、肾,治疗周期长,则多为内伤咳嗽。

2. 辨咳嗽　根据咳嗽的时间节律、声音、加重因素等来辨别证型。若白天咳嗽较多,多为外感实证、内伤实证;午后、黄昏咳嗽加重,多为阴虚;早晨咳嗽,痰出后咳减,多为痰湿。若咳嗽声重,多为风寒;咳声重浊,多为痰热;咳声嘶哑,病程短,多为风热;咳声嘶哑,病程长,多为阴虚。若单声咳嗽,轻微短促,多为风燥、阴虚;连声咳嗽,声音重浊,多为痰湿。若因寒热变化、异味而加重,多为风盛挛急;饮食肥甘生冷后加重,多为痰湿;郁怒后加重,多为肝火。

3. 辨痰　根据痰的量、色、质、气味来辨别证型。若痰白,多为风、寒、湿;痰黄,多为热;痰中带血,多为痰热、阴虚。若痰液稀薄,多为风寒;痰黏,多为风热、痰热、肝火、阴虚;痰稠厚,多为痰湿、痰热。若干咳少痰,多为风燥、风盛挛急、肝火、阴虚;咳嗽痰多,多为痰湿、痰热。若痰液味道热腥,多为痰热;味甜,多为痰湿;味咸,多为阴虚。

（二）证候分型

1. 外感咳嗽

（1）风寒袭肺证

［主要证候］咳嗽声重，气急，咽痒，咳白稀痰，常伴有鼻塞，流清涕，头痛，肢体酸痛，恶寒发热，无汗；舌苔薄白，脉浮紧。

［证候分析］风寒束表，内袭于肺，肺气失宣，故咳嗽声重，气急，咽痒；寒邪郁肺，气不布津，凝聚为痰，故咳白稀痰；寒束于表，腠理闭塞，阻遏经络，故头痛，肢体酸痛；卫阳被郁，正邪相争，故恶寒发热；舌苔薄白，脉浮紧，均为风寒袭肺之象。

［护治原则］疏风散寒，宣肺止咳。

［常用方剂］三拗汤合止嗽散。

（2）风热犯肺证

［主要证候］咳嗽频剧，气粗或咳声嘶哑，喉燥咽痛，咳痰不爽，痰黏稠或色黄，常伴有鼻流黄涕，口渴，头痛，恶风，身热；舌红，苔薄黄，脉浮数。

［证候分析］风热犯肺，肺失清肃，故咳嗽频剧，气粗或咳声音哑；肺热伤津，煎熬津液，故喉燥咽痛，口渴，咯痰不爽，痰黏稠或色黄，鼻流黄涕；风热外袭，卫表失和，故恶风，身热；风热上犯于头，故头痛；舌红，苔薄黄，脉浮数，均为风热犯表之象。

［护治原则］疏风清热，宣肺止咳。

［常用方剂］桑菊饮。

（3）风燥伤肺证

［主要证候］干咳无痰，或痰少而黏，不易咳出，或痰中带有血丝，咽喉干痛，口鼻干燥，初起或伴有少许恶寒，身热头痛；舌尖红，苔薄白或薄黄而干，脉小而数。

［证候分析］燥邪伤肺，肺失清肃，故干咳无痰，或痰少而黏，不易咳出；燥热灼伤肺络，故痰中带有血丝；燥胜则干，故咽喉干痛，口鼻干燥；风燥侵袭，卫气被遏，故初起或伴有恶寒，身热，头痛；舌尖红，苔薄白或薄黄而干，脉小而数，均为风燥伤肺之象。

［护治原则］疏风清肺，润燥止咳。

［常用方剂］桑杏汤。

（4）风盛挛急证

［主要证候］干咳无痰或少痰，咽痒，痒即咳嗽，或呛咳阵作，气急，遇外界寒热变化、异味等因素突发或加重，多于夜卧晨起时咳剧，呈反复性发作；舌苔薄白，脉弦。

［证候分析］风邪犯肺，邪客肺络，气道挛急，肺气失宣，故干咳无痰或少痰；风性开泄，风盛则动，故咽痒，痒即咳嗽，或呛咳阵作，气急；风邪善行而数变，故呈反复性发作；舌苔薄白，脉弦，均为风盛挛急之象。

［护治原则］疏风宣肺，解痉止咳。

［常用方剂］苏黄止咳汤。

2. 内伤咳嗽

（1）痰湿蕴肺证

［主要证候］咳嗽反复发作，咳声重浊，因痰而嗽，痰出则咳缓，痰多色白，黏腻或稠厚成块，每

于晨起或食甘甜油腻物后加重,胸闷脘痞,纳差乏力,大便时溏;舌苔白腻,脉濡滑。

[证候分析]脾湿生痰,上渍于肺,痰湿蕴肺,肺失宣降,故咳嗽反复发作,咳声重浊,痰多色白,黏腻或稠厚成块;脾失健运,运化无力,故纳差,大便时溏;痰湿中阻,气机不畅,故胸闷脘痞;舌苔白腻,脉濡滑,均为痰湿内蕴之象。

[护治原则]燥湿化痰,理气止咳。

[常用方剂]二陈汤合三子养亲汤。

（2）痰热郁肺证

[主要证候]咳嗽气粗,喉中可闻及痰声,痰多黄稠或黏厚,咯吐不爽,或有热腥味,或夹有血丝,胸胁胀满,咳时引痛,常伴有面赤,或有身热,口干欲饮;舌红,苔薄黄腻,脉滑数。

[证候分析]痰热郁肺,肺失清肃,故咳嗽气粗,痰多黄稠或黏厚,咯吐不爽;痰热蕴蒸,热伤肺络,故痰有热腥味,夹有血丝;痰热壅盛,气机不畅,故胸胁胀满,咳时引痛;肺热内郁,故面赤,身热,口干欲饮;舌红,苔薄黄腻,脉滑数,均为痰热内蕴之象。

[护治原则]清热化痰,肃肺止咳。

[常用方剂]清金化痰汤。

（3）肝火犯肺证

[主要证候]咳嗽阵作,咳时面红目赤,引胸胁作痛,咽干口苦,常感痰滞咽喉而咯之难出,量少质黏,或痰如絮条,症状可随情绪波动而增减;舌红,苔薄黄少津,脉弦数。

[证候分析]肝火犯肺,肺失肃降,故气逆咳嗽阵作;肝火上炎,故咳时面红目赤,咽干口苦;胁肋为肝经循行之区域,故咳引胸胁作痛;木火刑金,炼液成痰,故常感痰滞咽喉而咯之难出,量少质黏,或痰如絮条;舌红,苔薄黄少津,脉弦数,均为肝火内盛之象。

[护治原则]清肺泻肝,化痰止咳。

[常用方剂]黄芩泻白散合黛蛤散。

（4）肺阴亏虚证

[主要证候]干咳,咳声短促,痰少质黏色白,或痰中见血,或声音逐渐嘶哑,口干咽燥,午后潮热,颧红盗汗,常伴有日渐消瘦,神疲乏力;舌红少苔,脉细数。

[证候分析]肺失滋润,肃降无权,故干咳,咳声短促,痰少质黏色白;热伤肺络,故痰中见血;金破不鸣,故声音逐渐嘶哑;阴虚失于濡润,故口干咽燥;虚热内灼,故午后潮热,颧红盗汗;阴精不能充养,故日渐消瘦;舌红少苔,脉细数,均为阴虚之象。

[护治原则]养阴清热,润肺止咳。

[常用方剂]沙参麦冬汤。

三、护理措施

对于咳嗽病的病人,应观察咳嗽的诱因、发作季节、发作时间、持续时间、声音特点;痰的量、色、质、气味,痰中是否夹有血丝。观察伴随症状,比如恶寒、发热、汗出、胸闷、胸痛、消瘦。若病人出现高热不退,咳嗽加剧,伴胸痛,或口中有血腥味,痰中带血,应立即报告医生。

（一）辨证施护

1. 风寒袭肺证

（1）生活起居护理　居室温暖安静,空气新鲜,阳光充足,不可有强风、对流风。多休息,注意背部保暖。

（2）饮食护理　食物宜温热。可饮紫苏叶茶、柚核糖水。宜食宣肺散寒的食物,如生姜、葱白、杏仁。戒烟限酒,不宜食生冷、酸收、肥甘的食物。

（3）情志护理　护士可运用语言开导疗法,向病人讲解头身疼痛的发生原因和缓解方法,安抚病人紧张的情绪,鼓励其配合治疗。

（4）用药护理　中药汤剂应武火快煎,饭后热服。服后进食热饮、热粥,加盖衣被,使其微微汗出,热退后更衣。不可大汗和汗出当风。

（5）操作技术　① 拔罐疗法:取肺俞、风门、大杼,留罐10分钟,隔日1次。② 敷贴疗法:取大椎、肺俞、风门;用白芥子75 g,白芷10 g,研磨成粉后与蜂蜜调成糊状,加热后敷贴,早晚各换药1次。③ 穴位按摩法:取肺俞、列缺、太渊、合谷、太阳,用拇指揉法,按摩至局部发热或有酸麻重胀感,每日1次;孕妇禁用。④ 药熨疗法:用苏子、白芥子、香附、芜荑各30 g,细辛10 g,食盐30 g,食醋少许;翻炒至芳香灼手后装入软布袋,制成温度为60~70℃的中药热罨包,在脊柱或啰音密集处隔衣推熨,或待布袋温度下降后直接熨于皮肤,每次20分钟,每日2次;孕妇腰骶部禁用。

2. 风热犯肺证

（1）生活起居护理　居室凉爽避风,光线柔和。衣被宜薄。卧床休息。保持口腔清洁,饭后用金银花甘草液漱口。若汗多,应及时擦干,并换掉湿衣被。若发热,不可使用冷敷法。

（2）饮食护理　多饮水,可饮雪梨汁、西瓜汁、甘蔗汁、竹沥,或饮金银花茶、菊花茶。宜食疏风清热的食物,如白萝卜、枇杷、藕、荸荠、丝瓜。食疗方:鱼腥草猪肺汤、薄荷豆腐。戒烟限酒,不宜食辛辣、香燥的食物。

（3）情志护理　护士可运用语言开导疗法和移情易性疗法,向病人讲解发热和头痛的发生原因、缓解方法,安抚病人焦灼的情绪,并适时转移病人的注意力。

（4）用药护理　薄荷后下。中药汤剂应武火快煎,饭后温服。用药后观察汗出情况和体温,以微汗、热退、脉静、身凉为佳。

（5）操作技术　① 拔罐疗法:取肺俞、膻中、大椎,留罐10分钟,隔日1次。② 穴位按摩疗法:取肺俞、中府、列缺、太渊、曲池、尺泽,用拇指揉法,按摩至局部发热或有酸麻重胀感,每日1次;孕妇禁用。③ 刺血疗法:取大椎、曲池,皮肤消毒后揉按局部使其充血,用三棱针的3毫米针尖,快速刺入并出针,放出1.0 mL以下的血液,用无菌干棉球擦拭或按压;适用于高热不退者。

3. 风燥伤肺证

（1）生活起居护理　居室湿润舒适,安静避风。多休息,不要高声讲话。若干咳剧烈,可取坐位或半仰卧位,用舌尖抵住上腭,以减轻咳嗽。

（2）饮食护理　饮食宜清淡、滑软。多饮水,少量频饮以润喉,可饮桑叶茶。宜食疏风润燥的食物,如白萝卜、枇杷、蜂蜜、甘蔗、番茄。忌浓茶、咖啡、烟酒,不宜食辛辣、香燥、质地粗糙的食物。

（3）情志护理　护士可运用语言开导疗法,向病人讲解干咳的发生原因和缓解方法,安抚病人的情绪。

（4）用药护理　中药汤剂应武火快煎,饭后少量频饮,温服或偏凉服,服后卧床休息。

（5）操作技术　① 雾化吸入疗法:用桑杏汤,将药汤加入雾化装置,以43℃中药蒸汽吸入呼吸道,每次10分钟,每日1~2次。② 穴位按摩法:取肺俞、中府、列缺、太渊、太溪、照海,用拇指揉法,按摩至局部发热或有酸麻重胀感,每日1次;孕妇禁用。

4. 风盛挛急证

（1）生活起居护理　居室温暖湿润,空气新鲜,光线柔和,不可有强风、对流风。多休息,外出时戴口罩。若呛咳剧烈,取坐位或半仰卧位,适时屏息,以减轻咳嗽。在呛咳发作时,家属或护士应扶住病人,防止其摔倒,并用手掌在其背部由上至下轻轻推擦。若病人在呛咳后流出大量唾液,应及时清理。

（2）饮食护理　饮食宜清淡、滑软。多饮水,少量频饮以润喉,可用乌梅1颗泡水代茶饮。宜食益气润燥的食物,如山药、猪瘦肉、西瓜、橘子、雪梨。可用5~7粒白果与猪肉一起蒸食。忌烟酒、发物,不宜食辛辣、香燥、质地粗糙的食物。

（3）情志护理　护士可运用语言开导疗法,向病人讲解呛咳的发生原因和缓解方法,安抚其恐惧的情绪,鼓励病人积极配合治疗。

（4）用药护理　中药汤剂应饭后少量多次温服。携带润喉片,时时噙化。

（5）操作技术　① 点穴疗法:取天突,在呛咳发作时,用指按法,病人适时屏息。② 雾化吸入疗法:用苏黄止咳汤,以43℃中药蒸汽吸入呼吸道,每次10分钟,每日1~2次。③ 噙化疗法:用西瓜霜含片、草珊瑚含片或银黄含片,时时噙在口中含化。④ 灸法:取大椎、风门、外关,用温和灸,艾条燃着端悬于施灸部位上,距离皮肤2~3厘米,灸至病人有温热舒适无灼痛的感觉,皮肤稍有红晕,每日1次。

5. 痰湿蕴肺证

（1）生活起居护理　居室温暖干燥,安静舒适,空气新鲜。多休息,定时翻身、拍背。当病情平稳时,可适量锻炼,以不疲劳为度。若痰多,可用吸痰器吸出。

（2）饮食护理　饮食有节,少食多餐,不可暴饮暴食。可饮热白萝卜汁、陈皮茶。宜食健脾化痰的食物,如柚子、莱菔子、山药。食疗方:柠檬叶猪肺汤、风栗猪瘦肉汤、松塔豆腐汤。不宜食糯米甜食及生冷、肥甘、厚味的食物,如肥肉、奶油、花生。

（3）情志护理　病人病程较长,容易思虑过度,护士可运用语言开导疗法和暗示解惑疗法,耐心开导病人,抚慰和鼓励病人,帮助病人正确认识病情,保持心情舒畅。

（4）用药护理　中药汤剂应饭后温服,少量频服。

（5）操作技术　① 灸法:取大椎、肺俞、膏肓、足三里,用温和灸,艾条燃着端悬于施灸部位上,距离皮肤2~3厘米,灸至病人有温热舒适无灼痛的感觉,皮肤稍有红晕,每日1次;或用督灸,取大椎至腰俞,用3斤生姜末和9~11个7厘米长的艾炷,每次连灸3壮,每月1次,2~3次为一个疗程;孕妇禁用。② 耳压疗法:取气管、肺、脾、肾等耳穴,用耳穴压丸贴片贴压,每日按揉4~5次,以局部发热泛红为度,留置2~4日;孕妇禁用。③ 穴位按摩法:取肺俞、中府、列缺、太渊、足三里、丰隆,用拇指揉法,按摩至局部发热或有酸麻重胀感,每日1次;孕妇禁用。

6. 痰热郁肺证

（1）生活起居护理　居室凉爽安静,空气新鲜。多休息,定时翻身、拍背,可进行适量锻炼。注意口腔护理,饭后用金银花甘草液漱口。若痰中带血,咳后可用生理盐水漱口,以保持口腔的舒适感。若咳嗽时胸胁疼痛,可在咳嗽时用手按住疼痛处,减少胸廓活动度,以减轻疼痛。

(2)饮食护理　若咳吐血痰,应禁食。待症状消失后,进食半流食。可饮竹沥、白萝卜汁、鲜芦根茶。宜食清热化痰的食物,如荸荠、雪梨、薏苡仁、藕。忌烟酒、浓茶、咖啡,不宜食肥甘、辛辣、香燥的食物。

(3)情志护理　因症状较重,且可能伴有咳吐血痰,病人可能感到焦虑、恐惧。护士可运用语言开导疗法,与病人及家属共同评估其忧虑程度,多与病人沟通,安慰和鼓励病人,介绍治疗效果较好的同种病人互相交流,以增强病人的信心,避免恐惧、思虑。

(4)用药护理　中药汤剂应饭后温服或偏凉服。

(5)操作技术　① 电离子导入疗法:取肺部听诊湿啰音处,用紫草液或鱼腥草液,进行药物离子导入,每次 20 分钟,每日 1 次;孕妇禁用。② 敷贴疗法:取涌泉、孔最、膈俞,用冰片 3 g,研磨成粉后与大蒜泥 9 g 调匀,制成大拇指指面大小的药饼,敷贴于腧穴上,用胶布固定,每次 2 小时,每日 1 次。

7. 肝火犯肺证

(1)生活起居护理　居室凉爽湿润,安静舒适,光线柔和,空气新鲜。可进行适量锻炼,以微微出汗为宜。

(2)饮食护理　多饮水,可饮绿豆汁、藕汁、雪梨汁、菊花茶、丝瓜花茶。宜食清肝泻火的食物,如丝瓜、芹菜、香菇。戒烟限酒,不宜食辛辣、香燥的食物。

(3)情志护理　病人常有情绪波动,护士可运用语言开导疗法、移情易性疗法和顺意疗法,告诉病人不良的情绪会加重病情,要求病人忌怒;用读书、听音乐等方法使病人感到放松;不聊有争议性的话题,避免不良的人际关系影响病人的情绪。

(4)用药护理　蛤壳先煎。中药汤剂应饭后温服或偏凉服。

(5)操作技术　① 雾化吸入疗法:用黄芩泻白散,以 43℃ 中药蒸汽吸入呼吸道,每次 10 分钟,每日 1~2 次。② 穴位按摩法:取肺俞、太渊、行间、鱼际、血海,用拇指揉法,按摩至局部发热或有酸麻重胀感,每日 1 次;孕妇禁用。③ 耳压疗法:取心、神门等耳穴,用耳穴压丸贴片贴压,每日按揉 4~5 次,以局部发热泛红为度,留置 2~4 日;孕妇禁用。

8. 肺阴亏虚证

(1)生活起居护理　居室凉爽湿润,安静舒适,光线柔和,空气新鲜,不可有强风、对流风。卧床休息,定时翻身、拍背。睡眠充足,偶尔进行轻缓的运动,如散步、打太极拳。若盗汗,应及时擦干,并换掉湿衣被。若痰中带血,咳痰后用生理盐水漱口。不要熬夜、过劳、剧烈咳嗽、长时间高声讲话。

(2)饮食护理　若咳吐血痰,应禁食。待症状缓解后,可进食半流食。鼓励进食,经常变换菜品,少食多餐。可饮薏苡仁茶。五汁蜜膏:雪梨、白萝卜各 1 000 g,生姜、炼乳、蜂蜜各 250 g;雪梨(去核)、白萝卜、生姜分别捣碎绞挤取汁;将雪梨汁、白萝卜汁合而煮至膏状,加入生姜汁、炼乳、蜂蜜,急搅令匀后煮沸,冷却后装瓶;每次取 1 汤匙,用沸水冲调,每日 2 次。宜食滋阴润肺的食物,如银耳、百合、藕、莲子、柿饼、燕窝、鳖肉。忌烟酒、浓茶、咖啡,不宜食肥甘、辛辣、香燥的食物。

(3)情志护理　病人痰中带血,病程较长,经常感到疲乏,可能出现恐惧、消沉的情绪,护士可运用语言开导疗法和移情易性疗法,多关心和鼓励病人,用看电视、聊天等方法转移其注意力,介绍治疗效果较好的同种病人互相交流,以增强病人的信心,消除不良情绪。

（4）用药护理　中药汤剂宜饭前温服,少量频服。

（5）操作技术　① 穴位按摩法：取肺俞、中府、列缺、太渊、膏肓、太溪,用拇指揉法,按摩至局部发热或有酸麻重胀感,每日1次;孕妇禁用。② 敷贴疗法：取涌泉,用大蒜泥制成大拇指指面大小的药饼敷贴,每次2小时,每日1次。

（二）健康教育

居室向阳避风,空气新鲜。注意保暖,防止感冒。适当进行体育锻炼,以增强体质。进行自我保健按摩,可每日揉按风池10分钟,以局部有发热感或酸麻重胀感为佳。

饮食宜清淡、营养、易消化。多吃新鲜的水果和蔬菜。忌烟酒、发物,不宜食辛辣、肥腻、过甜的食物,如带鱼、黄鱼、胡椒、辣椒、大蒜、大葱、韭菜。

保持精神愉快。指导病人自我调节,避免忧虑、恼怒。

服用止咳化痰药后,不要立即饮水,以免冲淡药液而降低疗效。服用散剂时,用温水调服,禁止干服,以防粉末呛入气管而加重咳嗽。

鼓励病人有效咳痰：饮少量水湿润咽部,缓慢深吸气,屏气1~2秒后再用力咳嗽,将深部的痰咳出。若痰黏难咳,协助病人取半仰卧位,定时翻身;用空心掌自下而上、由外向内轻叩病人背部,并配合有效咳痰,以促进排痰。

若病人有百日咳、肺结核等传染性疾病,应严格执行呼吸道隔离。室内空气定期消毒,痰液消毒后方可倾倒。

Section 2   Cough

Cough is a lung system disease mainly characterized by cough and expectoration of phlegm. It is caused by failure of lung qi to disperse and descend and subsequent adverse rising of lung qi, which are due to invasion of the lung by six external pathogenic factors, stimulation of harmful gases, internal damage of zang-fu organs, lung and spleen qi deficiency, phlegm and retained fluid accumulating in the lung, invasion of the lung by liver fire, or chronic illness with deficiency of qi and yin. It includes cough caused by external pathogens and internal damage. This section may be referred to for the nursing of diseases with cough as the main manifestation in Western medicine, such as acute trachea-bronchitis, chronic bronchitis, and cough variant asthma.

ETIOLOGY AND PATHOGENESIS

The etiology includes affection by external pathogens and internal damage. The six pathogenic factors enter the body from the mouth, nose, skin or hair, and fetter lung qi, resulting in failure of lung qi to disperse and descend, and adverse rising of qi causes sounds in the airway, hence cough occurs. Wind is the chief of six excesses and cough due to external affection is mostly induced by wind. Internal damage of zang-fu organs is mainly caused by diseases of the lung or those of other zang-organs that involve the lung. For example, the lung suffers from several kinds of prolonged diseases that consume lung qi, scorch lung yin, and cause failure of lung qi to disperse and descend; overstrain, spleen and stomach damage, and failure of the spleen to transport and transform produce internal phlegm and dampness that upward stain the lung; improper diet and predilection for cigarette and alcohol assist fire to scorch the lung and stomach; or long-time emotional stimulation and failure of the liver to act freely generate fire that upward invades the lung.

The pathogenesis is pathogens invading the lung, leading to failure of lung qi to disperse and descend, which causes counterflow of lung qi. The disease is located in the lung and relates to the liver, spleen and kidney. Cough due to external affection belongs to excess syndrome while cough due to internal damage may be deficiency-excess in complexity, predominant by pathogens, or by deficiency of healthy qi.

COMMON SYNDROMES

Key Points in Syndrome Differentiation

1. Differentiation of External Affection from Internal Damage

The differentiation is based on the length of disease course, severity of condition, and location of disease. Cough due to external affection is featured by acute onset, short course, mild condition and localized lesion in the lung, and is easily cured. Cough due to internal damage is marked by long course, repeated occurrence, severe condition, lesion mainly in the lung but involving the liver, spleen and kidney, and long treatment cycle.

2. Differentiation of Cough

The differentiation is based on the occurrence pattern, sound and aggravating factors. If cough mostly occurs during the daytime, it indicates excess syndrome of external affection or internal damage. If cough aggravates in the afternoon or at dusk, it means yin deficiency. If cough occurs in the morning and is relieved after expectoration, it pertains to phlegm dampness. Heavy sound indicates wind-cold type while heavy turbid sound, phlegm heat. Hoarse sound and short course of disease means wind-heat type whereas hoarse sound and long course of disease, yin deficiency. Single cough with slight shortness and hastiness means wind-dryness and yin deficiency whereas repeated cough with heavy turbid sound, phlegm dampness. Cough worsened with variance of cold and heat and peculiar smell relates to wind exuberance that causes airway contraction. Cough worsened after eating fatty, too-sweet, raw and cold foods links with phlegm dampness. And cough aggravated after depressed anger means liver fire.

3. Differentiation of Phlegm

The differentiation is based on the amount, color, texture and smell phlegm. White phlegm means wind, cold and dampness. Yellow phlegm shows heat. Phlegm with blood indicates phlegm heat and yin deficiency. Clear thin phlegm means wind-cold; sticky phlegm indicates wind-heat, phlegm heat, liver fire, and yin deficiency; thick phlegm symbolizes phlegm dampness and phlegm heat. Dry cough with scanty phlegm links with wind-dryness, wind exuberance that causes airway contraction, liver fire and yin deficiency. Cough with profuse phlegm relates to phlegm-heat and phlegm-dampness. Foul-smelling, sweet and salty phlegm suggest phlegm-heat, phlegm-dampness and yin deficiency, respectively.

Syndrome Differentiation

1. Cough due to External Affection

(1) Wind-Cold Attacking the Lung Syndrome

[Clinical Manifestations] Cough with heavy sound, rapid breathing, itching throat, white thin phlegm, often accompanied by nasal congestion, thin nasal discharge, headache, aching limbs, aversion to cold, fever, absence of sweating, white thin tongue coating, and floating tight pulse.

[Manifestations Analysis] Wind-cold fettering the exterior causes failure of lung qi to disperse and descend, so cough occurs with heavy sound, rapid breathing, and itching throat. Cold pathogen depressing the lung makes qi unable to distribute body fluids, which are condensed into phlegm, so white thin phlegm is coughed. Cold fettering the exterior blocks striae and interstice as well as meridians, leading to headache and aching limbs. Defensive yang is constrained and healthy qi struggles with pathogenic qi, so aversion to cold and fever occur. White thin tongue coating and floating tight pulse are signs of wind-cold attacking the lung.

[Nursing Principle] Dispersing wind and dissipating cold; ventilating lung and relieving cough.

[Suggested Formula] San'ao Decoction and Zhisou Powder.

(2) Wind-Heat Invading the Lung Syndrome

[Clinical Manifestations] Frequent severe cough, rough breathing, cough with hoarseness, dry and sore throat, difficult expectoration, sticky thick phlegm or yellow phlegm, often accompanied by yellow nasal discharge, thirst, headache, aversion to wind, fever, red tongue with thin yellow coating, and floating rapid pulse.

[Manifestations Analysis] Wind-heat invading the lung causes failure of lung qi to disperse and descend, leading to frequent severe cough, rough breathing, and cough with hoarseness. Lung heat consumes body fluids, so such symptoms appear as dry and sore throat, thirst, difficult expectoration, sticky thick phlegm or yellow phlegm, and yellow nasal discharge. External invasion of wind-heat causes disharmony of defensive exterior, so aversion to wind and fever occur. Wind-heat upward invades the head, so headache happens. Red tongue with thin yellow coating and floating rapid pulse are manifestations of wind-heat invading the lung.

[Nursing Principle] Dispersing wind and clearing heat; ventilating lung and relieving cough.

[Suggested Formula] Sangju Drink.

(3) Wind-Dryness Damaging the Lung Syndrome

[Clinical Manifestations] Dry cough without phlegm, or scanty sticky phlegm, difficult expectoration, or blood-streaked phlegm, dry and sore throat, dry mouth and nose, possible companion of slight aversion to cold, fever and headache at the early stage, red tongue tip, thin white tongue coating or thin yellow and dry coaking, and small rapid pulse.

[Manifestations Analysis] Pathogenic dryness damaging the lung cause failure of lung qi to disperse and descend, leading to dry cough without phlegm, or scanty sticky phlegm, and difficult expectoration. Dryness-heat scorches lung collaterals, so there is blood-streaked phlegm. Dominance of dryness brings about dry and sore throat, and dry mouth and nose. Wind-dryness constrains defense qi, therefore, there occur possible companion of slight aversion to cold, fever and headache at the early stage. Red tongue tip, thin white tongue coating or thin yellow and dry coating, and small rapid pulse are manifestations of wind-dryness damaging the lung.

[Nursing Principle] Dispersing wind and clearing the lung; moistening dryness and relieving cough.

[Suggested Formula] Sangxing Decoction.

(4) Wind Exuberance and Airway Contraction Syndrome

[Clinical Manifestations] Dry cough with no or scanty phlegm, itching throat with concomitant cough, or paroxysmal choking cough, rapid breathing, cough suddenly occurring or worsened with variance of cold and heat and peculiar smell, repeated severe cough often at night when sleeping or in the morning when getting up, white thin tongue coating, and wiry pulse.

[Manifestations Analysis] Pathogenic wind invades the lung and intrudes into lung collaterals, which causes the airway to contract and failure of lung qi to disperse and descend, leading to dry cough with no or scanty phlegm. Wind pathogen is characterized by opening, dispersing and mobile, so present symptoms such as itching throat with concomitant cough, or paroxysmal choking cough, and rapid breathing. Wind is mobile and changeable, so cough occurs repeatedly. White thin tongue coating and wiry pulse are signs of wind exuberance and airway contraction.

[Nursing Principle] Dispersing wind and ventilating the lung; arresting convulsions and relieving cough.

[Suggested Formula] Suhuang Zhike Decoction.

2. Cough due to Internal Damage

(1) Phlegm-Dampness Accumulating in the Lung Syndrome

[Clinical Manifestations] Repeated cough with heavy turbid sound, cough caused by phlegm and alleviated after expectoration, profuse white sticky phlegm or thick phlegm clots, aggravation in the morning when getting up or after intake of too-sweet and greasy foods, chest oppression, gastric stuffiness, poor appetite, lassitude, frequent loose stool, white slimy tongue coating, and soggy slippery pulse.

[Manifestations Analysis] Spleen dampness generates phlegm that stains the lung, and phlegm-dampness accumulates in the lung, leading to failure of lung qi to disperse and descend, so the symptoms occur including repeated cough with heavy turbid sound, profuse white phlegm that is sticky or forms thick clots. Dysfunction of the spleen in transportation and transformation explains poor appetite and frequent loose stool. Phlegm-dampness obstructs the middle energizer and inhibits qi movement, so chest oppression and gastric stuffiness are felt. White slimy tongue coating and soggy slippery pulse are signs of internal accumulation of phlegm-dampness.

[Nursing Principle] Drying dampness and resolving phlegm; regulating qi and relieving cough.

[Suggested Formula] Erchen Decoction and Sanzi Yangqin Decoction.

(2) Phlegm-Heat Depressing the Lung Syndrome

[Clinical Manifestations] Cough with rough breathing, phlegm sound in the throat, profuse yellow sticky or thick phlegm, difficult expectoration, or foul-smelling phlegm, blood-streaked phlegm, chest and hypochondriac fullness and distention, chest and hypochondriac pain when coughing, red complexion, or fever, dry mouth with desire to drink, red tongue with thin yellow and slimy coating, and slippery rapid pulse.

[Manifestations Analysis] Phlegm-heat depressing the lung causes failure of lung qi to disperse and descend, leading to cough with rough breathing, profuse yellow sticky or thick phlegm, and difficult expectoration. Phlegm-heat accumulates in the lung and steams lung collaterals, so foul-smelling phlegm or blood-streaked phlegm is produced. Phlegm-heat exuberance inhibits qi movement, so the patients feel chest and hypochondriac fullness and distention, or chest and hypochondriac pain when coughing. Interior depression of lung heat leads to red complexion, fever, and dry mouth with desire to drink. Red tongue with thin yellow and slimy coating and slippery rapid pulse suggest interior accumulation of phlegm-heat.

[Nursing Principle] Clearing heat and resolving phlegm; descending lung qi and relieving cough.

[Suggested Formula] Qingjin Huatan Decoction.

(3) Liver-Fire Invading the Lung Syndrome

[Clinical Manifestations] Paroxysmal cough with red face and eyes, chest and hypochondriac pain when coughing, dry throat, bitter taste in the mouth, difficult expectoration with sensation of phlegm stagnating in the throat, scanty sticky or flocculent phlegm, symptoms changing with emotional fluctuation, red tongue with thin yellow coating and scanty fluids, and wiry rapid pulse.

[Manifestations Analysis] Liver-fire invading the lung causes failure of lung qi to disperse and descend, leading to counterflow of qi and paroxysmal cough. Liver fire flames upward, resulting in red face and eyes when coughing, dry throat, and bitter taste in the mouth. Hypochondriac area is in the course of liver meridian, so chest and hypochondriac are painful when coughing. Wood fire tormenting metal and scorching fluids results in difficult expectoration with sensation of phlegm stagnating in the throat as well as scanty sticky or flocculent phlegm. Red tongue with thin yellow coating and scanty fluids, and wiry rapid pulse manifest exuberance of liver fire.

[Nursing Principle] Clearing the lung and draining the liver; resolving phlegm and relieving cough.

[Suggested Formula] Huangqin Xiebai Powder and Daige Powder.

(4) Lung-Yin Depletion Syndrome

[Clinical Manifestations] Dry cough with shortness and hastiness, white scanty and sticky phlegm, or blood-streaked phlegm, or gradual hoarseness of voice, dry mouth and throat, afternoon tidal fever, hectic cheeks, night sweat, often accompanied by gradual emaciation, mental and physical fatigue, red tongue with scanty coating, and thready rapid pulse.

[Manifestations Analysis] The lung lacking nourishment causes failure of lung qi to disperse and descend, leading to dry cough with shortness and hastiness as well as white scanty and sticky phlegm. Heat damaging lung collaterals explains blood-streaked phlegm. Broken metal failing to sound causes gradual hoarseness of voice. Yin deficiency cannot moisten the lung, so dry mouth and throat is felt. Deficiency heat scorching fluids results in afternoon tidal fever, hectic cheeks, and night sweat. Yin essence cannot fill and nourish the body, so gradual emaciation is developed. Red tongue with scanty coating, and thready rapid pulse symbolize yin deficiency.

[Nursing Principle] Nourishing yin and clearing heat; moistening lung and relieving cough.

[Suggested Formula] Shashen Maidong Decoction.

NURSING MEASURES

For patients with cough, nurses should observe the inducing factor; the season, time and duration of onset; the sound characteristics of cough; the amount, color, texture and smell of phlegm; and the presence of blood streak in phlegm. They should check the accompanied symptoms, such as aversion to cold, fever, sweating, chest oppression, chest pain and emaciation. If the patient has unabating high fever and worsening cough, accompanied with chest pain, blood taste in the mouth, or blood in phlegm, report to the doctor immediately.

Syndrome-Based Nursing Measures

1. Wind-Cold Attacking the Lung Syndrome

(1) Daily life nursing. The ward should be warm, quiet, and full of fresh air and adequate sunshine, and avoid strong and convective wind. The patients should take more rest, and keep the back of the trunk warm.

(2) Diet nursing. Foods should be warm. Zisuye (leaf of purple perilla) tea or pomelo seed sugar water is recommended. The patients may eat foods that ventilate the lung and dissipate cold, such as shengjiang (fresh ginger), congbai (scallion white), and xingren (apricot kernel). They should refrain from smoking, drinking and eating foods that are raw, cold, sour, astringent, greasy and sweet.

(3) Emotion nursing. Nurses may use verbal enlightenment therapy to impart patients the pathogenesis and relieving methods of headache and generalized pain, calm their nerves and encourage them to cooperate in treatment.

(4) Medication nursing. Decoction should be prepared fast with strong fire and taken hot after meals. The patients should eat hot porridge or hot rice soup, tuck themselves in to perspire slightly after taking the decoction. When the sweating is over, change the wet clothes timely. Profuse sweating and sweating in the wind are prohibited.

(5) Manipulation techniques. ① Cupping therapy: select Feishu (BL 13), Fengmen (BL 12), and Dazhu (BL 11); retain the cup on the acupoints for 10 minutes, once every other day. ② Paste application therapy: select Dazhui (GV 14), Feishu (BL 13), and Fengmen (BL 12); grind into powder baijiezi (white mustard seed) 75 g and baizhi (angelica root) 10 g, blend the powder with honey to make paste, and apply the paste on the acupoints once in the morning and once in the evening. ③ Acupressure therapy: select Feishu (BL 13), Lieque (LU 7), Taiyuan (LU 9), Hegu (LI 4) and Taiyang (EX − HN5); apply thumb kneading manipulation on each of the acupoints until the area turns hot or the patient has the feelings of soreness, numbness, heaviness and distension in the area, once per day. And it is contraindicated in pregnancy. ④ Medicated ironing therapy: take suzi (perilla fruit) 30 g, baijiezi (white mustard seed) 30 g, xiangfu (cyperus rhizome) 30 g, wuyi (elm cake) 30 g, xixin (Manchurian wild ginger) 10 g, salt 30 g and some vinegar; stir-fry the above materials until they are fragrant and hot, and put them into a cloth bag for medicated ironing at a temperature of 60~70℃; put

the bag on the spinal cord or above the rale region of the lung through clothes and move the bag constantly, or put the bag directly on the skin and move along when the temperature becomes warm; 20 minutes each time, twice per day. And it cannot be applied on the lumbosacral region of pregnant women.

2. Wind-Heat Invading the Lung Syndrome

(1) Daily life nursing. The ward should be cool, full of gentle light, and away from wind. The coverings should be thin. The patients should stay in bed, pay attention to oral hygiene, and rinse the mouth after meals with jinyinhua gancao (honeysuckle flower and licorice root) liquid. For the patients with profuse sweating, wipe the sweat away and change the wet clothes and bedding timely. For the patients with fever, cold application therapy is prohibited.

(2) Diet nursing. The patients should drink more water. They may drink snow pear juice, watermelon juice, sugarcane juice, zhuli (bamboo sap), jinyinhua (honeysuckle flower) tea or juhua (chrysanthemum flower) tea. They may eat foods that disperse wind and clear heat, such as white radishes, loquats, lotus root, biqi (waternuts) and luffa. Food therapy: yuxingcao zhufei (heartleaf houttuynia and pig lung) soup, and bohe doufu (field mint stewed with tofu). They should refrain from smoking and drinking, and avoid pungent, spicy, fragrant and dry-natured foods.

(3) Emotion nursing. Nurses may use verbal enlightenment therapy as well as emotional transference and dispositional change therapy to impart patients the causes and relieving methods of fever and headache, calm their nerves, and distract their attention when necessary.

(4) Medication nursing. Bohe (field mint) should be decocted later. Decoction should be prepared fast with strong fire and taken warm after meals. After taking medicine, observe the condition of sweating and body temperature. Slight sweating, fever abatement, pacified pulse and cool skin are preferred conditions.

(5) Manipulation techniques. ① Cupping therapy: select Feishu (BL 13), Danzhong (CV 17) and Dazhui (GV 14); retain the cup on the acupoints for 10 minutes, once every other day. ② Acupressure therapy: select Feishu (BL 13), Zhongfu (LU 1), Lieque (LU 7), Taiyuan (LU 9), Quchi (LI 11) and Chize (LU 5); apply thumb kneading manipulation on each of the acupoints until the area turns hot or the patient has the feelings of soreness, numbness, distension and heaviness in the area; once per day. And it is contraindicated in pregnancy. ③ Blood-letting therapy: select Dazhui (GV 14) and Quchi (LI 11); after the skin is disinfected, rub the local area to make it hyperemic, use a three-edged needle to quickly pierce the skin at a depth of 3 millimeters, remove the needle to release blood less than 1.0 mL, and wipe or press the pierced point with a sterile dry cotton ball. This therapy is suitable for patients with persistent high fever.

3. Wind-Dryness Damaging the Lung Syndrome

(1) Daily life nursing. The ward should be moist, cool, quiet and away from wind. The patients should take more rest and avoid speaking loudly. For patients with severe dry cough, take a sitting or semi-supine position, and hold the tongue tip against the upper palate to ease the cough.

(2) Diet nursing. The diet should be light, slippery and soft. The patients should drink more water, multiple times in small portions to moist the throat, and may drink sangye (mulberry leaf) tea. They may eat foods that disperse wind and moist dryness, such as white radishes, loquats, honey, sugarcanes, and tomatoes. They should refrain from drinking strong tea coffee and alcohol, smoking and eating foods that are pungent, spicy, fragrant, dry-natured and coarse.

(3) Emotion nursing. Nurses may use verbal enlightenment therapy to impart patients the causes and relieving methods of dry cough to soothe them.

(4) Medication nursing. Decoction should be prepared fast with strong fire and taken warm or slightly cool after meals, multiple times with small portions. After taking medicine, the patients should take a rest in the bed.

(5) Manipulation techniques. ① Spray inhalation therapy: inhale the steam of Sangxing Decoction into respiratory tract at a temperature of 43℃, 10 minutes each time, 1~2 times per day. ② Acupressure therapy: select Feishu (BL 13), Zhongfu (LU 1), Lieque (LU 7), Taiyuan (LU 9), Taixi (KI 3) and Zhaohai (KI 6); apply thumb kneading manipulation on each of the acupoints until the area turns hot or the patient has the feelings of soreness, numbness, distension and heaviness in the area; once per day. And it is contraindicated in pregnancy.

4. Wind Exuberance and Airway Contraction Syndrome

(1) Daily life nursing. The ward should be warm, moist and full of fresh air and gentle light, and avoid strong and convective wind. The patients should take more rest and wear a mask when going outside. For patients with severe choking cough, take a sitting or semi-supine position and hold the breath timely to ease the cough. During choking cough, family members or the nurses should support the patients with hands to prevent falls, and do the palm-pushing and scrubbing manipulations gently on their back from top to bottom. If there is large amount of saliva after choking cough, it should be cleaned in time.

(2) Diet nursing. The diet should be light, slippery and soft. The patients should drink more water, multiple times in small portions to moist the throat, or make tea using a wumei (smoked plum) and drink it. They may eat foods that replenish qi and moist dryness, such as shanyao (common yam rhizome), lean pork, watermelons, oranges and snow pears. Food therapy: 5~7 baiguo (ginkgo nuts) steamed with pork. The patients should refrain from smoking, drinking, and eating foods that induce or aggravate disease, and those that are pungent, spicy, fragrant, dry-natured and coarse.

(3) Emotion nursing. Nurses may use verbal enlightenment therapy to impart patients the causes and relieving methods of chocking cough to soothe the terrified patients and encourage them to cooperate in treatment.

(4) Medication nursing. Medicinals should be decocted for a short time with strong fire and taken warm after meals, multiple times with small portions. The patients should take with them throat tablets at all times, and have one in the mouth constantly.

(5) Manipulation techniques. ① Acupoint-pressing therapy: select Tiantu (CV 22); apply finger-

pressing manipulation on the acupoint when choking cough happens; the patients should hold the breath at the same time. ② Spray inhalation therapy: inhale the steam of Suhuang Zhike Decoction at a temperature of 43℃ into the respiratory tract, 10 minutes each time, once or twice a day. ③ Mouth dissolving therapy: use Xiguashuang (watermelon frost) Buccal Tablet, Caoshanhu (Sarcandra glabra) Buccal Tablet or Yinhuang Buccal Tablet; dissolve the tablet in mouth constantly. ④ Moxibustion therapy: select Dazhui (GV 14), Fengmen (BL 12) and Waiguan (TE 5); place the moxa stick 2~3 centimeters away from the skin to perform mild moxibustion on each of the acupoints until the area turns red and the patient feels warm and comfortable without the sensation of burning pain, once per day.

5. Phlegm-Dampness Accumulating in the Lung Syndrome

(1) Daily life nursing. The ward should be warm, dry, quiet, comfortable and full of fresh air. The patients should take more rest, and have regular turning-over and back-patting. When the condition is stabilized, the patients should take moderate exercise and avoid getting tired. For patients with profuse phlegm, sputum aspirator may be used.

(2) Diet nursing. The patients should follow a regular and moderate diet, and have small frequent meals without being too full. They may drink hot white radish juice or chenpi (aged tangerine peel) tea, and eat foods that invigorate spleen and resolve phlegm, such as pomelos, laifuzi (radish seed) and shanyao (common yam rhizome). Food therapy: lemon leaf pig lung soup, dried Chinese chestnut lean pork soup, or pinecone tofu soup. The patients should refrain from eating foods made of glutinous rice and foods that are raw, cold, fatty and sweet, such as fatty meat, butter and peanuts.

(3) Emotion nursing. Because of a long disease course, the patients may worry too much. To help the patients understand the condition and maintain a good mood, nurses may use verbal enlightenment therapy as well as suggestive and doubts-dispelling therapy to patiently enlighten, comfort and encourage them, so that they can better understand the disease and have a good mood.

(4) Medication nursing. Decoction should be taken warm after meals, multiple times in small portions.

(5) Manipulation techniques. ① Moxibustion therapy: select Dazhui (GV 14), Feishu (BL 13), Gaohuang (BL 43) and Zusanli (ST 36); place the moxa stick 2~3 centimeters away from the skin to perform mild moxibustion on each of the acupoints until the area turns red and the patient feels warm and comfortable without the sensation of burning pain, once per day. Or select the area between Dazhui (GV 14) and Yaoshu (GV 2); use mashed fresh ginger 1 500 g and 9~11 moxa cones of 7 centimeters long to apply governor vessel moxibustion, three moxa cones each time, once per month, and 2~3 sessions as a course of treatment. And it is contraindicated in pregnancy. ② Articular pressure therapy: select the auricular acupoints of trachea (CO16), lung (CO14), spleen (CO13) and kidney (CO10); apply specialized pasters on the points, knead each of them till the area turns hot and red, 4~5 times per day, and keep the pasters for 2~4 days. And it is contraindicated in pregnancy. ③ Acupressure therapy: select Feishu (BL 13), Zhongfu (LU 1), Lieque (LU 7), Taiyuan (LU 9), Zusanli (ST 36) and Fenglong

（ST 40）; apply thumb kneading manipulation on each of the acupoints until the area turns hot or the patient has the feelings of soreness, numbness, distension and heaviness in the area; once per day. And it is contraindicated in pregnancy.

6. Phlegm-Heat Depressing the Lung Syndrome

（1）Daily life nursing. The ward should be cool, quiet, and full of fresh air. The patients should take more rest, have regular turning-over and back-patting, do moderate exercise, pay attention to oral hygiene, and rinse the mouth after meals with jinyinhua gancao（honeysuckle flower and licorice root）liquid. For patients with bloody phlegm, rinse the mouth with normal saline after cough to keep the patients comfortable. For patients with chest and rib-side pain during cough, press the painful location to reduce the range of thoracic motion to ease the pain.

（2）Diet nursing. For patients with bloody phlegm, they are fasted and allowed to have semi-liquid diet when the symptom disappears. The patients may drink Zhuli（bamboo sap）, white radish juice, or xianlugen（fresh reed root）tea, and eat foods that clear heat and resolve phlegm, such as biqi （waternuts）, snow pears, yiyiren（coix seed）and lotus root. The patients should refrain from smoking and drinking alcohol, strong tea and coffee and eating foods that are fatty, sweet, pungent, spicy, fragrant and dry-natured.

（3）Emotion nursing. Because the symptoms are severe and possibly accompanied with bloody phlegm, the patients may feel anxious and frightened. To enhance patients' confidence and eliminate their fear and anxiety, nurses may evaluate the degree of anxiety with the patients and their family members, use verbal enlightenment therapy to comfort and encourage them, and organize communication with patients of the same disease who have shown better treatment effect.

（4）Medication nursing. Decoction should be taken warm or slightly cool after meals.

（5）Manipulation techniques. ① Electrical iontophoresis therapy: select the moist rale areas of the lung, and use zicao（arnebia root）or yuxingcao（heartleaf houttuynia）decoction for electrical iontophoresis therapy, 20 minutes each time, once per day. And it is contraindicated in pregnancy. ② Paste application therapy: select Yongquan（KI 1）, Kongzui（LU 6）and Geshu（BL 17）; grind 3 g of bingpian（borneol）into powder, blend it with 9 g of ground garlic to make thumb-pulp-sized medicated cakes, apply the cakes on the acupoints, and fix them with adhesive tapes, 2 hours each time, once per day.

7. Liver-Fire Invading the Lung Syndrome

（1）Daily life nursing. The ward should be cool, moist, quiet, comfortable, and full of gentle light and fresh air. The patients may do moderate exercise, with slight sweating preferred.

（2）Diet nursing. The patients should drink more water. They may drink lüdou（mung bean）juice, lotus root juice, snow pear juice, juhua（chrysanthemum flower）tea or luffa flower tea, and eat foods that clear liver and purge fire, such as luffa, celery, and lentinus edodes. They should refrain from smoking, drinking and eating foods that are pungent, spicy, fragrant and dry-natured.

（3）Emotion nursing. The patients often suffers from mood fluctuations, so nurses may use verbal enlightenment therapy to tell the patients that a bad mood would aggravate the disease and they should avoid being angry; adopt emotional transference and dispositional change therapy to advise them to read or listen to music for relaxation; and employ submission therapy to avoid controversial topics and influence of bad interpersonal relationship.

(4) Medication nursing. Geqiao (clam shell) should be decocted earlier. Decoction should be taken warm or slightly cool after meals.

(5) Manipulation techniques. ① Spray inhalation therapy: decoct Huangqin Xiebai Powder, and inhale the steam of the decoction into respiratory tract at a temperature of 43℃, 10 minutes each time, 1~2 times per day. ② Acupressure therapy: select Feishu (BL 13), Taiyuan (LU 9), Xingjian (LR 2), Yuji (LU 10) and Xuehai (SP 10); apply thumb kneading manipulation on each of the acupoints until the area turns hot or the patient has the feelings of soreness, numbness, distension and heaviness in the area; once per day. And it is contraindicated in pregnancy. ③ Auricular pressure therapy: select the auricular points of heart (CO15) and shenmen (TF4); apply specialized pasters on the points, knead each of them till the area turns hot and red, 4~5 times per day, and keep the pasters for 2~4 days. And it is contraindicated in pregnancy.

8. Lung-Yin Depletion Syndrome

(1) Daily life nursing. The ward should be cool, moist, quiet, comfortable, and full of gentle light and fresh air, and avoid strong and convective wind. The patients should stay in bed, have regular turning-over and back-patting, ensure sufficient sleep, and do moderate exercise occasionally, such as walking and Taiji. For the patients with night sweat, wipe the sweat away and change the wet clothes and bedding timely. For patients with bloody phlegm, rinse the mouth with normal saline after expectoration. Avoid staying up late, overstrain, severe cough and long-time loud speaking.

(2) Diet nursing. For patients with bloody phlegm, they are fasted and allowed to have semi-liquid diet after the symptom is alleviated. Encourage the patients to have small frequent meals, and serve them a variety of dishes constantly. Yiyiren (coix seed) tea is recommended. Wuzhimi Extract: prepare snow pears 1 000 g, white radishes 1 000 g, shengjiang (fresh ginger) 250 g, condensed milk 250 g and honey 250 g; squash the snow pears (without core), white radishes and shengjiang (fresh ginger) separately to get the juice; blend the snow pear juice with white radish juice and boil them into condensed extract, add in shengjiang (fresh ginger) juice, condensed milk and honey, quickly stir and boil, and then bottle the extract after coolling; take one spoon of the extract and melt with boiling water each time, twice per day. The patients may eat foods that nourish yin and moist the lung, such as yin'er (tremella), baihe (lily bulb), lotus root, lianzi (lotus seed), dried persimmon, bird's nest and meat of soft-shelled turtles. They should refrain from smoking, alcohol, strong tea, coffee and foods that are fatty, sweet, pungent, spicy, fragrant and dry-natured.

(3) Emotion nursing. Because of bloody phlegm, a long course of disease, and frequent fatigue, the patients may experience fear or depression. To enhance patients' confidence and prevent bad moods, nurses may use verbal enlightenment therapy as well as emotional transference and dispositional change

therapy to care for and encourage them as much as possible, distract their attention by watching TV or chatting, and organize communication with patients of the same disease who have shown better treatment effect.

(4) Medication nursing. Decoction should be taken warm before meals, multiple times in small portions.

(5) Manipulation techniques. ① Acupressure therapy: select Feishu (BL 13), Zhongfu (LU 1), Lieque (LU 7), Taiyuan (LU 9), Gaohuang (BL 43) and Taixi (KI 3); apply thumb kneading manipulation on each of the acupoints until the area turns hot or the patient has the feelings of soreness, numbness, distension and heaviness in the area; once per day. And it is contraindicated in pregnancy. ② Paste application therapy: select Yongquan (KI 1); shape mashed garlic into thumb-pulp-sized cakes, and apply the cakes on the acupoints, 2 hours each time, once per day.

Patient Education

The room should face the sun and away from wind. The patients should keep warm so as to avoid catching cold and do moderate exercise to enhance the health. Healthcare massage therapy is recommended: apply kneading and pressing manipulation on Fengchi (GB 20) until the area turns hot or the patient has the feelings of soreness, numbness, heaviness and distension in the area; 10 minutes every day.

The diet should be light, nutritious and digestible. Fresh fruit and vegetables should be supplemented. The patients should refrain from smoking, drinking and eating foods that induce or aggravate disease, and those that are pungent, spicy, greasy and too-sweet, such as hairtail, yellow croaker, hujiao (pepper fruit), chili, garlic, scallions and Chinese chives.

The patients should have a good mood. Nurses should instruct them how to adjust the mood so as to avoid anxiety and irritation.

After taking the medicine that resolve phlegm and relieve cough, avoid drinking water right away so as not to dilute the decoction and reduce the efficacy. When taking dry medical powder, use warm water to dissolve it before taking, to prevent aspiration into the trachea and aggravating cough.

Nurses should instruct the patients how to expectorate effectively: drink small amount of water to moist the throat, slowly take a deep breath, and hold the breath for 1～2 seconds, then cough vigorously to expel the phlegm from deep inside the lung. For patients with sticky phlegm that is difficult to expectorate, nurses may assist them to take a semi-supine position, turn over their body regularly, and use hollow palm to pat the back gently from bottom to top and from outside to inside, and simultaneously require the patients to cough effectively so as to promote expectoration.

For patients with infectious diseases, such as pertussis and pulmonary tuberculosis, strict respiratory tract quarantine should be implemented. Sterilize the indoor air regularly, and phlegm should be disinfected before poured out.

第三节 哮 病

哮病，是指因禀赋不足，由粉尘或刺激性气体激发，或由外邪、劳累、饮食不节、情志失调等因素诱发，而引动宿痰留饮，导致痰气交阻、气道挛急，以发作前可见鼻痒、喷嚏、咳嗽、胸闷等先兆症状，突发呼吸急促，喉中哮鸣有声，不得平卧为临床特征的反复发作性的肺系病。西医的支气管哮喘可参照本节进行护理。

一、病因病机

哮病的病因包括脏腑虚弱、外邪侵袭、饮食不当、情志失宜、劳倦太过。病人先天禀赋不足，易受邪气侵袭，或因病损伤肺、脾、肾，痰饮留伏。或外感风寒、风热、暑湿之邪，邪蕴于肺，肺气不能散布津液，或嗅吸花粉、烟尘，肺气失布，聚液成痰。病人过食生冷伤脾，脾阳不足，痰饮内生，或嗜食酸咸肥甘厚味，痰热内蕴，或进食鱼腥虾蟹，引动宿痰。病人抑郁、惊恐、恼怒，伤及情志，或剧烈运动、过劳，皆可使气机失调，肺失宣肃，痰气交阻，壅塞气道，发为哮病。

哮病的病机为痰阻气道，肺失宣降。病位在肺，与脾、肾有关。发作期以实证为主，缓解期以虚证为主。

二、常见证型

（一）辨证要点

1. 辨虚实　根据发作期与缓解期来辨别。发作期：呼吸急促，喉中哮鸣有声，痰液咳吐不利，甚则张口抬肩，不能平卧，胸膈满闷如室，烦闷不安。缓解期：肺虚者，语声低微，自汗畏风，咳痰清稀色白；脾虚者，食少便溏，痰多；肾虚者，平素息促短气，动则为甚，呼多吸少，耳鸣腰酸。

2. 辨寒热　根据哮鸣的声音、痰的颜色和质地等来辨别。若喉中哮鸣如水鸡声，痰液清稀色白，多为寒哮。若喉中痰鸣如吼，胸高气粗，痰液黏浊稠厚，咯吐不利，则多为热哮。

（二）证候分型

1. 发作期

（1）寒哮证

[主要证候] 呼吸急促，喉中哮鸣如水鸡声，胸膈满闷如塞；咳不甚，痰稀薄色白，咳吐不爽，面色晦滞带青，天冷或受寒易发；初起多兼恶寒，发热，头痛；舌苔白滑，脉弦紧或浮紧。

[证候分析] 痰气搏击于气道，故呼吸急促，喉中哮鸣有声；肺气闭郁，故胸膈满闷如塞；阴盛于内，阳气失宣，故面色晦滞带青；外寒引动内饮，故天冷或受寒易发；若风寒束表，则恶寒，发热，头痛；舌苔白滑，脉弦紧或浮紧，均为寒盛之象。

［护治原则］宣肺散寒,化痰平喘。

［常用方剂］射干麻黄汤。

（2）热哮证

［主要证候］气粗息涌,咳呛阵作,喉中哮鸣如吼,胸高胁胀,烦闷不安;汗出、口渴喜饮,面赤口苦,咳痰色黄,黏浊稠厚,咳吐不利,不恶寒;舌质红,苔黄腻,脉滑数。

［证候分析］肺气上逆,痰气搏击,故气粗息涌,咳呛阵作,喉中哮鸣,胸高胁胀,烦闷不安;热蒸炼液成痰,痰热交结,故咳痰色黄,黏浊稠厚,咳吐不利;痰火郁蒸,热伤津液,故汗出,口渴喜饮,面赤口苦;舌质红,苔黄腻,脉滑数,均为实热之象。

［护治原则］清热宣肺,化痰定喘。

［常用方剂］定喘汤。

2. 缓解期

（1）肺虚证

［主要证候］喘促气短,语声低微,面色白,自汗畏风;咳痰清稀色白,多因天气变化而诱发,发前喷嚏频作,鼻塞,流清涕;舌淡苔白,脉细弱或虚大。

［证候分析］肺气虚弱,气不化津,痰饮蕴肺,故喘促气短,咳痰清稀色白;肺气虚弱,腠理不固,故自汗畏风,多因天气变化而诱发;肺气失宣,窍道不利,故发前喷嚏频作,鼻塞,流清涕;语声低微,面色白,舌淡苔白,脉细弱或虚大,均为肺气虚弱之象。

［护治原则］补肺益气。

［常用方剂］玉屏风散。

（2）脾虚证

［主要证候］痰多而黏,咳吐不爽,胸脘满闷,恶心纳呆;或食油腻后易腹泻,每因饮食不当而诱发哮病;倦怠无力,食少便溏,面色萎黄无华;舌质淡,苔白滑或腻,脉细弱。

［证候分析］脾气亏虚,聚湿生痰,上贮于肺,故痰多而黏;脾虚运化无权,故食少便溏;脾虚中气不足,故倦怠无力;面色萎黄无华,舌质淡,苔白滑或腻,脉细弱,均为脾气虚弱之象。

［护治原则］健脾益气。

［常用方剂］六君子汤。

（3）肾虚证

［主要证候］平素息促气短,动则为甚,呼多吸少;咳痰质黏起沫,脑转耳鸣,腰酸腿软,心慌,不耐劳累;或五心烦热,颧红,口干;或畏寒肢冷,面色苍白;舌淡苔白质胖,或舌红少苔,脉沉细或细数。

［证候分析］肾虚摄纳失常,故平素息促气短,动则为甚,呼多吸少;肾精亏乏,不能充养,故脑转耳鸣,腰酸腿软,心慌,不耐劳累;若肾阴不足,则五心烦热,颧红,口干,舌红少苔,脉细数;若肾阳虚衰,则畏寒肢冷,面色苍白,舌淡苔白质胖,脉沉细。

［护治原则］补肾纳气。

［常用方剂］金匮肾气丸或七味都气丸。

三、护理措施

对于哮病的病人，应密切观察发作期的开始时间、持续时间、加重时间，以及昼夜变化的规律；呼吸的频率、节律、深浅；咳嗽的性质、程度、持续时间、发作规律；咳痰的难易程度；痰液的量、色、质；胸闷的性质、持续时间。注意观察心率、神志、面色、汗出、体温、脉象，以及口唇和肢端的发绀程度。询问诱发因素。在晚饭后至次日上午10点之间加强巡视，留意发作的先兆症状。若出现发作先兆，或急性发作，或发作持续24小时以上，伴胸闷如窒，汗出肢冷，面青唇紫，烦躁不安，或伴神昏嗜睡，脉大无根，应立即报告医生。

（一）辨证施护

1. 寒哮证

（1）生活起居护理　居室温暖避风，湿度适中，光线明亮，空气新鲜，避免烟尘和其他刺激性气味。绝对卧床，取端坐位或半仰卧位。注意保暖，尤其是背部保暖。加强夜间巡视，保持呼吸道通畅，及时清除口鼻分泌物。发作时予吸氧。若痰不易咳出，可轻拍其背部。病人不可吸烟，室内不可放置地毯、毛绒玩具。

（2）饮食护理　急性发作时禁食。病情平稳后，可食温肺豁痰的食物，如葱白、白胡椒。食疗方：干姜茯苓粥、杏苏莱菔粥。不宜食发物和生冷、油腻的食物。

（3）情志护理　急性发作时症状较重，病人多惊恐万分，护士应沉着冷静，运用语言开导疗法，多关心和安慰病人及其家属，向病人介绍疾病的相关知识，使病人保持情绪稳定，积极配合治疗。

（4）用药护理　中药汤剂宜热服。将汤剂的两煎药汁混匀后分成4份，日服3次，夜服1次。若发作有规律，可在发作前1小时服用。服药后观察心率、血压和汗出情况。

（5）操作技术　① 敷贴疗法：取肺俞、定喘、天突、内关，用天雄、川乌、附子、桂枝、细辛、川椒、干姜各等分，研磨成粉与芝麻油调成糊状敷贴，3日1次。② 灸法：取定喘、肺俞、天突、风门、膻中、大椎，用温和灸，艾条燃着端悬于施灸部位上，距离皮肤2~3厘米，灸至病人有温热舒适无灼痛的感觉，皮肤稍有红晕，每日1次；或取少商，用艾炷灸，适用于急性发作时。③ 穴位按摩法：取膻中，用一指禅推法，按摩至局部发热或有酸麻重胀感，每日1次；适用于胸闷者，孕妇禁用。④ 耳压疗法：取心、胸、神门、小肠、内分泌、皮质下等耳穴，用耳穴压丸贴片贴压，每日按揉4~5次，以局部发热泛红为度，留置2~4日；孕妇禁用。

2. 热哮证

（1）生活起居护理　居室凉爽安静，空气新鲜，不可有强风、对流风。绝对卧床，取半仰卧位或端坐位。加强夜间巡视，记录出入量，发作时予吸氧。保持口腔清洁、湿润，经常用菊花茶漱口。保持皮肤清洁干燥。若出汗较多，应及时擦干，并换掉湿衣被。若持续咳嗽，可频饮温开水。若痰黏难以咯出，予拍背，或遵医嘱进行中药雾化吸入。若烦躁不安，可加床栏，以防止跌仆。

（2）饮食护理　急性发作时禁食。多饮水，可饮水果汁、荸荠汁、藕汁。宜食清热化痰的食物，如豆腐、枇杷、鱼腥草、海蜇、丝瓜。食疗方：猪肺白萝卜汤。多吃高纤维的蔬菜，以保持大便通畅。不宜食辛辣、油腻的食物。

（3）情志护理　急性发作时症状较重，病人可能会极度烦躁，护士可运用语言开导疗法，告知病人情志因素对于疾病的影响,以使病人配合治疗。限制探视,以避免不良的情绪刺激。

(4)用药护理　中药汤剂宜温服或偏凉服。若发作有规律,可在发作前1小时服用。一旦出现鼻喉作痒、喷嚏、咳嗽等先兆症状,应立即遵医嘱给药。

(5)操作技术　① 刮痧疗法:取背部、胸部和上肢部,自大椎至至阳、自大杼至膈俞、自天突至膻中进行刮痧,点刮中府、定喘、尺泽;若痰多,加刮足三里至丰隆;以皮肤出现潮红或起痧为度;两次刮痧之间宜间隔3~6日,女性月经期或妊娠期禁用。② 拔罐疗法:取肺俞、大椎、天突、定喘、膻中,留罐10分钟,隔日1次。③ 穴位按摩法:取肺俞、天突、定喘、膻中、曲池、合谷、尺泽,用拇指揉法、一指禅推法,按摩至局部发热或有酸麻重胀感,每日1次;孕妇禁用。

3. 肺虚证

(1)生活起居护理　居室温暖避风,空气新鲜。注意保暖,预防感冒。若病情平稳,可适量运动,如慢跑、打太极拳,以不疲劳为度。避免异味刺激,室内不可有花草。

(2)饮食护理　宜食益气补肺的食物,如柿饼、猪肺、薏苡仁、鳖肉。人参粥:人参末5 g,生姜汁15 g,米100 g,煮粥,空腹温服。

(3)情志护理　因病情反复,病人容易产生悲观的情绪,护士可运用语言开导疗法,关心安慰病人,鼓励其积极配合治疗。

(4)用药护理　中药汤剂宜文火久煎,饭前温服。

(5)操作技术　① 敷贴疗法:取肺俞、脾俞、肾俞、天突、膻中、气海、膏肓、定喘;用白芥子、细辛各21 g,延胡索、甘遂各12 g,人工麝香10~15 g,研磨成粉后与生姜汁调匀,做成小圆薄饼;在夏季三伏天,分3次敷贴,每次1~2小时,10日1次;孕妇禁用。② 穴位按摩法:取大椎、肺俞、足三里、定喘、天突、风门、膻中,用拇指揉法、一指禅推法,按摩至局部发热或有酸麻重胀感,每日1次;孕妇禁用。

4. 脾虚证

(1)生活起居护理　居室温暖干燥,光线明亮,空气新鲜。鼓励病人翻身,经常予拍背。若病情平稳,可于无风处晒太阳,适量运动,经常做腹式呼吸和缩唇呼吸,以不疲劳为度。

(2)饮食护理　餐食宜温热软烂,进食宜缓慢,少食多餐。宜食健脾益气的食物,如乳鸽、茯苓、大枣、百合。食疗方:柚子肉炖鸡、参芪粥、莲子银耳羹。忌过饥、过饱,不宜食生冷、油腻、辛辣的食物,如肥肉、奶油、冷饮。

(3)情志护理　病人的病程较长,护士可运用顺意疗法,鼓励病人多表达,耐心倾听病人的倾诉,为病人提供心理支持。

(4)用药护理　中药汤剂宜文火久煎,饭前温服,少量频服。

(5)操作技术　① 穴位按摩法:取脾俞、中脘、肺俞、足三里、阴陵泉、三阴交,用拇指揉法、一指禅推法,按摩至局部发热或有酸麻重胀感,每日1次;孕妇禁用。② 耳压疗法:取肺、脾、肾、内分泌、肝、皮质下、交感等耳穴,用耳穴压丸贴片贴压,每日按揉4~5次,以局部发热泛红为度,留置2~4日;孕妇禁用。

5. 肾虚证

(1)生活起居护理　居室温暖避风,安静舒适,空气新鲜。起居有常。经常做深呼吸训练。不可熬夜,节制性行为。若病情平稳,可适量运动,如散步,以不疲劳为度。不宜剧烈运动,以防止跌仆。

（2）饮食护理　宜食补肺益肾的食物，如乌鸡、杏仁、黑豆、百合、黑木耳、桑椹。食疗方：白果核桃粥。肾阳虚者，可食羊脊骨粥：羊脊骨 1 具捣碎，肉苁蓉 50 g 切片，草果 3 个，荜茇 9 g，水煎成汁，滤去渣，入葱白，作粥食之。

（3）情志护理　病人体虚久病，护士可运用语言开导疗法，解除病人的思想负担，帮助病人树立战胜疾病的信心。

（4）用药护理　中药汤剂宜文火久煎，饭前温服，可用淡盐水送服。遵医嘱坚持长期用药。

（5）操作技术　① 敷贴疗法：取涌泉，用补骨脂 10 g，研磨成粉后与生姜汁调成糊状敷贴，每次 2~8 小时，每日 1 次。② 保健按摩疗法：取合谷、后溪、昆仑、涌泉，用拇指揉法，常自行按之，按摩至局部发热或有酸麻重胀感；孕妇禁用。③ 灸法：取大椎，用温和灸，艾条燃着端悬于施灸部位上，距离皮肤 2~3 厘米，灸至病人有温热舒适无灼痛的感觉，皮肤稍有红晕，从上午 9 点到上午 10 点，每日 1 次。

（二）健康教育

居室干净温暖，空气新鲜。防寒保暖，预防感冒。加强锻炼，以不疲劳为度。天气骤然变冷或花粉飞扬之季，应减少户外活动。避免接触刺激性气体和工业有机尘。居室内禁放鲜花，禁养猫、狗等宠物。

饮食宜清淡、营养、易消化，少食多餐。多吃新鲜的水果和蔬菜。若对寒凉水果不适应，可用温水浸泡后食用。适量多进食蛋白质，如猪瘦肉。戒烟限酒，不宜食过酸、过咸、生冷、肥甘、辛辣的食物，如辣椒、花椒、芥末。忌发物，如带鱼、黄鱼、蚶子、蛤蜊、螃蟹、虾、猪头肉、公鸡、羊肉、狗肉、驴肉、马肉、韭菜、春笋、大葱、大蒜、甜酒酿。

保持心情舒畅，避免不良情绪刺激。

遵医嘱坚持用药，不可自行减药或停药。病人平时须随身携带急救吸入制剂。若体质虚弱，可遵医嘱服用扶正固本的药物。

积极寻找发病诱因。检测、识别与规避过敏源。

Section 3 Wheezing

Wheezing is a recurrent lung system disease clinically characterized by sudden rapid and difficult breathing, wheezing sound in the throat, inability to lie flat, such possible premonitory symptoms as itching nose, sneezing, coughing and chest oppression. It is caused by inhalation of pollen and dust and irritating smell, on top of a weak body constitution. It may also be induced by external pathogenic factors, overstrain, unhealthy diet and emotional fluctuation, which trigger the hidden phlegm and cause it to ascend with qi, leading to airway spasm. This section may be referred to for the nursing of bronchial asthma in Western medicine.

ETIOLOGY AND PATHOGENESIS

The etiology includes deficiency of zang-fu organs, external affection of pathogenic factors, improper diet, emotional fluctuation and overstrain. Specifically speaking, a weak constitution is vulnerable to attack from pathogenic factors, or impairment of the lung, spleen and kidney causes hidden phlegm and fluid retention. Wind-cold, wind-heat and summerheat-dampness pathogens accumulate in the lung that makes lung qi fail to distribute body fluids, or inhalation of pollen and dust causes lung qi unable to distribute body fluids, leading to transformation of fluids into phlegm. Excessive ingestion of raw and cold foods injures spleen yang and results in interior phlegm and fluid retention, or predilection for sour, salty, fatty, and too-sweet foods causes phlegm-heat to accumulate in the interior, or eating fish, shrimps and crabs triggers hidden phlegm. Emotional fluctuation caused by depression, fear and anger, strenuous exercise, and overstrain, can all lead to disorder of qi movement and failure of lung qi to disperse and descend, causes phlegm to bind with qi and obstructs the airway, resulting in wheezing.

The pathogenesis is phlegm obstructing airway and failure of lung qi to disperse and descend. The disease is located in the lung but relates to the spleen and kidney. The onset stage is mainly excess syndrome while the remission stage mainly deficiency syndrome.

COMMON SYNDROMES

Key Points in Syndrome Differentiation
1. Differentiation of Deficiency Syndrome from Excess Syndrome
The differentiation is based on the onset and remission stages. At onset stage, such symptoms occur as rapid breathing, wheezing sound in the throat, difficult expectoration, even breathing with raised

shoulders and open mouth, inability to lie flat, chest fullness and oppression, and dysphoria. At remission stage, patients with lung deficiency have low voice, spontaneous sweating, aversion to wind, and clear thin and white phlegm; patients with spleen deficiency have reduced appetite, loose stool and profuse phlegm; and patients with kidney deficiency have rapid and short breathing aggravated with physical exertion, exhalation more than inhalation, tinnitus and aching lumbus.

2. Differentiation of Cold Syndrome from Heat Syndrome

The differentiation is based on the wheezing sound, and color and texture of phlegm. Frog rale in the throat, and clear thin and white phlegm means cold wheezing. Roaring wheezing sound in the throat, raised chest, rough breathing, sticky thick and turbid phlegm, and difficult expectoration indicate heat wheezing.

Syndrome Differentiation

1. Onset Stage

（1）Cold Wheezing Syndrome

[Clinical Manifestations] Rapid breathing, frog rale in the throat, chest fullness and oppression, mild cough, clear thin and white phlegm, difficult expectoration, dark bluish complexion, easy occurrence in cold weather or when attacked by cold, mostly accompanied with aversion to wind, fever and headache at the initial stage, white slippery tongue coating, and wiry tight or floating tight pulse.

[Manifestations Analysis] Phlegm binding with qi obstructs the airway, leading to rapid breathing and wheezing sound in the throat. Lung qi depression is responsible for chest fullness and oppression. Interior yin exuberance constrains yang qi, so dark bluish complexion can be seen. Exterior affection of cold pathogen stirs interior hidden fluid-retention, that is the reason why wheezing easily occurs in cold weather or when attacked by cold. If wind-cold fetters the exterior, aversion to wind, fever and headache thus appear. White slippery tongue coating and wiry tight or floating tight pulse are manifestations of cold exuberance.

[Nursing Principle] Ventilating the lung and dissipating cold; resolving phlegm and relieving dyspnea.

[Suggested Formula] Shegan Mahuang Decoction.

（2）Heat Wheezing Syndrome

[Clinical Manifestations] Rough breathing, paroxysmal choking cough, roaring wheezing sound in the throat, raised chest, hypochondriac distension, dysphoria, sweating, thirst with desire to drink, red complexion, bitter taste in the mouth, sticky thick and turbid phlegm of yellow color, difficult expectoration, no aversion to cold, red tongue with yellow slimy coating, and slippery rapid pulse.

[Manifestations Analysis] Counter-flowing lung qi that binds with phlegm obstructs the airway, leading to rough breathing, paroxysmal choking cough, wheezing sound in the throat, raised chest, hypochondriac distension, and dysphoria. Heat scorches fluids into phlegm that in turn binds with heat, resulting in sticky thick and turbid phlegm of yellow color, and difficult expectoration. Phlegm, fire and heat damage fluids, causing sweating, thirst with desire to drink, red complexion, and bitter taste in the mouth. Red tongue with yellow slimy coating and slippery rapid pulse are signs of excess heat.

［Nursing Principle］Clearing heat and ventilating the lung; resolving phlegm and relieving dyspnea.

［Suggested Formula］Dingchuan Decoction.

2. Remission Stage

（1）Lung Deficiency Syndrome

［Clinical Manifestations］Panting, shortness of breath, low voice, white complexion, spontaneous sweating, fear of wind, clear white phlegm, wheezing often induced by weather change, frequent sneezing before wheezing, nasal congestion, thin nasal discharge, pale tongue with white coating, and thready weak pulse or feeble large pulse.

［Manifestations Analysis］Lung qi deficiency causes failure of qi to transform fluids, which leads to accumulation of phlegm and fluid-retention in the lung, so there appear panting, shortness of breath, and clear white phlegm. Lung qi deficiency leads to insecurity of striae and interstice, so the patients suffer from spontaneous sweating, fear of wind, and wheezing often induced by weather change. Failure of lung qi to disperse and descend causes obstruction of orifices, resulting in frequent sneezing before wheezing, nasal congestion, and thin nasal discharge. Low voice, white complexion, pale tongue with white coating, and thready weak pulse or feeble large pulse, are all signs of lung qi deficiency.

［Nursing Principle］Tonifying the lung and replenishing qi.

［Suggested Formula］Yupingfeng Powder.

（2）Spleen Deficiency Syndrome

［Clinical Manifestations］Profuse sticky phlegm, difficult expectoration, chest and epigastric fullness and oppression, nausea, anorexia, diarrhea after eating greasy foods, wheezing often induced by improper diet, lassitude, reduced appetite, loose stool, sallow lusterless complexion, pale tongue with white slippery or slimy, and thready weak pulse.

［Manifestations Analysis］Due to spleen qi deficiency, dampness accumulates and generates phlegm that stays in the lung, so there is profuse sticky phlegm. Deficient spleen fails to transport and transform, so reduced appetite and loose stool occur. Spleen deficiency leads to insufficiency of middle qi, therefore, lassitude is felt. Sallow lusterless complexion, pale tongue with white slippery or slimy coating, and thready weak pulse, are all signs of spleen deficiency.

［Nursing Principle］Invigorating the spleen and replenishing qi.

［Suggested Formula］Liujunzi Decoction.

（3）Kidney Deficiency Syndrome

［Clinical Manifestations］Usual rapid and short breathing that aggravates with physical exertion, exhalation more than inhalation, sticky and foamy phlegm, dizziness, tinnitus, aching lumbus and weak legs, flusteredness, fatigue intolerance, or vexing heat in chest, palms and soles, hectic cheeks, dry mouth, or fear of cold, cold limbs, pale complexion, pale enlarged tongue with white coating, or red tongue with scanty coating, sunken thready pulse or thready rapid pulse.

［Manifestations Analysis］Deficient kidney fails to receive qi, so such symptoms occur as usual rapid and short breathing that aggravates with physical exertion, and exhalation more than inhalation. The kidney with essence depletion cannot nourish the body, so the patients show dizziness, tinnitus, aching lumbus and weak legs, flusteredness, and fatigue intolerance. Kidney yin deficiency may show vexing heat in chest, palms and soles, hectic cheeks, dry mouth, red tongue with scanty coating, and thready rapid pulse. Kidney yang deficiency may lead to fear of cold, cold limbs, pale complexion, pale enlarged tongue with white coating, and sunken thready pulse.

［Nursing Principle］Tonifying the kidney and improving qi reception.

［Suggested Formula］Jin'gui Shenqi Pills or Qiwei Duqi Pills.

NURSING MEASURES

For patients with wheezing, nurses should closely observe the following: the onset time, duration, aggravating time and the changing pattern during the day and night; the frequency, rhythm and depth of breath; the nature, degree, duration and pattern of cough; the difficulty level of expectoration; the amount, color and texture of phlegm; and the nature and duration of chest oppression. Nurses should also observe heart rate, mental status, complexion, sweating, body temperature, pulse, and cyanosis degree of lips and four extremities. They should also ask about the inducing factors. Moreover, nurses should increase the inspection frequency between supper and 10 a.m. of the next day, and be cautious about the prodrome. If there is wheezing prodrome or sudden onset, or duration lasts for over 24 hours, accompanied by asphyxia with chest oppression, sweating and cold limbs, cyanosis of lips and face, dysphoria, or unconsciousness and somnolence, rootless and large pulse, report to the doctor immediately.

Syndrome-Based Nursing Measures

1. Cold Wheezing Syndrome

（1）Daily life nursing. The ward should be warm with moderate humidity, bright light, fresh air, and away from wind, smoke, dust and other irritating smell. The patients should stay in bed absolutely, take a sitting or semi-supine position, and keep themselves warm, especially on the back of the trunk. Increase the inspection frequency at night, keep the respiratory track clear, clean oral and nasal discharge timely, and give oxygen inhalation during wheezing. For patients with sticky phlegm that is hard to be expectorated, pat on their back gently. The patients should refrain from smoking. Avoid placing carpets or fluffy toys in the ward.

（2）Diet nursing. Fasting is required at the acute onset of wheezing. When the condition is stabilized, the patients may eat foods that warm the lung and eliminate phlegm, such as congbai (scallion white) and baihujiao (white pepper). Food therapy: ganjiang fuling (dried ginger rhizome and poria) porridge, and xingsu (apricot kernels perilla seeds and perilla leaves) laifu (radish seeds) porridge. They should refrain from eating foods that induce or aggravate disease and foods that are cold, raw and greasy.

（3）Emotion nursing. The symptoms are severe at sudden onset, and the patients often experience extreme fright and terror. Nurses should stay calm and use verbal enlightenment therapy to constantly care for and comfort the patients and their family members, and impart them relevant knowledge about wheezing to keep them calm and cooperative.

(4) Medication nursing. Decoction should be taken hot. Decoct the medicinals two times and blend the two portions of decoction together, then divide it into four equal servings. Take three servings during the day and one at night. If the onset of wheezing is regular, take the decoction one hour before the onset. After taking medicine, heart rate, blood pressure and sweating should be observed.

(5) Manipulation techniques. ① Paste application therapy: select Feishu (BL 13), Dingchuan (EX－B1), Tiantu (CV 22) and Neiguan (PC 6); grind into powder equal amount of tianxiong (Aconitum carmichaeli Debx. root), chuanwu (common monkshood mother root), fuzi (monkshood), guizhi (cinnamon twig), xixin (Manchurian wild ginger), chuanjiao (pricklyash peel) and ganjiang (dried ginger rhizome); blend the powder with sesame oil to make pastes, apply them on the acupoints, and change the pastes every three days. ② Moxibustion therapy: select Dingchuan (EX－B1), Feishu (BL 13), Tiantu (CV 22), Fengmen (BL 12), Danzhong (CV 17) and Dazhui (GV 14); place the moxa stick 2~3 centimeters away from the skin to perform mild moxibustion on each of the acupoints until the area turns red and the patient feels warm and comfortable without the sensation of burning pain, once per day. Or select Shaoshang (LU 11); apply moxa cone moxibustion therapy on the acupoint, and it is suitable for acute onset. ③ Acupressure therapy: select Danzhong (CV 17); apply one-finger pushing manipulation on it until the area turns hot or the patient has the feelings of soreness, numbness, distension and heaviness in the area; once per day for patients with chest oppression. And it is contraindicated in pregnancy. ④ Auricular pressure therapy: select the auricular points of heart (CO15), chest (AH10), shenmen (TF4), small intestine (CO6), endocrine (CO18) and subcortex (AT4); apply specialized pasters on the points, knead each of them till the area turns hot and red, 4~5 times per day, and keep the pasters for 2~4 days. And it is contraindicated in pregnancy.

2. Heat Wheezing Syndrome

(1) Daily life nursing. The ward should be cool, quiet and full of fresh air, and avoid strong and convective wind. Nurses should make more rounds of the wards at night, take records of 24-hour intake and output, and apply oxygen inhalation during an episode of wheezing. Patients should stay in bed absolutely, take a semi-supine or sitting position, keep the mouth clean and moist, constantly rinse the mouth with juhua (chrysanthemum flower) tea, and keep the skin clean and dry. For patients with profuse sweating, wipe the sweat away and change the wet clothes and bedding timely. For patients with persistent cough, frequently drink warm boiled water. For patients with sticky phlegm that is hard to expectorate, give regular back-patting, or follow the doctor's advice to use spray inhalation therapy. For patients with dysphoria, use bed rails to prevent falls.

(2) Diet nursing. During the acute episode of wheezing, fast is required. The patients should drink more water. They may drink fruit juice, biqi (waternut) juice and lotus root juice, and eat foods that clear heat and resolve phlegm, such as tofu, loquats, yuxingcao (heartleaf houttuynia), jellyfish and

luffa. Food therapy: pig lung white radish soup. They should supplement vegetables rich in fiber to keep a normal bowel movement and avoid pungent, spicy, and greasy foods.

（3）Emotion nursing. The symptoms are severe in the acute episode of wheezing, and the patients may have extreme dysphoria. Nurses may use verbal enlightenment therapy to tell them the emotional impact over the disease to promote their cooperation in treatment. Restrict visits to patients to avoid undesirable emotional stimulation.

（4）Medication nursing. Decoction should be taken warm or slightly cool. If the episode of wheezing has a regular pattern, take the decoction one hour before the onset. Once the prodromes of wheezing occur, such as itching sensation of nose and throat, sneezing and cough, follow the doctor's advice to administrate the medicine to the patients immediately.

（5）Manipulation techniques. ① Scraping therapy: select the areas on the back, chest and upper extremities, from Dazhui（GV 14）to Zhiyang（GV 9）, from Dazhu（BL 11）to Geshu（BL 17）, and from Tiantu（CV 22）to Danzhong（CV 17）; apply scraping therapy on the areas. Or select Zhongfu（LU 1）, Dingchuan（EX－B1）and Chize（LU 5）; apply point scraping therapy on the acupoints; and for patients with profuse phlegm, add the area between Zusanli（ST 36）and Fenglong（ST 40）; apply scraping therapy on it. Keep scraping till the area turns red or *qi sha*（rashes occur）. An interval of 3~6 days is preferred between two sessions. And it should be avoided during menstruation or pregnancy. ② Cupping therapy: select Feishu（BL 13）, Dazhui（GV 14）, Tiantu（CV 22）, Dingchuan（EX－B1）and Danzhong（CV 17）; retain the cup on the acupoints for 10 minutes, once every other day. ③ Acupressure therapy: select Feishu（BL 13）, Tiantu（CV 22）, Dingchuan（EX－B1）, Danzhong（CV 17）, Quchi（LI 11）, Hegu（LI 4）and Chize（LU 5）; apply thumb kneading and one-finger pushing manipulations on each of the acupoints until the area turns hot or the patient has the feelings of soreness, numbness, distension and heaviness in the area; once per day. And it is contraindicated in pregnancy.

3. Lung Deficiency Syndrome

（1）Daily life nursing. The ward should be warm, full of fresh air, and away from wind. The patients should keep themselves warm to prevent common cold. When the condition is stabilized, they may do moderate exercise, such as jogging and Taiji. Stimulating odor and indoor flowers and plants should be avoided.

（2）Diet nursing. The patients may eat foods that replenish qi and tonify the lung, such as dried persimmon, pig lung, yiyiren（coix seed）and meat of soft-shelled turtles. Renshen（ginseng）porridge is recommended: use renshen（ginseng）5 g, shengjiang（fresh ginger）juice 15 g and rice 100 g to cook a porridge, and take the porridge warm on an empty stomach.

（3）Emotion nursing. Because of the reoccurrences of the disease, the patients may be pessimistic. Nurses may use verbal enlightenment therapy to care for and comfort them, and encourage them to cooperate in the treatment.

（4）Medication nursing. Decoction should be prepared slowly over low heat and taken warm before meals.

(5) Manipulation techniques. ① Paste application therapy: select Feishu (BL 13), Pishu (BL 20), Shenshu (BL 23), Tiantu (CV 22), Danzhong (CV 17), Qihai (CV 6), Gaohuang (BL 43) and Dingchuan (EX‑B1); grind into powder baijiezi (white mustard seed) 21 g, xixin (Manchurian wild ginger) 21 g, yanhusuo (corydalis rhizome) 12 g, gansui (gansui root) 12 g, and man-made shexiang (musk) 10~15 g; blend the powder with shengjiang (fresh ginger) juice to make thin small round medicated cakes; apply the medicated cakes on the acupoints during the dog days (on the first or second day of the three ten-day periods after the summer solstice) for three times, 1~2 hours each time, once every ten days. And it is contraindicated in pregnancy. ② Acupressure therapy: select Dazhui (GV 14), Feishu (BL 13), Zusanli (ST 36), Dingchuan (EX‑B1), Tiantu (CV 22), Fengmen (BL 12) and Danzhong (CV 17); apply thumb kneading and one-finger pushing manipulations on each of the acupoints until the area turns hot or the patient has the feelings of soreness, numbness, distension and heaviness in the area; once per day. And it is contraindicated in pregnancy.

4. Spleen Deficiency Syndrome

(1) Daily life nursing. The ward should be warm, dry, and full of bright light and fresh air. Encourage the patients to turn over and give them back-patting frequently. For patients with stable condition, take a sun bath in windless environment, do moderate exercise, and often practice moderate diaphragmatic breathing and pursed lip breathing.

(2) Diet nursing. The diet should be warm, soft and mushy. The patients should have small frequent meals slowly and take foods that invigorate the spleen and replenish qi, such as squab, fuling (poria), dazao (Chinese date), and baihe (lily bulb). Food therapy: chicken stewed with grapefruit, shenqi (ginseng and astragalus root) porridge, and lianzi yin'er (lotus seed and tremella) thick soup. The patients should avoid being too hungry or too full, and refrain from eating raw, cold, greasy, pungent and spicy foods, such as fatty meat, butter and cold drinks.

(3) Emotion nursing. Because the disease course is long, nurses may use submission therapy to encourage the patients to express themselves, listen to them patiently, and provide them with psychological support.

(4) Medication nursing. Decoction should be prepared slowly over low heat and taken warm before meals, multiple times in small portions.

(5) Manipulation techniques. ① Acupressure therapy: select Pishu (BL 20), Zhongwan (CV 12), Feishu (BL 13), Zusanli (ST 36), Yinlingquan (SP 9) and Sanyinjiao (SP 6); apply thumb kneading and one-finger pushing manipulations on each of the acupoints until the area turns hot or the patient has the feelings of soreness, numbness, distension and heaviness in the area; once per day. And it is contraindicated in pregnancy. ② Auricular pressure therapy: select the auricular points of lung (CO14), spleen (CO13), kidney (CO10), endocrine (CO18), liver (CO12), subcortex (AT4) and sympathetic (AH6a); apply specialized pasters on the points, knead each of them till the area turns hot and red, 4~5 times per day, and keep the pasters for 2~4 days. And it is contraindicated in pregnancy.

5. Kidney Deficiency Syndrome

（1）Daily life nursing. The ward should be warm, quiet, comfortable, full of fresh air and away from wind. The patients should live a regular life, practize deep breathing frequently, avoid staying up late and value sexual abstinence. For patients with stable condition, they may do moderate exercise such as walking, and avoid getting tired. They should not engage in strenuous activity to prevent falls.

（2）Diet nursing. The patients may eat foods that tonify the lung and replenish the kidney, such as black-boned chicken, xingren (apricot kernel), heidou (black soybean), baihe (lily bulb), heimuer (black fungus) and sangshen (mulberry). Food therapy: baiguo hetao (ginkgo nut and walnut) porridge. For patients with kidney yang deficiency, sheep backbone porridge is recommended: prepare a mashed sheep backbone, 50 g of sliced roucongrong (desert cistanche), three grains of caoguo (tsaoko fruit), and 9 g of biba (long pepper fruit), boil them together to get the soup, filter and remove the dregs, and add in congbai (scallion white) to make porridge.

（3）Emotion nursing. Because the patients are weak with a long disease course, nurses may use verbal enlightenment therapy to reduce their mental stress and provide reassurance in winning the battle against the disease.

（4）Medication nursing. Decoction should be prepared slowly over low heat and taken warm before meals with or without dilute saline. Follow the doctor's advice to stick to long-time medication.

（5）Manipulation techniques. ① Paste application therapy: select Yongquan (KI 1); blend ground buguzhi (psoralea fruit) 10 g with shengjiang (fresh ginger) juice to make pastes, and apply them on the acupoint, 2~8 hours each time, once per day. ② Healthcare massage therapy: select Hegu (LI 4), Houxi (SI 3), Kunlun (BL 60) and Yongquan (KI 1); the patients frequently apply thumb kneading manipulation on each of the acupoints until the area turns hot or the patient has the feelings of soreness, numbness, distension and heaviness in the area; once per day. And it is contraindicated in pregnancy. ③ Moxibustion therapy: select Dazhui (GV 14); place the moxa stick 2~3 centimeters away from the skin to perform mild moxibustion on the acupoint from 9 a.m. to 10 a.m. until the area turns red and the patient feels warm and comfortable without the sensation of burning pain, once per day.

Patient Education

The room should be clean, warm, and full of fresh air. The patients should keep themselves warm to prevent common cold, and take moderate exercise. When the weather suddenly turns cold, or when the pollen season comes, they should reduce outdoor activities. Moreover, minimize exposure to irritant gases and organic industrial dust. Avoid placing flowers indoors and keeping pets such as cats and dogs.

The diet should be light, nutritious and digestible. The patients should have small frequent meals. Eat more fresh fruit and vegetables. For patients who are intolerant to cold fruit, immerse the fruit in warm water before eating. Proteins should be supplemented, such as lean pork. The patients should refrain from smoking and drinking. They should also refrain from eating too-sour, too-salty, raw, cold, greasy, pungent and spicy foods, such as chili, huajiao (pricklyash peel) and mustard, and also foods that induce or aggravate the disease, such as ribbon fish, yellow croakers, clams, crabs, shrimp, pig's head meat, rooster, mutton, dog meat, donkey meat, horse meat, Chinese chives, spring bamboo shoots, scallion, garlic, and sweet fermented glutinous rice.

Stay good-humored, and avoid negative emotional stimuli.

In medication, the patients should follow the doctor's advice strictly and don't reduce the dosage or stop the medicine by themselves. They should take with them emergency inhalation preparations at all times. For patients with a weak constitution, follow the doctor's advice to take medicines that reinforce healthy qi and consolidate the constitution.

Find out the inducing factors actively. Detect, identify and avoid the allergens.

第四节　喘　病

喘病,是指因外感风寒,邪热束肺,或因痰浊壅肺,导致痰气交结,肃降无权,或因先天不足,久咳伤肺,导致肾不纳气,以气短喘促,呼吸困难,稍动尤甚,甚则张口抬肩,鼻翼翕动,不得平卧,伴见咳嗽、痰多、胸闷、紫绀、胸高胁胀为临床特征的肺系病。西医的慢性阻塞性肺疾病、肺源性心脏病、心源性哮喘,以及肺结核、矽肺发生呼吸困难时,可参照本节进行护理。

一、病因病机

喘病的病因包括外邪侵袭、饮食不节、七情失调、劳倦久病、痰饮瘀血。外邪侵袭,如风寒外袭皮毛,内阻肺气,或风热侵袭肺卫,火热内迫,或燥邪由口鼻而入,损伤肺金,或暑热侵袭,灼伤肺气,均可致肺气上逆,引发喘病。病人过食厚味,或恣食生冷,或嗜酒伤中,可伤脾生痰,上干于肺,致肺气上逆。病人悲忧伤肺,或郁怒伤肝,或惊恐伤肾,均可使气机逆乱,肺气上逆。病人过劳伤脾,或纵欲伤肾,或久病伤肺,均可使气失所主,肺气上逆。或因其他疾病产生痰饮瘀血,可使肺气壅塞,上逆发为喘病。

喘病的病机为:实喘者邪犯于肺,肺气上逆;虚喘者肺不主气,肾失摄纳。病位在肺、肾,与肝、脾、心有关。实喘者为实证。虚喘者以虚证为主,亦可出现虚实夹杂之证。

二、常见证型

(一)辨证要点

1. **辨虚实**　根据体质、病因、呼吸、脉象等来辨别。若病人既往体健,由外邪侵袭、饮食不节、情志失调所致,起病急,症见呼吸深长有余,呼出为快,气粗声高,脉数有力,多为实证。若病人既往体虚,由久病迁延或劳欲损伤所致,起病徐缓,时轻时重,症见呼吸短促难续,深吸为快,气怯声低,脉微弱或浮大无根,则多为虚证。

2. **辨寒热**　根据痰色、痰质、面色、舌脉等来辨别。若痰液色白清稀,面色青灰,四肢不温,口不渴,舌质淡,苔白滑,脉浮紧或沉细,多为寒证。若痰黄黏稠,面赤身热,口渴而喜冷饮,尿赤便秘,舌质红,苔黄,脉数,则多为热证。

3. **辨病位**　根据病位等来辨别。若因外邪、痰浊、肝气郁结所致,则实证居多,病位在肺。若因久病劳欲,肺肾气机出纳失常而致,则虚证居多,或为虚实夹杂,病位在肺、肾。

(二)证候分型

1. 实喘

(1)风寒犯肺证

[主要证候]喘息咳逆,呼吸急促,胸部胀闷;痰多、色白清稀,恶寒无汗,头痛鼻塞;或有发热,

口不渴;舌苔薄白而滑,脉浮紧。

[证候分析]外感风寒,内闭于肺,肺气上逆,故喘息咳逆,呼吸急促,胸部胀闷;肺气失宣,津聚为痰,故痰多、色白清稀;风寒束表,皮毛闭塞,故恶寒无汗,或有发热;寒凝气机不利,故头痛;肺气失宣,肺窍不利,故鼻塞;舌苔薄白而滑,脉浮紧,均为风寒之象。

[护治原则]宣肺散寒。

[常用方剂]麻黄汤合华盖散。

（2）表寒里热证

[主要证候]喘逆上气,息粗鼻翕,胸胀或痛;咳而不爽,吐痰稠黏,伴形寒身痛,身热烦闷;有汗或无汗,口渴;舌苔薄白或薄黄,舌边红,脉浮数或滑。

[证候分析]外寒束表,肺有郁热,肺气上逆,故喘逆上气,息粗鼻翕,胸胀或痛;热郁于肺,灼津为痰,故咳而不爽,吐痰稠黏;寒邪束表,故形寒身痛;里热内盛,故身热烦闷;热伤津液,故口渴;舌苔薄白或薄黄,舌边红,脉浮数或滑,均为表寒里热之象。

[护治原则]解表清里,化痰平喘。

[常用方剂]麻杏石甘汤。

（3）痰热郁肺证

[主要证候]喘咳气涌,胸部胀痛,痰多、质黏色黄,或夹血痰;伴胸中烦闷,身热有汗,口渴而喜冷饮;面赤咽干,尿赤便秘;舌质红,苔黄腻,脉滑数。

[证候分析]痰热郁遏,肺气肃降无权,故喘咳气涌,胸部胀痛;痰热内盛,热伤肺络,故痰多、质黏色黄,或夹血痰;痰热郁蒸于肺,故胸中烦闷,身热有汗,口渴而喜冷饮;热伤津液,故面赤咽干,尿赤便秘;舌质红,苔黄腻,脉滑数,均为痰热内蕴之象。

[护治原则]清热化痰,宣肺平喘。

[常用方剂]桑白皮汤。

（4）痰浊阻肺证

[主要证候]喘咳痰鸣,胸中满闷,甚则胸盈仰息;痰多、黏腻色白,咯吐不利;呕恶纳呆,口黏不渴;舌质淡,苔厚腻色白,脉滑。

[证候分析]脾失健运,积湿成痰,痰浊塞肺,气机不畅,肃降失职,肺气上逆,故喘咳痰鸣,胸中满闷,甚则胸盈仰息,痰多、黏腻色白,咯吐不利;痰湿蕴中,脾胃不和,故呕恶纳呆,口黏不渴;舌质淡,苔厚腻色白,脉滑,均为痰湿之象。

[护治原则]祛痰降逆,宣肺平喘。

[常用方剂]二陈汤合三子养亲汤。

（5）肝气乘肺证

[主要证候]每遇情志刺激而诱发,突然呼吸短促,息粗气憋;胸胁闷痛,咽中如窒,但喉中痰鸣不明显;平素多忧思抑郁,或失眠,心悸;或心烦易怒,面红目赤;舌质淡或红,苔薄白或薄黄,脉弦或弦数。

[证候分析]郁怒伤肝,肝气冲逆乘肺,肺气不降,故呼吸短促,息粗气憋;肝气不舒,肺气郁闭,故胸胁闷痛,咽中如窒,但喉中痰鸣不明显;心肝气郁,心神不安,故忧思抑郁,或失眠,心悸,或心烦易怒,面红目赤;舌质淡或红,苔薄,脉弦,均为肝气郁结之象。

［护治原则］解郁降气平喘。

［常用方剂］五磨饮子。

（6）水凌心肺证

［主要证候］喘咳气逆,倚息难以平卧,咳痰稀白,心悸,全身浮肿,尿少;怯寒肢冷,面色瘀暗,唇甲青紫;舌淡胖或胖暗,或有瘀斑、瘀点,舌下青筋显露,苔白滑,脉沉细或涩。

［证候分析］肾阳衰弱,水邪干肺,故喘咳气逆,倚息难以平卧,咳痰稀白;水气凌心,心阳受损,故心悸;喘促日久,肺脾肾俱虚,气化不利,阳虚水泛,故全身浮肿,尿少;阳虚不温四肢,故怯寒肢冷;心阳受损,不能鼓动血脉运行,血行瘀滞,故面色瘀暗,唇甲青紫,舌胖暗,有瘀斑、瘀点,舌下青筋显露;舌淡胖,苔白滑,脉沉细或涩,均为阳虚水停之象。

［护治原则］温阳利水,泻肺平喘。

［常用方剂］真武汤合葶苈大枣泻肺汤。

2. 虚喘

（1）肺虚证

［主要证候］喘促短气,气怯声低,喉有鼾声;肺气不足,咳声低弱,痰吐稀薄,自汗畏风;或咳呛,痰少质黏,烦热口干,咽喉不利,面颧潮红;舌淡红,或舌红少苔,脉软弱或细数。

［证候分析］肺气不足,故喘促短气,气怯声低,喉有鼾声;肺气不足,气不化津,故咳声低弱,痰吐稀薄;卫外不固,故自汗畏风;舌淡红,脉软弱,均为肺气虚弱之象。若肺阴不足,虚火上炎,则咳呛,痰少质黏,烦热口干,咽喉不利,面颧潮红,舌红少苔,脉细数。

［护治原则］补肺益气。

［常用方剂］生脉散合补肺汤。

（2）肾虚证

［主要证候］喘促日久,动则喘甚,呼多吸少,气不得续;形瘦神惫,跗肿,汗出肢冷,面青唇紫;或见喘咳,面红烦躁,口咽干燥,足冷,汗出如油;舌淡苔白或黑润,或舌红少津,脉沉弱或细数。

［证候分析］久病肺虚及肾,气失摄纳,故喘促日久,动则喘甚,呼多吸少,气不得续;肾精亏耗,形神失养,故形瘦神惫;阳虚卫外不固,故汗出;阳虚气不化水,故跗肿;阳虚失于温煦,故肢冷;舌淡苔白或黑润,脉沉弱,均为肾阳虚衰之象。或肾阴衰竭,阴不敛阳,阳气浮越,则喘咳,面红烦躁,口咽干燥,足冷,汗出如油,舌红少津,脉细数。

［护治原则］补肾纳气。

［常用方剂］金匮肾气丸合参蛤散。

（3）喘脱证

［主要证候］喘逆剧甚,张口抬肩,鼻翼翕动,不能平卧,稍动则咳喘欲绝;或有痰鸣,心悸烦躁,四肢厥冷,面青唇紫,汗出如珠;脉浮大无根,或脉微欲绝。

［证候分析］肺肾衰竭,气失所主,气不归根,故喘逆剧甚,张口抬肩,鼻翼翕动,不能平卧,稍动则咳喘欲绝;心阳虚脱,虚阳躁动,故心悸烦躁;阳脱血脉失于温运,则四肢厥冷,面青唇紫;阳脱阴液外泄,故汗出如珠;脉浮大无根,或脉微欲绝,均为阳脱阴竭之象。

［护治原则］扶阳固脱,镇摄肾气。

［常用方剂］参附汤送服黑锡丹。

三、护理措施

对于喘病的病人,应密切观察喘促的诱因、发作时间、持续时间;呼吸的频率、节律、深度,以及呼气与吸气的时间比例;咳嗽的性质、程度、发作时间、持续时间;咳痰的难易程度;痰的量、色、质。观察神志、体温、心率、血压、面色、尿量、出汗情况,以及有无发绀。对于水气凌心的病人,应记录24小时出入量。若病人出现神志恍惚,面青唇紫,汗出如珠,四肢厥冷,血压骤降,脉浮大无根或脉微欲绝,应立即报告医生,并配合抢救。

（一）辨证施护

1. 风寒犯肺证

（1）生活起居护理 居室温暖避风,安静舒适,阳光充足,空气新鲜。卧床休息,适当抬高床头,帮助病人勤换体位。低流量吸氧,保持呼吸道的通畅,协助拍背,或指导病人有效咳嗽、咳痰和深呼吸。做好胸背部保暖。若发热,不可使用冷敷法。限制探视时间,不宜疲劳及过量运动。

（2）饮食护理 宜食温肺散寒的食物,如生姜、葱白。可食灵芝汤,每周2~3次。或食紫苏粥:粳米100 g,紫苏叶20 g,白糖少许;将紫苏叶捣碎,加水煎取浓汁,入粳米煮粥,佐餐温服。不宜食生冷瓜果。

（3）情志护理 疾病新起,症状较重,护士可运用语言开导疗法,讲解疾病的成因与预后,以消除病人恐惧的情绪。

（4）用药护理 中药汤剂宜武火快煎,饭后热服。服药后马上进食热粥,加盖衣被,使其微微汗出。

（5）操作技术 ① 推拿疗法:取背部膀胱经,用擦法,以透热为度;孕妇禁用。② 拔罐疗法:取大椎、肺俞,留罐10分钟,每日1次。③ 穴位按摩法:取肺俞、心俞、膈俞、膻中、列缺、风门,用拇指揉法、一指禅推法,按摩至局部发热或有酸麻重胀感,每日1次;孕妇禁用。

2. 表寒里热证

（1）生活起居护理 居室温暖避风,空气新鲜。卧床休息,适当抬高床头。低流量吸氧,保持呼吸道通畅,指导病人有效咳嗽,协助翻身、拍背,遵医嘱进行中药雾化吸入。若痰液黏稠,可频饮温开水。若发热,不可使用冷敷法。

（2）饮食护理 宜食解表清里的食物,如莴笋、雪梨、甘蔗、藕。可食芦根粥:鲜芦根45 g,煎煮40分钟后去渣,加入大米30 g,煮成粥食用。

（3）情志护理 疾病新起,护士可运用语言开导疗法,缓解病人的焦虑。

（4）用药护理 生石膏先煎。中药汤剂宜饭后温服,服后以微汗为宜。用药后观察体温和汗出情况。

（5）操作技术 ① 拔罐疗法:取大椎、风门、肺俞、心俞、膏肓,每次选择2~4个腧穴,留罐10分钟,隔日1次。② 刮痧疗法:取大椎、风池、肺俞、脾俞,以皮肤出现潮红或起痧为度;两次刮痧之间宜间隔3~6日,女性月经期或妊娠期禁用。

3. 痰热郁肺证

（1）生活起居护理 居室凉爽避风,空气新鲜。卧床休息,适当抬高床头。保持口腔清洁,饭后用金银花甘草液漱口。低流量吸氧,鼓励病人缓慢深呼吸。保持呼吸道通畅,遵医嘱进行中药雾化吸入。若发热,可用温水擦浴。若出汗较多,应及时擦干,并换掉湿衣被。

（2）饮食护理　多饮水,可饮荸荠汁、西瓜汁。若痰液黏稠,可饮竹沥。多吃高纤维的水果和蔬菜,以保持大便通畅。宜食清热化痰的食物,如柿饼、荸荠、丝瓜、白萝卜、百合。不宜食煎炸、燥热、辛辣的食物。

（3）情志护理　病人症状较重,护士可运用移情易性疗法,鼓励病人之间多交流疾病的防治经验,以减轻其精神负担,避免焦虑、抑郁。

（4）用药护理　中药汤剂宜饭后温服或偏凉服。

（5）操作技术　① 穴位按摩法:取膻中、列缺、肺俞、丰隆、定喘、天突,用拇指揉法、一指禅推法,按摩至局部发热或有酸麻重胀感,每日 1 次;孕妇禁用。② 耳压疗法:取肺、气管、神门、皮质下、肾上腺、交感等耳穴,用耳穴压丸贴片贴压,每日按揉 4~5 次,以局部发热泛红为度,留置 2~4 日;孕妇禁用。

4. 痰浊阻肺证

（1）生活起居护理　居室温暖干燥,安静避风,空气新鲜。卧床休息,适当抬高床头。注意保暖。低流量吸氧,保持呼吸道通畅,指导病人清晨起床后,深吸气咳出宿痰。病情平稳后,适量体育锻炼,以不疲劳为度。

（2）饮食护理　少食多餐。宜食健脾化痰的食物,如生姜、丝瓜、肉桂、茯苓、白萝卜、山药、枇杷。食疗方:橘皮杏仁饮、雪梨银耳百合汤、杏仁豆腐汤。杏仁豆腐汤:用杏仁 15 g,豆腐 120 g,共煮 1 小时,去药渣,吃豆腐喝汤,早晚各 1 次,连服 4~5 天。不宜食过甜、生冷、肥腻的食物。

（3）情志护理　病情缠绵反复,护士可运用顺意疗法,多与病人交流,鼓励病人多表达,及时疏导不良情绪,使病人情绪稳定。

（4）用药护理　中药汤剂宜饭后热服,少量频服。

（5）操作技术　① 灸法:取肺俞、肾俞、膏肓、气海、足三里、内关,用温和灸,艾条燃着端悬于施灸部位上,距离皮肤 2~3 厘米,灸至病人有温热舒适无灼痛的感觉,皮肤稍有红晕,每日 2~3 次;孕妇腹部及腰骶部禁用。② 拔罐疗法:取足三里、中脘、内关,留罐 10 分钟,隔日 1 次;孕妇腹部禁用。③ 水针疗法:取定喘、肺俞、膏肓、列缺、合谷或夹脊,每次选择两侧的同一个腧穴,用胎盘注射液或维生素 B_{12} 注射液进行穴位注射。④ 耳压疗法:取脾、胃、三焦、胰胆等耳穴,用耳穴压丸贴片贴压,每日按揉 4~5 次,以局部发热泛红为度,留置 2~4 日;孕妇禁用。

5. 肝气乘肺证

（1）生活起居护理　居室安静舒适,空气新鲜。卧床休息,适当抬高床头,低流量吸氧。起居有常,不可熬夜。指导病人使用放松技术,如练气功,读书,听音乐,缓慢地深呼吸,放松全身肌肉。

（2）饮食护理　可饮玫瑰花茶。宜食行气解郁的食物,如柚子、佛手。食疗方:橘皮粥。不宜食滋腻、易产气的食物,如红薯。

（3）情志护理　病人应保持情绪稳定,忌怒。护士可运用语言开导疗法,告诉病人及家属情绪与病情之间的关系。或运用移情易性疗法,转移病人的注意力,鼓励病人适量参加社交活动与体育锻炼。

（4）用药护理　代赭石先煎,旋覆花包煎,沉香后下。中药汤剂不宜久煎,应饭后温服。中病即止,不可久服。

（5）操作技术　① 穴位按摩法：取肺俞、大椎、风门、列缺、合谷、足三里,用拇指揉法,按摩至局部发热或有酸麻重胀感,每日 1 次;孕妇禁用。② 耳压疗法：取肺、肝、气管等耳穴,用耳穴压丸贴片贴压,于发作前轻按,以局部发热泛红为度;孕妇禁用。

6. 水凌心肺证

（1）生活起居护理　居室温暖安静,空气新鲜,不可有强风、对流风。卧床休息,适当抬高床头,定时翻身,低流量吸氧。睡眠充足,注意保暖,避免受凉。不可剧烈运动、剧烈咳嗽。

（2）饮食护理　限制钠盐和水的摄入。餐食宜温热,进食宜缓慢,少食多餐。宜食温阳化饮的食物,如赤小豆、山楂。不宜食生冷、油腻的食物。

（3）情志护理　病情较重,护士可运用语言开导疗法,向病人介绍疾病知识,鼓励病人积极防治,避免产生消极、悲观情绪。

（4）用药护理　附子先煎,葶苈子包煎。中药汤剂宜饭后温服,少量频服。

（5）操作技术　① 灸法：取定喘、膻中、肺俞、大椎、合谷,用温和灸,每次选择 3~5 个腧穴,艾条燃着端悬于施灸部位上,距离皮肤 2~3 厘米,灸至病人有温热舒适无灼痛的感觉,皮肤稍有红晕,每日 2~3 次。② 穴位按摩法：取尺泽、孔最、内关、经渠、足三里、丰隆,用拇指揉法,按摩至局部发热或有酸麻重胀感,每日 1 次;孕妇禁用。

7. 肺虚证

（1）生活起居护理　居室温暖避风,安静舒适,空气新鲜。起居有常,不可熬夜。注意保暖,避免受凉。坚持长期氧疗。当病情平稳时,适量运动,以不疲劳为度。

（2）饮食护理　宜食补肺健脾的食物,如鲤鱼、百合。食疗方：猪肺白萝卜汤、山药薏苡仁粥。猪肺白萝卜汤：猪肺 300 g,白萝卜 250 g,加盐、生姜炖熟。山药薏苡仁粥：山药、薏苡仁各 60 g,加入大米,煮粥食用。不宜食生冷的食物。

（3）情志护理　病人久病体虚,护士可运用顺意疗法,经常巡视病房,了解病人所需,尽可能地满足病人的合理要求。

（4）用药护理　中药汤剂宜文火久煎,饭前温服,少量频服。服药后卧床休息片刻。

（5）操作技术　① 保健按摩疗法：取天突、膻中,自行轻轻揉按;或用手自下而上轻轻拍打脊柱两旁的腧穴;或横擦前胸上部及背部心俞、肺俞区,每日数次;孕妇禁用。② 气功锻炼：可练凝神松肌功;阳虚者意守丹田或命门,少放多守;阴虚者意守涌泉,多放少守;每日 30 分钟。③ 敷贴疗法：取颈百劳、肺俞、膏肓,用白芥子、延胡索、细辛、甘遂等份研粉,与生姜汁调成糊状,捏饼敷贴,用胶布固定,每次 0.5~2 小时,每日 1 次。④ 灸法：取肺俞、膏肓,用温和灸,艾条燃着端悬于施灸部位上,距离皮肤 2~3 厘米,灸至病人有温热舒适无灼痛的感觉,皮肤稍有红晕,每周 1 次。

8. 肾虚证

（1）生活起居护理　居室安静舒适,空气新鲜。床单整洁干燥。起居有常,睡眠充足。注意皮肤护理,可用温水轻柔擦拭,每日用红花乙醇溶液按摩受压部位。密切观察血压、脉搏的变化,防止喘脱。若卧床不起,应定时翻身。病情平稳时,可适量运动,以不疲劳为度。运动时,应有人陪伴,以防止跌仆。若咳痰无力,可用吸痰器吸出。若二便失禁,应进行会阴部护理。节制性行为,不可过劳。

（2）饮食护理　低盐饮食,进食高热量、高维生素、高蛋白的食物。宜食补益肾精的食物,如羊肉、核桃仁、黑芝麻、猪肾、鳖肉。

（3）情志护理　病人久病体虚,护士可运用语言开导疗法,关心病人,耐心倾听病人的倾诉,认同病人的感受,鼓励其坚持治疗。

（4）用药护理　附子先煎,蛤蚧尾研末冲服。中药汤剂宜文火久煎,饭前温服。

（5）操作技术　① 推拿疗法:直擦背部督脉,横擦腰部肾俞、命门,以透热为度;孕妇禁用。② 穴位按摩法:取膏肓、肺俞、气海、肾俞、足三里、太渊、太溪,用拇指揉法、摩法、一指禅推法,按摩至局部发热或有酸麻重胀感,每日1次;孕妇禁用。③ 灸法:取脊柱段上的督脉,用督灸法,涂抹生姜汁,撒上督灸粉,覆盖桑皮纸,厚铺生姜泥,在姜泥上放置艾绒,点燃艾绒,每次连续灸3遍;每月1～2次;孕妇禁用。

9. 喘脱证

（1）生活起居护理　居室温暖安静,空气新鲜。衣物宽松。绝对卧床,取端坐位,遵医嘱吸氧。定时翻身、拍背,遵医嘱进行中药雾化吸入。护士每15～20分钟巡视1次,观察神志、呼吸、皮肤黏膜的颜色,记录出入量,备齐抢救设备。

（2）饮食护理　鼻饲流食。可食鹌鹑蛋。

（3）情志护理　安慰和鼓励病人及家属,使其保持情绪稳定,避免产生畏惧、恐慌情绪。

（4）用药护理　附子先煎,人参另煎。中药汤剂宜急煎,黑锡丹用淡盐水送服,或用温水溶化后鼻饲。注意观察用药后的反应,以防用药过量。

（5）操作技术　① 水针疗法:取曲池、足三里、尺泽、丰隆,用卡介菌多糖核酸注射液进行穴位注射。② 灸法:取肺俞、肾俞、命门、膏肓、气海、足三里,用温和灸,艾条燃着端悬于施灸部位上,距离皮肤2～3厘米,灸至病人有温热舒适无灼痛的感觉,皮肤稍有红晕,每日1次;孕妇腹部及腰骶部禁用。

（二）健康教育

居室应避风,空气新鲜,不可寒冷、干燥或有异味、灰尘、花粉。起居有常,劳逸适度,睡眠充足。注意保暖,勿汗出当风,以预防感冒。病情稳定时,进行锻炼和保健,如叩齿、慢走、打太极拳、按摩足底。定时进行深呼吸、腹式呼吸和缩唇呼吸训练。节制性行为,不可熬夜及过劳。

饮食宜清淡、营养、易消化。饮食有节,少食多餐,烹饪以蒸、煮为宜,进食高蛋白、高维生素的食物,多吃水果和绿叶蔬菜。宜食化痰的食物,如冬瓜、陈皮、雪梨、枇杷。忌烟酒、发物,不宜食辛辣、肥腻、煎炸、过甜、过咸、易产气的食物。

保持情绪稳定。本病缠绵难愈,病人可能精神负担较重,易出现焦虑、抑郁的情绪,护士可指导病人自我调节,鼓励家属常伴左右,以调畅情志,树立战胜疾病的信心。

定期复诊,遵医嘱按时服药,积极治疗原发病。病人平时须随身携带急救吸入制剂。查找过敏原,并避免接触过敏原。若有慢性严重缺氧,应遵医嘱长期低流量、低浓度氧疗,以提高生活质量。

Section 4   Dyspnea

Dyspnea is a lung system disease clinically characterized by shortness of breath, panting, difficult breathing aggravated with slight physical exertion, even breathing with raised shoulders and open mouth, flaring nostrils and inability to lie flat, accompanied with cough, profuse phlegm, chest oppression, cyanosis, raised chest, and hypochondriac distension. The nursing of dyspnea also applies to some diseases in Western medicine that present with dyspnea, such as chronic obstructive pulmonary disease, pulmonary heart disease and cardiogenic asthma, as well as difficult breathing in tuberculosis and silicosis.

ETIOLOGY AND PATHOGENESIS

The etiology includes invasion of external pathogenic factors, improper diet, emotional disorder, overstrain, chronic disease, phlegm and fluid-retention as well as blood stasis. Invasion of external pathogenic factors may induce adverse rising of lung qi, leading to dyspnea, for example, wind-cold attacks the exterior skin and hair and obstructs the interior lung qi, wind-heat attacks lung-defense and forces fire-heat into the interior, pathogenic dryness enters the body from the mouth and nose and damages the lung, or summer-heat scorches lung qi. Overeating rich, raw and cold foods or alcohol addiction may damage the spleen and produce phlegm that may induce adverse rising of lung qi. Emotional disorders, such as sorrow and anxiety damaging the lung, depressed anger damaging the liver or fright damaging the kidney, may disturb qi movement and induce adverse rising of lung qi. Factors such as overstrain damaging the spleen, sexual indulgence consuming kidney essence, or chronic disease impairing lung qi, may all cause failure to govern qi and induce adverse rising of lung qi. Illness-caused phlegm, fluid-retention and blood stasis congest lung qi and induce its adverse rising, leading to dyspnea.

The pathogenesis for excess dyspnea is that pathogenic factors invade the lung, inducing adverse rising of lung qi. On the contrary, the pathogenesis for deficiency dyspnea is that the lung fails to govern qi and the kidney fails to hold and receive qi. The disease is located in the lung and kidney but relates to the liver, spleen and heart. Excess dyspnea belongs to excess syndrome. Deficiency dyspnea is mostly deficiency syndrome, but sometimes it may be syndrome of deficiency-excess in complexity.

COMMON SYNDROMES

Key Points in Syndrome Differentiation

1. Differentiation of Deficiency Syndrome from Excess Syndrome

The differentiation is based on body constitution, disease cause, respiration and pulse manifestation. For previously robust patients who have acute onset caused by external pathogens, improper diet, or emotional disorder, there are symptoms like deep and long breathing, fast exhalation, rough and high voice, and rapid and powerful pulse, which is excess syndrome. On the contrary, for previously weak patients who show gradual development and unstable condition triggered by overstrain or prolonged illness, there are symptoms like discontinuous and rapid breathing, fast inhalation, soft and low voice, weak pulse or floating, large and rootless pulse, which is deficiency syndrome.

2. Differentiation of Cold Syndrome from Heat Syndrome

The differentiation is based on the color and texture of phlegm, complexion, and tongue and pulse manifestations. White clear phlegm, bluish or grayish complexion, cold limbs, no thirst, pale tongue with white slippery coating, and floating tight pulse or sunken thready pulse indicate cold syndrome. Yellow thick and sticky phlegm, red complexion, fever, thirst with desire for cold drinks, dark urine, constipation, red tongue with yellow coating, and rapid pulse suggest heat syndrome.

3. Differentiation of Disease Location

The differentiation is based on the disease location. If the disease is caused by external pathogens, phlegm turbidity, and liver qi depression, it mostly belongs to excess syndrome and is located in the lung. And if the disease is induced by overstrain or prolonged illness that causes abnormal movement of lung qi and kidney qi, it is primarily deficiency syndrome and located in the lung and kidney.

Syndrome Differentiation

1. Excess Dyspnea

(1) Wind-Cold Invading the Lung Syndrome

[Clinical Manifestations] Dyspnea, cough with counterflow of lung qi, rapid breathing, chest distention and oppression, profuse white clear phlegm, aversion to cold, no sweating, headache, nasal congestion, or fever, no thirst, thin white tongue coating, and floating tight pulse.

[Manifestations Analysis] Exterior wind-cold blocks in the lung causes counterflow of lung qi, leading to dyspnea, cough with counterflow of lung qi, rapid breathing, and chest distention and oppression. Failure of lung qi to disperse causes fluid to accumulate and generate phlegm, so the patients have profuse white clear phlegm. Wind-cold fettering the exterior causes skin and pores occlusion that explains aversion to cold and absence of sweating or presence of fever. Cold coagulation hinders qi movement, so headache is felt. Failure of lung qi to disperse is responsible for nasal congestion. Thin white and slippery tongue coating and floating tight pulse are manifestations of wind-cold.

[Nursing Principle] Ventilating the lung and dissipating cold.

［Suggested Formula］Mahuang Decoction and Huagai Powder.

（2）Exterior Cold and Interior Heat Syndrome

［Clinical Manifestations］Dyspnea with counterflow of lung qi, rough breathing, flaring nostrils, chest distention or pain, cough with difficult expectoration, thick sticky phlegm, accompanied with cold body and generalized pain, fever and dysphoria, sweating or absence of sweating, thirst, thin white or thin yellow tongue coating, red tongue margins, and floating rapid pulse or slippery pulse.

［Manifestations Analysis］Wind-cold fettering the exterior leads to depressed heat in the lung and counterflow of lung qi, resulting in dyspnea with counterflow of qi, rough breathing, flaring nostrils, and chest distention or pain. Depressed heat in the lung scorches and transform fluids into phlegm, leading to thirst, cough with difficult expectoration, and thick sticky phlegm. Wind-cold fettering the exterior explains cold body and generalized pain. Exuberance of interior heat contributes to fever and dysphoria. Heat consumes fluids and causes thirst. Thin white or thin yellow tongue coating, red tongue margins, and floating rapid pulse or slippery pulse indicate exterior cold and interior heat.

［Nursing Principle］Releasing exterior and clearing interior; resolving phlegm and relieving dyspnea.

［Suggested Formula］Maxing Shigan Decoction.

（3）Phlegm-Heat Depressing the Lung Syndrome

［Clinical Manifestations］Dyspnea and cough with overflow of qi, chest distention and pain, profuse yellow sticky phlegm or phlegm with blood streak, accompanied with dysphoria, fever, sweating, thirst with desire for cold drinks, red complexion and dry throat, dark urine, constipation, red tongue with yellow slimy coating, and slippery rapid pulse.

［Manifestations Analysis］Depression of phlegm-heat causes failure of lung qi to disperse and descend, leading to dyspnea and cough with overflow of qi as well as chest distention and pain. Interior phlegm-heat exuberance damages lung collaterals, so phlegm is profuse, sticky, yellow or blood-streaked. Phlegm-heat steaming the lung is the cause of dysphoria, fever, sweating, and thirst with desire for cold drinks. Heat consuming fluids contributes to red complexion and dry throat, dark urine, and constipation. Red tongue with yellow slimy coating and slippery rapid pulse suggest interior accumulation of phlegm-heat.

［Nursing Principle］Clearing heat and resolving phlegm; ventilating the lung and relieving dyspnea.

［Suggested Formula］Sangbaipi Decoction.

（4）Phlegm-Turbidity Obstructing the Lung Syndrome

［Clinical Manifestations］Dyspnea and cough with gurgling phlegm sound, chest fullness and oppression, even suffocating sensation with inability to lie flat, profuse white sticky phlegm, difficult expectoration, nausea, vomiting, anorexia, sticky mouth, no thirst, pale tongue with white thick slimy coating, and slippery pulse.

［Manifestations Analysis］Dysfunction of the spleen in transportation and transformation generates phlegm-dampness that congests the lung and hinders qi movement, leading to failure of lung qi to disperse and descend, causing counterflow of lung qi with such symptoms as dyspnea and cough with gurgling phlegm sound, chest fullness and oppression, even suffocating sensation with inability to lie flat, profuse white sticky phlegm, and difficult expectoration. Phlegm-dampness accumulates in the middle energizer and causes spleen-stomach disharmony, resulting in nausea, vomiting, anorexia, sticky mouth, and no thirst. Pale tongue with white thick slimy coating and slippery pulse indicate phlegm-dampness.

[Nursing Principle] Dispelling phlegm and descending adverse qi; ventilating the lung and relieving dyspnea.

[Suggested Formula] Erchen Decoction and Sanzi Yangqin Decoction.

(5) Liver Qi Overwhelming the Lung Syndrome

[Clinical Manifestations] Dyspnea is always triggered by emotional stimulation, with such symptoms as short rapid and rough breathing, chest and hypochondriac oppression and pain, suffocating sensation in the throat without obvious gurgling phlegm sound, anxiety and depression, or insomnia, palpitation, heart vexation, irritability, red complexion and eyes, pale or red tongue with thin white or thin yellow coating, and wiry pulse or wiry rapid pulse.

[Manifestations Analysis] Depressed anger damaging the liver makes liver qi rush upward to overwhelm the lung and causes failure of lung qi to disperse and descend, leading to short rapid and rough breathing. Dual depression of liver qi and lung qi is the cause of chest and hypochondriac oppression and pain, and suffocating sensation in the throat without obvious gurgling phlegm sound. Dual depression of liver qi and heart qi along with heart-spirit fidgety induces anxiety and depression, or insomnia, palpitation, heart vexation, irritability, and red complexion and eyes. Pale or red tongue with thin coating and wiry pulse suggest depression of liver qi.

[Nursing Principle] Relieving depression, descending qi, and relieving dyspnea.

[Suggested Formula] Wumo Yinzi Decoction.

(6) Water Intimidating the Heart and Lung Syndrome

[Clinical Manifestations] Dyspnea and cough with counterflow of qi, propped breathing and inability to lie flat, thin white phlegm, palpitation, generalized edema, scanty urine, fear of cold, cold limbs, dull complexion, cyanotic lips and nails, pale enlarged or dark enlarged tongue, possibly with ecchymoses or petechia, obvious sublingual veins, white slippery tongue coating, and sunken thready pulse or unsmooth pulse.

[Manifestations Analysis] Kidney yang weakness and disturbance of the lung by water pathogen lead to dyspnea and cough with counterflow of qi, propped breathing and inability to lie flat, and thin white phlegm. Water pathogen intimidating the heart impairs heart yang, causing palpitation. Chronic panting with deficiency of the lung, spleen and kidney causes dysfunction of qi transformation, yang deficiency and water overflow, leading to generalized edema and scanty urine. Deficient yang cannot warm the four limbs, so fear of cold and cold limbs are felt. Impaired heart yang cannot propel the movement of blood and leads to sluggish blood circulation, so such symptoms occur as dull complexion, cyanotic lips and nails, dark enlarged tongue, possibly with ecchymoses or petechia, and obvious sublingual veins. Pale enlarged tongue with white slippery coating and sunken thready pulse or unsmooth pulse are signs of yang deficiency with water retention.

[Nursing Principle] Warming yang and promoting urination; purging the lung and relieving dyspnea.

[Suggested Formula] Zhenwu Decoction and Tingli Dazao Xiefei Decoction.

2. Deficiency Dyspnea

(1) Lung Deficiency Syndrome

[Clinical Manifestations] Dyspnea, shortness of breath, weak qi with low voice, snoring sound in the throat, lung qi insufficiency, weak cough, thin clear phlegm, spontaneous sweating, fear of wind, or choking cough, scanty sticky phlegm, heat vexation, dry mouth and sore throat, flushed face, pale red tongue or red tongue with scanty coating, and soft weak or thready rapid pulse.

[Manifestations Analysis] Lung qi insufficiency is the cause of dyspnea, shortness of breath, weak qi with low voice, and snoring sound in the throat. Lung qi insufficiency and failure of qi to transform fluids contributes to weak cough and thin clear phlegm. Insecurity of defensive exterior explains spontaneous sweating and fear of wind. Pale red tongue and soft weak pulse are signs of lung qi deficiency. If lung yin is insufficient, deficiency fire flames up. Then there appear choking cough, scanty sticky phlegm, heat vexation, dry mouth and sore throat, flushed face, red tongue with scanty coating, and thready rapid pulse.

[Nursing Principle] Tonifying the lung and replenishing qi.

[Suggested Formula] Shengmai Powder and Bufei Decoction.

(2) Kidney Deficiency Syndrome

[Clinical Manifestations] Chronic dyspnea that aggravates with physical exertion, exhalation more than inhalation, discontinuous breathing, emaciation, lassitude, foot edema, sweating, cold limbs, bluish complexion and purple lips, or cough with dyspnea, red complexion, dysphoria, dry mouth and throat, cold feet, oily sweat, pale tongue with white coating or black moist coating, or red tongue with scanty fluids, and sunken weak pulse or thready rapid pulse.

[Manifestations Analysis] Chronic illness with lung deficiency causes failure of kidney to receive qi, leading to chronic dyspnea that aggravates with physical exertion, exhalation more than inhalation, and discontinuous breathing. Depleted kidney essence fail to nourish the body and spirit, resulting in emaciation and lassitude. Insecurity of defensive exterior due to yang deficiency is the cause of sweating. Failure of qi to transform water due to yang deficiency results in foot edema. Deficient yang cannot warm the body, causing cold limbs. Pale tongue with white coating or black moist coating and sunken weak pulse are signs of kidney yang deficiency. Or kidney yin exhaustion makes yin fail to constrain yang, and yang qi floats outward, then such symptoms appear as cough with dyspnea, red complexion, dysphoria, dry mouth and throat, cold feet, oily sweat, red tongue with scanty fluids, and thready rapid pulse.

[Nursing Principle] Tonifying the kidney and receiving qi.

［Suggested Formula］Jin'gui Shenqi Pills and Shen'ge Powder.

（3）Dyspnea with Collapse Syndrome

［Clinical Manifestations］Severe dyspnea, breathing with open mouth and raised shoulders, flaring nostrils, inability to lie flat, life-threatening dyspnea with slight physical exertion, gurgling phlegm sound, palpitation, dysphoria, cold limbs, bluish complexion and purple lips, profuse pearly sweat, floating large and rootless pulse, or extremely faint pulse.

［Manifestations Analysis］Lung and kidney failure causes inability to govern and receive qi, leading to severe dyspnea, breathing with open mouth and raised shoulders, flaring nostrils, inability to lie flat, and life-threatening dyspnea with slight physical exertion. Heart yang collapse causes the restlessness of deficiency yang, so palpitation and dysphoria are felt. Yang collapse causes inability to warm the blood and vessels, resulting in cold limbs, bluish complexion and purple lips. Yang collapse makes external leakage of yin fluids, so profuse pearly sweat appears. Floating large and rootless pulse or extremely faint pulse are signs of yang collapse and yin exhaustion.

［Nursing Principle］Reinforcing yang and stopping collapse; consolidating and astringing kidney qi.

［Suggested Formula］Shenfu Decoction and Heixi Pellets.

NURSING MEASURES

For patients with dyspnea, nurses should closely observe the inducing factor, onset time and duration of panting; the frequency, rhythm and depth of breath; the duration ratio of exhalation to inhalation; the nature, degree, onset time and duration of cough; the difficulty level of expectoration; the amount, color and texture of phlegm. They should check the mental status, body temperature, heart rate, blood pressure, complexion, urine volume, sweating and the presence of cyanosis of patients. For patients with water pathogen attacking the heart, the 24-hour intake and output should be recorded. If the patient shows unconsciousness, face and lips cyanosis, profuse pearly sweat, cold limbs, suddenly decline of blood pressure, and floating, large and rootless pulse, or extremely faint pulse, report to the doctor immediately and assist in emergency treatment.

Syndrome-Based Nursing Measures

1. Wind-Cold Invading the Lung Syndrome

（1）Daily life nursing. The ward should be warm, quiet, comfortable, full of adequate sunshine and fresh air, and away from wind. The patients should rest in bed with the head of the bed slightly raised. Nurses assist the patients to turn over timely, apply low flow oxygen inhalation with the patients' respiratory tract clear, pat on their back gently, guide them to practize efficient coughing, expectoration and deep breathing, and keep their chest and back warm. For patients with fever, cold application therapy is prohibited. Restrict visits to patients and avoid overstrain and excessive exercise.

（2）Diet nursing. The patients may eat foods that warm the lung and dissipate cold, such as shengjiang（fresh ginger）and congbai（scallion white）, and take lingzhi（glossy ganoderma）soup 2~3 times per week. They may also eat zisu (purple perilla) porridge: prepare jingmi (polished round-grained rice) 100 g, zisuye (leaf of purple perilla) 20 g, and some white sugar; boil the squashed zisuye (leaf of purple perilla) to get the thick juice, put the rice into the juice, boil to make porridge, and eat the porridge warm during meals. Cold and raw vegetables and fruit should be avoided.

(3) Emotion nursing. Because the disease shows severe symptoms at onset, nurses may use verbal enlightenment therapy to impart patients the causes and prognosis of disease to eliminate their fright.

(4) Medication nursing. Decoction should be prepared fast with strong fire and taken hot after meals. After taking medicine, the patients should eat hot porridge and tuck themselves in to perspire slightly.

(5) Manipulation techniques. ① Tuina therapy: select the bladder meridian of foot-taiyang on the back of the trunk; apply scrubbing manipulation until the area turns hot. And it is contraindicated in pregnancy. ② Cupping therapy: select Dazhui (GV 14) and Feishu (BL 13); retain the cup on the acupoints for 10 minutes, once per day. ③ Acupressure therapy: select Feishu (BL 13), Xinshu (BL 15), Geshu (BL 17), Danzhong (CV 17), Lieque (LU 7) and Fengmen (BL 12); apply thumb kneading and one-finger pushing manipulations on each of the acupoints until the area turns hot or the patient has the feelings of soreness, numbness, distension and heaviness in the area; once per day. And it is contraindicated in pregnancy.

2. Exterior Cold and Interior Heat Syndrome

(1) Daily life nursing. The ward should be warm, full of fresh air and away from wind. The patients should take a rest in bed with the head of the bed slightly raised. Nurses apply low flow oxygen inhalation with the patients' respiratory tract clear, guide them to practize efficient coughing, assist them to turn over, pat on their back, and follow the doctor's advice to give spray inhalation therapy with Chinese medicine. For patients with sticky phlegm, drink warm water frequently. For patients with fever, cold application therapy is prohibited.

(2) Diet nursing. The patients may eat foods that relive exterior and clear heat, such as lettuces, snow pears, sugarcane, and lotus root. Lugen (reed rhizome) porridge is recommended: prepare xianlugen (fresh reed rhizome) 45 g, boil it for 40 minutes and remove the residue, put rice 30 g into the decoction, and boil to make porridge.

(3) Emotion nursing. Because the disease is newly onset, nurses may use verbal enlightenment therapy to ease anxiety of the patients.

(4) Medication nursing. Shengshigao (raw gypsum) should be decocted earlier. Decoction should be taken warm after meals. After taking medicine, perspiring slightly is preferred, and nurses should observe the body temperature and sweating condition.

(5) Manipulation techniques. ① Cupping therapy: select Dazhui (GV 14), Fengmen (BL 12), Feishu (BL 13), Xinshu (BL 15) and Gaohuang (BL 43); retain the cup on the acupoints for 10 minutes, 2~4 acupoints each time, once every other day. ② Scraping therapy: select Dazhui (GV 14), Fengchi (GB 20), Feishu (BL 13) and Pishu (BL 20) ; repeat the scraping manipulation till the area

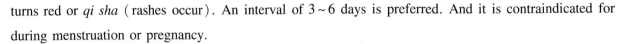

turns red or *qi sha* (rashes occur). An interval of 3～6 days is preferred. And it is contraindicated for during menstruation or pregnancy.

3. Phlegm-Heat Depressing the Lung Syndrome

(1) Daily life nursing. The ward should be cool, moist, quiet, full of fresh air and away from wind. The patients should rest in bed with the head of the bed slightly raised, keep oral hygiene, and rinse the mouth with jinyinhua gancao (honeysuckle flower and licorice root) liquid after meals. Nurses apply low flow oxygen inhalation with the patients' respiratory tract clear, guide them to practize slow deep breathing, and follow the doctor's advice to give spray inhalation therapy with Chinese medicine. For patients with fever, take a warm sponge bath. For patients with profuse sweating, wipe the sweat away and change the wet clothes and bedding timely.

(2) Diet nursing. The patients should drink more water and may drink biqi (waternut) juice, and watermelon juice. For patients with sticky phlegm, zhuli (bamboo sap) is recommended. They should eat fruit and vegetables rich in fiber to keep a normal bowel movement, and have foods that clear heat and resolve phlegm, such as dried persimmon, biqi (waternut), luffa, white radishes and baihe (lily bulb). Avoid fried, dry- or heat-natured, pungent and spicy foods.

(3) Emotion nursing. Because the patients are suffering from severe symptoms, nurses may use emotional transference and dispositional change therapy to encourage them to share their experience in disease prevention and treatment to reduce their mental stress, so as to avoid anxiety and depression.

(4) Medication nursing. Decoction should be taken warm or slightly cool after meals.

(5) Manipulation techniques. ① Acupressure therapy: select Danzhong (CV 17), Lieque (LU 7), Feishu (BL 13), Fenglong (ST 40), Dingchuan (EX－B1) and Tiantu (CV 22); apply thumb kneading and one-finger pushing manipulations on each of the acupoints until the area turns hot or the patient has the feelings of soreness, numbness, distension and heaviness in the area; once per day. And it is contraindicated in pregnancy. ② Auricular pressure therapy: select the auricular points of lung (CO14), trachea (CO16), shenmen (TF4), subcortex (AT4), adrenal gland (TG2p) and sympathetic (AH6a); apply specialized pasters on the points, knead each of them till the area turns hot and red, 4～5 times per day, and keep the pasters for 2～4 days. And it is contraindicated in pregnancy.

4. Phlegm-Turbidity Obstructing the Lung Syndrome

(1) Daily life nursing. The ward should be warm, dry, quiet, full of fresh air, and away from wind. The patients should take a rest in bed with the head of the bed slightly raised. They should keep themselves warm. Nurses apply low flow oxygen inhalation with the patients' respiratory tract clear, and guide them to take a deep breath after getting up in the morning to expectorate the retained phlegm. When the condition is stabilized, the patients may do moderate exercise and avoid getting tired.

(2) Diet nursing. The patients should have small frequent meals, and take foods that invigorate the spleen and dissolve phlegm, such as shengjiang (fresh ginger), luffa, rougui (cinnamon bark), fuling (poria), white radishes, shanyao (common yam rhizome) and loquat. Food therapy: jupi xingren (tangerine peel and apricot kernel) drink, xueli yin'er baihe (snow pears, tremella and lily bulb) soup,

and xingren doufu (apricot kernel and tofu) soup. Xingren doufu soup: take apricot kernel 15 g and tofu 120 g, boil them together for one hour, remove the residue, eat the tofu and drink the soup, once in the morning and once in the evening for 4~5 days in a row. Avoid too-sweet, raw, cold and greasy foods.

(3) Emotion nursing. Because the disease recurs persistently, nurses may use submission therapy to communicate with the patients as much as possible and encourage them to express themselves to eliminate undesirable feelings in time and keep them calm.

(4) Medication nursing. Decoction should be taken hot after meals, multiple times in small portions.

(5) Manipulation techniques. ① Moxibustion therapy: select Feishu (BL 13), Shenshu (BL 23), Gaohuang (BL 43), Qihai (CV 6), Zusanli (ST 36) and Neiguan (PC 6); place the moxa stick 2~3 centimeters away from the skin to perform mild moxibustion on each of the acupoints until the area turns red and the patient feels warm and comfortable without the sensation of burning pain, once per day. And it cannot be applied on the abdomen and lumbosacral region of pregnant women. ② Cupping therapy: select Zusanli (ST 36), Zhongwan (CV 12) and Neiguan (PC 6); retain the cup on the acupoints for 10 minutes, once every other day. And it cannot be applied on the abdomen of pregnant women. ③ Water acupuncture therapy: select Dingchuan (EX － B1), Feishu (BL 13), Gaohuang (BL 43), Lieque (LU 7), Hegu (LI 4) or Jiaji (EX － B2), the same acupoint on both side; inject placenta injection or Vitamin B_{12} injection into the acupoints, one acupoint (bilateral) each time. ④ Auricular pressure therapy: select the auricular points of spleen (CO13), stomach (CO10), triple energizer (CO17) and pancreas-gallbladder (CO11); apply specialized pasters on the points, knead each of them till the area feels hot and turns red, 4~5 times per day, and keep the pasters for 2~4 days. And it is contraindicated in pregnancy.

5. Liver Qi Overwhelming the Lung Syndrome

(1) Daily life nursing. The ward should be quiet, comfortable, and full of fresh air. The patients should rest in bed with the head of the bed slightly raised, have low flow oxygen inhalation, live a regular life, and avoid staying up late. Nurses guide the patients to do relaxing practice, such as practicing Qigong, reading, listening to music, and taking a slow deep breath to relax muscles.

(2) Diet nursing. The patients may drink meiguihua (rose flower) tea, and eat foods that move qi and relieve depression, such as pomelo and foshou (finger citron fruit). Food therapy: jupi (tangerine peel) porridge. Avoid greasy and flatulent foods, such as sweet potatoes.

(3) Emotion nursing. The patients should stay calm and avoid being angry. Nurses may use verbal enlightenment therapy to tell them and their family the association between emotion and disease, or use emotional transference and dispositional change therapy to distract their attention and encourage them to moderately take part in social activities and sports.

(4) Medication nursing. Daizheshi (hematite) should be decocted earlier, xuanfuhua (inula flower) wrap-boiled, and chenxiang (aquilaria wood) decocted later. The decoction should be prepared for a short time and taken warm after meals. Stop taking the medicine immediately after the disease is cured.

(5) Manipulation techniques. ① Acupressure therapy: select Feishu (BL 13), Dazhui (GV 14), Fengmen (BL 12), Lieque (LU 7), Hegu (LI 4) and Zusanli (ST 36); apply thumb kneading manipulation on each of the acupoints until the area turns hot or the patient has the feelings of soreness, numbness, distension and heaviness in the area; once per day. And it is contraindicated in pregnancy. ② Auricular pressure therapy: select the auricular points of lung (CO14), liver (CO12) and trachea (CO16); apply specialized pasters on the points, gently knead each of them before an episode of dyspnea till the area turns hot and red. And it is contraindicated in pregnancy.

6. Water Intimidating the Heart and Lung Syndrome

(1) Daily life nursing. The ward should be warm, quiet and full of fresh air, and avoid strong and convective wind. The patients should rest in bed with the head of the bed slightly raised, turn over regularly, and have low flow oxygen inhalation. They should also have adequate sleep, keep themselves warm to prevent colds, and avoid strenuous exercise and severe cough.

(2) Diet nursing. Limit the intake of sodium salt and water. The patients should eat warm foods in small frequent meals at a slow speed, and take foods that warm yang and resolve fluid-retention, such as chixiaodou (adzuki beans) and shanzha (hawthorn fruit). Avoid raw, cold and greasy foods.

(3) Emotion nursing. Because of the severe condition, nurses may use verbal enlightenment therapy to impart patients the knowledge about the disease and encourage them to actively prevent and treat the disease to avoid pessimism.

(4) Medication nursing. Fuzi (monkshood) should be decocted earlier and tinglizi (pepperweed seed) wrap-boiled. Decoction should be taken warm after meals, multiple times in small portions.

(5) Manipulation techniques. ① Moxibustion therapy: select Dingchuan (EX - B1), Danzhong (CV 17), Feishu (BL 13), Dazhui (GV 14) and Hegu (LI 4); place the moxa stick 2~3 centimeters away from the skin to perform mild moxibustion on each of the acupoints until the area turns red and the patient feels warm and comfortable without the sensation of burning pain, 3~5 acupoints each time, 2~3 times per day. ② Acupressure therapy: select Chize (LU 5), Kongzui (LU 6), Neiguan (PC 6), Jingqu (LU 8), Zusanli (ST 36) and Fenglong (ST 40); apply thumb kneading manipulation on each of the acupoints until the area turns hot or the patient has the feelings of soreness, numbness, distension and heaviness in the area; once per day. And it is contraindicated in pregnancy.

7. Lung Deficiency Syndrome

(1) Daily life nursing. The ward should be warm, quiet, comfortable, full of fresh air, and away from wind. The patients should live a regular life, avoid staying up late, keep themselves warm to prevent colds, and have long-term oxygen inhalation. When the condition is stabilized, they may do moderate exercise and avoid getting tired.

(2) Diet nursing. The patients may eat foods that tonify the lung and invigorate the spleen, such as carps and baihe (lily bulb). Food therapy: pig lung white radish soup and shanyao yiyiren (common yam rhizome and coix seed) porridge. Pig lung white radish soup: stew together pig lung 300 g, white radishes 250 g, some salt and shengjiang (fresh ginger). Shanyao yiyiren porridge: boil 60 g of common

yam rhizome and 60 g of coix seed with rice to make porridge. Avoid cold and raw foods.

(3) Emotion nursing. Because the patients are weak with a long course of disease, nurses may use submission therapy and frequently make the rounds of the wards, learn about their demands, and meet their reasonable needs as much as possible.

(4) Medication nursing. Decoction should be prepared slowly over low heat and taken warm before meals, multiple times in small portions. After taking medicine, the patients should take a rest in bed.

(5) Manipulation techniques. ① Healthcare massage therapy: select Tiantu (CV 22) and Danzhong (CV 17); apply gentle kneading and pressing manipulations on the acupoints by the patients' themselves; or apply gentle patting on the acupoints along the spinal cord from bottom to top; or apply transverse-scrubbing manipulation on the upper chest and the areas around xinshu (BL 15) and shenshu (BL 13) on the back; several times per day. And it is contraindicated in pregnancy. ② Qigong therapy: practize spirit-concentration and muscle-relaxation exercise; for patients with yang deficiency, concentrate on Dantian (cinnabar field, a Taoist term used in the practice of inner alchemy) or Mingmen (GV 4), with more concentration than relaxation; for patients with yin deficiency, concentrate on Yongquan (KI 1), with more relaxation than concentration; 30 minutes each time, once per day. ③ Paste application therapy: select Jingbailao (EX - HN15), Feishu (BL 13) and Gaohuang (BL 43); grind into powder equal amount of baijiezi (white mustard seed), yanhusuo (corydalis rhizome), xixin (Manchurian wild ginger) and gansui (gansui root), blend the powder with shengjiang (fresh ginger) juice to make pastes, apply them on the acupoints, and fix them with adhesive tapes; 0.5~2 hours each time, once per day. ④ Moxibustion therapy: select Feishu (BL 13) and Gaohuang (BL 43); place the moxa stick 2~3 centimeters away from the skin to perform mild moxibustion on each of the acupoints until the area turns red and the patient feels warm and comfortable without the sensation of burning pain, once per week.

8. Kidney Deficiency Syndrome

(1) Daily life nursing. The ward should be quiet, comfortable, and full of fresh air. Keep the bedding tidy and dry. The patients should live a regular life, take adequate sleep, pay attention to skin hygiene, gently scrub the skin with warm water, and massage the compression part with honghua (safflower) ethanol solution every day. Nurses should observe closely the patients' change of blood pressure and pulse to prevent dyspnea collapse. For patients who are completely bedridden, nurses should turn them over regularly. When the condition is stabilized, the patients may do moderate exercise under close watch to prevent tiredness and falls. For patients with forceless expectoration, use sputum aspirator to suck it out. For patients with urinary and fecal incontinence, apply perineal care. Patients should value sexual abstinence and avoid overstrain.

(2) Diet nursing. The patients may have a low-salt diet, eat foods high in calorie, vitamin and protein, as well as those that tonify kidney essence, such as mutton, hetaoren (walnut), heizhima (black sesame), pig kidneys and meat of soft-shelled turtles.

(3) Emotion nursing. Because the patients are weak with a long course of disease, nurses may use

verbal enlightenment therapy to care for and listen to them patiently, acknowledge their feelings and encourage them to stick with the treatment.

(4) Medication nursing. Fuzi (monkshood) should be decocted earlier, and gejiewei (gecko tail) should be finely ground and blended with water for oral taking. Decoction should be prepared slowly over low heat and taken warm before meals.

(5) Manipulation techniques. ① Tuina therapy: select the area along the governor vessel on the back of the trunk, and apply longitudinal scrubbing manipulation until the area turns hot; select the area around Shenshu (BL 23) and Mingmen (GV 4), and apply transverse scrubbing manipulation until the area turns hot. And it is contraindicated in pregnancy. ② Acupressure therapy: select Gaohuang (BL 43), Feishu (BL 13), Qihai (CV 6), Shenshu (BL 23), Zusanli (ST 36), Taiyuan (LU 9) and Taixi (KI 3); apply thumb kneading, palm flat pushing and one-finger pushing manipulations on each of the acupoints until the area turns hot or the patient has the feelings of soreness, numbness, distension and heaviness in the area; once per day. And it is contraindicated in pregnancy. ③ Moxibustion therapy: select the area along the governor vessel on the back of the trunk and apply governor vessel moxibustion therapy: smear shengjiang (fresh ginger) juice on the area, dust the juice with medicated powder, cover with mulberry paper, spread a thick layer of fresh ginger mud on the paper, and put moxa on the mud. Light the moxa for moxibustion, three consecutive times per session, 1~2 sessions every month. And it is contraindicated in pregnancy.

9. Dyspnea with Collapse Syndrome

(1) Daily life nursing. The ward should be warm, quiet, and full of fresh air. Loose-fitting clothing is preferred. The patients should stay absolutely in bed with a sitting position, and follow the doctor's advice to have oxygen inhalation. They should have regular turning-over and back-patting, and take spray inhalation therapy with Chinese medicine. Nurses should go the rounds of the wards every 15~20 minutes, observe the patients' mental status, respiration and the color of skin and mucosa, take records of intake and output and get ready the rescue equipment.

(2) Diet nursing. Give liquid diet by nasal feeding. Quail eggs are recommended.

(3) Emotion nursing. Nurses should comfort and encourage the patients and their family, so that they can stay calm and away from fear and panic.

(4) Medication nursing. Fuzi (monkshood) should be decocted earlier, and renshen (ginseng) separately. Decoction should be boiled quickly. Heixi Pellets should be taken with dilute saline, or dissolved in warm water and taken by nasal feeding. Nurses should closely observe the patients after medication to prevent overdose.

(5) Manipulation techniques. ① Water acupuncture therapy: select Quchi (LI 11), Zusanli (ST 36), Chize (LU 5) and Fenglong (ST 40); and inject bcg-psn injection into the acupoints. ② Moxibustion therapy: select Feishu (BL 13), Shenshu (BL 23), Mingmen (GV 4), Gaohuang (BL 43), Qihai (CV 6) and Zusanli (ST 36); place the moxa stick 2~3 centimeters away from the skin to perform mild moxibustion on each of the acupoints until the area turns red and the patient feels

warm and comfortable without the sensation of burning pain, once per day. And it cannot be applied on the abdomen and lumbosacral region of pregnant women.

Patient Education

The room should be warm and moist, full of fresh air, away from wind, and without peculiar smell, dust or pollen. The patients should live a regular life, balance work and rest, have adequate sleep, keep themselves warm, and avoid exposure to wind after sweating to prevent colds. When the condition is stabilized, the patients should do health care exercise, such as clicking teeth, slow walking, Taiji and foot massage. They may regularly practize deep breathing, diaphragmatic breathing and pursed lip breathing. They should value sexual abstinence, and avoid staying up late and overstrain.

The diet should be light, nutritious and digestible. Steaming and boiling are the preferred cooking methods. The patients should follow a moderate diet, have small frequent meals, eat fresh fruit and vegetables, and take high-protein and high-vitamin foods and those that revolve phlegm, such as wax gourd, chenpi (aged tangerine peel), snow pears and loquat. They should refrain from smoking, drinking and eating foods that induce or aggravate disease. Avoid pungent, spicy, greasy, fried, too-sweet, too-salty and flatulent foods.

The patients should stay calm. Since the disease tends to reoccur frequently, the patients may have mental stress, anxiety and depression. Nurses may guide the patients to adjust their state of mind, and encourage their family to be with them as much as possible to regulate their emotions and help them restore confidence in winning the battle against disease.

The patients should return to the hospital regularly, follow the doctor's advice in medication, treat primary disease actively, and carry emergency inhalation preparation all the time. Find out the allergen to avoid it. For patients with chronic severe anoxia, follow the doctor's advice to take long-term, low-flow and low-concentration oxygen inhalation to improve the quality of life.

第五节　心　　悸

　　心悸,是指因气虚血弱,导致心失所养,或因情绪刺激,外邪直中心络,或因痰饮、瘀血痹阻心脉而引起的,以自觉心脏异常跳动,心慌不安,或时作时止为临床特征的心系病。西医的心律失常、心力衰竭,以心悸为主要表现的,可参照本节进行护理。

一、病因病机

　　心悸的病因包括感受外邪、情志所伤、饮食不节、体质虚弱、药物所伤。病人外感温热邪毒,逆传心包,耗气伤阴,心神失养;或外感风寒湿邪,侵袭体表,痹阻血脉,心脉不畅,均可发为心悸。病人思虑过度,劳伤心脾,心血暗耗,化源不足,心失所养;或恼怒伤肝,气滞血瘀,心脉瘀阻;或气郁化火,炼液成痰,痰火扰心;或素体心虚胆怯,暴受惊恐,心气逆乱,均可发为心悸。病人嗜食肥甘醇酒,蕴热化火生痰,痰火扰心;或饮食不节,损伤脾胃,脾虚生痰,痹阻心脉,可发为心悸。病人素体禀赋不足,阴阳失调,气血失和,心脉不畅;或素体脾胃虚弱,化源不足,或年老体衰,久病失养,劳欲过度,气血阴阳亏虚,心失所养;或水肿日久,或脾肾阳虚,水饮内停,继而水饮凌心,均可发为心悸。用药不当,或药物毒性较剧,损及于心,亦可发为心悸。

　　心悸的病机是气血阴阳亏虚,心失所养;或邪扰心神,心神不宁。病位在心,与肝、脾、肺、肾有关。心悸以虚证居多,也可因虚致实,形成虚实夹杂之证。

二、常见证型

　　(一)辨证要点

　　1. 辨轻重　根据病因、病势、病程等来辨别。若由惊恐、恼怒、紧张引起,起病急,持续时间短,则多病情较轻。若由体虚或脏腑功能受损引起,过劳即发,起病缓,持续时间长,则多病情较重。

　　2. 辨虚实　虚者,包括血虚、阴虚、阳虚。实者,包括水饮、痰火、瘀血。若心悸头晕,面色无华,多为血虚;心悸盗汗,口干潮热,多为阴虚;心悸肢冷,畏寒气短,多为阳虚。若心悸,舌苔水滑,肢体浮肿,小便短少,多为水饮;心悸体丰,口苦纳呆,舌苔黄腻,多为痰火;心悸唇暗,舌有瘀斑,脉结代,多为血瘀。

　　(二)证候分型

　　1. 心虚胆怯证

　　[主要证候]心悸不宁,善惊易恐,坐卧不安,失眠多梦而易惊醒,恶闻声响,食少纳呆;苔薄白,脉细数或细弦。

［证候分析］心为神舍,心虚则心不藏神,神摇不安,故心悸不宁,失眠多梦;胆怯则善惊易恐,故坐卧不安,寐中容易惊醒,恶闻声响;母病及子,脾失健运,故食少纳呆;苔薄白,脉细数或细弦,均为心神不安,气血逆乱之象。

［护治原则］镇惊定志,养心安神。

［常用方剂］安神定志丸。

2. 心血不足证

［主要证候］心悸气短,头晕目眩,失眠健忘,面色无华,倦怠乏力,纳呆食少;舌淡红,脉细弱。

［证候分析］思虑劳心暗耗心血,或脾气亏虚,气血生化不足,皆可致心神失养,故心悸,失眠;血虚不能濡养脑髓,故头晕目眩,健忘;血虚不能上荣肌肤,故面色无华;脾气虚弱,故倦怠乏力,纳呆食少;舌淡红,脉细弱,均为心血不足之象。

［护治原则］补血养心,益气安神。

［常用方剂］归脾汤。

3. 阴虚火旺证

［主要证候］心悸易惊,心烦失眠,五心烦热,口干,盗汗,思虑劳心则症状加重,伴耳鸣腰酸,头晕目眩,急躁易怒;舌红少津,苔少或无,脉细数。

［证候分析］肾阴不足,水不济火,致心阴不足,心火亢旺,扰动心神,故心悸易惊,心烦失眠;肾阴亏虚,腰为肾之府,故腰酸;肾虚髓海不足,故耳鸣,头晕目眩;思虑劳心,阴血暗耗,故症状加重;五心烦热,口干,盗汗,舌红少津,苔少或无,脉细数,均为阴虚火旺之象。

［护治原则］滋阴清火,养心安神。

［常用方剂］天王补心丹合朱砂安神丸。

4. 心阳不振证

［主要证候］心悸不安,胸闷气短,动则尤甚,面色苍白,形寒肢冷;舌淡苔白,脉虚弱或沉细无力。

［证候分析］心阳虚衰,无以温养心神,故心悸不安;胸中阳气不足,宗气运转无力,故胸闷气短,动则尤甚;心阳虚衰,血液运行迟缓,肢体失于温煦,故面色苍白,形寒肢冷;舌淡苔白,脉虚弱或沉细无力,为心阳不振、鼓动无力之象。

［护治原则］温补心阳,安神定悸。

［常用方剂］桂枝甘草龙骨牡蛎汤合参附汤。

5. 水饮凌心证

［主要证候］心悸眩晕,胸闷痞满,渴不欲饮,小便短少,或下肢浮肿,形寒肢冷,伴恶心,欲吐,流涎;舌淡胖,苔白滑,脉弦滑,或沉细而滑。

［证候分析］阳虚不能蒸水化气,水饮上凌于心,故心悸;饮阻于中,清阳不升,故眩晕;中焦气机不利,故胸闷痞满;气化不利,水液内停,故渴不欲饮,下肢浮肿;阳气虚衰,膀胱气化失司,故小便短少;阳气不能达于四肢、充于肌表,故形寒肢冷;饮邪上逆,故恶心呕吐,流涎;舌淡胖,苔白滑,脉弦滑,或沉细而滑,均为水饮内停之象。

［护治原则］振奋心阳,化气利水,宁心安神。

［常用方剂］苓桂术甘汤。

6. 痰火扰心证

[主要证候] 心悸时发时止,受惊易作,胸闷烦躁,失眠多梦,口干苦,大便秘结,小便短赤;舌红,苔黄腻,脉弦滑。

[证候分析] 痰浊阻滞,心神被扰,故心悸;气机不畅,故胸闷;痰郁化火,故口干,大便秘结,小便短赤;舌红,苔黄腻,脉弦滑,均为痰热之象。

[护治原则] 清热化痰,宁心安神。

[常用方剂] 黄连温胆汤。

7. 瘀阻心脉证

[主要证候] 心悸不安,胸闷不舒,心痛时作,痛如针刺,唇甲青紫;舌质紫暗或有瘀斑,脉涩或结或代。

[证候分析] 血瘀气滞,心脉瘀阻,心神失养,故心悸不宁;心神失养,心络挛急,故心痛时作;脉络瘀阻,故唇甲青紫;舌质紫暗或有瘀斑,脉涩或结或代,均为瘀阻心脉之象。

[护治原则] 活血化瘀,理气通络。

[常用方剂] 桃仁红花煎。

三、护理措施

对于心悸的病人,应观察心率、心律、脉搏、血压、呼吸、体温。注意观察情绪、面色、汗出、纳食、二便情况。询问病人有无胸闷、胸痛。对于病情较重者,应密切观察病情的变化,若心率持续低于40次/分或超过120次/分,脉结代,伴气短,面色苍白,烦躁不安,或伴胸中绞痛,大汗淋漓,四肢厥冷,应立即报告医生,并配合抢救。

（一）辨证施护

1. 心虚胆怯证

（1）生活起居护理　居室安静舒适,护士应说话轻、操作轻、走路轻、关门轻,不可有动力施工、重物坠地、大声喧哗和高频尖厉的声响。起居有常,23点钟以前入眠,不可熬夜。病情平稳后应加强运动,比如练习气功、打太极拳。日常应回避恐怖的电视、小说或旅游场景。

（2）饮食护理　宜食养心安神的食物,如莲子、龙眼肉、大枣、荔枝、猪心、蛋类。酸枣仁粥:粳米100 g,酸枣仁末15 g,先把粳米煮成粥,粥将熟时放入酸枣仁末。

（3）情志护理　当病人惊恐发作时,应有人陪伴、安慰、关怀病人,使病人放松和有所依靠。当病情平稳后,护士可运用语言开导疗法,向病人讲解心悸的病因,帮助病人认识疾病,指导病人设法避开病因,以保持心情愉快。护士应与病人家属进行沟通,为病人营造良好的环境,避免情绪刺激。

（4）用药护理　磁石、龙齿先煎,琥珀粉冲服。中药汤剂宜饭前温服。

（5）操作技术　①足浴疗法:选用镇惊定志、养心安神的中药,煎煮后待水温降至37~42℃时洗按足部,每次20分钟,每日1次;血压过低者慎用。②敷贴疗法:取涌泉、神阙,用黄连、肉桂、吴茱萸、酸枣仁,按1:0.5:0.5:1.5的比例,研磨成粉后与大蒜汁调匀,制成2厘米见方的药膏,睡前敷贴,晨起取下,每日1次。③穴位按摩法:取内关、神门、郄门、厥阴俞、膻中、心俞、胆俞,用拇指揉法、一指禅推法,按摩至局部发热或有酸麻重胀感,每日1次;孕妇禁用。④耳压疗法:取交感、神门、心、肝、胰胆等耳穴,用耳穴压丸贴片贴压,每日按揉 4~5 次,以局部发热泛红为度,留置 2~4 日。孕妇禁用。

2. 心血不足证

(1) 生活起居护理　居室温暖干燥,安静舒适,光线明亮。多休息,起居有常,劳逸适度。对于年老体弱、长期卧床、活动无耐力者,可由护士协助其生活起居。注意皮肤护理,预防压疮。可在床上擦浴,不宜淋浴。睡前避免不良刺激,不可熬夜及思虑劳倦。

(2) 饮食护理　食物宜清淡、营养、易消化,少食多餐。宜食养心健脾的食物,如龙眼肉、猪肉、猪肝、茯苓、鸽肉、乌鸡、荔枝、芡实、山药、莲子、大枣。食疗方:清蒸茶鲫鱼,党参当归炖猪心。党参当归炖猪心:猪心 1 只,党参 10 g,当归 6 g,炖熟,去药后食之,2~3 日 1 次。不宜食辛辣、甜腻的食物。

(3) 情志护理　病人体虚久病,可能会有消沉的情绪,护士可运用移情易性疗法,转移病人的注意力,避免因思虑伤脾而加重病情。

(4) 用药护理　中药汤剂宜文火久煎,饭前温服,少量频服。

(5) 操作技术　① 足浴疗法:选用健脾养心、安神定志的中药,煎煮后待水温降至 37~42℃时洗按足部,每次 20 分钟,每日 1 次;血压过低者慎用。② 穴位按摩法:取内关、神门、心俞、脾俞,用拇指揉法,按摩至局部发热或有酸麻重胀感,每日 1 次;孕妇禁用。③ 耳压疗法:取交感、神门、心、脾、肾等耳穴,用耳穴压丸贴片贴压,每日按揉 4~5 次,以局部发热泛红为度,留置 2~4 日;孕妇禁用。

3. 阴虚火旺证

(1) 生活起居护理　居室凉爽安静,湿润舒适,光线柔和。卧床休息。发作期避免性行为,缓解期节制性行为。不可熬夜及过劳。若盗汗,应及时擦干,并换掉湿衣被。

(2) 饮食护理　少食多餐。可遵医嘱饮西洋参茶、玉竹茶。宜食滋阴降火的食物,如雪梨、桑椹、鸭肉、鳖肉、牡蛎。食疗方:枸杞肉丝、银耳百合莲子羹、紫菜猪心。酸枣仁粉 10~15 g,睡前冲服。不宜食辛辣、炙煿、助热生火的食物。

(3) 情志护理　病人虚热躁扰,兼有耳鸣,容易有烦躁的情绪,护士可运用移情易性疗法,转移其注意力,营造安静的休息环境。

(4) 用药护理　中药汤剂宜文火久煎,饭前温服,少量频服。遵医嘱用药,朱砂安神丸中含有朱砂,服药时间不能过长。

(5) 操作技术　① 穴位按摩法:取膻中、中庭、巨阙、心俞,用一指禅推法,每个位置按摩 2 分钟;再取至阳,用掌心振法按摩 1 分钟,以传至心脏为度;再取周荣,用指揉法按摩 1 分钟,由轻到重;再取神门,用指按法按摩 1 分钟;再取通里,用掐法按摩 2~3 下,力道以病人能忍受为度;每日 1 次;孕妇禁用。② 耳压疗法:取神门、交感、心、皮质下、小肠、肾等耳穴,用耳穴压丸贴片贴压,每日睡前按揉 3~5 分钟,以局部发热泛红为度,留置 2~4 日;孕妇禁用。

4. 心阳不振证

(1) 生活起居护理　居室温暖干燥,安静舒适,光线明亮,空气新鲜。卧床休息,注意防寒保暖,可进行日光浴。洗澡、如厕时须有人协助。注意皮肤护理,防止压疮。限制探视时间,不可过劳。房间内应备齐抢救设备。

（2）饮食护理　饮食宜温热，少食多餐，不可过饱。宜食温补心阳的食物，如黄牛肉、羊肉、韭菜、肉桂、龙眼肉，可用大葱、干姜或大蒜调味。食疗方：桂心人参蒸羊心。不宜食生冷、油腻的食物。

（3）情志护理　病人病情较重，护士应加强巡视，运用语言开导疗法，安慰和鼓励病人，向病人解释卧床的原因，使病人积极配合治疗。

（4）用药护理　龙骨、牡蛎、附子先煎，人参另煎。中药汤剂宜浓煎热服，少量频服。

（5）操作技术　①灸法：取心俞，用温和灸，艾条燃着端悬于施灸部位上，距离皮肤2~3厘米，灸至病人有温热舒适无灼痛的感觉，皮肤稍有红晕，每日1次。②敷贴疗法：取膻中或胸闷点，用川芎、冰片、乳香，按1∶0.5∶1的比例打粉后与大蒜汁调匀，制成2厘米见方的药膏敷贴，每次8小时，每日1次。③足浴疗法：选用温补心阳、安神定悸的中药，煎煮后待水温降至37~42℃时洗按足部，每次20分钟，每日1次；血压过低者慎用。④穴位按摩法：取内关、神门、膻中、肾俞、大陵，用拇指揉法、一指禅推法，按摩至局部发热或有酸麻重胀感，每日1次；孕妇禁用。

5. 水饮凌心证

（1）生活起居护理　居室温暖干燥，安静舒适，光线明亮，空气新鲜。绝对卧床，取坐位、半仰卧位或垂足坐位，以减缓心悸。注意皮肤护理，经常变换体位，预防压疮。待症状好转后，可逐渐恢复活动，不可过劳。注意胃脘部保暖。若呼吸困难，可予低流量吸氧和心电监护。

（2）饮食护理　饮食宜温热，少食多餐，不可过饱，限制饮水量和钠盐的摄入量。可饮白萝卜生姜茶。宜食温阳化饮的食物，如茯苓、鲤鱼、海参、羊肉、鸡肉，加适量的小葱、生姜、大蒜调味。食疗方：冬瓜鲢鱼汤、八宝莲子粥。不宜食生冷、油腻的食物。

（3）情志护理　病人病情较重，发作期绝对卧床，可能会有焦虑的情绪，护士可运用语言开导疗法，在病情平稳时向病人讲解心悸的病因和缓解方法，以稳定病人的情绪，使其积极配合治疗。

（4）用药护理　中药汤剂宜浓煎热服，少量频服。

（5）操作技术　①敷贴疗法：取劳宫、涌泉，用生天南星3g，川乌3g，研磨成粉后与熔化的蜂蜡调成糊状敷贴；每日1次，夜敷晨取；孕妇禁用。②穴位按摩法：取间使、神门、心俞、巨阙、脾俞，用拇指揉法、一指禅推法，按摩至局部发热或有酸麻重胀感，每日1次；孕妇禁用。

6. 痰火扰心证

（1）生活起居护理　居室凉爽安静，光线柔和，空气新鲜。心悸发作时，绝对卧床休息。待症状好转后，可逐渐恢复活动，以保持大便通畅。

（2）饮食护理　可饮竹沥。宜食清热化痰的食物，如荸荠、枇杷、马齿苋。食疗方：银耳莲子羹。不宜食肥甘、辛辣、煎炸、炙煿、助热生火的食物，如韭菜、小茴香、肉桂。

（3）情志护理　病人病情较重，需绝对卧床，且实火扰心，可能会烦躁、恐惧，护士可运用移情易性疗法，转移病人的注意力，使其保持情绪稳定。

（4）用药护理　中药汤剂宜饭后温服或偏凉服。

（5）操作技术　①点穴疗法：取内关，用指按法推拿1分钟，适用于心悸严重者。②水针疗法：取内关、心俞、督俞、厥阴俞、足三里、丰隆，每次选择2~3个腧穴，用5%当归注射液进行穴位注射。③足浴疗法：选用清热化痰、宁心安神的中药，煎煮后待水温降至37~42℃时洗按足部，每次20分钟，每日1次；血压过低者慎用。

7. 瘀阻心脉证

（1）生活起居护理　居室温暖安静，光线明亮，空气新鲜。卧床休息。病情稳定后可适量活动。若病人年老体弱、长期卧床，护士应协助其生活起居。注意皮肤护理，预防压疮。若胸痛，面唇色暗，应予吸氧和心电监护。护士应加强巡视，若病人出现剧烈心痛，面色苍白，汗出肢冷，脉结代，应立即报告医生，并配合抢救。

（2）饮食护理　可饮玫瑰花茶。宜食活血化瘀的食物，如山楂、韭菜。食疗方：红花炖羊心。不宜食肥甘的食物。

（3）情志护理　护士可运用语言开导疗法、顺意疗法，帮助病人保持调畅的情绪，避免因忧郁、悲观导致肝气郁结而加重血瘀。

（4）用药护理　中药汤剂宜饭后温服。

（5）操作技术　① 水针疗法：取心俞、脾俞、肾俞、肝俞、内关、神门、足三里、三阴交，每次选择2~3个腧穴，用复方当归注射液或复方丹参注射液进行穴位注射。② 足浴疗法：选用理气活血、解郁安神的中药，煎煮后待水温降至37~42℃时洗按足部，每次20分钟，每日1次；血压过低者慎用。③ 穴位按摩法：取内关、神门、郄门、血海、膈俞，用拇指揉法，按摩至局部发热或有酸麻重胀感，每日1次；孕妇禁用。④ 耳压疗法：取交感、神门、心、肝、三焦等耳穴，用耳穴压丸贴片贴压，每日按揉4~5次，以局部发热泛红为度，留置2~4日；孕妇禁用。

（二）健康教育

起居有常，睡眠充足，睡前避免过度兴奋。保持大便通畅，养成定时排便的习惯，排便时避免过于用力。适量进行体育锻炼，不可剧烈运动及过劳，包括久看电视、小说，以及长时间从事需要高度集中注意力的工作。避开嘈杂、寒冷的环境。

饮食有节，少食多餐，不可过饥、过饱。宜食清淡、营养的食物，如蔬菜、豆类、猪肝。可常吃龙眼肉、莲子、大枣。早晚服蜂蜜1匙，以保持大便通畅。忌烟酒、浓茶、咖啡，不宜食辛辣、肥甘、厚味、煎炸、炙煿的食物。

保持情绪稳定，不要忧虑、紧张、恼怒。心悸发作时应有人陪伴，予以心理安慰。若长时间情绪不佳，可进行情绪疏导，如采用移情易性疗法、音乐疗法、歌吟疗法等。

长病程者应坚持遵医嘱用药，积极治疗原发病。

在恢复期可行保健按摩疗法，取内关、外关、神门、合谷、足三里、膻中、大椎，自行揉按，以局部有发热或酸麻重胀感为佳。睡前或晨起时按摩腹部，以保持大便通畅。

Section 5　Palpitation

Palpitation refers to a heart system disease clinically characterized by conscious intermittent abnormal heartbeat, flusteredness and restlessness. It is caused by malnourishment of the heart due to deficiency of qi and blood, or direct attack of heart collaterals by external pathogens due to emotional stimulation, or heart vessel obstruction by phlegm, fluid-retention and blood stasis. The nursing of palpitation also applies to some diseases in Western medicine that present with palpitation as the main manifestation, such as arrhythmia and heart failure.

ETIOLOGY AND PATHOGENESIS

The etiology includes affection of external pathogenic factors, emotional stimulation, improper diet, weak constitution, and medicine. As for affection of external pathogenic factors, reverse transmission of pathogenic warm and heat into the pericardium consumes qi and yin, which causes malnourishment of heart spirit; or pathogenic wind, cold and dampness invade the exterior, and obstruct blood vessels which impedes heart vessel and results in palpitation. As for emotional stimulation, all the following factors might induce palpitation, for example, excessive contemplation damages the heart and spleen and consumes heart blood, which leads to insufficient source of qi and blood and malnourishment of the heart; anger damaging the liver causes qi stagnation and blood stasis as well as obstruction of heart vessels; qi depression transforms into fire that scorches fluids into phlegm, thus, phlegm and fire disturb the heart; or constitutional heart deficiency with timidity, sudden fright and counterflow of heart qi leads to palpitation. As for diet, predilection for fatty sweet foods and alcohol accumulates heat-fire and phlegm that in turn disturb the heart; improper diet damages the spleen and stomach, thus spleen deficiency produces phlegm that obstructs heart vessels; the two aspects above might subsequently lead to palpitation. Weak constitution and imbalance of yin and yang causes disharmony of qi and blood; congenital spleen and stomach weakness leads to insufficient source of qi and blood; worn out with age, loss of nourishment due to illness, overstrain and over-indulgence may result in deficiency of qi, blood, yin and yang, failing to nourish the heart; chronic edema or internal water and fluid-retention due to yang deficiency of the spleen and kidney causes water pathogen to attack the heart, hence palpitation occurs. Inappropriate use of medicine or serious drug toxicity also damages the heart and causes palpitation.

The pathogenesis is deficiency of qi, blood, yin and yang that cannot nourish the heart spirit, or disturbance of the heart spirit by pathogenic factors and the subsequent restlessness. The disease is located in the heart but relates to the liver, spleen, lung and kidney. Palpitation mostly are deficiency syndrome but may also be deficiency-excess in complexity.

COMMON SYNDROMES

Key Points in Syndrome Differentiation

1. Differentiation of Severity of the Disease

The differentiation is based on the cause, tendency and course of disease. If caused by fright, anger and nervousness with acute onset, short duration and favorable prognosis, it is a mild case. However, if triggered by constitutional weakness or impairment of zang-fu organs with gradual onset or immediate onset after overstrain, long duration and unfavorable prognosis, it belongs to a severe case.

2. Differentiation of Deficiency Syndrome from Excess Syndrome

Deficiency syndrome usually refers to deficiency of blood, yin and yang whereas excess syndrome is caused by water, fluid-retention, phlegm fire, and blood stasis. Palpitation with vertigo and lusterless complexion often indicates blood deficiency. Palpitation with night sweat, dry mouth and tidal fever often means yin deficiency. Palpitation with cold limbs, intolerance of cold and shortness of breath often occurs in yang deficiency. Palpitation, slippery tongue coating, swollen limbs and scanty urine often indicate fluid-retention. Palpitation, fatty figure, bitter taste in the mouth, anorexia, yellow and greasy tongue coating often mean phlegm fire. Palpitation, dark lips, tongue with ecchymosis, and irregularly or regularly intermittent pulse often occur in blood stasis.

Syndrome Differentiation

1. Heart Deficiency with Timidity Syndrome

[Clinical Manifestations] Palpitation, susceptibility to fear and fright, restlessness, insomnia, dreaminess, easy wake-up, aversion to sound, anorexia, thin white tongue coating and thready rapid pulse or thready wiry pulse.

[Manifestations Analysis] Heart is the house of spirit and deficient heart cannot store the spirit, leading to palpitation, restlessness, insomnia, and dreaminess. Timidity is the causes of susceptibility to fear and fright, restlessness, easy wake-up, and aversion to sound. Disorder of mother-organ affects child-organ, and leads to failure of the spleen on transport and transform, resulting in anorexia. Thin white tongue coating and thready rapid pulse or thready wiry pulse are signs of restlessness of heart spirit.

[Nursing Principle] Calming fright and stabilizing mind; nourishing the heart and tranquilizing mind.

[Suggested Formula] Anshen Dingzhi Wan.

2. Heart Blood Insufficiency Syndrome

[Clinical Manifestations] Palpitation, shortness of breath, dizziness, insomnia, forgetfulness, lusterless complexion, lassitude, anorexia, pale red tongue and thready weak pulse.

[Manifestations Analysis] Either excessive contemplation consuming heart blood or failure of the spleen to provide sufficient qi and blood due to spleen qi deficiency may lead to malnourishment of heart spirit, so palpitation and insomnia occur. Insufficient blood cannot nourish the brain marrow, so dizziness, insomnia and forgetfulness are felt. And it cannot upward nourish the skin, so lusterless complexion occurs. Spleen qi deficiency is responsible for lassitude and anorexia. Pale red tongue and thready weak pulse indicate insufficiency of heart blood.

[Nursing Principle] Tonifying blood and nourishing the heart; replenishing qi and tranquilizing mind.

[Suggested Formula] Guipi Decoction.

3. Yin Deficiency with Effulgent Fire Syndrome

[Clinical Manifestations] Palpitation, susceptibility to fright, heart vexation, insomnia, vexing heat in chest, palms and soles, dry mouth, night sweat, aggravation with anxiety and contemplation, accompanied by tinnitus, aching lumbus, dizziness, vertigo, irritability, red tongue with scanty fluids and coating or even no coating, and thready rapid pulse.

[Manifestations Analysis] With kidney yin insufficiency, water fails to support and restrict fire, which causes heart yin inadequacy, and effulgent heart fire disturbs heart spirit, leading to palpitation, susceptibility to fright, heart vexation, and insomnia. Lumbus is the house of the kidney, so when kidney yin is deficient, aching lumbus is felt. The deficient kidney cannot fill the sea of marrow i.e., the brain, so tinnitus, dizziness and vertigo occur. Anxiety and contemplation wears the heart out and consumes yin blood insidiously, so the symptoms aggravate. Vexing heat in chest, palms and soles, dry mouth, night sweat, red tongue with scanty fluids and coating or even no coating, thready rapid pulse, are all signs of yin deficiency with effulgent fire.

[Nursing Principle] Nourishing yin and clearing fire; nourishing the heart and tranquilizing mind.

[Suggested Formula] Tianwang Buxin Pellets and Zhusha Anshen Pills.

4. Heart Yang Devitalization Syndrome

[Clinical Manifestations] Palpitation, restlessness, chest oppression and shortness of breath that aggravates on exertion, pale complexion, cold body and limbs, pale tongue with white coating, and weak pulse or sunken thready and forceless pulse.

[Manifestations Analysis] Deficient heart yang cannot warm and nourish heart spirit, leading to palpitation and restlessness. Deficient yang qi in the chest cannot promote pectoral qi to flow vigorously, resulting in chest oppression and shortness of breath that aggravates on exertion. Deficient heart yang deficiency cannot propel the blood in normal speed to warm the limbs, causing pale complexion, cold feeling, and cold limbs. Pale tongue with white coating and weak pulse or sunken thready and forceless pulse indicate devitalization of heart yang.

[Nursing Principle] Warming and tonifying heart yang; tranquilizing mind and stabilizing palpitation.

[Suggested Formula] Guizhi Gancao Longgu Muli Decoction and Shenfu Decoction.

5. Water and Fluid-Retention Attacking the Heart Syndrome

[Clinical Manifestations] Palpitation, vertigo, chest oppression and fullness, thirst with no desire to drink, scanty urine, or edema of lower limbs, cold body and limbs, accompanied with nausea, vomiting and sialorrhea, pale enlarged tongue with white slippery coating, wiry slippery pulse or sunken thready and slippery pulse.

[Manifestations Analysis] Deficient yang cannot transform qi and evaporate water, so water pathogen upward attacks the heart, hence palpitation occurs. Fluid-retention obstructs the middle energizer, which causes clear yang to fail to ascend, leading to dizziness and vertigo. Inhibition of qi movement in the middle energizer is the cause of chest oppression and fullness. Failure of qi transformation and interior accumulation of water and fluid-retention contribute to thirst with no desire to drink and edema of lower limbs. Yang qi deficiency causes dysfunction of the bladder in qi transformation, resulting in scanty urine. Yang qi cannot reach to the four limbs and the exterior, causing cold body and limbs. Fluid-retention goes upward, therefore, nausea, vomiting and sialorrhea occur. Pale enlarged tongue with white slippery coating, wiry slippery pulse or sunken thready and slippery pulse indicate internal accumulation of water and fluid-retention.

[Nursing Principle] Vitalizing heart yang, transforming qi and evaporating water, and calming the heart and tranquilizing mind.

[Suggested Formula] Linggui Zhugan Decoction.

6. Phlegm-Fire Harassing the Heart Syndrome

[Clinical Manifestations] Intermittent palpitation easily triggered by fright, chest oppression, dysphoria, insomnia, dreaminess, dry mouth with bitter taste, constipation, scanty dark urine, red tongue with yellow slimy coating, and wiry slippery pulse.

[Manifestations Analysis] Phlegm turbidity disturbs heart spirit, causing palpitation. Inhibition of qi movement causes chest oppression. Phlegm depression transforms into fire, so there appear symptoms of dry mouth, constipation, and scanty dark urine. Red tongue with yellow slimy coating and wiry slippery pulse means phlegm-heat.

[Nursing Principle] Clearing heat and resolving phlegm; calming the heart and tranquilizing mind.

[Suggested Formula] Huanglian Wendan Decoction.

7. Stasis Obstructing Heart Vessel Syndrome

[Clinical Manifestations] Palpitation, restlessness, chest oppression and discomfort, frequent stabbing pain in the heart, cyanotic lips and nails, dark purple tongue or possibly with ecchymosis, and unsmooth pulse, or irregularly intermittent pulse, or regularly intermittent pulse.

[Manifestations Analysis] Qi stagnation and blood stasis leads to obstruction of heart vessel and malnourishment of heart spirit, so palpitation and restlessness occur. Malnourishment of heart spirit brings about spasm of heart collateral, so there is frequent stabbing pain in the heart. Obstruction of vessel and collateral is responsible for cyanotic lips and nails. Dark purple tongue or possibly with ecchymosis, and unsmooth pulse, or irregularly intermittent pulse, or regularly intermittent pulse, are all signs of heart vessel obstruction.

[Nursing Principle] Activating blood and resolving stasis; regulating qi and dredging collateral.

［Suggested Formula］Taoren Honghua Decoction.

NURSING MEASURES

For patients with palpitation, nurses should closely observe the heart rate, heart rhythm, pulse, blood pressure, respiration and body temperature. They should check the mood, complexion, sweating, appetite, urine and feces of the patient, and inquire about the presence of chest oppression and pain. For patients with severe symptoms, the change of condition should be closely observed. If the patient has a heart rate below 40 beats per minute or over 120 beats per minute, and regularly or irregularly intermittent pulse, accompanied with shortness of breath, pale complexion, dysphoria, or with angina pectoris, profuse dripping sweat and reversal cold of four limbs, report to the doctor immediately and assist in emergency treatment.

Syndrome-Based Nursing Measures

1. Heart Deficiency with Timidity Syndrome

（1）Daily life nursing. The ward should be quiet and comfortable. Nurses should speak, operate, walk and close the door quietly. There should be no various kinds of noises such as construction noise, loud talking, high frequency sharp sound, and noises from falling heavy objects. The patients should live a regular life, go to sleep before 11 p.m. and avoid staying up late. When the condition is stabilized, they should do physical exercise, such as Qigong and Taiji, and avoid scary TV shows, novels and tour scenes.

（2）Diet nursing. The patients may eat foods that nourish the heart and tranquilize mind, such as lianzi（lotus seed）, longyanrou（longan）, dazao（Chinese date）, lychee, pig heart, and eggs. Suanzaoren（spiny date seed）porridge is recommended：jingmi（rice fruit）100 g and suanzaoren（spiny date seed）powder 15 g. Boil the rice into porridge, then add in suanzaoren powder when the porridge is almost done.

（3）Emotion nursing. During the episode of panic, there should be someone to accompany, comfort and care for the patients, so that they can relax and have some support. When the condition is stabilized, nurses may use verbal enlightenment therapy to impart patients the causes of palpitation to help them understand the disease, stay away from the causes and stay in a happy mood. Nurses should communicate with patients' family to creat a good environment for the patients and avoid emotional stimulation.

（4）Medication nursing. Cishi（magnetite）and longchi（fossilized teeth）should be decocted earlier, and hupo（amber）powder should be mixed with water for oral taking. Decoction should be taken warm before meals.

（5）Manipulation techniques. ① Foot bath therapy：decoct medicinals that calm fright, stabilize mind, nourish the heart and tranquilize mind；wash the feet with the decoction at a temperature of 37～42℃ and massage, 20 minutes each time, once per day. And it should be used with caution for patients with hypotension. ② Paste application therapy：select Yongquan（KI 1）and Shenque（CV 8）；grind into powder huanglian (coptis rhizome), rougui (cinnamon bark), wuzhuyu (medicinal evodia fruit) and suanzaoren (spiny date seed) in a ratio of 1 : 0.5 : 0.5 : 1.5; blend the powder with dasuan (garlic) juice to make pastes 2 centimeters long and wide, apply the pastes on the acupoints before sleep, and remove them the next morning, once per day. ③ Acupressure therapy: select Neiguan (PC 6), Shenmen (HT 7), Ximen (PC 4), Jueyinshu (BL 14), Danzhong (CV 17), Xinshu (BL 15) and Danshu (BL19); apply thumb kneading and one-finger pushing manipulations on each of the acupoints until the area turns hot or the patient has the feelings of soreness, numbness, distension and heaviness in the area; once per day. And it is contraindicated in pregnancy. ④ Auricular pressure therapy: select the auricular points of sympathetic (AH6a), shenmen (TF4), heart (CO15), liver (CO12) and pancreas-gallbladder (CO11); apply specialized pasters on the points, knead each of them till the area turns hot and red, 4 ~ 5 times per day, and keep the pasters for 2 ~ 4 days. And it is contraindicated in pregnancy.

2. Heart Blood Insufficiency Syndrome

(1) Daily life nursing. The ward should be warm, dry, quiet, comfortable, and full of bright light. The patients should take more rest, live a regular life, and balance work and rest. For patients who are old, weak, long-time bedridden and activity intolerant, nurses should assist with their daily living and pay attention to their skin hygiene to prevent pressure sores. In-bed sponge bath is recommended while shower bath is prohibited. The patients should avoid unfavorable stimulation before sleep, overstrain, over thinking, and staying up late.

(2) Diet nursing. The diet should be light, nutritious and digestible with small frequent meals. The patients may eat foods that nourish the heart and invigorate the spleen, such as longyanrou (longan), pork, pig liver, fuling (poria), pigeon meat, black-boned chicken, lychee, qianshi (euryale seed), shanyao (common yam rhizome), lianzi (lotus seed) and dazao (Chinese date). Food therapy: crucian steamed with green tea; or dangshen danggui (codonopsis root and Chinese angelica) stewed pig heart: one pig heart, dangshen (codonopsis root) 10 g and danggui (Chinese angelica) 6 g, stew them together, remove the dregs, and eat the pig heart once every 2 ~ 3 days. Avoid pungent, spicy, sweet and greasy foods.

(3) Emotion nursing. Because the patients are weak with a long course of disease, they may feel downhearted. Nurses may use emotional transference and dispositional change therapy to distract their attention and prevent over-thought from damaging the spleen and aggravating the disease.

(4) Medication nursing. Decoction should be prepared slowly over low heat and taken warm before meals, multiple times in small portions.

(5) Manipulation techniques. ① Foot bath therapy: decoct medicinals that invigorate the spleen, nourish the heart and tranquilize mind; wash the feet with the decoction at a temperature of 37 ~ 42℃ and massage, 20 minutes each time, once per day. And it should be used with caution for patients with hypotension. ② Acupressure therapy: select Neiguan (PC 6), Shenmen (HT 7), Xinshu (BL 15) and Pishu (BL 20); apply thumb kneading manipulation on each of the acupoints until the area turns hot the

patient has the feelings of soreness, numbness, distension and heaviness in the area; once per day. And it is contraindicated in pregnancy. ③ Auricular pressure therapy: select the auricular points of sympathetic (AH6a), shenmen (TF4), heart (CO15), spleen (CO13) and kidney (CO10); apply specialized pasters on the points, knead each of them till the area turns hot and red, 4~5 times per day, and keep the pasters for 2~4 days. And it is contraindicated in pregnancy.

3. Yin Deficiency with Effulgent Fire Syndrome

(1) Daily life nursing. The ward should be cool, quiet, moist, comfortable and full of gentle light. The patients should take adequate rest in bed, avoid sexual intercourse during the onset stage, value sexual abstinence during the remission stage, and keep away from overstrain and staying up late. For patients with night sweating, wipe the sweat away and change the wet clothes and bedding timely.

(2) Diet nursing. The patients should have small frequent meals, and follow the doctor's advice to drink xiyangshen (American ginseng) tea, or yuzhu (fragrant solomonseal rhizome) tea. They may eat foods that nourish yin and reduce fire, such as snow pears, sangshen (mulberry), duck meat, meat of soft-shelled turtles and oysters. Food therapy: gouqi (Chinese wolfberry) stir-fried with shredded pork, yin'er baihe lianzi (tremella, lily bulb and lotus seed) thick soup, and laver stewed with pig heart. Suanzaoren power is recommended: take suanzaoren (spiny date seed) power 10~15 g, blend it with water, and drink it before sleep. Avoid pungent, spicy, fried and roasted foods that generates heat and fire.

(3) Emotion nursing. Since the patients suffer from agitation due to deficient heat, as well as tinnitus, they may have dysphoria. Nurses may use emotional transference and dispositional change therapy to distract their attention and create a quiet environment for them to rest.

(4) Medication nursing. Decoction should be prepared slowly over low heat and taken warm before meals, multiple times in small portions. Following the doctor's advice in medication. Avoid long-term use of this medication because there is zhusha (cinnabar) in Zhusha Anshen Pills.

(5) Manipulation techniques. ① Acupressure therapy: select Danzhong (CV 17), Zhongting (CV 16), Juque (CV 14) and Xinshu (BL 15) to apply single-finger pushing therapy on the acupoints, 2 minutes for each acupoint; then select Zhiyang (GV 9) to apply palm-center vibrating manipulation for 1 minute until the vibration conducts to the heart; then select Zhourong (SP 20) to apply thumb kneading manipulation for 1 minute, with the kneading strength gradually increased; then select Shenmen (HT 7) to apply thumb kneading manipulation for 1 minute; then select Tongli (HT 5) to apply nipping manipulation for 2 ~ 3 times with the strength the patients can tolerate; once per day. And it is contraindicated in pregnancy. ② Auricular pressure therapy: select the auricular points of shenmen (TF4), sympathetic (AH6a), heart (CO15), subcortex (AT4), small intestine (CO6) and kidney (CO10); apply specialized pasters on the points, knead each of them for 3~5 minutes before sleep till the area turns hot and red, once per day, and keep the pasters for 2~4 days. And it is contraindicated in pregnancy.

4. Heart Yang Devitalization Syndrome

(1) Daily life nursing. The ward should be warm, dry, quiet, comfortable, full of bright light and fresh air, and equipped with first aid equipments. The patients should rest in bed, keep themselves warm, and may take sunbath sometimes. They should be assisted when taking a shower and going to the toilet, and pay attention to skin hygiene to prevent pressure sores. Limit the visiting time to avoid overstrain.

(2) Diet nursing. The diet should be warm. The patients should have small frequent meals and take foods that warm and tonify heart yang, such as beef, mutton, Chinese chives, rougui (cinnamon bark) and longyanrou (longan), which may be seasoned with scallion, ganjiang (dried ginger rhizome) or dasuan (garlic). Food therapy: guixin renshen (tender cinnamon bark and ginseng) steamed with lamb heart. Avoid cold, raw and greasy foods.

(3) Emotion nursing. Because the symptoms are severe, nurses should increase the frequency of making rounds of the ward and use verbal enlightenment therapy to comfort and encourage the patients, and impart them the knowledge about the disease to get their cooperation with treatment.

(4) Medication nursing. Longgu (dinosaur bone), muli (oyster shell) and fuzi (monkshood) should be decocted earlier, and renshen (ginseng) separately. Decoction should be concentrated and taken hot in multiple times in small portions.

(5) Manipulation techniques. ① Moxibustion therapy: select Xinshu (BL 15); place the moxa stick 2~3 centimeters away from the skin to perform moxibustion on the acupoint until the area turns red and the patient feels warm and comfortable without the sensation of burning pain, once per day. And it cannot be applied on the abdomen and lumbosacral region of pregnant women. ② Paste application therapy: select Danzhong (CV 17) or the chest oppression point; grind into powder chuanxiong (Sichuan lovage root), bingpian (borneol) and ruxiang (frankincense) in a ratio of 1 : 0.5 : 1; blend the powder with dasuan (garlic) juice to make pastes 2 centimeters long and wide, and apply the pastes on the points, 8 hours once every day. ③ Foot bath therapy: decoct medicinals that warm and tonify heart yang, tranquilize mind and ease palpitation; wash the feet with the decoction at a temperature of 37~42℃ and massage, 20 minutes each time, once per day. And it should be used with caution for patients with hypotension. ④ Acupressure therapy: select Neiguan (PC 6), Shenmen (HT 7), Danzhong (CV 17), Shenshu (BL 23) and Daling (PC 7); apply thumb kneading and one-finger pushing manipulations on each of the acupoints until the area turns hot or the patient has the feelings of soreness, numbness, distension and heaviness in the area; once per day. And it is contraindicated in pregnancy.

5. Water and Fluid-Retention Attacking the Heart Syndrome

(1) Daily life nursing. The ward should be warm, dry, quiet, comfortable, and full of bright light and fresh air. The patients should absolutely stay in bed in a sitting, semi-supine or feet-hanging-down sitting position to relieve palpitation, pay attention to skin hygiene, change positions constantly to prevent pressure sores and keep the epigastric region warm. When the condition is stabilized, the patients could gradually increase physical activities, but avoid overstain. For patients with dyspnea, apply low

flow oxygen inhalation and ECG monitoring.

（2）Diet nursing. The diet should be warm. The patients should have small frequent meals, reduce the intake of water and sodium salt, and may drink bailuobo shengjiang（white radishes and fresh ginger）tea and eat foods that warm yang and resolve fluid-retention, such as fuling（poria）, carp, haishen（sea cucumber）, mutton and chicken, which are seasoned with spring onion, shengjiang（fresh ginger）and dasuan（garlic）. Food therapy: donggua lianyu（Chinese waxgourd and silver carp）soup, babao lianzi（lotus seed）porridge. Avoid cold, raw and greasy foods.

（3）Emotion nursing. Because the patients have severe symptoms and are required to absolutely rest in bed during the onset stage, they may feel anxious. Nurses may use verbal enlightenment therapy to impart the patients the causes and relieving methods of palpitation to make them calm and cooperative with treatment.

（4）Medication nursing. Decoction should be concentrated and taken hot, multiple times in small portions.

（5）Manipulation techniques. ① Paste application therapy: select Laogong（PC 8）and Yongquan（KI 1）; grind into powder shengtiannanxing（raw jackinthepulpit tuber）3 g and chuanwu（common monkshood mother root）3 g; blend the powder with melted beeswax to make pastes, and apply the pastes on the acupoints; once per day, from the evening to the next morning. And it is contraindicated in pregnancy. ② Acupressure therapy: select Jianshi（PC 5）, Shenmen（HT 7）, Xinshu（BL 15）, Juque（CV 14）and Pishu（BL 20）; apply thumb kneading and one-finger pushing manipulations on each of the acupoints until the area turns hot or the patient has the feelings of soreness, numbness, distension and heaviness in the area; once per day. And it is contraindicated in pregnancy.

6. Phlegm-Fire Harassing the Heart Syndrome

（1）Daily life nursing. The ward should be cool, quiet, and full of gentle light and fresh air. During the onset stage, the patients should absolutely stay in bed. When the condition is stabilized, the patients could gradually increase physical activities to guarantee a normal bowel movement.

（2）Diet nursing. The patients may drink zhuli（bamboo sap）and eat foods that clear heat and resolve phlegm, such as biqi（waternut）, loquat and machixian（purslane）. Food therapy: yin'er lianzi（tremella and lotus seed）thick soup. Avoid fatty, sweet, pungent, spicy, fried, roasted foods that generate heat and fire, such as Chinese chives, xiaohuixiang（fennel）and rougui（cinnamon bark）.

（3）Emotion nursing. With severe symptoms, the patients are bedridden with excess fire disturbing the heart, they may have dysphoria and fear. Nurses may use emotional transference and dispositional change therapy to distract their attention so they can stay calm.

（4）Medication nursing. Decoction should be taken warm or slightly cool after meals.

（5）Manipulation techniques. ① Acupoint-pressing therapy: select Neiguan（PC 6）; apply finger-pressing manipulation on the point for 1 minute; it is suitable for patients with severe palpitation. ② Water acupuncture therapy: select Neiguan（PC 6）, Xinshu（BL 15）, Dushu（BL 16）, Jueyinshu（BL 14）, Zusanli（ST 36）and Fenglong（ST 40）; inject 5% Danggui（Chinese angelica）Injection into the acupoints, 2 ~ 3 acupoints each time. ③ Foot bath therapy: decoct medicinals that clear heat, resolve phlegm, calm the heart and tranquilize mind; wash the feet with the decoction at a temperature of 37 ~ 42℃ and massage, 20 minutes each time, once per day. And it should be used with caution for patients with hypotension.

7. Stasis Obstructing Heart Vessel Syndrome

(1) Daily life nursing. The ward should be warm, quiet, and full of bright light and fresh air. The patients should rest in bed. When the condition is stabilized, they may do moderate exercise. For patients who are old, weak or long-time bedridden, nurses should assist with the daily living, and pay attention to skin hygiene to prevent pressure sores. For patients with chest pain, dark lips and complexion, apply oxygen inhalation and ECG monitoring. Nurses should increase the frequency of going the rounds of the wards. In case of severe cardiac pain, pale complexion, sweating, cold limbs, regular or irregular intermittent pulse, report to the doctor immediately and assist in emergency treatment.

(2) Diet nursing. The patients may drink meiguihua (rose flower) tea and eat foods that activate blood and resolve stasis, such as shanzha (Chinese hawthorn fruit) and Chinese chives. Food therapy: honghua (safflower) stewed with lamb heart. Avoid fatty and sweet foods.

(3) Emotion nursing. Nurses may use verbal enlightenment therapy and submission therapy to help patients keep a good mood to prevent liver qi depression and blood stasis aggravation caused by sorrow and depression.

(4) Medication nursing. Decoction should be taken warm after meals.

(5) Manipulation techniques. ① Water acupuncture therapy: select Xinshu (BL 15), Pishu (BL 20), Shenshu (BL 23), Ganshu (BL 18), Neiguan (PC 6), Shenmen (HT 7), Zusanli (ST 36) and Sanyinjiao (SP 6); inject Compound Danggui (Chinese angelica) Injection or compound Danshen (danshen root) Injection into the acupoints, 2 ~ 3 acupoints each time. ② Foot bath therapy: decoct medicinals that regulate qi, activate blood, relieve depression and tranquilize mind; wash the feet with the decoction at a temperature of 37 ~ 42℃ and massage, 20 minutes each time, once per day. And it should be used with caution for patients with hypotension. ③ Acupressure therapy: select Neiguan (PC 6), Shenmen (HT 7), Ximen (PC 4), Xuehai (SP 10) and Geshu (BL 17); apply thumb kneading manipulation on each of the acupoints until the area turns hot or the patient has the feelings of soreness, numbness, distension and heaviness in the area; once per day. And it is contraindicated in pregnancy. ④ Auricular pressure therapy: select the auricular points of sympathetic (AH6a), shenmen (TF4), heart (CO15), liver (CO12) and triple energizer (CO17); apply specialized pasters on the points, knead each of them till the area turns hot and red, 4 ~ 5 times per day, and keep the pasters for 2 ~ 4 days. And it is contraindicated in pregnancy.

Patient Education

The patients should live a regular life, have adequate sleep without being overexcited before sleep. They should also keep a normal bowel movement, go to the bathroom at fixed time without overexertion in defecation, and do moderate non-strenuous exercise. Moreover, they should avoid noisy and cold environments as well as overstrain, such as watching TV, reading a novel engage in highly focused work for a long time.

The patients should follow a moderate diet and have small frequent meals, without being too hungry or too full. They can eat longyanrou (longan), lianzi (lotus seed) and dazao (Chinese date), and light and nutritious foods such as vegetables, beans, and pig liver, and take one spoon of honey every night and morning to maintain a normal bowel movement. Moreover, they should refrain from smoking and drinking alcohol, coffee and strong tea as well as eating foods that are pungent, spicy, fatty, sweet, rich, fried, and roasted.

The patients should stay calm without being worried, nervous or angry. During an episode of palpitation, they should be accompanied and comforted. For patients with long-time bad mood, use some methods to adjust their emotions, such as emotional transference and dispositional change therapy, music therapy, singing and chanting therapy.

For patients with a long course of disease, follow the doctor's advice in medication and treat the primary disease actively.

For patients in the remission stage, healthcare massage therapy is recommended: select Neiguan (PC 6), Waiguan (SJ 5), Shenmen (HT 7), Hegu (LI 4), Zusanli (ST 36), Danzhong (CV 17) and Dazhui (GV 14); apply kneading and pressing manipulations by themselves until the area turns hot or the patient has the feelings of soreness, numbness, heaviness and distension in the area. Moreover, massage the abdomen before sleep and in the morning to maintain a normal bowel movement.

第六节　胸　　痹

　　胸痹,是指因胸阳不振,阴寒、痰浊、血瘀等留踞胸廓,或因心气不足,鼓动乏力,导致气血痹阻,心失血养,以胸闷、气短、发作性心胸疼痛为临床特征的心系病。轻者仅膻中或胸部憋闷、疼痛,可伴有心悸,称为厥心痛。重者心痛彻背,背痛彻心,疼痛剧烈且持续不能缓解,四肢厥逆,面色苍白,冷汗淋漓,脉微欲绝,旦发夕死,夕发旦死,称为真心痛。西医的冠状动脉粥样硬化性心脏病引起的心绞痛和心肌梗死可参照本节进行护理。

一、病因病机

　　胸痹的病因包括素体虚弱、外邪侵袭、饮食失节、情志失调、劳逸失当,常由劳累、饱餐、寒冷或情绪激动而诱发。病人先天不足,或年迈体虚,或久病过劳,使气血阴阳不足,脉络受损。或遇到天气骤变,六淫犯肺,尤以风冷暴寒最为常见,逆传心包,损伤脉络,发为胸痹。病人过食肥甘,或饮食生冷,或饥饱无度,或嗜酒成癖,损伤脾胃,运化失司,气血生化乏源,心脉失养;脾胃损伤,聚湿生痰,上犯心胸,心气不畅,脉络闭阻;痰浊停聚,化热结瘀,蕴毒损伤心络。或郁怒伤肝,疏泄失常,气滞血瘀,或忧思伤脾,气结生痰,阻塞心脉。病人久坐少动,气郁血停,滞而成瘀,或过逸伤脾,痰湿内生,痹阻胸阳,亦可发为胸痹。

　　胸痹的病机为心脉痹阻。病位在心,与肝、肺、脾、肾有关。胸痹多为虚实夹杂之证。

二、常见证型

（一）辨证要点

　　1. 辨脏腑　根据病因、疼痛部位、舌脉等来辨别。若痛在胸背肩胛间,伴胸闷,则病位在心。若因饮食无度而起,病人形体丰满,伴胸闷、脉滑、苔腻,则病位在心、脾。若由暴怒忧思而起,痛在胸与胁下,容易走窜,胸闷,闷较重而痛较轻,伴胸胁胀满,则病位在心、肝。若病重,心痛彻背,喘不得卧,则病位在心、肺。若病危,汗出肢冷,脉微欲绝,则病位在心、肾。

　　2. 辨虚实　根据年龄、疼痛的性质及发作时间、舌脉等来辨别。若年壮初痛,多为实证;久病年老,多为虚证。若胸闷较重而心痛较轻,伴身重困倦,脘痞纳呆,苔腻脉滑,多为痰浊;痛如针刺,固定不移,入夜痛甚,舌紫暗有瘀斑,脉涩,多为血瘀;因感寒或于寒冷季节发生或加重,心痛彻背,背痛彻心,伴形寒肢冷,脉沉紧,多为寒凝心脉。若心胸隐痛,休息可稍缓解,伴气短乏力,神疲懒言,脉细弱,多为气虚;胸闷胸痛,伴虚烦不寐,口干盗汗,舌红少苔或有剥裂,脉细数,多为阴虚;胸闷心痛,伴四肢不温,舌淡胖,苔薄白,脉沉细迟,多为阳虚。

　　3. 辨病情轻重　根据疼痛的发作频率、持续时间、缓解因素等来辨别。若反复发生,已成规律,病症特点和诱因等稳定不变,则病情较轻;首次发生,或病症特点和诱因较以往有明显变化,则病情较重。若疼痛程度较轻,持续时间短,休息后可缓解,则病情较轻;疼痛程度较重,甚则心痛彻背,背痛彻心,持续不解,则病情较重。若症状发作时,伴有汗出肢冷,气不得续,唇甲青紫,甚则晕厥,则多属危重。

(二)证候分型

1. 痰浊内阻证

[主要证候]胸闷较重而心痛较轻;伴有身重困倦,脘痞纳呆,口黏恶心,咯吐痰涎;苔白腻或白滑,脉滑。

[证候分析]饮食不节,恣食肥甘,或忧思伤脾,运化失司,聚湿成痰,痰为阴邪,痹阻胸阳,故胸闷较重而心痛较轻;痰湿困脾,脾失健运,故身重困倦,脘痞纳呆,口黏恶心,咯吐痰涎;苔白腻或白滑,脉滑,均为痰浊内阻之象。

[护治原则]通阳泄浊,豁痰开结。

[常用方剂]瓜蒌薤白半夏汤。

2. 气滞心胸证

[主要证候]胸痛时作,痛无定处;时欲太息,情志抑郁可诱发或加重,或兼有脘腹胀闷,得嗳气或矢气则舒;苔薄或薄腻,脉弦。

[证候分析]情志抑郁,或郁怒伤肝,肝郁气滞,心脉痹阻,故胸痛时作,痛无定处,时欲太息,情志抑郁可诱发或加重;肝郁乘脾,气机不利,故脘腹胀闷,得嗳气或矢气则舒;苔薄或薄腻,脉弦,均为肝气郁结之象。

[护治原则]疏肝理气,调畅心脉。

[常用方剂]柴胡疏肝散。

3. 心血瘀阻证

[主要证候]心胸疼痛,心痛如刺,痛处固定,入夜更甚;唇舌紫暗,舌有瘀斑,苔薄,脉涩或结代。

[证候分析]血瘀内停,心脉瘀阻,故心胸疼痛,心痛如刺,痛处固定;血属阴,夜亦属阴,故入夜更甚;唇舌紫暗,舌有瘀斑,苔薄,脉涩或结代,均为瘀血内停之象。

[护治原则]活血化瘀,通络止痛。

[常用方剂]血府逐瘀汤合失笑散。

4. 寒凝心脉证

[主要证候]心痛彻背,背痛彻心,感寒痛甚,形寒肢冷,面色苍白,苔薄白,脉沉紧。

[证候分析]寒邪内侵,胸阳不振,心脉不畅,故心痛彻背,背痛彻心,感寒痛甚;阳气不能布达于外,故形寒肢冷,面色苍白;苔薄白,脉沉紧,均为阴寒凝结之象。

[护治原则]温经散寒,通阳止痛。

[常用方剂]瓜蒌薤白桂枝汤合当归四逆汤。

5. 心气亏虚证

[主要证候]心胸隐痛,气短心悸,动则益甚;神疲懒言;舌质淡,苔薄白,脉细弱。

[证候分析]心气不足,鼓动无力,心脉不畅,故心胸隐痛,气短心悸,动则益甚;气虚则神疲懒

言;舌质淡,苔薄白,脉细弱,均为气虚之象。

[护治原则]补益心气,畅脉止痛。

[常用方剂]保元汤。

6. 心阴不足证

[主要证候]心胸隐痛;五心烦热,心悸怔忡,头晕耳鸣,口燥咽干;舌红少津,苔少或花剥,脉细数。

[证候分析]心阴不足,心脉失养,故心胸隐痛;心阴虚,虚火扰神,故心悸怔忡;水不涵木,肝阳偏亢,故头晕耳鸣;五心烦热,口燥咽干,舌红少津,苔少或花剥,脉细数,均为阴虚之象。

[护治原则]滋阴养心,润脉止痛。

[常用方剂]生脉散合天王补心丹。

7. 心肾阳虚证

[主要证候]胸闷心痛,心悸怔忡;神倦怯寒,面色㿠白,四肢不温;舌质淡胖,苔薄白,脉沉细迟。

[证候分析]心肾阳虚,失于温运,胸阳不振,故胸闷心痛,心悸怔忡;肾阳虚衰,阳气不达四肢,不充肌肤,故神倦怯寒,面色㿠白,四肢不温;舌质淡胖,苔薄白,脉沉细迟,均为阳虚之象。

[护治原则]补肾助阳,温通心脉。

[常用方剂]参附汤合桂枝甘草汤。

三、护理措施

对于胸痹的病人,应密切观察疼痛的部位、性质、发生时间、持续时间、发作次数、诱因、缓解和加重的因素。注意观察面色、神志、呼吸、血压、脉象、心律、心率。若疼痛剧烈,护士应每隔 3~5 分钟询问病人 1 次,并备齐抢救设备。若疼痛剧烈,持续超过 30 分钟,有压榨感、窒息感、濒死感,伴面色苍白,汗出肢冷,唇甲青紫,脉微欲绝,应立即报告医生,并配合抢救。

(一)辨证施护

1. 痰浊内阻证

(1)生活起居护理　居室温暖向阳,安静干燥,空气新鲜。卧床休息,注意胃脘部保暖。若痰黏难咯,重病者宜侧卧,必要时吸痰或遵医嘱进行中药雾化吸入。不可过劳。

(2)饮食护理　可饮荷叶茶。少食多餐,多吃新鲜的水果和蔬菜。宜食健脾化痰的食物,如茯苓、山药、薏苡仁、玉米、木瓜。食疗方:陈皮鱼片、萝卜豆腐汤、双菇冬瓜汤。双菇冬瓜汤:鲜香菇、鲜蘑菇各 5 只,洗净,入油中稍煸,加水适量,旺火煮沸,加入切成小块的冬瓜,煮熟后食之。不宜食生冷、油腻的食物。

(3)情志护理　病人应保持情绪稳定,避免因过思伤脾生痰而加重病情。护士可运用语言开导疗法,向病人解释情志和饮食对于疾病的影响,说明忧虑、受凉、过饱是本病的诱因。

(4)用药护理　中药汤剂宜饭后温服,少量频服。

(5)操作技术　穴位按摩法:取心俞、厥阴俞、膻中、内关、丰隆、肺俞、间使,用拇指揉法、一指禅推法,按摩至局部发热或有酸麻重胀感,每日 1 次;孕妇禁用。

2. 气滞心胸证

(1)生活起居护理　居室安静开阔,空气新鲜。卧床休息,注意保持大便通畅。

(2)饮食护理　可饮红花茶、玫瑰花茶。宜食行气活血的食物,如山楂、白萝卜、佛手、陈皮。不宜食易产气的食物,如红薯。

(3)情志护理　护士可运用语言开导疗法,向病人解释情志因素对于疾病的影响,指导病人学会控制情绪,平和地表达内心感受,避免发怒。

(4)用药护理　中药汤剂宜饭后温服。

(5)操作技术　穴位按摩法:取心俞、厥阴俞、膻中、内关、太冲,用拇指揉法、一指禅推法,按摩至局部发热或有酸麻重胀感,每日1次;孕妇禁用。

3. 心血瘀阻证

(1)生活起居护理　居室温暖安静,空气新鲜,不可有强风、对流风。卧床休息,根据天气变化及时增减衣被,注意保暖。

(2)饮食护理　宜食活血化瘀的食物,如黑木耳、茄子、山楂、红糖、火麻仁。不宜食生冷、酸收的食物。

(3)情志护理　护士可运用语言开导疗法,向病人解释情志因素对于疾病的影响。或运用移情易性疗法,比如赏花、听音乐,转移病人的注意力,使其保持情绪稳定。

(4)用药护理　蒲黄、五灵脂包煎。中药汤剂宜饭后温服。

(5)操作技术　① 电离子导入疗法:取心俞、厥阴俞、膻中,用当归、丹参、红花、桃仁、钩藤、络石藤、羌活煎汤,用药物离子导入仪进行导入,每次20分钟,每日1次;孕妇禁用。② 足浴疗法:用当归、红花,煎煮后待水温降至37~42℃时洗按足部,每次20分钟,每日1次;血压过低者慎用。③ 敷贴疗法:取膻中、鸠尾,用伤湿止痛膏,撒少许七厘散敷贴;每日1次,连用2周。④ 穴位按摩法:取心俞、厥阴俞、膻中、内关、血海、三阴交,用拇指揉法、一指禅推法,按摩至局部发热或有酸麻重胀感,每日1次;孕妇禁用。

4. 寒凝心脉证

(1)生活起居护理　居室温暖安静,光线明亮,空气新鲜,不可有强风、对流风。卧床休息,根据天气变化及时增减衣被,特别注意夜间保暖。

(2)饮食护理　食物宜温热。宜食通阳散寒的食物,如龙眼肉、羊肉、韭菜、山楂,可用干姜、花椒调味,或饮少量米酒。薤白粥:薤白15 g,粳米100 g,水1升,煮稀粥食之。不宜食生冷、寒凉的食物。

(3)情志护理　护士可运用移情易性疗法,经常巡视,关心、鼓励病人,使病人感到温暖,保持心情愉悦。

(4)用药护理　中药汤剂宜饭后热服。

(5)操作技术　① 药熨疗法:取背部,用川芎、细辛,研磨炒热后装入布袋中,制成温度为60~70℃的中药热罨包,药熨20分钟,每日1次;孕妇腰骶部禁用。② 热敷疗法:取膻中、心俞、巨阙、内关、通里,用50~60℃的砭石热敷,每次20分钟,每日1次。

5. 心气亏虚证

(1)生活起居护理　居室温暖安静,空气新鲜,不可有强风、对流风。绝对卧床,注意保暖。保持大便通畅。不可过劳。

（2）饮食护理　宜食益气活血的食物，如牛肉、蛇肉、山药、百合、大枣。食疗方：红薯鱼肉饼、黄芪莲子大枣粥、海蜇煲猪蹄。黄芪莲子大枣粥：黄芪 15 g，莲子 10 g，大枣 10 粒，加水后用文火煮 20 分钟，去黄芪，加粳米 50 g，煮粥食之。海蜇煲猪蹄：泡发的海蜇头、泡发的猪蹄筋各 200 g，与黑木耳、胡萝卜片、笋片一起放入锅中，加水慢炖 20 分钟，每日早晚温热服用。不宜食油腻的食物。

（3）情志护理　病人体虚久病，护士可运用语言开导疗法和暗示解惑疗法，经常鼓励和安慰病人，为其介绍同证型的康复病人，使其产生战胜疾病的信心。

（4）用药护理　中药汤剂宜文火久煎，饭前温服。

（5）操作技术　① 灸法：取心俞、厥阴俞、膻中、气海、足三里，用温和灸，艾条燃着端悬于施灸部位上，距离皮肤 2~3 厘米，灸至病人有温热舒适无灼痛的感觉，皮肤稍有红晕，每日 1 次；孕妇腹部禁用。② 水针疗法：取心俞、足三里、丰隆，用黄芪注射液或丹参注射液进行穴位注射。

6. 心阴不足证

（1）生活起居护理　居室凉爽安静，空气新鲜，不可有强风、对流风。卧床休息，起居有常，不可过劳和熬夜。若病人盗汗，应及时擦干，并换掉湿衣被。若便秘，可教病人进行腹部按摩：顺时针按摩，每次 20~30 圈，每日 2~3 次。

（2）饮食护理　可饮酸枣仁茶、西洋参茶。宜食滋阴养心的食物，如鳖肉、鸭肉、银耳、百合、兔肉、大枣、黑芝麻、桑椹、猪皮。食疗方：木耳鱼片、山药煲猪肾。山药煲猪肾：猪肾 1 对切丁，山药 50 g 切片；先煸山药，再另起油锅，取大葱、生姜稍煸，入猪肾爆炒，加黄酒、细盐少许，入山药片，旺火煮令熟，食之。不宜食辛辣、燥烈的食物。

（3）情志护理　病人虚火妄动，可能会焦虑、急躁，护士可运用移情易性疗法，转移病人的注意力，以保持情绪平和。

（4）用药护理　中药汤剂宜饭前温服，少量频服。

（5）操作技术　① 穴位按摩法：取心俞、厥阴俞、膻中、三阴交、太溪，用拇指揉法、一指禅推法，按摩至局部发热或有酸麻重胀感，每日 1 次；孕妇禁用。② 耳压疗法：取心、肾、小肠、交感、神门、皮质下、肾上腺等耳穴，用耳穴压丸贴片贴压，每日按揉 4~5 次，以局部发热泛红为度，留置 2~4 日；孕妇禁用。

7. 心肾阳虚证

（1）生活起居护理　居室温暖安静，光线明亮，不可有强风、对流风。卧床休息，注意保暖，不可过劳。

（2）饮食护理　宜食温补心肾的食物，如牛肉、洋葱、桑椹。食疗方：羊肉萝卜汤、茄子烧鳝鱼、羊肉核桃粥。羊肉核桃粥：羯羊肉 30 g，放葱白、生姜，煮至酥烂，加入粳米 30 g，煮成粥；核桃仁 1 个，灸熟后研细末，撒入粥中。不宜食生冷的食物。

（3）情志护理　病人久病阳虚，体弱难眠，可能会消沉、悲观，护士可运用语言开导疗法和音乐疗法，经常关心和鼓励病人，转移其注意力，以排解不良情绪。

（4）用药护理　附子先煎。中药汤剂宜饭前热服，少量频服。

（5）操作技术　① 灸法：取心俞、厥阴俞、膻中、关元、气海，用温和灸，艾条燃着端悬于施灸部位上，距离皮肤 2~3 厘米，灸至病人有温热舒适无灼痛的感觉，皮肤稍有红晕，每日 1 次；孕妇腹部禁用。② 敷贴疗法：取膻中、内关、心俞、虚里，用人参、黄芪、桂枝、肉桂、淫羊藿、枳实、瓜蒌、薤白、水蛭、全蝎、降香、桃仁、红花、川芎、延胡索、冰片，研磨成粉后与蜂蜜调成糊状敷贴，每日 1 次。

（二）健康教育

胸痹发作时，应立即停止活动，绝对卧床，取半仰卧位，高流量吸氧。避免不必要的翻身，限制探视。必要时予心电监护。控制输入液量及速度。预防压疮，定时更换体位，每 2 小时协助翻身 1 次，可使用气垫床，或用气圈或棉圈置于骨突部位下。

在缓解期应劳逸结合，可在上午 10~11 点或下午 3 点阳光充足时，适量运动，如气功疗法，以调息宁意，避免精神紧张。起居有常，睡眠充足，不可过劳。注意保暖。保持大便通畅，排便时避免过于用力。洗澡时水温适中，时长宜短，不要上锁，必要时应有人协助，须避开过饥、过饱的时候。

饮食宜清淡、营养、易消化。少食多餐。食物宜低盐、低糖、低脂肪、高维生素、高蛋白质、高钙。粗细粮搭配，多吃鱼、蔬菜、水果，少吃内脏、肥肉，以保持大便通畅。不可过饱，忌暴饮暴食，尤其晚餐量宜少。戒烟限酒，忌浓茶，不宜食辛辣、肥甘的食物。

保持情绪稳定。安心静养，避免过于激动或喜怒忧思无度。若病人恐惧、惊慌，须有人陪伴、关怀病人。护士应多巡视，勤观察，安慰和鼓励病人，语气缓和平静，向病人及家属说明卧床休息和保持心情平和的重要性。

遵医嘱坚持治疗，中药与西药的服药时间应间隔 30 分钟以上。病人平时须随身携带急救药品。

Section 6   Chest Impediment

Chest impediment is a heart system disease clinically characterized by chest oppression, shortness of breath and paroxysmal pain in the heart and chest. It is caused by chest yang devitalization with retention of yin cold, phlegm turbidity, and blood stasis in the chest, or by insufficiency of heart qi with weak propelling function that causes obstruction of qi and blood as well as malnourishment of the heart. The mild case, known as precordial pain with cold limbs, only presents pain and oppression sensation in the chest or Danzhong (CV 17) area, possibly accompanied by palpitation. The serious case, known as real heart pain, shows heart pain radiating to the back and back pain radiating to the heart, severe persistent pain that cannot be alleviated, reversal cold of limbs, profuse cold sweating, and faint pulse verging on expiry, with occurrence in the morning causing death in the evening or vice versa. The nursing of chest impediment also applies to some diseases in Western medicine that present with chest impediment as the main manifestation such as angina pectoris and myocardial infarction due to coronary atherosclerotic heart disease.

ETIOLOGY AND PATHOGENESIS

The etiology includes constitutional weakness, invasion by external pathogens, improper diet, emotional disorder, and imbalance between work and rest. Chest impediment is usually induced by fatigue, overeating, cold or emotional excitement. Constitutional weakness, being worn out with age, or chronic disease with overstrain causes insufficiency of qi, blood, yin and yang as well as damages vessel and collateral. With sudden weather change and invasion of the lung by six excesses, especially wind-cold and sudden cold, the pathogens are reversely transmitted to the pericardium and damage vessel and collateral. Overeating fatty, sweet, raw and cold foods, being extremely full or hungry, or predilection for alcohol damages the spleen and stomach, which leads to dysfunction of the spleen in transportation and transformation, insufficient source of qi and blood generation and transformation, and ultimately, malnourishment of heart vessel. Impairment of the spleen and stomach accumulates dampness and generates phlegm that attacks the heart and chest, which triggers inhibition of heart qi and obstruction of vessel and collateral. Accumulated phlegm-turbidity transforms into heat, binds with blood stasis, and accumulates toxin to injure the heart vessel. Depressed anger may damage the liver and affect the liver's function in regulating the free flow of qi, leading to qi stagnation and blood stasis; or overanxiety and contemplation may damage the spleen and cause spleen qi stagnation and generation of phlegm, which later obstructs heart vessel. Long-time sitting causes qi depression and blood stagnation that eventually leads to blood stasis; or excessive idleness damages the spleen and generates phlegm, which later obstructs chest yang and induces chest impediment.

The pathogenesis is heart vessel obstruction. The disease is located in the heart but relates to the liver, lung, spleen and kidney. It mostly belongs to deficiency-excess in complexity.

COMMON SYNDROMES

Key Points in Syndrome Differentiation

1. Differentiation of Zang-Fu Organs

The differentiation is based on the cause of disease, pain location, tongue and pulse manifestations. If the pain is in the chest, back and shoulder blades accompanied with chest oppression, the location of disease is in the heart. If the pain is triggered by improper diet and the patients have a plump figure accompanied with chest oppression, slippery pulse and slimy tongue coating, the location is in the heart and spleen. If the pain is in the chest and below the costal region and triggered by rage or overanxiety and contemplation, and the patients have severe chest oppression and mild wandering pain accompanied with chest and hypochondriac fullness and distention, the location is in the heart and liver. If the condition is severe with heart pain radiating to the back, panting and inability to lie flat, the location is in the heart and lung. If the condition is critical with sweating, cold limbs and faint pulse verging on expiry, the location is in the heart and kidney.

2. Differentiation of Deficiency from Excess

The differentiation is based on the age, the nature and onset time of the pain, and tongue and pulse manifestations. Sudden pain in the young are usually excess syndrome while pain in the old with prolonged illness are mostly deficiency syndrome. Phlegm-turbidity syndrome shows severe chest oppression with mild heart pain, generalized heavy sensation, lassitude, gastric stuffiness, anorexia, slimy tongue coating, and slippery pulse. Blood stasis syndrome exhibits stabbing pain with fixed location that aggravates at night, cyanotic tongue with ecchymosis, and unsmooth pulse. Cold coagulation in heart vessel syndrome presents heart pain radiating to the back and back pain radiating to the heart, pain occurring or worsening with affection of cold or in cold season, cold body and limbs, and sunken tight pulse. Qi deficiency displays dull pain in the heart and chest alleviated with rest, shortness of breath, lassitude, no desire to speak, and thready weak pulse. Yin deficiency manifests heart pain with chest oppression, vacuity vexation and insomnia, dry mouth, night sweat, red tongue with scanty or peeling coating, and thready rapid pulse. And yang deficiency presents heart pain with chest oppression, cold limbs, pale enlarged tongue with thin white coating, and sunken thready and slow pulse.

3. Differentiation of Severity of the Disease

The differentiation is based on the frequency, duration and alleviation factors of pain. If the case occurs repeatedly and regularly with stable characteristics and inducing factors, the condition is relatively mild. If the case occurs for the first time or the characteristics and inducing factors have obvious changes, the condition is more severe. If the pain is mild with short duration and is relieved after rest, the disease is relatively mild. If the case has severe pain, even heart pain radiating to the back and back pain radiating to the heart, with a long duration, the condition is more serious. If the case is accompanied by sweating, cold limbs, discontinuous breathing, cyanotic lips and nails, and even syncope, the disease is mostly critical.

Syndrome Differentiation

1. Syndrome of Internal Obstruction of Phlegm-Turbidity

[Clinical Manifestations] Severe chest oppression with mild heart pain, accompanied with generalized heavy sensation, lassitude, gastric stuffiness, anorexia, sticky mouth, nausea, expectoration of phlegm and saliva, white slimy or white slippery tongue coating, and slippery pulse.

[Manifestations Analysis] Improper diet, overeating fatty sweet foods or over-contemplation damages the spleen, which causes dysfunction of the spleen in transportation and transformation, leading to dampness accumulation and phlegm generation. Phlegm is a yin pathogen, and when it obstructs chest yang, there occurs severe chest oppression with mild heart pain. Phlegm-dampness encumbers the spleen and causes its dysfunction in transportation, leading to generalized heavy sensation, lassitude, gastric stuffiness, anorexia, sticky mouth, nausea, and expectoration of phlegm and saliva. White slimy or white slippery tongue coating and slippery pulse indicate internal obstruction by phlegm-turbidity.

[Nursing Principle] Unblocking yang and discharging turbidity; eliminating phlegm and opening knots.

[Suggested Formula] Gualou Xiebai Banxia Decoction.

2. Syndrome of Qi Stagnation in the Heart and Chest

[Clinical Manifestations] Frequent onset of heart pain without fixed location, frequent sigh, ocurring or aggravating with emotional depression, possibly accompanied with abdominal distension and oppression that is alleviated with belching or flatus, thin tongue coating or thin slimy coating, and wiry pulse.

[Manifestations Analysis] Emotional depression or depressed anger damages the liver, which brings about liver depression and qi stagnation as well as obstruction of heart vessel, so such symptoms exhibit as frequent onset of heart pain without fixed location, frequent sigh, ocurring or aggravating with emotional depression. Liver depression overwhelming the spleen causes inhibition of qi movement, leading to epigastric and abdominal distension and oppression that is alleviated with belching or flatus. Thin tongue coating or thin slimy coating and wiry pulse are signs of liver qi depression.

[Nursing Principle] Soothing the liver and regulating qi; adjusting and unblocking heart vessel.

[Suggested Formula] Chaihu Shugan Powder.

3. Heart Blood Obstruction Syndrome

[Clinical Manifestations] Stabbing pain in the heart and chest with fixed location that aggravates at night, cyanotic lips and tongue with ecchymosis and thin tongue coating, and unsmooth pulse or irregularly or regularly intermittent pulse.

[Manifestations Analysis] Internal retention of blood stasis obstructs heart vessel, so there is stabbing pain in the heart and chest with fixed location. Both blood and night pertain to yin in nature, so the pain aggravates during night. Cyanotic lips and tongue with ecchymosis and thin coating, and unsmooth pulse or irregularly or regularly intermittent pulse, are all signs of internal retention of blood stasis.

[Nursing Principle] Activating blood and resolving stasis; unblocking collateral and relieving pain.

[Suggested Formula] Xuefu Zhuyu Decoction and Shixiao Powder.

4. Syndrome of Cold Coagulation in Heart Vessel

[Clinical Manifestations] Heart pain radiating to the back and back pain radiating to the heart, pain worsened with cold, cold body and limbs, pale complexion, thin white tongue coating, and sunken tight pulse.

[Manifestations Analysis] Interior invasion of pathogenic cold devitalizes chest yang and inhibits heart vessel, so the patients feel heart pain radiating to the back and back pain radiating to the heart and pain worsened with cold. Yang qi cannot reach the exterior, leading to cold limbs, and pale complexion. Thin white tongue coating and sunken tight pulse are signs of yin-cold coagulation.

[Nursing Principle] Warming meridians and dissipating cold; unblocking yang and relieving pain.

[Suggested Formula] Gualou Xiebai Guizhi Decoction and Danggui Sini Decoction.

5. Heart Qi Deficiency Syndrome

[Clinical Manifestations] Dull pain in the heart and chest, shortness of breath and palpitation aggravating with exertion, lassitude, no desire to speak, pale tongue with thin white coating, and thready weak pulse.

[Manifestations Analysis] Heart qi insufficiency leads to weak propelling function of the heart and inhibition of heart vessel, leading to dull pain in the heart and chest as well as shortness of breath and palpitation aggravating with exertion. Qi deficiency is the cause of lassitude and no desire to speak. Pale tongue with thin white coating and thready weak pulse indicate qi deficiency.

[Nursing Principle] Tonifying and replenishing heart qi; unblocking vessel and relieving pain.

[Suggested Formula] Baoyuan Decoction.

6. Heart Yin Insufficiency Syndrome

[Clinical Manifestations] Dull pain in the heart and chest, vexing heat in chest, palms and soles, palpitation, fearful throbbing, dizziness, tinnitus, dry mouth and throat, red tongue with scanty fluids, scanty coating or peeling coating, and thready rapid pulse.

[Manifestations Analysis] Insufficient heart yin cannot nourish heart vessel, so dull pain in the heart and chest is felt. Heart yin insufficiency causes deficiency-fire harassing spirit, leading to palpitation and fearful throbbing. Insufficient kidney yin failing to nourish the liver leads to ascendant hyperactivity of liver yang, causing dizziness and tinnitus. Vexing heat in chest, palms and soles, dry mouth and throat, red tongue with scanty fluids, scanty or peeling coating, and thready rapid pulse, are all signs of yin deficiency.

[Nursing Principle] Tonifying yin and nourishing the heart; moistening vessel and relieving pain.

[Suggested Formula] Shengmai Powder and Tianwang Buxin Pellets.

7. Heart-Kidney Yang Deficiency Syndrome

[Clinical Manifestations] Heart pain with chest oppression, palpitation, fearful throbbing, lassitude, fear of cold, bright white bloodless complexion, cold limbs, pale enlarged tongue with thin white coating, and sunken thready and slow pulse.

[Manifestations Analysis] Heart-kidney yang deficiency with warming dysfunction devitalizes chest yang, leading to chest oppression, palpitation, and fearful throbbing. Kidney yang deficiency makes yang qi unable to reach four limbs and the skin, resulting in lassitude, fear of cold, bright white and bloodless complexion, cold limbs. Pale enlarged tongue with thin white coating and sunken thready and slow pulse are signs of yang deficiency.

[Nursing Principle] Tonifying the kidney and assisting yang; warming and dredging heart vessel.

[Suggested Formula] Shenfu Decoction and Guizhi Gancao Decoction.

NURSING MEASURES

For patients with chest impediment, nurses should closely observe the location, nature, onset time, duration, frequency and inducing, relieving and aggravating factors of pain. They should also check the complexion, mental status, respiration, blood pressure, pulse, heart rhythm and rate of the patients. For those with severe chest pain, nurses should ask the patients every 3~5 minutes about the pain and ensure the rescue equipment is prepared. If severe chest pain lasts for over 30 minutes with the sensation of crushing, suffocating or nearly dying, accompanied by pale complexion, sweating, cold limbs, lips and face cyanosis, and faint pulse verging on expiry, report to the doctor immediately and assist in emergency treatment.

Syndrome-Based Nursing Measures

1. Syndrome of Internal Obstruction of Phlegm-Turbidity

(1) Daily life nursing. The ward should be warm and sunny, quiet, dry, and full of fresh air. The patients should rest in bed and keep the epigastric region warm. For patients who are badly ill and suffer from sticky phlegm that is hard to be expectorated, take a lateral recumbent position, and receive sputum aspiration or spray inhalation therapy when necessary. Avoid overstrain.

(2) Diet nursing. Heye (lotus leaf) tea is recommended. The patients should have small frequent meals, have more fresh fruit and vegetables, and may eat foods that invigorate the spleen and resolve phlegm, such as fuling (poria), shanyao (common yam rhizome), yiyiren (coix seed), corn and mugua (Chinese quince fruit). Food therapy: chenpi (aged tangerine peel) stewed with fish slice, white radish bean curd soup, or shuanggu donggua soup. Shuanggu donggua (double mushroom and Chinese waxgourd) soup: take 5 fresh xianggu (lentinus edodes) and five fresh mogu (mushroom), stir-fry

them in oil for a short time, then add in some water, boil with strong fire, add in small cubes of Chinese waxgourd, cook them together and eat the soup. Avoid raw, cold and greasy foods.

(3) Emotion nursing. The patients should stay calm, and avoid over-thought that damages the spleen, generates phlegm and aggravates the disease. Nurses may use verbal enlightenment therapy to impart patients the impact of emotion and diet over the disease, and explain that being worried, cold or too full are the inducing factors of the disease.

(4) Medication nursing. Decoction should be taken warm after meals, multiple times in small portions.

(5) Manipulation techniques. Acupressure therapy: select Xinshu (BL 15), Jueyinshu (BL 14), Danzhong (CV 17), Neiguan (PC 6), Fenglong (ST 40), Feishu (BL 13) and Jianshi (PC 5); apply thumb kneading and one-finger pushing manipulations on each of the acupoints until the area turns hot the patient has the feelings of soreness, numbness, distension and heaviness in the area; once per day. And it is contraindicated in pregnancy.

2. Syndrome of Qi Stagnation in the Heart and Chest

(1) Daily life nursing. The ward should be quiet, spacious, and full of fresh air. The patients should rest in bed, and keep a normal bowel movement.

(2) Diet nursing. The patients may drink honghuang (safflower) tea and meiguihua (rose flower) tea, and eat foods that move qi and activate blood, such as shanzha (Chinese hawthorn fruit), white radishes, foshou (finger citron fruit), and chenpi (aged tangerine peel). Avoid flatulent foods like sweet potatoes.

(3) Emotion nursing. Nurses may use verbal enlightenment therapy to tell patients the relationship between emotion and disease, teach them to control the emotion, express inner feelings peacefully, and avoid getting angry.

(4) Medication nursing. Decoction should be taken warm after meals.

(5) Manipulation techniques. Acupressure therapy: select Xinshu (BL 15), Jueyinshu (BL 14), Danzhong (CV 17), Neiguan (PC 6) and Taichong (LR 3); apply thumb kneading and one-finger pushing manipulations on each of the acupoints until the area turns hot or the patient has the feelings of soreness, numbness, distension and heaviness in the area; once per day. And it is contraindicated in pregnancy.

3. Heart Blood Obstruction Syndrome

(1) Daily life nursing. The ward should be warm, quiet and full of fresh air, and avoid strong and convective wind. The patients should take rest in bed, timely adjust the clothing and bedding according to weather changes, and keep themselves warm.

(2) Diet nursing. The patients may eat foods that activate blood and resolve blood stasis, such as heimuer (black fungus), eggplant, shanzha (Chinese hawthorn fruit), brown sugar, and huomaren (hemp seed). Avoid raw, cold, sour and astringent foods.

(3) Emotion nursing. Nurses may use verbal enlightenment therapy to impart patients the impact of

emotion over the disease, or use emotional transference and dispositional change therapy, such as enjoying flowers and listening to music, to distract their attention and keep them calm.

(4) Medication nursing. Puhuang (cattail pollen) and wulingzhi (flying squirrel faeces) should be wrap-boiled. Decoction should be taken warm after meals.

(5) Manipulation techniques. ① Electrical iontophoresis therapy: select Xinshu (BL 15), Jueyinshu (BL 14), and Danzhong (CV 17); prepare danggui (Chinese angelica), danshen (danshen root), honghua (safflower), taoren (peach kernel), gouteng (gambir plant), luoshiteng (Chinese star jasmine stem) and qianghuo (notoptetygium root); decoct the above medicinals and then use medicinal iontophoresis apparatus to conduct the medicinal ions of the decoction into the acupoints, 20 minutes each time, once per day. And it is contraindicated in pregnancy. ② Foot bath therapy: decoct danggui (Chinese angelica) and honghua (safflower); wash the feet with the decoction at a temperature of 37~ 42℃ and massage, 20 minutes each time, once per day. And it should be used with caution for patients with hypotension. ③ Paste application therapy: select Danzhong (CV 17) and Jiuwei (CV 15); spray a little Qili Powder on the acupoints, tape them with Shangshi Zhitong Plaster, and change the medicine once per day for consecutive 2 weeks. ④ Acupressure therapy: select Xinshu (BL 15), Jueyinshu (BL 14), Danzhong (CV 17), Neiguan (PC 6), Xuehai (SP 10) and Sanyinjiao (SP 6); apply thumb kneading and one-finger pushing manipulations on each of the acupoints until the area turns hot or the patient has the feelings of soreness, numbness, distension and heaviness in the area; once per day. And it is contraindicated in pregnancy.

4. Syndrome of Cold Coagulation in Heart Vessel

(1) Daily life nursing. The ward should be warm, quiet, and full of bright light and fresh air, and avoid strong and convective wind. The patients should take rest in bed, adjust the clothing and bedding according to weather changes, and keep themselves warm, especially at night.

(2) Diet nursing. The food should be warm. The patients may drink a little rice wine and eat foods that activate yang and dissipate cold, such as longyanrou (longan), mutton, Chinese chives and shanzha (Chinese hawthorn fruit), which may be seasoned with a little ganjiang (dried ginger rhizome) and huajiao (pricklyash peel). Xiebai (long stamen onion bulb) porridge is recommended: xiebai (long stamen onion bulb) 15 g, jingmi (rice fruit) 100 g, and one liter of water; boil them together to make porridge. Avoid raw, cold and cool-natured foods.

(3) Emotion nursing. Nurses may use emotional transference and dispositional change therapy to constantly tour in the ward to care and encourage the patients as much as possible to make them feel warm and keep a good mood.

(4) Medication nursing. Decoction should be taken warm after meals.

(5) Manipulation techniques. ① Medicated ironing therapy: choose back of the trunk; grind into powder chuanxiong (Sichuan lovage root) and xixin (Manchurian wild ginger), stir-fry the powder and put it into a cloth bag for medicated ironing at a temperature of 60~70℃; 20 minutes each time, once per day. And it cannot be applied on the lumbosacral region of pregnant women. ② Hot compress

therapy: choose Danzhong (CV 17), Xinshu (BL 15), Juque (CV 14), Neiguan (PC 6) and Tongli (HT 5); apply hot compresses with healing stones of 50~60℃ to the acupoints, 20 minutes each time, once per day.

5. Heart Qi Deficiency Syndrome

(1) Daily life nursing. The ward should be warm, quiet and full of fresh air, and avoid strong and convective wind. The patients should absolutely rest in bed, keep themselves warm, maintain a normal bowel movement, and avoid overstrain.

(2) Diet nursing. The patients may eat foods that replenish qi and activate blood, such as beef, snake meat, shanyao (common yam rhizome), baihe (lily bulb) and dazao (Chinese date). Food therapy: sweet potato fish cakes; huangqi lianzi dazao (astragalus root, lotus seed and Chinese date) porridge: prepare huangqi (astragalus root) 15 g, lianzi (lotus seed) 10 g and 10 dazao (Chinese dates), brew them with water over low heat for 20 minutes, remove huangqi (astragalus root) residue, add in jingmi (rice fruit) 50 g, and boil them to make porridge; jellyfish stewed with pig's feet: prepare soaked jellyfish head 200 g, soaked pig's feet tendon 200 g, some heimuer (black fungus), carrot slice and bamboo shoot slice, brew them slowly with water over low heat for 20 minutes; eat the food warm every night and morning. Avoid raw, cold and greasy foods.

(3) Emotion nursing. Because the patients are weak with a long course of disease, nurses may use verbal enlightenment therapy as well as suggestive and doubts-dispelling therapy to constantly encourage and comfort the patients, and introduce patients of the same syndrome with better treatment results to help them restore the confidence of winning the battle against disease.

(4) Medication nursing. Decoction should be prepared slowly over low heat and taken warm before meals.

(5) Manipulation techniques. ① Moxibustion therapy: select Xinshu (BL 15), Jueyinshu (BL 14), Danzhong (CV 17), Qihai (CV 6) and Zusanli (ST 36); place the moxa stick 2~3 centimeters away from the skin to perform mild moxibustion on each of the acupoints until the area turns red and the patient feels warm and comfortable without the sensation of burning pain, once per day. And it cannot be applied on the abdomen of pregnant women. ② Water acupuncture therapy: select Xinshu (BL 15), Zusanli (ST 36) and Fenglong (ST 40); inject Huangqi (astragalus root) Injection or Danshen (danshen root) Injection into the acupoints.

6. Heart Yin Insufficiency Syndrome

(1) Daily life nursing. The ward should be cool, quiet and full of fresh air, and avoid strong and convective wind. The patients should rest in bed, live a regular life, and avoid staying up late and overstrain. For patients with night sweat, wipe the sweat away and change the wet clothes and bedding timely. For patients with constipation, teach them to do abdomen massage: massage the abdomen clockwise for 20~30 circles, and 2~3 times per day.

(2) Diet nursing. The patients may drink suanzaoren (spiny date seed) tea or xiyangshen (American ginseng) tea and eat foods that tonify yin and nourish the heart, such as meat of soft-shelled

turtles, duck meat, yin'er (tremella), baihe (lily bulb), rabbit meat, dazao (Chinese date), heizhima (black sesame), sangshen (mulberry) and pigskin. Food therapy: muer (wood ear) stir-fried with fish slices; shanyao (common yam rhizome) stewed with pig kidneys: chop one pair of pig kidneys into small cubes, cut shanyao (common yam rhizome) 50 g into slices, stir-fry shanyao slices, then slightly stir-fry some scallion and shengjiang (fresh ginger) in another pot and add in the pig kidneys, a little yellow wine and fine salt for further stir-frying with strong fire, then add in the shanyao slices, and boil them with strong fire until cooked. Avoid pungent, spicy, and dry-natured foods.

(3) Emotion nursing. Because the patients have frenetic stirring of deficiency fire, they may feel anxious and irritable, and nurses may use emotional transference and dispositional change therapy to distract their attention and make them stay calm.

(4) Medication nursing. Decoction should be taken warm before meals, multiple times in small portions.

(5) Manipulation techniques. ① Acupressure therapy: select Xinshu (BL 15), Jueyinshu (BL 14), Danzhong (CV 17), Sanyinjiao (SP 6) and Taixi (KI 3); apply thumb kneading and one-finger pushing manipulations on each of the acupoints until the area turns hot or the patient has the feelings of soreness, numbness, distension and heaviness in the area; once per day. And it is contraindicated in pregnancy. ② Auricular pressure therapy: select the auricular points of heart (TF4), kidney (CO10), small intestine (CO6), sympathetic (AH6a), shenmen (TF4), subcortex (AT4) and adrenal gland (TG2p); apply specialized pasters on the points, press on each of them till the area turns hot and red, 4 ~5 times per day, and keep the pasters for 2~4 days. And it is contraindicated in pregnancy.

7. Heart-Kidney Yang Deficiency Syndrome

(1) Daily life nursing. The ward should be warm, quiet and full of bright light, and avoid strong and convective wind. The patients should rest in bed, keep themselves warm, and avoid overstrain.

(2) Diet nursing. The patients may eat foods that warm and tonify the heart and kidney, such as beef, onion and mulberry. Food therapy: mutton white radish soup; eggplants stewed with ricefield eels; mutton walnut porridge: brew meat of castrated sheep 30 g with some congbai (scallion white) and shengjiang (fresh ginger) until the meat becomes mushy, add in jingmi (rice fruit) 30 g for further brewing to make porridge, and scatter into the porridge the powder of one grain of quick-boiled hetaoren (walnut). Avoid raw and cold foods.

(3) Emotion nursing. Because the patients are weak and sleepless with yang deficiency and a long course of disease, they may feel depressed and pessimistic. Nurses may use verbal enlightenment therapy and music therapy to care for and encourage them as much as possible in order to distract their attention and eliminate undesirable feelings.

(4) Medication nursing. Fuzi (monkshood) should be decocted earlier. Decoction should be taken hot before meals, multiple times in small portions.

(5) Manipulation techniques. ① Moxibustion therapy: select Xinshu (BL 15), Jueyinshu (BL 14), Danzhong (CV 17), Guanyuan (CV 4) and Qihai (CV 6); place the moxa stick 2~3 centimeters

away from the skin to perform mild moxibustion on each of the acupoints until the area turns red and the patient feels warm and comfortable without the sensation of burning pain, once per day. And it cannot be applied on the abdomen of pregnant women. ② Paste application therapy: select Danzhong (CV 17), Neiguan (PC 6), Xinshu (BL 15) and Xuli (apical pulsation); grind into powder renshen (ginseng), huangqi (astragalus root), guizhi (cinnamon twig), rougui (cinnamon bark), yinyanghuo (aerial part of epimedium), zhishi (immature bitter orange), gualou (snakegourd fruit), xiebai (long stamen onion bulb), shuizhi (leech), quanxie (scorpion), jiangxiang (rosewood), taoren (peach kernel), honghua (safflower), chuanxiong (Sichuan lovage root), yanhusuo (corydalis rhizome) and bingpian (borneol); blend 4 g of the powder with honey to make pastes, and apply them on the acupoints, once per day.

Patient Education

During an episode of chest impediment, the patients should stop any movement immediately, absolutely rest in bed in a semi-supine position, and have high flow oxygen inhalation. They should avoid unnecessary turning-over, and restrict visits to them. Nurses should apply ECG monitoring if necessary, and control the volume and speed of infusion. To prevent pressure sores, the patients should turn over regularly, or nurses should assist with turning-over every 2 hours, use an air cushion bed, or put an air cushion or cotton cushion under the bone protruding part.

The patients should balance work and rest during the remission stage. Around 10~11 a.m. or 3 p.m. when the sunshine is bright, they may do moderate exercise, such as Qigong to regulate breathing, tranquilize mind, and reduce stress. They should live a regular life, have adequate sleep and avoid overstrain. They should keep themselves warm, maintain a normal bowel movement, and avoid overexertion in defecation. They may have a bath at a moderate temperature for a short time with the door unlocked. The patients may be assisted during bath if necessary. Don't take a bath when too hungry or too full.

The diet should be light, nutritious and digestible, with a balance between coarse and refined grains. The patients should have small frequent meals, and take foods with low salt, low sugar, low fat, high vitamin, high protein and high calcium. Fish, fresh fruit and vegetables should be supplemented while animal innards and fat meat should be reduced in order to keep a normal bowel movement. Moreover, they should not be too hungry or too full, choose a small meal for supper, and should refrain from smoking and drinking alcohol and strong tea, and eating foods that are pungent, spicy, fatty and sweet.

The patients should stay calm, take more rest, and avoid overexcitation, overjoy, fierce anger, severe distress and excessive pensiveness. For patients with fear and panic, always accompany and care for them with patience. Nurses should often make rounds of the ward, observe their condition, comfort and encourage them with a calm voice, and tell them and their family the importance of resting in bed and keeping calm.

The patients should follow the doctor's advice in medication. Chinese and Western medicine should be administered at an interval of more than 30 minutes. They should take with them emergency medicine at all times.

第七节　中　风

中风,泛指因年老或脏腑虚衰,情志变动,外因诱发,导致风痰入络,或因气血逆乱,导致脑络痹阻,或因血溢于脑而引起的,以突然昏仆,或半身不遂、口眼喝斜、肢体麻木、舌謇难言为临床特征的一类急慢性颅脑病。急性期指发病2周以内,神昏者可延长至发病4周,恢复期指发病2周至6个月,后遗症期指发病6个月以后。西医的急性脑血管疾病可参照本节进行护理。

一、病因病机

中风的病因包括气血亏虚、劳欲过度、情志过极、饮食不节、天气变化。病人年迈气虚,不能行血,脑脉瘀滞不通;或重病久病,阴血亏虚,水不涵木,肝风夹痰夹瘀,阻于清窍。或烦劳过度,亢奋不敛,引动风阳;或房劳伤阴,阴虚阳亢,均可发为中风。病人七情失调,肝郁血滞,瘀阻脑脉;或暴怒伤肝,肝阳上亢;或心火暴盛,血随气逆,上犯于脑。或嗜食肥甘醇酒,脾虚生痰,郁久化热,引动肝风,夹痰上扰,均可发为中风。天气骤变,或于冬季寒凝血瘀,或因春季转暖,引动肝风,亦可导致中风。

中风的病机为阴阳失调,气血逆乱,上犯清窍。病位在脑,与心、肝、脾、肾有关。中风的急性期以实证为主,恢复期及后遗症期以虚实夹杂为主。

二、常见证型

(一)辨证要点

1. 辨中经络与中脏腑　根据发病后有无神志改变等来辨别。若仅有偏身麻木,肢体力弱,口舌喝斜,言謇不语,而无神识昏蒙,则属轻证,多为中经络。若既有半身不遂,口舌喝斜,舌强不语,又有神识恍惚,或神志昏愦,则属重证,多为中脏腑。

2. 辨闭证与脱证　根据口、手、二便的状态等来辨别。若神识恍惚,牙关紧闭,两手握拳,肢体拘紧,大小便闭,多为闭证。若神志昏愦,口张不闭,手撒肢软,二便自遗,脉微欲绝,则多为脱证。脱证多由闭证恶化而成,预后较差。

(二)证候分型

1. 急性期

(1)中经络

1)风痰阻络证

[主要证候]肌肤不仁,甚则半身不遂,口舌喝斜;言语不利,或謇涩或不语;头晕目眩,痰多而黏;舌质暗淡,舌苔白腻,脉弦滑。

［证候分析］中年以后,肝阴虚则内风易动,脾气虚则痰湿内生,肝风夹痰上扰清窍,脑脉痹阻,经络不畅,故肌肤不仁,甚则半身不遂、口舌㖞斜、言语不利,或謇涩或不语;痰浊中阻,清阳不升,故头晕目眩;舌质暗淡,舌苔白腻,脉弦滑,均为风痰阻络之象。

［护治原则］熄风化痰,活血通络。

［常用方剂］化痰通络汤。

2）风阳上扰证

［主要证候］半身不遂,口舌㖞斜,舌强言謇或不语,偏身麻木;眩晕头痛,面红目赤,口苦咽干,心烦易怒,尿赤便干;舌红,苔黄,脉弦数。

［证候分析］肝郁化火,阳亢风动,风火相煽,直冲犯脑,故半身不遂,口舌㖞斜,舌强言謇或不语,偏身麻木;上扰清窍,故眩晕头痛,面红目赤;肝经郁热,故口苦咽干;肝火扰心,故心烦易怒;舌红,苔黄,脉弦数,均为风阳上扰之象。

［护治原则］清肝泻火,熄风潜阳。

［常用方剂］天麻钩藤饮。

3）痰热腑实证

［主要证候］半身不遂,口舌㖞斜,言语謇涩或不语,偏身麻木;腹胀,便干便秘,头痛目眩,咯痰或痰多;舌质红,苔黄腻,脉弦滑。

［证候分析］痰热上扰清窍,故半身不遂,口舌㖞斜,言语謇涩或不语,偏身麻木;痰热阻滞中焦,腑气不通,故腹胀,便干便秘;痰热阻滞中焦,清阳不升,故头痛目眩,咯痰或痰多;舌质红,苔黄腻,脉弦滑,均为痰热腑实之象。

［护治原则］清热化痰,通腑泻浊。

［常用方剂］星蒌承气汤。

（2）中脏腑

1）痰热内闭证

［主要证候］突然昏仆,不省人事;牙关紧闭,两手握固,大小便闭,肢体强痉,兼有面赤身热,气粗口臭,躁扰不宁;舌苔黄腻,脉弦滑而数。

［证候分析］痰热闭阻清窍,神机失用,故突然昏仆,不省人事,牙关紧闭,两手握固,肢体强痉;痰火内结阳明,腑气不通,故大便秘结;痰火上扰,故气粗口臭,躁扰不宁;舌苔黄腻,脉弦滑而数,均为痰热内闭之象。

［护治原则］清热化痰,醒神开窍。

［常用方剂］羚羊角汤合安宫牛黄丸。

2）痰蒙清窍证

［主要证候］突然昏倒,不省人事;牙关紧闭,两手握固,大小便闭,肢体强痉;面白唇暗,四肢不温,静卧不烦;舌苔白腻,脉沉滑。

［证候分析］湿痰内蕴,夹内生之风,蒙塞清窍,故突然昏倒,不省人事,牙关紧闭,两手握固,大小便闭,肢体强痉;卫阳之气不充肌肤,故面白唇暗;湿为阴邪,易伤阳气,故四肢不温;脑髓血脉受损,神气伏匿不出,故静卧不烦;舌苔白腻,脉沉滑,均为痰蒙清窍之象。

［护治原则］温阳化痰,醒神开窍。

［常用方剂］涤痰汤合苏合香丸。

3）元气败脱证

［主要证候］突然昏仆,不省人事,目合口张,鼻鼾息微,手撒遗尿;汗多不止,四肢冰冷;舌痿,脉微欲绝。

［证候分析］脏腑精气衰竭,阴阳离决,正气将脱,心神颓败,故突然昏仆,不省人事,目合口张,鼻鼾息微,手撒遗尿;汗多不止,四肢冰冷,舌痿,脉微欲绝,均为元气败脱之象。

［护治原则］回阳救阴,益气固脱。

［常用方剂］参附汤。

2. 恢复期

（1）气虚血瘀证

［主要证候］半身不遂,口舌㖞斜,言语謇涩或不语,偏身麻木;面色㿠白,气短乏力,自汗出,心悸,便溏,手足肿胀;舌质暗淡,有齿痕,舌苔白腻,脉沉细。

［证候分析］正气不足,血行不畅,瘀阻经络,故半身不遂,口舌㖞斜,言语謇涩或不语,偏身麻木;中气不足,血不上荣,故面色㿠白;气虚不摄,故气短乏力,自汗出;心脉失养,故心悸;脾气虚弱,故便溏;气虚血瘀,手足筋脉、肌肤失于温煦、濡养,故手足肿胀;舌质暗淡,有齿痕,舌苔白腻,脉沉细,均为气虚血瘀之象。

［护治原则］益气活血。

［常用方剂］补阳还五汤。

（2）阴虚风动证

［主要证候］半身不遂,口舌㖞斜,言语謇涩或不语,偏身麻木;眩晕耳鸣,手足心热,咽干口燥;舌质红且舌体瘦,少苔或无苔,脉弦细数。

［证候分析］肝肾阴虚,阴不制阳,内风翕动,气血逆乱,上犯虚损之脑脉,故半身不遂,口舌㖞斜,言语謇涩或不语,偏身麻木;肾精不足,脑髓不充,故眩晕耳鸣;阴虚生内热,虚热内扰,故手足心热,咽干口燥;舌质红且舌体瘦,少苔或无苔,脉弦细数,均为阴虚之象。

［护治原则］育阴熄风,活血通络。

［常用方剂］育阴通络汤。

三、护理措施

对于中风的病人,应监测生命体征,密切观察体温、神志、瞳孔、呼吸、痰鸣音、心率、血压、血氧饱和度、出汗、舌脉。观察病人头昏、头痛的情况;眩晕的发作次数、持续时间、程度,有无呛咳;痰、大便、小便的量、色、质;患侧肢体的肌力、肌张力、关节活动度的变化;语言功能情况;情绪变化。若病人出现烦躁不安,面白肢冷,汗出淋漓,喉中痰鸣,咳痰不畅,呼吸急促,考虑为痰阻气道,引起窒息;若病人出现头痛,呕吐加剧,面白肢冷,呼吸不规则,双侧瞳孔不等大,考虑为脑疝;若病人出现血压骤升,脉搏缓慢,呼吸变深,考虑为颅内出血;若病人出现血压骤降,瞳孔散大,对光反射消失,肢冷,脉微欲绝,考虑为阴阳离绝。以上情况均应立即报告医生,并配合抢救。

（一）辨证施护

1. 风痰阻络证

（1）生活起居护理　居室安静温暖，光线柔和。卧床休息，定时变换体位，动作宜慢，保持良肢位，每日进行 2~3 次患肢锻炼，下床活动时需有人陪伴。将病人的常用物品放在易取处，不可深低头、旋转，以防止摔倒。保持皮肤清洁，床单干燥平整，以预防压疮。保持呼吸道通畅，定时翻身、拍背，及时清除口腔分泌物，饭前、饭后、睡前用金银花甘草液漱口。若痰多而黏，可遵医嘱进行中药雾化吸入，操作动作要轻柔。

（2）饮食护理　饮食宜清淡，少食多餐。可饮玫瑰花茶、菊花茶。宜食熄风化痰的食物，如山楂、橘皮、茯苓、黑木耳、昆布、荞麦、玉米、芋头、炸全蝎、金橘。食疗方：乌蛇天麻汤、莲子发菜瘦肉汤、鲜蘑萝卜条、兔肉紫菜豆腐汤。不宜食肥甘、辛辣、生湿酿痰的食物，如酒、羊肉、狗肉、海虾、海蟹、糯米、甜食、生冷瓜果。

（3）情志护理　病人新病且有眩晕，护士可运用语言开导疗法，向病人讲解眩晕的发生机制，指导病人避开诱因。病人言语謇涩，护士应教给病人自我调适的方法，以保持心态平和，避免因急躁易怒而加重病情。

（4）用药护理　中药汤剂宜饭后温服。

（5）操作技术　① 穴位按摩法：取水沟、百会、太阳、风池、内关、极泉、尺泽、委中、三阴交、足三里、丰隆、合谷，用拇指揉法，每次共 30 分钟，每日 4~5 次；孕妇禁用。② 拍击疗法：取脊柱两侧的足太阳膀胱，用虚掌由下往上、由外向内轻扣，每次 3~5 分钟，每日 2~3 次；根据痰液的多少，调整力度、时间和次数。

2. 风阳上扰证

（1）生活起居护理　居室凉爽安静，光线柔和。眩晕发作时应卧床休息，定时变换体位，保持良肢位。减少探视。做好口腔护理，若口唇干裂，可外涂润滑油。若病情平稳，可适量运动，以保证睡眠质量和大便通畅。

（2）饮食护理　饮食宜清淡。多饮水，可饮菊花茶。宜食熄风清热的食物，如炸全蝎、绿豆、香菇、冬瓜、黄瓜、雪梨、莲子。食疗方：芹菜菊花粥、天麻炖甲鱼。忌烟酒、浓茶、咖啡，不宜食煎炸、辛辣、肥甘、油腻、辛香燥烈的食物，如羊肉、狗肉、韭菜、大蒜、大葱。

（3）情志护理　病人新病且为实热证，容易紧张、焦虑，护士可运用语言开导疗法，主动介绍医院环境，了解病人的需要和生活习惯，帮助病人解决问题，多做解释工作，以消除病人的不良情绪。

（4）用药护理　中药汤剂宜饭后温服或偏凉服。

（5）操作技术　① 穴位按摩法：取水沟、百会、内关、极泉、尺泽、委中、三阴交、足三里、太冲、行间，用拇指揉法，每次共 30 分钟，每日 4~5 次；孕妇禁用。② 耳压疗法：取神门、肝、脾、肾、心、交感等耳穴，用耳穴压丸贴片贴压，每日按揉 4~5 次，以局部发热泛红为度，留置 2~4 日；孕妇禁用。

3. 痰热腑实证

（1）生活起居护理　居室凉爽安静，光线柔和。卧床休息，定时变换体位，保持良肢位，衣被宜薄。起居有常，减少探视。定时排便，排便时不可久蹲或过于用力。保持呼吸道通畅。保持口腔清洁。若病情平稳，可适量运动。

（2）饮食护理　饮食宜清淡，少食多餐。多饮水，可饮竹沥。多吃新鲜的水果和蔬菜。宜食清热化痰的食物,如西瓜、蜂蜜、薏苡仁、莲子、山药、丝瓜、茯苓、白萝卜、芹菜。食疗方:荸荠炖海蜇。忌烟酒、浓茶、咖啡,不宜食辛辣、炙煿、油腻、肥甘的食物。

(3)情志护理 病人严重便秘,护士可运用语言开导疗法,告诉病人若配合治疗,顺利排便,就可缓解病情。帮助病人调畅情志,克服对于排便的焦虑感。

(4)用药护理 生大黄后下,芒硝冲服。中药汤剂宜饭后温服。中病即止,以免耗伤正气。服用泻下药后,护士应观察用药后的反应,若病人在3~5小时内排出2~3次稀便,则不需再服药。若服药后仍未解大便,可报告医生,继续服药。

(5)操作技术 ① 穴位按摩法:取水沟、百会、内关、极泉、尺泽、委中、三阴交、足三里、曲池、内庭、胃俞、脾俞、丰隆、中脘、关元、涌泉,用拇指揉法、一指禅推法,每次共30分钟,每日4~5次;孕妇禁用。② 耳穴压豆:取神门、心、肾、交感等耳穴,用耳穴压丸贴片贴压,每日按揉4~5次,以局部发热泛红为度,留置2~4日;适用于失眠者,孕妇禁用。

4. 痰热内闭证

(1)生活起居护理 居室凉爽安静,光线稍暗。病房宜靠近护士站,加强巡视。病人宜卧床,定时变换体位,保持良肢位,头部抬高15°~20°,头偏向一侧。安排专人守护,避免搬动。对躁动不安者进行保护性约束,以避免损伤或坠床。若牙关紧闭,可用乌梅擦牙,或取下假牙后使用开口器,以防止咬伤舌头。遵医嘱吸氧,做好口腔护理,保持呼吸道通畅。若高热,可遵医嘱采用中药擦浴,或冷敷头部及大血管经过的表浅部位(腋窝、腹股沟等处)。

(2)饮食护理 昏迷病人予鼻饲低盐、低脂的流食。饮食宜清淡、营养、易消化。可鼻饲二角三汁饮、白萝卜汁、米汤、牛奶、藕粉。宜食清热化痰的食物,如雪梨、香蕉。遵医嘱使用荷叶麻仁粥:鲜薄荷叶、鲜荆芥穗各30 g,水煎取汁,与炒火麻仁50 g、粳米75 g煮成稀粥,过筛后分次鼻饲。不宜食肥甘、辛香燥烈、易产气的食物,如辣椒、大蒜、羊肉。

(3)情志护理 鼓励家属多陪伴病人,为病人提供心理支持。

(4)用药护理 羚羊角粉冲服,生石决明、龟板先煎。中药汤剂若为灌服,应徐徐喂服,听到药汁咽下声后才能继续,以防发生呛咳。中药丸剂宜用温水溶化后频频鼻饲,每6~8小时服1丸。

(5)操作技术 穴位按摩法:取水沟、素髎、百会、内关、曲池、大椎、合谷、太冲,用拇指揉法,每次共30分钟,每日4~5次;孕妇禁用。

5. 痰蒙清窍证

(1)生活起居护理 居室温暖干燥,安静舒适,光线稍暗,空气新鲜,不可有强风、对流风。病人应卧床,定时变换体位,保持良肢位,头部稍抬高且偏向一侧,注意保暖。舌后坠者,用拉舌钳固定。遵医嘱吸氧,做好口腔护理。遵医嘱留置导尿管。使用便器时动作宜轻缓,保持会阴部清洁干燥,及时更换被污染的床单及衣裤。

(2)饮食护理 昏迷病人予鼻饲低盐、低脂的流食,遵医嘱进行肠内营养补充。食物的温度宜温。可鼻饲竹沥、生姜汁。宜食温性、豁痰开窍的食物,如葱白、山楂、南瓜。可遵医嘱食石菖蒲猪肾粥,过筛后分次鼻饲。不宜食肥甘、生冷、易产气的食物。

(3)情志护理 鼓励家属多陪伴病人,为病人提供心理支持。

(4)用药护理 中药汤剂宜温热鼻饲。中药丸剂宜用温水溶化后频频鼻饲,每6~8小时服1丸。

（5）操作技术 ① 敷贴疗法：取肺俞、膏肓、定喘、天突，遵医嘱将温阳化痰、醒神开窍的中药打粉后与生姜汁调成糊状敷贴，每次8小时，每日1次。② 药枕疗法：取风池、风府、哑门、大椎，遵医嘱使用装有醒脑开窍中药的药枕。③ 穴位按摩法：取水沟、素髎、百会、内关、合谷、太冲，用拇指揉法，每次共30分钟，每日4~5次；孕妇禁用。

6. 元气败脱证

（1）生活起居护理 居室温暖安静，光线较暗，空气新鲜。病人应卧床，定时变换体位，头侧向一边，以防呕吐物及口腔内的痰液吸入呼吸道。遵医嘱吸氧。若汗多，应及时擦干，并换掉湿衣被。若眼睑不能闭合，可覆盖生理盐水纱布或涂金霉素眼膏。若张口呼吸，可覆盖生理盐水纱布。做好口腔护理，保持呼吸道通畅。保持会阴部清洁干燥。遵医嘱留置导尿管。备齐抢救设备，做好气管切开准备。

（2）饮食护理 予鼻饲低盐、低脂的流食，遵医嘱进行肠内营养补充。食物的温度宜温。鼻饲足够的水和富于营养的流食，如果汁、米汤、牛奶、菜汤、肉汤。宜食补气止脱的食物，如牡蛎、山药、粳米、大枣、番茄、豆腐、桑椹、菠菜、黑木耳、山楂。可食人参粥：人参3g，冰糖适量，粳米50~100g，煮成软烂的稀粥，过筛后分次鼻饲。

（3）情志护理 护士应与家属沟通，嘱家属不要惊慌、焦虑，应配合医院的治疗。

（4）用药护理 人参另煎兑服，附子先煎。中药汤剂应急煎，频频鼻饲。

（5）操作技术 ① 灸法：取神阙、气海、关元、百会、三阴交、足三里，用温和灸，艾条燃着端悬于施灸部位上，距离皮肤2~3厘米，灸至病人有温热舒适无灼痛的感觉，皮肤稍有红晕，每日1次；孕妇腹部禁用。② 穴位按摩法：取水沟、素髎、百会、内关、肾俞、八髎、足三里、天枢，用拇指揉法，每次共30分钟，每日4~5次；孕妇禁用。

7. 气虚血瘀证

（1）生活起居护理 居室温暖安静，空气新鲜，不可有强风、对流风。病情稳定后，尽早开始康复治疗。定时更换体位，每2小时协助翻身、拍背1次，用红花乙醇溶液按摩骨突部位。保持皮肤清洁，定期用温水擦浴。保持呼吸道通畅，教病人有效咳嗽，以避免痰液潴留。若痰液黏稠，遵医嘱进行中药雾化吸入。进行腹部按摩，以保持大便通畅。

（2）饮食护理 可予普食，少食多餐，进食宜慢，避免呛咳。食物的温度宜温。宜食补气通络的食物，如薏苡仁、黄芪、莲子、白菜、冬瓜、丝瓜、木耳、赤小豆、山楂。多吃血肉有情的食物，如牛肉、羊肉。可食松子仁、黑芝麻，以润肠通便。食疗方：羊肚煲山药，枸杞核桃仁鸡丁。不可峻补，不宜食生冷、油腻、肥甘的食物。

（3）情志护理 病人已进入恢复期，护士应鼓励病人在耐力范围内，进行日常生活活动和运动，以增强病人的自我价值感。

（4）用药护理 中药汤剂宜饭前温服，少量频服。

（5）操作技术 ① 熏洗疗法：取络石藤30g，当归、川芎、红花、桑枝各15g，川乌、草乌各9g；煎汤后取1~2升药液，水温50~70℃时熏蒸患侧手部，水温降至37~40℃时浸泡、淋洗胀大的手部及患侧的肢体，每次20分钟，每日2次；适用于恢复期手胀者。② 灸法：取关元、天枢、神阙、气海，用温和灸，每次选择1~2个腧穴，艾条燃着端悬于施灸部位上，距离皮肤2~3厘米，灸至病人有温热舒适无灼痛的感觉，皮肤稍有红晕，每日1次；孕妇腹部禁用。③ 保健按摩疗法：取平卧位，以肚脐为中心,顺时针按揉腹部,以腹内有热感为宜,每次 20~30 圈,每日 2~3 次;适用于便秘者。④ 热敷疗法:用热水袋热敷少腹部;适用于尿潴留者,孕妇禁用。⑤ 塞鼻疗法:用川乌、草乌、细辛、三七、皂角各等份,共研细末,每次 2 g,塞于鼻中(向左斜者塞右鼻、向右斜者塞左鼻);适用于中风后口眼㖞斜者,孕妇禁用。

8. 阴虚风动证

(1)生活起居护理 居室凉爽安静,光线较暗,空气新鲜,不可有强风、对流风。病情稳定后,尽早开始康复治疗。定时更换体位,每 2 小时协助翻身、拍背 1 次。起居有常,睡眠充足,减少探视,不可熬夜。将常用物品放在病人易取处。注意保持皮肤清洁。每晚睡前用热水泡脚。若口唇干裂,可外涂润滑油。

(2)饮食护理 饮食宜清淡,少食多餐。多饮水,多吃新鲜的水果和蔬菜。可饮荸荠豆浆。宜食益阴养血的食物,如枸杞子、银耳、黑芝麻、木耳、黑米、海参、鳖肉、乌鸡、鸭肉。食疗方:天麻猪脑粥、百合莲子薏仁粥、玉兰鱼球、大蒜烧茄子。可食酸枣仁膏、牛奶,以促进睡眠。可食香蕉、蜂蜜,以促进排便。忌浓茶、咖啡,不宜食辛辣动火的食物。

(3)情志护理 病人阴虚久病,容易心烦,护士可运用语言开导疗法,向病人讲解不良的情绪会加重病情,要学会调节情绪。或运用移情易性疗法,如听轻音乐,以转移病人的注意力,稳定情绪,促进睡眠。护士应与医生及家属多沟通,尽量帮助病人解决实际困难,协助减轻病人的医疗负担,从而避免病人忧思。

(4)用药护理 生龙骨、生牡蛎、代赭石、龟板先煎,钩藤后下。中药汤剂宜饭前温服,少量频服。

(5)操作技术 ① 敷贴疗法:取涌泉,用大蒜捣泥外敷,每晚 1 次,适用于失眠者;蓖麻叶捣烂敷患侧,或用僵蚕 30 g,白附子、蝎尾各 15 g,研磨成粉后与黄酒调匀敷贴,适用于口眼㖞斜处,孕妇禁用。② 穴位按摩法:取神门、百会、三阴交、劳宫、涌泉,每日睡前用拇指揉法,按摩至局部发热或有酸麻重胀感;孕妇禁用。③ 水针疗法:取肩井、曲池、内关、风市、足三里,每次选择 2~3 个腧穴,用复方丹参注射液进行穴位注射。④ 鳝血疗法:大鳝鱼 2 条,用针刺取鳝鱼头部血,适用于口眼㖞斜处左斜者涂右,右斜者涂左,每次 30 分钟,3 日 1 次。

(二)健康教育

居室安静舒适,光线柔和。起居有常,劳逸适度,不可过劳及熬夜。可于无风的晴天,在阳光里短时散步或轻微运动。运动时应有人陪伴,以防止跌仆。变换体位和转头时动作宜慢,避免做引起颅内压增高的动作。鼓励病人开口说话,尽早制订康复计划并及时调整训练方案。注意患肢保暖。根据天气变化及时增减衣服,勿受凉吹风,以预防感冒。保持大便通畅,定时排便,排便时不可久蹲或过于用力。做好皮肤护理,定时变换体位,用温水擦洗,以预防压疮。为病人系好安全手腕带,以利于走失时寻找。

饮食宜清淡、营养、易消化。进食低脂、低盐、高碳水、高纤维、高蛋白的食物。吃饭时不要说话,进食速度宜慢,鼓励病人自己用餐,保持环境安静,减少干扰因素。若病人有吞咽障碍,食物应为糊状,少量多次进食。勿过饥、过饱,忌烟酒、浓茶、咖啡,忌发物,如公鸡肉、猪头肉、海鲜。不宜食辛辣、油腻、生冷、肥甘、炙煿的食物。

保持心情舒畅,避免焦虑、恼怒、忧思、孤独。鼓励家属多陪伴病人,为病人提供心理支持,注意保护病人的自尊心。同病人交谈时要有耐心,态度和蔼,经常安慰、劝导、鼓励病人,帮助其建立信心。对于中风后情绪低落或有情绪波动的病人,应及时发现和治疗,以预防自伤、自杀。

遵医嘱服药,切忌自行服药或停药。若用药后感到不适,应及时向医护人员反映。中药汤剂宜少量多次频服,以防止呛咳。对于神志昏迷的病人应采用鼻饲法,密切观察病人服药后有无异常反应。

病人可经常按摩百会、四神聪、神庭、极泉、尺泽、肩髃、合谷、太溪、神门、委中、阳陵泉、足三里,用揉法、点法、搓法,按摩至局部发热或有酸麻重胀感。可遵医嘱选用舒筋通络、活血化瘀、温经散寒的中药,煎汤后熏洗患肢。

病人出院后应定期门诊复查,积极治疗原发病,以预防再次中风或中风后痴呆、抑郁、癫病的发生。注意血压的变化,如有头痛、眩晕、呕吐、血压升高或肢体麻木加重,为中风先兆症状,应立即由家属协助到医院进行治疗。

Section 7   Wind Stroke

Wind stroke is a kind of acute or chronic craniocerebral disease mainly characterized by sudden collapse or hemiplegia, facial palsy, numbness of the limbs, stiff tongue and sluggish speech, etc. It is generally caused by aging, debilitation of zang-fu organs, emotional disorder, and external pathogens that cause wind phlegm to invade collaterals, by qi and blood counterflow that causes impediment and obstruction of brain collaterals, or by cerebral hemorrhage. The acute phase refers to the period of time owithin two weeks after onset of the disease, and the period can be extended to four weeks in cases of coma. The recovery phase refers to two weeks to six months after the onset, and the sequelae phase refers to six months after the onset. This section may be referred to for the nursing of acute cerebrovascular diseases in Western medicine.

ETIOLOGY AND PATHOGENESIS

The etiology includes deficiency of qi and blood, overstrain and sexual overindulgence, being over emotional, improper diet and weather change. In old patients, qi deficiency fails to promote blood flow and subsequently leads to blood stasis and stagnation in brain collaterals. Serious or prolonged disease consuming yin-blood makes water fail to moisten wood, and consequently, liver wind carrying phlegm and stasis stirs upward to block clear orifices. Overstrain causes yang hyperactivity and wind stirring. Sexual overindulgence damages yin and subsequently induces yin deficiency with yang hyperactivity. Seven emotional disorders bring about liver depression and blood stasis that stagnates in brain collaterals; violent rage damages the liver and subsequently causes ascendant hyperactivity of liver yang. Exuberance of heart fire makes blood go upward following qi counterflow to invade the brain. Excessive intake of fatty sweet foods and alcohol results in spleen deficiency and phlegm generation. Depressed heat stirs liver wind that carries phlegm to upward harass clear orifices. All these may cause wind stroke. Sudden weather change, or cold coagulation and blood stasis in winter, or internal stirring of liver wind due to spring turning warm may also induce wind stroke.

The pathogenesis is yin-yang disharmony that causes qi and blood counterflow to upward invade clear orifices. The disease is located in the brain but connected to the heart, liver, spleen and kidney. Most of the cases at the acute phase belong to excess syndrome whereas most are deficiency-excess in complexity at the recovery and sequelae phases.

COMMON SYNDROMES

Key Points in Syndrome Differentiation

1. Differentiation of Meridian Stroke from Zang-Fu Organ Stroke

The differentiation is based on the mental status. The mild conditions are called meridian stroke characterized by hemiplegia, lack of strength in the affected limb, deviated mouth and tongue, and sluggish speech without unconsciousness. The severe conditions are called zang-fu organ stroke featured by hemiplegia, deviated mouth and tongue, stiff tongue and sluggish speech, and mental confusion or unconsciousness.

2. Differentiation of Block Syndrome from Collapse Syndrome

The differentiation is based on the status of mouth, hands, urine and stool. Block syndrome shows mental confusion, trismus, clenched fist, convulsion, anuria and constipation. Collapse syndrome exhibits unconsciousness, opened mouth, loose hands, weak limbs, incontinence of urine and stool, and faint pulse verging on expiry. Collapse syndrome is usually deteriorated from block syndrome and has a poor prognosis.

Syndrome Differentiation

1. Acute Phase

（1）Meridian Stroke

1）Wind-Phlegm Obstructing Collateral Syndrome

[Clinical Manifestations] Numbness of skin, even hemiplegia, deviated mouth and tongue, slurred or sluggish speech or loss of speech, dizziness, profuse sticky phlegm, dark tongue with white slimy coating, and wiry slippery pulse.

[Manifestations Analysis] After middle age, liver yin deficiency brings on internal stirring of liver wind, and spleen qi deficiency results in internal phlegm-dampness. Liver wind with phlegm upward disturbs clear orifices and obstructs brain collaterals and meridians, leading to numbness of skin, even hemiplegia, deviated mouth and tongue, slurred or sluggish speech or loss of speech. Phlegm-turbidity obstructing the middle makes clear yang fail to ascend, causing dizziness. Dark tongue with white slimy coating and wiry slippery pulse are signs of wind-phlegm obstructing collaterals.

[Nursing Principle] Extinguishing wind and resolving phlegm; activating blood and dredging collateral.

[Suggested Formula] Huatan Tongluo Decoction.

2）Wind Yang Stirring Upward Syndrome

[Clinical Manifestations] Hemiplegia, deviated mouth and tongue, stiff tongue and sluggish speech or loss of speech, hemilateral numbness, dizziness, headache, red face and eyes, bitter taste in mouth, dry throat, heart vexation, irritability, dark urine, dry stool, red tongue with yellow coating, and wiry rapid pulse.

[Manifestations Analysis] Liver depression transforms into fire and hyperactive liver yang stirs liver wind. The fire and wind join each other to upward invade the brain, leading to hemiplegia, deviated mouth and tongue, stiff tongue and sluggish speech or loss of speech, and hemilateral numbness. They upward disturb clear orifices, causing dizziness, headache, and red complexion and eyes. Heat depression in liver meridian causes bitter taste in the mouth and dry throat. Liver fire harassing the heart explains heart vexation and irritability. Red tongue with yellow coating and wiry rapid pulse are signs of wind yang stirring upward.

[Nursing Principle] Clearing the liver and reducing fire; extinguishing wind and subduing yang.

[Suggested Formula] Tianma Gouteng Drink.

3) Phlegm Heat and Fu-Organ Excess Syndrome

[Clinical Manifestations] Hemiplegia, deviated mouth and tongue, sluggish speech or loss of speech, hemilateral numbness, abdominal distention, dry stool, constipation, headache, dizziness, expectoration or profuse phlegm, red tongue with yellow slimy coating, and wiry slippery pulse.

[Manifestations Analysis] Phlegm heat upward stirring clear orifices leads to hemiplegia, deviated mouth and tongue, sluggish speech or loss of speech, and hemilateral numbness. Phlegm heat obstructing the middle energizer induces the obstruction of fu-organ qi, causing abdominal distention, dry stool and constipation. Phlegm heat obstructing the middle energizer also makes clear yang fail to ascend, leading to headache, dizziness and expectoration or profuse phlegm. Red tongue with yellow slimy coating and wiry slippery pulse are manifestations of phlegm heat and fu-organ excess.

[Nursing Principle] Clearing heat and resolving phlegm; dredging fu-organs and discharging turbidity.

[Suggested Formula] Xinglou Chengqi Decoction.

(2) Zang-Fu Organ Stroke

1) Syndrome of Internal Block of Phlegm-Heat

[Clinical Manifestations] Sudden collapse, unconsciousness, trismus, clenched fist, anuria and constipation, stiffness and spasm in the affected limb, accompanied with red complexion, generalized fever, rough breathing, foul breath, restlessness, yellow slimy tongue coating, and wiry, slippery and rapid pulse.

[Manifestations Analysis] Phlegm heat blocking clear orifices leads to failure of vital activity, causing sudden collapse, unconsciousness, trismus, clenched fist, and stiffness and spasm in the affected limb. Internal binding of phlegm to fire in yangming meridian causes the obstruction of fu-organ qi, resulting in constipation. Phlegm fire harassing upward results in rough breathing, foul breath and restlessness. Yellow slimy tongue coating and wiry, slippery and rapid pulse are manifestations of internal block of phlegm-heat.

[Nursing Principle] Clearing heat and resolving phlegm; restoring consciousness and opening orifice.

[Suggested Formula] Lingyangjiao Decoction and Angong Niuhuang Pills.

2）Phlegm Clouding Clear Orifice Syndrome

［Clinical Manifestations］Sudden collapse, unconsciousness, trismus, clenched fist, anuria and constipation, stiffness and spasm in the affected limb, pale complexion, dark lips, cold limbs, lying quietly without vexation, white slimy tongue coating, and sunken slippery pulse.

［Manifestations Analysis］Internal accumulation of dampness-phlegm carrying internal wind clouds and blocks clear orifices, leading to sudden collapse, unconsciousness, trismus, clenched fist, anuria and constipation, and stiffness and spasm in the affected limb. Defense yang fails to fill the skin, causing pale complexion and dark lips. Dampness is yin pathogen and tends to damage yang qi, so the limbs become cold. Brain marrow and blood vessels are damaged and spirit qi hides latently inside, so the patients lie quietly without vexation. White slimy tongue coating and sunken slippery pulse are signs of phlegm clouding clear orifice.

［Nursing Principle］Warming yang and resolving phlegm; restoring consciousness and opening orifice.

［Suggested Formula］Ditan Decoction and Suhexiang Pills.

3）Primordial Qi Collapse Syndrome

［Clinical Manifestations］Sudden collapse, unconsciousness, closed eyes and opened mouth, snore with faint breath, loose hands, incontinence of urine, nonstop profuse sweating, cold limbs, atrophic tongue, faint pulse verging on expiry.

［Manifestations Analysis］Debilitation and exhaustion of essential qi of zang-fu organs and separation of yin and yang from each other cause collapse of healthy qi and decline of heart spirit, leading to sudden collapse, unconsciousness, closed eyes and opened mouth, snore with faint breath, loose hands, and incontinence of urine. Nonstop profuse sweating, cold limbs, atrophic tongue and faint pulse verging on expiry are signs of primordial qi collapse.

［Nursing Principle］Restoring yang and saving yin; replenishing qi and stopping collapse.

［Suggested Formula］Shenfu Decoction.

2. Recovery Phase

（1）Qi Deficiency and Blood Stasis Syndrome

［Clinical Manifestations］Hemiplegia, deviated mouth and tongue, sluggish speech or loss of speech, hemilateral numbness, bright white complexion, shortness of breath, lack of strength, spontaneous sweating, palpitation, loose stool, swollen hands and feet, dark tongue with teeth marks and white slimy coating, and sunken thready pulse.

［Manifestations Analysis］Healthy qi insufficiency and unsmooth blood flow cause the obstruction of meridians and collaterals, leading to hemiplegia, deviated mouth and tongue, sluggish speech or loss of speech, and hemilateral numbness. Middle qi insufficiency makes blood fail to upward nourish the face, so there is bright white complexion. Failure of qi in its controlling function due to qi deficiency explains shortness of breath, lack of strength and spontaneous sweating. Malnourishment of heart vessels causes palpitation. Spleen qi weakness results in loose stool. Qi deficiency and blood stasis make muscles and tendons of hands, feet and skin unable to be warmed and nourished, so there are swollen hands and feet. Dark tongue with teeth marks and white slimy coating, and sunken thready pulse are signs of qi deficiency and blood stasis.

[Nursing Principle] Replenishing qi and activating blood.

[Suggested Formula] Buyang Huanwu Decoction.

(2) Yin Deficiency Stirring Wind Syndrome

[Clinical Manifestations] Hemiplegia, deviated mouth and tongue, sluggish speech or loss of speech, hemilateral numbness, dizziness, tinnitus, feverish sensation in palms and soles, dry throat and mouth, red thin tongue with scanty or no coating, and wiry, thready and rapid pulse.

[Manifestations Analysis] Liver-kidney yin deficiency causes failure of yin to control yang and stirring of internal wind, which subsequently leads to qi and blood counterflow upward to invade brain vessels, resulting in hemiplegia, deviated mouth and tongue, sluggish speech or loss of speech, and hemilateral numbness. Insufficiency of both kidney essence and brain marrow brings on dizziness and tinnitus. Yin deficiency generates internal deficiency heat that stirs internally, leading to present feverish sensation in palms and soles, and dry throat and mouth. Red thin tongue with scanty or no coating and wiry, thready and rapid pulse are signs of yin deficiency.

[Nursing Principle] Fostering yin and extinguishing wind; activating blood and dredging collateral.

[Suggested Formula] Yuyin Tongluo Decoction.

NURSING MEASURES

For patients with wind stroke, nurses should monitor the vital signs, and closely observe the body temperature, mental status, pupil, respiration, phlegm sound in the throat, heart rate, blood pressure, oxygen saturation of blood, sweating, tongue and pulse of the patients. They should also check the condition of vertigo and headache; the frequency, duration and degree of dizziness; the presence of chocking cough; the amount, color and texture of phlegm, stool and urine; the muscle force, muscle tone, and range of motion of the affected limb; the language ability; and changes in emotion of the patients. If the patient shows dysphoria, white complexion, cold limbs, profuse sweating, phlegm sound in the throat, unsmooth expectoration and rapid breathing, asphyxia caused by phlegm blocking the airway may be indicated; if the patient presents with headache, aggravated vomiting, white complexion, cold limbs, irregular breath and anisocoria, brain hernia may be implied; if the patient experiences suddenly raised blood pressure, slow pulse and deep breath, intracranial hemorrhage may be considered; if the patient manifests suddenly dropped blood pressure, dilated pupils, absent pupillary reaction to light, cold limbs, and faint pulse verging on expiry, departure of yin and yang may be indicated. In case of the above conditions, report to the doctor immediately and assist in emergency treatment.

Syndrome-Based Nursing Measures

1. Wind-Phlegm Obstructing Collateral Syndrome

(1) Daily life nursing. The ward should be warm, quiet and full of gentle light. The patients should

rest in bed, turn over regularly, move slowly, keep in a good limb position, take exercise of the affected limb 2~3 times a day, and be accompanied when getting off bed for activities. Put daily-used items near the patients. The patients should avoid bowing head deeply and turning around to prevent falls. Pay attention to skin hygiene, and make sure the sheets are dry and neat to prevent pressure sores. Keep the respiratory tract clean, pat on the patients' back regularly, remove the oral excretion timely, and rinse the mouth with jinyinhua gancao (honeysuckle flower and licorice root) liquid before and after meals, and before sleep. For patients with profuse sticky phlegm, take spray inhalation therapy with Chinese medicine by gentle manipulation.

(2) Diet nursing. The diet should be light. Meiguihua (rose flower) tea and juhua (chrysanthemum flower) tea are recommended. The patients should have small frequent meals and eat foods that extinguish wind and resolve dampness, such as shanzha (Chinese hawthorn fruit), jupi (tangerine peel), fuling (poria), heimuer (black fungus), kelp, buckwheat, corn, taro, fried scorpion and kumquat. Food therapy: wushe tianma (black-tail snake and tall gastrodis tuber) soup, lianzi facai shourou (lotus seed, hair weeds and lean pork) soup, xianmo luobotiao (fresh mushroom and white radish strip), and turou zicai doufu (rabbit meat, laver and tofu) soup. However, fatty, sweet, pungent, spicy, and dampness-generating foods should be avoided, such as liquor, mutton, dog meat, sea shrimp, sea crab, glutinous rice, sweet foods, and cold and raw fruit.

(3) Emotion nursing. Because the disease attacks suddenly with vertigo, nurses may use verbal enlightenment therapy to impart patients the pathogenesis of vertigo to help them to avoid the causes of disease in the future. Since the patients have difficulty in speaking, nurses should help them to do self-psychological adjustment in order to maintain mental health and prevent irritability from aggravating the disease.

(4) Medication nursing. Decoction should be taken warm after meals.

(5) Manipulation techniques. ① Acupressure therapy: select Shuigou (GV 26), Baihui (GV 20), Taiyang (EX − HN5), Fengchi (GB 20), Neiguan (PC 6), Jiquan (HT 1), Chize (LU 5), Weizhong (BL 40), Sanyinjiao (SP 6), Zusanli (ST 36), Fenglong (ST 40) and Hegu (LI 4); apply thumb kneading manipulation on each of the acupoints, 30 minutes each time, 4~5 times per day. And it is contraindicated in pregnancy. ② Patting therapy: select the bladder meridian of foot-taiyang along the side of spinal cord; apply gentle patting from bottom to top and outside to inside, 3~5 minutes each time, 2~3 times a day; and adjust the strength, duration and frequency of patting based on the amount of phlegm.

2. Wind Yang Stirring Upward Syndrome

(1) Daily life nursing. The ward should be cool, quiet, and full of gentle light. When vertigo occurs, the patients should rest in bed, turn over regularly, keep in a good limb position, reduce the visiting time and keep oral hygiene. For patients with dry lips, smear moisturizer on the lips. When the condition is stabilized, the patients should do moderate exercise to maintain sleep quality and a normal bowel movement.

（2）Diet nursing. The diet should be light. Juhua（chrysanthemum flower）tea is recommended. The patients should drink more water and eat foods that extinguish wind and clear heat, such as fried scorpion, lüdou（mung bean）, xianggu（lentinus edodes）, Chinese waxgourd, cucumber, snow pears and lianzi（lotus seed）. Food therapy: qincai juhua（celery and chrysanthemum flower）porridge, tianma（tall gastrodis tuber）stewed with jiayu（meat of soft-shelled turtles）. The patients should refrain from smoking, drinking alcohol, strong tea and coffee, and eating foods that are fried, pungent, spicy, sweet, greasy, fragrant, and dry-natured, such as mutton, dog meat, Chinese chives, garlic and scallion.

（3）Emotion nursing. Because the patients are newly ill and have excess heat syndrome, they may feel nervous and anxious. Nurses may use verbal enlightenment therapy to introduce them the environment in the hospital, know about their daily life habits and basic needs, help them solve problems, and make more explanation to eliminate their undesirable emotion.

（4）Medication nursing. Decoction should be taken warm or slightly cool after meals.

（5）Manipulation techniques. ① Acupressure therapy: select Shuigou（GV 26）, Baihui（GV 20）, Neiguan（PC 6）, Jiquan（HT 1）, Chize（LU 5）, Weizhong（BL 40）, Sanyinjiao（SP 6）, Zusanli（ST 36）, Taichong（LR 3）and Xingjian（LR 2）; apply thumb kneading manipulation on each of the acupoints, 30 minutes each time, 4～5 times per day. And it is contraindicated in pregnancy. ② Auricular pressure therapy: select the auricular points of shenmen（TF4）, liver（CO12）, spleen（CO13）, kidney（CO10）, heart（CO15）and sympathetic（AH6a）; apply specialized pasters on the points, press on each of them till the area turns hot and red, 4～5 times per day, and keep the pasters for 2～4 days. And it is contraindicated in pregnancy.

3. Phlegm Heat and Fu-Organ Excess Syndrome

（1）Daily life nursing. The ward should be cool, quiet, and full of gentle light. The patients should rest in bed, turn over regularly and keep in a good limb position with thin coverings. They should live a regular life with limited visiting time, and defecate regularly without overexertion and long-time squatting. Keep the respiratory tract clean and oral hygiene. When the condition is stabilized, they may do moderate exercise.

（2）Diet nursing. The diet should be light. Zhuli（bamboo sap）is recommended for frequent drinking. The patients should have small frequent meals, drink more water, and eat more fresh fruit and vegetables as well as foods that clear heat and resolve phlegm, such as watermelon, honey, yiyiren（coix seed）, lianzi（lotus seed）, shanyao（common yam rhizome）, luffa, fuling（poria）, white radishes and celery. Food therapy: biqi（waternut）stewed with jellyfish. The patients should refrain from smoking, drinking alcohol, coffee and strong tea, and eating foods that are pungent, spicy, fried, roasted, greasy and sweet.

（3）Emotion nursing. Because the patients have severe constipation, nurses may use verbal enlightenment therapy to tell them that the condition may be improved if they cooperate in treatment and maintain a normal bowel movement. Nurses should also help them adjust emotion to overcome the anxiety over defecation.

（4）Medication nursing. Shengdahuang（raw rhubarb root and rhizome）should be decocted later. Mangxiao（sodium sulphate）should be dissolved in water and taken. Decoction should be taken warm after meals. Stop taking the medicine once the disease is cured, to avoid consume the healthy qi. After taking purgative medicine, nurses should observe the therapeutic effect. If the patient has loose stool for 2~3 times within 3~5 hours, the medication should be stopped. If the patient fails to defecate, nurses should report to the doctor for further medication.

（5）Manipulation techniques. ① Acupressure therapy: select Shuigou（GV 26）, Baihui（GV 20）, Neiguan（PC 6）, Jiquan（HT 1）, Chize（LU 5）, Weizhong（BL 40）, Sanyinjiao（SP 6）, Zusanli（ST 36）, Quchi（LI 11）, Neiting（ST 44）, Weishu（BL 21）, Pishu（BL 20）, Fenglong（ST 40）, Zhongwan（CV 12）, Guanyuan（CV 4）and Yongquan（KI 1）; apply thumb kneading and one-finger pushing manipulations on each of the acupoints, 30 minutes each time, 4~5 times per day. And it is contraindicated in pregnancy. ② Auricular pressure therapy: select the auricular points of shenmen（TF4）, heart（CO15）, kidney（CO10）and sympathetic（AH6a）; apply specialized pasters on the points, press on each of them till the area turns hot and red, 4~5 times per day, and keep the pasters for 2~4 days. It is suitable for patients with insomnia and contraindicated in pregnancy.

4. Syndrome of Internal Block of Phlegm-Heat

（1）Daily life nursing. The ward should be cool and quiet with dim light, and near the nursing station. Nurses should increase the frequency of going rounds of the wards. The patients should rest in bed, turn over regularly, keep in a good limb position, with the head raised up 15° ~ 20° and side rotated. They should be cared by a specially-assigned person and avoid being moved about. For patients with dysphoria, make protective constraints to prevent injury and falling from bed. For patients with lockjaw, scrub teeth with smoked plums, or use mouth-gag with artificial teeth removed to prevent tongue biting. Follow the doctor's advice to apply oxygen inhalation, pay attention to oral hygiene, and keep the respiratory tract clean. For patients with high fever, apply a sponge bath with medicinal decoction, or cold compress on the head or above the major arteries（armpit, groin, etc.）.

（2）Diet nursing. For patients with unconsciousness, liquid diet should be given by nasal feeding. The diet should be light, nutritious, digestible and low in salt and fat. Erjiao Sanzhi Decoction, white radish juice, rice soup, milk and lotus root starch are recommended for nasal feeding. Eat foods that clear heat and resolve phlegm, such as snow pears and bananas. Follow the doctor's advice to eat heye maren（lotus leaf and hemp seed）porridge: decoct fresh leaves of field mint 30 g and fresh fineleaf schizonepeta spike 30 g, add stir-fried huomaren（hemp seed）50 g and jingmi（rice fruit）75 g into the decoction to make thin porridge, and remove the residue for nasal feeding for several times. Avoid fatty, too-sweet, pungent, aromatic, dry-natured and flatulent foods, such as chili, garlic, and mutton.

（3）Emotion nursing. Nurses should encourage patients' family members to accompany them as much as possible to provide psychological support.

（4）Medication nursing. Lingyangjiao（antelope horn）powder should be dissolved in water.

Shengshijueming (raw sea-ear shell) and guiban (tortoise plastron) should be decocted earlier. Decoction given by garage should be administered slowly, and medication can only continue after hearing the sound of swallowing to prevent choking cough. Pills should be dissolved in warm water before frequent nasal feeding in small amount, one pill every 6~8 hours.

(5) Manipulation techniques. Acupressure therapy: select Shuigou (GV 26), Suliao (GV 25), Baihui (GV 20), Neiguan (PC 6), Quchi (LI 11), Dazhui (GV 14), Hegu (LI 4) and Taichong (LR 3); apply thumb kneading manipulation, 30 minutes each time, 4~5 times per day. And it is contraindicated in pregnancy.

5. Phlegm Clouding Clear Orifice Syndrome

(1) Daily life nursing. The ward should be warm, dry, quiet, comfortable, dim-lighted and full of fresh air, and avoid strong and convective wind. The patients should rest in bed, keep warm, turn over regularly and keep in a good limb position with the head raised up slightly and side rotated. For patients with glossoptosis, fix the tongue with tongue pulling pliers. Follow the doctor's advice to apply oxygen inhalation, keep oral hygiene, and retain the urethral catheter. Be gentle and slow when using the bedpan, keep the perineal region clean and dry, and change contaminated sheets and clothes in time.

(2) Diet nursing. For patients in coma, liquid diet of low salt and fat should be given by nasal feeding. Follow the doctor's advice to supplement enteral nutrition. Food should be warm. Zhuli (bamboo sap) or shengjiang (fresh ginger) juice is recommended for nasal feeding. Eat warm-natured foods that eliminate phlegm and open orifice, such as congbai (scallion white), shanzha (Chinese hawthorn fruit), and pumpkins. Follow the doctor's advice to have shichangpu zhushen (grassleaf sweetflag rhizome and pig kidneys) porridge by nasal feeding, with the residue removed. Avoid fatty, too-sweet, raw, cold and flatulent foods.

(3) Emotion nursing. Nurses should encourage patients' family members to accompany them as much as possible to provide psychological support.

(4) Medication nursing. Decoction should be given warm by nasal feeding. Pills should be dissolved in warm water before frequent nasal feeding in small amount, one pill every 6~8 hours.

(5) Manipulation techniques. ① Paste application therapy: select Feishu (BL 13), Gaohuang (BL 43), Dingchuan (EX - B1) and Tiantu (CV 22); follow the doctor's advice to grind into powder medicinals that warm yang, resolve phlegm, restore consciousness and open orifices; mix the powder with shengjiang (fresh ginger) juice to make pastes, and apply them on the acupoints, 8 hours each time, once per day. ② Medicated pillow therapy: select Fengchi (GB 20), Fengfu (GV 16), Yamen (GV 15) and Dazhui (GV 14); follow the doctor's advice to use a medicated pillow filled with medicinals that awaken the brain and open the orifices. ③ Acupressure therapy: select Shuigou (GV 26), Suliao (GV 25), Baihui (GV 20), Neiguan (PC 6), Hegu (LI 4) and Taichong (LR 3); apply thumb kneading manipulation on each of the acupints, 30 minutes each time, and 4~5 times per day. And it is contraindicated in pregnancy.

6. Primordial Qi Collapse Syndrome

（1）Daily life nursing. The ward should be warm and quiet with dim light and fresh air. The patients should rest in bed, turn over regularly with the head turning to one side to prevent chocking caused by vomitus or oral phlegm from being inhaled into the respiratory tract. Follow the doctor's advice to apply oxygen inhalation. For patients with profuse sweat, wipe the sweat away and change the wet clothes and bedding timely. For patients with opened eyelids, cover the eyes with normal saline-soaked gauze, or smear chlortetracycline hydrochloride eye ointment. For patients breathing through opened mouth, cover the mouth with normal saline-soaked gauze. Pay attention to oral hygiene. Keep the respiratory tract clear, and the perineal region clean and dry. Follow the doctor's advice to retain the urethral catheter. Prepare the rescue equipment, and be ready to assist with tracheotomy.

（2）Diet nursing. Give liquid diet of low salt and fat by nasal feeding. Follow the doctor's advice to supplement enteral nutrition. Diet should be warm. Give adequate water and nutritious liquid foods by nasal feeding, such as fruit juice, rice soup, milk, vegetable soup and meat soup. Eat foods that replenish qi and stop collapse, such as oyster, shanyao (common yam rhizome), jingmi (rice fruit), dazao (Chinese date), tomato, tofu, mulberry, spinach, heimuer (black fungus) and shanzha (Chinese hawthorn fruit). Renshen (ginseng) porridge is recommended: use renshen (ginseng) 3 g, some crystal sugar, jingmi (rice fruit) 50~100 g, boil them together to make a mushy porridge, and remove the residue for nasal feeding.

（3）Emotion nursing. Nurses should communicate with patients' family members, and tell them not to be scared and anxious, but cooperate in treatment.

（4）Medication nursing. Renshen (ginseng) should be decocted separately, and then mix with the main decoction. Fuzi (monkshood) should be decocted earlier. Decoction should be prepared rapidly for frequently nasal feeding.

（5）Manipulation techniques. ① Moxibustion therapy: select Shenque (CV 8), Qihai (CV 6), Guanyuan (CV 4), Baihui (GV 20), Sanyinjiao (SP 6) and Zusanli (ST 36); place the moxa stick 2~3 centimeters away from the skin to perform mild moxibustion on each of the acupoints until the area turns red and the patient feels warm and comfortable without the sensation of burning pain, once per day. And it cannot be applied on the abdomen of pregnant women. ② Acupressure therapy: select Shuigou (GV 26), Suliao (GV 25), Baihui (GV 20), Neiguan (PC 6), Shenshu (BL 23), Baliao (BL 31~34), Zusanli (ST 36) and Tianshu (ST 25); apply thumb kneading manipulation on each of the acupoints, 30 minutes each time, 4~5 times per day. And it is contraindicated in pregnancy.

7. Qi Deficiency and Blood Stasis Syndrome

（1）Daily life nursing. The ward should be warm, quiet and full of fresh air, and avoid strong and convective wind. When the condition is stabilized, the patients should start rehabilitation therapy as early as possible. The patients should turn over regularly. Nurses should assist with the turn-over and back-patting every two hours, and massage on the bone protruding region with honghua (safflower) ethanol solution. Pay attention to skin hygiene and take regular warm sponge bath. Keep the respiratory tract clear. Teach the patients to practise efficient coughing to prevent phlegm retention. For patients with sticky phlegm, follow the doctor's advice to give spray inhalation therapy with Chinese medicine. Apply abdomen massage to maintain a normal bowel movement.

（2）Diet nursing. The patients may have general diet in small frequent meals. They should eat slowly to prevent chocking cough. Diet should be warm. Eat foods that replenish qi and dredge collateral, such as yiyiren（coix seed）, huangqi（astragalus root）, lianzi（lotus seed）, Chinese cabbage, Chinese waxgourd, luffa, muer（wood ear）, chixiaodou（adzuki bean）and shanzha（Chinese hawthorn fruit）. Meat should be supplemented, such as mutton and beef. Songziren（pine nut）and heizhima（black sesame）are recommended to moisten the intestine and relieve constipation. Food therapy: sheep stomach stewed with shanyao（common yam rhizome）, gouqi hetaoren jiding（Chinese wolfberry fruit, walnut, and diced chicken meat）. Avoid strong tonics and foods that are raw, cold, fatty and too-sweet.

（3）Emotion nursing. Since patients are recovering, nurses should encourage the patients to do moderate daily life activities and exercise that they can tolerate to reinforce their sense of self-worth.

（4）Medication nursing. Decoction should be taken warm before meals, multiple times in small portions.

（5）Manipulation techniques. ① Fumigating and washing therapy: luoshiteng（Chinese star jasmine stem）30 g, danggui（Chinese angelica）15 g, chuanxiong（Sichuan lovage root）15 g, honghua（safflower）15 g, sangzhi（mulberry twig）15 g, chuanwu（common monkshood mother root）9 g, and caowu（kusnezoff monkshood root）9 g; decoct the above ingredients and obtain 1~2 liters of decoction for fumigating the affected hand at a temperature of 50~70℃, and for washing the affected hand and swollen limb at a temperature of 37~40℃, 20 minutes each time, twice per day. This therapy is suitable for patients with swollen hands at recovery phase. ② Moxibustion therapy: select Guanyuan（CV 4）, Tianshu（ST 25）, Shenque（CV 8）and Qihai（CV 6）, choose 1~2 acupoint(s) each time; place the moxa stick 2~3 centimeters away from the skin to perform mild moxibustion on each of the acupoints until the area turns red and the patient feels warm and comfortable without the sensation of burning pain, once per day. And it cannot be applied on the abdomen of pregnant women. ③ Healthcare massage therapy: take a supine position, apply clockwise pressing and rubbing manipulations around the navel until there is heat sensation in the abdomen, 20~30 cycles each time, 2~3 times per day. It is suitable for patients with constipation. ④ Hot compress therapy: put a hot water bag on the lower abdomen. It is suitable for patients with uroschesis. And it is contraindicated in pregnancy. ⑤ Nose insertion therapy: grind into powder equal amount of chuanwu（common monkshood mother root）, caowu（kusnezoff monkshood root）, xixin（Manchurian wild ginger）, sanqi（pseudoginseng root）and zaojiao（Chinese honeylocust spine）; insert 2 g of the powder into the nostril（into the right nostril for cases with deviated mouth on the left-side, and vice versa）. It is suitable for patients with deviated mouth and eyes, and is contraindicated in pregnancy.

8. Yin Deficiency Stirring Wind Syndrome

（1）Daily life nursing. The ward should be cool, quiet, dim-lighted and full of fresh air, and avoid strong and convective wind. When the condition is stabilized, the patients should start rehabilitation therapy as early as possible. The patients should turn over regularly. Nurses should assist with the turn-over and back-patting every two hours. The patients should live a regular life, have adequate sleep, avoid staying up late, and reduce the visiting time. Put daily used items near the patients. Pay attention to skin hygiene. Take a hot foot bath every night before sleep. For patients with dry lips, smear moisturizer on the lips.

（2）Diet nursing. The diet should be light. The patients should have small frequent meals, drink more water, and eat more fresh fruit and vegetables. Biqi doujiang (waternut and soy bean milk) is recommended. Eat foods that replenish yin and nourish blood, such as gouqizi (Chinese wolfberry fruit), yin'er (tremella), heizhima (black sesame), muer (wood ear), black rice, haishen (sea cucumber), meat of soft-shelled turtles, black-boned chicken, and duck meat. Food therapy: tianma zhu'nao (tall gastrodis tuber and pig brain) porridge, baihe lianzi yiren (lily bulb, lotus seed, and coix seed) porridge, yulan (yulan magnolia) fish meat ball, garlic stewed with eggplant. They may eat suanzaoren (spiny date seed) extract or milk to improve sleep, and bananas or honey to keep a normal bowel movement. They should also refrain from drinking strong tea and coffee, and eating foods that are pungent, spicy and fire-generating.

（3）Emotion nursing. Because the patients have yin deficiency with a long course of disease, they may suffer from heart vexation. Nurses may use verbal enlightenment therapy to explain to the patients that undesirable emotion would aggravate the disease, so they should learn to regulate their emotion. Nurses may also use emotional transference and dispositional change therapy, such as listening to light music, to distract the patients' attention in order to ease their mind and improve sleep. Nurses should often communicate with doctors and patients' family, help patients solve difficulties, and assist with reducing the medical cost in order to ease their worries.

（4）Medication nursing. Shenglonggu (raw dinosaur bone), shengmuli (raw oyster shell), daizheshi (hematite) and guiban (tortoise plastron) should be decocted earlier. Gouteng (gambir plant) should be decocted later. Decoction should be taken warm before meals, multiple times in small portions.

（5）Manipulation techniques. ① Paste application therapy: select Yongquan (KI 1); apply smashed garlic on the acupoint, once per night; it is suitable for patients with insomnia. Apply smashed castor leaves on deviated parts on the face; or grind into fine powder jiangcan (stiff silkorm) 30 g, baifuzi (monkshood) 15 g, and xiewei (scorpion tail) 15 g, blend the powder with yellow wine to make a paste, and apply it on deviated part, of the face; it is contraindicated in pregnancy. ② Acupressure therapy: select Shenmen (HT 7), Baihui (GV 20), Sanyinjiao (SP 6), Laogong (PC 8) and Yongquan (KI 1); apply thumb kneading manipulation on each of the acupoints before sleep until the area turns hot or the patient has the feelings of soreness, numbness, distension and heaviness in the area; once per day. And it is contraindicated in pregnancy. ③ Water acupuncture therapy: select Jianjing (GB

21）, Quchi（LI 11）, Neiguan（PC 6）, Fengshi（GB 31）and Zusanli（ST 36）; inject compound danshen（danshen root）injection into the acupoints, 2～3 acupoints each time. ④ Ricefield eel blood therapy: prick the heads of two ricefield eels with a needle for blood, and smear the blood on the paralyzed side of the face（to smear the blood on the right side of the face for patients with the face deviated to the left, and vice versa）, 30 minutes each time, and once every three days. And it is suitable for patients with deviated mouth and eyes.

Patient Education

The ward should be quiet, comfortable, and full of gentle light. The patients should live a regular life, balance work and rest, and avoid overstrain and staying up late. Keep the paralyzed limb warm. The patients may take a short-time slow walk or do slight exercise in the sunlight when the day is sunny and windless. The movement should be slow during the change of body position or turning head. Avoid movements that may increase the intracranial pressure. Encourage the patients to talk, formulate the rehabilitation plan as early as possible and adjust it if necessary. The patients should be accompanied when moving around to prevent falls, adjust the clothing to match the change of weather and prevent colds, keep a normal bowel movement, and defecate regularly without overexertion and long-time squatting. Keep skin hygiene, change body position regularly, and take a warm sponge bath to prevent pressure sores. Tie an information wrist strap on patients' wrist so that the patients can be found easily in case they are missing.

The diet should be light, nutritious and digestible with low fat, low salt, high carbohydrate, high fiber, and high protein. Patients should eat slowly without talking. Encourage the patients to eat by themselves, keep the environment quiet, and reduce the disruptive factors. For patients with dysphagia, eat pasty foods for multiple times in small portions. The patients should not be too hungry or too full and should refrain from smoking, drinking alcohol, coffee and strong tea, and eating foods that induce or aggravate disease, such as rooster meat, pig's head meat, and seafood. Likewise, pungent, spicy, greasy, raw, cold, sweet, fried and roasted foods should be avoided.

The patients should stay in a happy mood, and avoid being anxious, angry, worried, or lonely. Encourage their family members to accompany them as much as possible, provide them with mental support, and try to protect their self-esteem. Always be patient and kind to the patients, and constantly comfort, advise and encourage them to help them rebuild confidence. For patients with depression or mood fluctuations after stroke, they should be noticed and treated at the first time to prevent suicide or self-mutilation.

In medication, the patients should follow the doctor's advice strictly and don't take or stop medicine without notice. For patients with discomfort after taking medicine, report to the doctors and nurses in time. Decoction should be taken multiple times in small portions to prevent choking cough. For patients with unconsciousness, use nasal feeding, and closely observe their reactions after taking medicine.

The patients could often massage Baihui（GV 20）, Sishencong（EX－HN1）, Shenting（EX－HN1）, Jiquan（HT 1）, Chize（LU 5）, Jianyu（LI 15）, Hegu（LI 4）, Taixi（KI 3）, Shenmen（HT

7）, Weizhong（BL 40）, Yanglingquan（GB 34）and Zusanli（ST 36）; apply kneading, pressing, and rolling manipulations on each of the acupoints until the area turns hot or the patient has the feelings of soreness, numbness, distension and heaviness in the area. Follow the doctor's advice to decoct medicinals that relax sinew, dredge collateral, activate blood, resolve blood stasis, warm meridian and dissipate cold to fumigate and bathe the paralyzed side.

After discharged from hospital, the patients should have regular reexamination and treat the primary disease actively to prevent the second attack of wind stroke, or wind stroke sequelae, such as dementia, depression, or depressive psychosis. Pay attention to the change of blood pressure. In case of headache, vertigo, vomiting, raised blood pressure, or aggravating limb numbness, it may be considered as the prodrome of wind stroke, and the patients should be sent to the hospital immediately by the family members.

第八节　呕　　吐

呕吐,是指因外感或内伤,或因头部损伤、妊娠、药物中毒等原因,导致胃失和降,胃气上逆,以胃内容物从口中吐出,或恶心作哕为临床特征的病证。西医的急性胃炎、慢性胃炎、病毒性肝炎、急性胰腺炎、急性胆囊炎、肠梗阻、尿毒症,以呕吐为主要表现的,可参照本节进行护理。

一、病因病机

呕吐的病因包括饮食失宜、情志失调、外邪犯胃、脾胃虚弱。病人暴饮暴食,过食生冷、辛辣、肥甘、油腻、腥秽的食物,嗜饮酒浆,或食用不洁食物,可损伤脾胃,使饮食停滞,阻滞气机,发为呕吐。急躁恼怒伤肝,肝郁横逆犯胃,或忧思抑郁伤脾,纳食不化,阻遏气机,可致胃气上逆,发为呕吐。风寒凝滞中阳,或暑湿阻滞中焦,均可因邪聚中焦,导致呕吐。病人素体脾虚,或久病过劳,损伤脾阳胃阴,亦可发为呕吐。

呕吐的病机为胃失和降,胃气上逆。病位在胃,与肝、脾有关。呕吐初起多为实证。若迁延日久,损伤脾胃,可由实转虚。

二、常见证型

(一)辨证要点

1. 辨虚实　根据病因、起病速度、病程长短,以及呕吐物的量、味等来辨别。若因外邪、饮食、气郁、痰饮而起,发病急,病程短,呕声响亮,呕吐量多,酸腐臭秽,脉实有力,多为实证。若因脾胃虚寒、胃阴不足所致,起病缓,病程长,呕声低微,呕吐量少,酸臭不甚,常伴有精神萎靡,倦怠乏力,脉弱无力,则多为虚证。

2. 辨呕吐物　根据呕吐物的颜色、质地、味道等来辨别证型。若呕吐物酸腐难闻,或为未消化的食物,则多为饮食停滞。若呕吐物为黄水,味苦,多为肝气犯胃。若呕吐物为清水痰涎,多为痰饮内阻。若无呕吐物,或呕吐物量少,则多为胃阴不足。

(二)证候分型

1. 外邪犯胃证

[主要证候]突发呕吐,脘腹满闷;若感受风寒,可兼有发热,恶寒,头痛,周身酸楚或酸痛,舌苔薄白,脉浮紧;若感受风热,可兼有恶风,头身疼痛,汗出,舌尖红,苔薄白或薄黄,脉浮数;若感受暑湿,可兼有胸脘痞闷,身热心烦,口渴,舌质红,苔黄腻,脉濡数。

[证候分析]外邪犯胃,胃失和降,胃气上逆,故突发呕吐,脘腹满闷;邪束肌表,营卫失和,故恶寒,发热,头身疼痛。

[护治原则] 疏邪解表,和胃降逆。

[常用方剂] 外感风寒,用藿香正气散;外感风热,用银翘散;外感暑湿,用黄连香薷饮。

2. 饮食停滞证

[主要证候] 呕吐酸腐量多,或吐出未消化的食物,嗳气厌食,脘腹胀满,得食更甚,吐后反快,大便秘结或溏泄,气味臭秽;舌苔厚腻,脉滑实有力。

[证候分析] 饮食不节,胃气壅滞,食随浊气上逆,故呕吐酸腐;食滞中焦,气机不利,故嗳气厌食,脘腹胀满;吐后气机得通,故吐后反快;中焦气机升降失常,大肠传导失司,故大便秘结或溏泄,气味臭秽;舌苔厚腻,脉滑实有力,均为饮食停滞之象。

[护治原则] 消食化滞,和胃降逆。

[常用方剂] 保和丸。

3. 肝气犯胃证

[主要证候] 呕吐吞酸,或干呕泛恶,脘胁胀痛,烦闷不舒,嗳气频频,每因情志不遂而发作或加重;舌边红,苔薄腻或微黄,脉弦。

[证候分析] 肝气郁结,横逆犯胃,其气上逆,故呕吐吞酸,嗳气频频;肝循两胁,胃居中脘,肝气犯胃,故脘胁胀痛;情志相激,肝郁加重,横犯胃土,故每因情志不遂而发作或加重;舌边红,苔薄腻或微黄,脉弦,均为肝气郁滞之象。

[护治原则] 疏肝和胃,降逆止呕。

[常用方剂] 四逆散合半夏厚朴汤。

4. 痰饮内阻证

[主要证候] 呕吐物多为清水痰涎,或胃部如囊裹水,胸脘痞闷,纳食不佳,头晕,心悸,或逐渐消瘦,或呕而肠鸣;舌苔白滑而腻,脉沉弦滑。

[证候分析] 痰饮内阻,胃气上逆,故呕吐痰涎清水,胸脘痞闷,或胃部如囊裹水;饮邪上犯,清阳不展,清窍失养,故头晕,心悸;舌苔白滑而腻,脉沉弦滑,均为痰饮内阻之象。

[护治原则] 温化痰饮,和胃降逆。

[常用方剂] 小半夏汤合苓桂术甘汤。

5. 脾胃虚寒证

[主要证候] 饮食稍多即欲呕吐,时发时止,食入难化,胸脘痞闷,不思饮食,面色㿠白,倦怠乏力,四肢不温,口干不欲饮或喜热饮,大便稀溏;舌质淡,苔薄白,脉濡弱或沉。

[证候分析] 脾虚不运,胃气上逆,故饮食稍多即易呕吐,时发时止;中阳不振,阳气不达四末,故面色㿠白,倦怠乏力,四肢不温;脾虚运化失常,故大便溏薄;舌质淡,苔薄白,脉濡弱或沉,均为脾胃虚寒之象。

[护治原则] 温中健脾,和胃降逆。

[常用方剂] 理中丸。

6. 胃阴不足证

[主要证候] 呕吐反复发作,或时作干呕,恶心,胃中嘈杂,似饥而不欲食,口燥咽干;舌红少津,苔少,脉细数。

[证候分析] 胃阴不足,不得润降,故呕吐反复发作,或时作干呕;胃阴亏虚,其受纳腐熟功能失

132

常,故胃中嘈杂,似饥而不欲食;胃阴不足,津液不能上承于口,故口燥咽干;舌红少津,苔少,脉细数,均为阴虚有热之象。

〔护治原则〕滋养胃阴,降逆止呕。

〔常用方剂〕麦门冬汤。

三、护理措施

对于呕吐的病人,应观察呕吐的次数、程度、持续时间;呕吐物的量、色、质、气味;腹胀的部位、程度、持续时间、诱发因素;腹痛的部位、程度、性质、次数、持续时间、诱发因素;有无恶心、嗳气、反酸、呛咳,以及腹部有无肠形包块。注意观察神志、面色、寒热、出汗、血压、舌脉。询问食量、胃口、二便、饮酒史以及情志状态。若呕吐物中带有咖啡样物或鲜血,或病人出现冷汗淋漓,面色苍白,烦躁不安,头痛,或病人出现发绀,均应立即报告医生。

(一)辨证施护

1. 外邪犯胃证

(1)生活起居护理　居室应避风。卧床休息,呕吐后用温开水漱口。保护脘腹,以避免复感外邪,可用手掌自上向下按摩胃脘部。外寒者,应注意保暖,可在脘腹部热敷。

(2)饮食护理　风寒者,可饮紫苏叶茶、生姜红糖水;宜食温中散寒的食物,如白胡椒、芥菜、小茴香、葱白;不宜食寒凉的食物,如鸭肉、螃蟹、香蕉。风热者,可饮银花茶、菊花茶;宜食疏风清热的食物,如白萝卜、薄荷叶。暑湿者,宜食清暑化湿的食物,如西瓜、荷叶、赤小豆、绿豆、白扁豆;不宜食辛辣、肥甘的食物。

(3)情志护理　护士可运用移情易性疗法,鼓励病人闭目养神,听轻音乐,以转移注意力。

(4)用药护理　中药汤剂宜武火快煎,饭后热服,少量频服,服后以微微出汗为宜。可在服药前将少许生姜汁滴于舌根以止呕。

(5)操作技术　①敷贴疗法:取中脘、内关,用荜茇、川椒,研磨成粉后与生姜汁调成糊状敷贴,每次12小时,每日1次;适用于外感风寒者。②穴位按摩法:取内关、中脘、胃俞、足三里、外关、大椎,用拇指揉法、摩法、一指禅推法,按摩至局部发热或有酸麻重胀感,每日1次;孕妇禁用。

2. 饮食停滞证

(1)生活起居护理　居室温暖干燥,空气新鲜,不可有强风、对流风。注意保持呼吸道通畅,取侧卧位,头可稍抬高。鼓励病人尽量将胃内容物吐出,可轻拍其背部,必要时使用吸引器。呕吐后用温水漱口,及时清理呕吐物,更换被污染的衣被。可进行适量锻炼,以不劳累为宜,以保持大便通畅。

(2)饮食护理　必要时禁食12~24小时。待呕吐停止后,酌情予半流食。清淡饮食,由素到荤,少量多次。可饮山楂麦芽茶、生姜焦米茶。宜食消食导滞的食物,如陈皮、白萝卜、米醋、金橘、萝卜缨、鸡内金。不宜食油腻、炙煿的食物,如肥肉、烤肉、油条。

(3)情志护理　病人症状较重,护士可鼓励家属多陪伴病人,安慰病人,以增加安全感,避免忧思、焦虑。

(4)用药护理　中药汤剂宜浓煎,饭后温服。

（5）操作技术　①敷贴疗法：取中脘、内关，用姜汁炒黄连、紫苏叶、白蔻仁、神曲，研磨成粉后与生姜汁调成糊状敷贴，每次12小时，每日1次。②涌吐法：以压舌板或羽毛刺激咽部，或饮温盐水后用手指探吐，以涌吐宿食；适用于欲吐不得吐者。③攻下法：遵医嘱用生大黄粉3~6 g吞服；适用于大便不通者，孕妇禁用。④穴位按摩法：取内关、中脘、胃俞、足三里、梁门、天枢，用拇指揉法、摩法、一指禅推法，按摩至局部发热或有酸麻重胀感，每日1次；孕妇禁用。

3. 肝气犯胃证

（1）生活起居护理　居室凉爽安静，空气新鲜。卧床休息，睡眠充足。

（2）饮食护理　若呕吐严重，可禁食4~6小时，待呕吐停止后，从流食、半流食、软食，逐渐过渡到普食，少食多餐。可饮玫瑰花茶、鲜芦根茶。宜食疏肝理气的食物，如金橘、橙子、佛手、白萝卜。戒烟限酒，不宜食油腻、辛辣、易产气的食物，如红薯。

（3）情志护理　由于病人每因情志不遂而发病或症状加重，所以保持情绪稳定非常重要。护士可运用移情易性疗法，转移其注意力。了解病人急躁、恼怒、郁闷的原因，鼓励家属多陪伴病人，引导病友间多沟通交流，营造轻松的氛围。

（4）用药护理　中药汤剂宜浓煎，饭后温服，少量频服。

（5）操作技术　①敷贴疗法：取中脘、足三里、神阙，用吴茱萸3 g，研磨成粉后与生姜汁调成糊状敷贴，每日1次；或取涌泉，用鲜地龙若干条，洗净泥土，撒上白砂糖，化为糊状后与面粉调成药饼敷贴。②点穴疗法：取内关，用力按1分钟；适用于呕吐剧烈时。③水针疗法：取单侧足三里，用维生素B$_6$注射液进行穴位注射；适用于嗳气剧烈者。④穴位按摩法：取内关、中脘、胃俞、足三里、太冲、期门，用拇指揉法、摩法、一指禅推法，按摩至局部发热或有酸麻重胀感，每日1次；孕妇禁用。

4. 痰饮内阻证

（1）生活起居护理　居室温暖干燥，空气新鲜，不可有强风、对流风。卧床休息，取坐位或半仰卧位，注意腹部保暖，呕吐时将头偏向一侧。

（2）饮食护理　生姜汁10~15 mL，频频用米汤送服以止呕。宜食健脾利湿的食物，如砂仁、红豆、荷叶、薏苡仁。不可饮酒，不宜食生冷、油腻的食物。

（3）情志护理　病人病程长，病情重，护士可运用语言开导疗法，耐心回答病人的疑问，以避免忧思、焦虑。

（4）用药护理　中药汤剂宜浓煎，饭后温服。

（5）操作技术　①敷贴疗法：取中脘、内关、神阙，用清半夏粉与生姜汁调成糊状敷贴，每次12小时，每日1次；孕妇禁用。②穴位按摩法：取内关、中脘、胃俞、足三里、丰隆、公孙，用拇指揉法、摩法、一指禅推法，按摩至局部发热或有酸麻重胀感，每日1次；孕妇禁用。

5. 脾胃虚寒证

（1）生活起居护理　居室温暖干燥，安静舒适，光线明亮，空气新鲜，不可有强风、对流风。卧床休息，注意腹部保暖。做好皮肤护理，每2小时协助翻身1次，以预防压疮。

（2）饮食护理　饮食宜多样化且色香味俱全，温热饮食，少食多餐。可饮生姜陈皮红糖水。宜食散寒和胃的食物，如莲子、芡实、茯苓、山药、薏苡仁。食疗方：猪肚粥、丁香姜糖。忌酒、韭菜、辣椒、咖啡，不宜食生冷、硬固的食物。

（3）情志护理　病人久病体虚，护士可运用语言开导疗法、顺意疗法、音乐疗法，向病人介绍本病的有关知识,关心体贴病人,满足其合理要求,请病人聆听舒缓的音乐,使之保持心情舒畅,避免悲观、消沉。

(4)用药护理 中药汤剂宜浓煎,饭前热服,少量频服。服药时可加生姜汁数滴,轻抚病人的背部。服药后静卧。

(5)操作技术 ①药熨疗法:取胃脘部,遵医嘱用温中健脾、和胃降逆的中药,研磨炒热后装入布袋中,制成温度为60~70℃的中药热罨包,药熨20分钟,每日1次;孕妇禁用。②灸法:取隐白、脾俞,用温和灸,艾条燃着端悬于施灸部位上,距离皮肤2~3厘米,灸至病人有温热舒适无灼痛的感觉,皮肤稍有红晕,每日1次。③穴位按摩法:取内关、中脘、胃俞、足三里、脾俞、公孙,用拇指揉法、摩法、一指禅推法,按摩至局部发热或有酸麻重胀感,每日1次;孕妇禁用。

6. 胃阴不足证

(1)生活起居护理 居室凉爽安静。卧床休息,不要过多翻身。遵医嘱留取呕吐物送检。保持口腔清洁,饭后及呕吐后用淡盐水或金银花甘草液漱口。睡眠充足,不看刺激性的书刊和电视节目。

(2)饮食护理 饮食宜清淡、细软、多汁。可饮香姜牛奶、甘蔗生姜汁、羊乳饮,或用鲜芦根30 g,铁皮石斛、麦冬各10 g,煎水代茶饮。宜食益胃养阴的食物,如荸荠、酸枣、莲子、百合、桑椹、藕节。食疗方:乌梅蜂蜜膏。若大便秘结,宜多吃高纤维的蔬菜以通便,不宜使用泻下剂。忌烟酒、大葱、韭菜、大蒜,不宜食肥甘、辛辣、香燥的食物。

(3)情志护理 病人有虚火且病程较长,护士可运用语言开导疗法和移情易性疗法,向病人解释病情,或转移病人的注意力,以避免恐惧、思虑,使其保持情绪稳定。

(4)用药护理 中药汤剂宜文火久煎、浓煎,饭前微温缓进,少量频服。服药前可进食少量易消化的食物,或在汤剂中滴入少许生姜汁,或嚼服生姜后再喝药。服药后静卧。

(5)操作技术 ①穴位按摩法:取内关、中脘、胃俞、足三里、脾俞、三阴交,用拇指揉法、摩法、一指禅推法,按摩至局部发热或有酸麻重胀感,每日1次;孕妇禁用。②保健按摩疗法:取胃脘部,用手掌顺时针方向摩至发热,每次10分钟,饭前及饭后进行。

(二)健康教育

居室安静避风,空气新鲜,避免强光及噪音刺激。起居有常,劳逸适度,适量锻炼,不可过劳。注意胃部保暖,谨防外感。

饮食宜清淡、营养、易消化。饮食有节,少食多餐,注意饮食卫生。进食宜慢,不可过饥、过饱。若对寒凉水果不适应,可用温水浸泡后食用。忌烟酒、浓茶、咖啡,不宜食生冷、肥腻、甜黏、辛辣、易产气的食物。

注意调畅情志,保持心情舒畅。

若频繁呕吐,应及时查明病因。

Section 8　Vomiting

Vomiting is a disease characterized by stomach contents being vomited out of the mouth or by nausea and retching. It is caused by stomach qi failing to descend but ascend instead due to external affection or internal damage as well as head damage, pregnancy or drug poisoning. This section may be referred to for the nursing of some diseases with vomiting as the main manifestation, such as acute and chronic gastritis, viral hepatitis, acute pancreatitis, acute cholecystitis, intestinal obstruction and uremia in Western medicine.

ETIOLOGY AND PATHOGENESIS

The etiology includes improper diet, emotional disorder, exogenous pathogen invading the stomach and spleen-stomach weakness. Improper diet, such as gluttony, overeating raw, cold, pungent, spicy, fatty, too-sweet, greasy and fishy foods, over-drinking alcohol, or eating contaminated foods, may damage the spleen and stomach, cause food retention and obstruction of qi movement, and subsequently lead to vomiting. Impatience and anger damage the liver and cause liver depression that transversely invades the stomach, or contemplation damages the spleen and causes food retention and obstruction of qi movement, all these may lead to stomach qi ascending counterflow and cause vomiting. Wind cold congealing middle yang, or summer-heat dampness obstructing the middle energizer, both may result in vomiting due to pathogen gathering in the middle energizer. Constitutional spleen deficiency, prolonged disease or overstrain, all may damage spleen yang and stomach yin, leading to vomiting.

The pathogenesis is stomach qi failing to descend but ascend instead. The disease is located in the stomach and involves the liver and spleen. In the initial phase, vomiting belongs to excess syndrome. It will transform from excess to deficiency syndrome as the disease becomes prolonged and damages the spleen and stomach.

COMMON SYNDROMES

Key Points in Syndrome Differentiation

1. Differentiation of Deficiency from Excess Syndrome

The differentiation is based on the causes, onset speed and course of disease as well as the amount and smell of the vomitus. Excess syndrome is usually caused by external pathogens, diet, qi depression, phlegm and fluid retention, and demonstrates acute onset, short course, vomiting with loud voice, large amount of vomitus, sour, putrid and foul-smelling odor, and replete forceful pulse. However, deficiency syndrome is usually caused by deficiency-cold of the spleen and stomach and stomach yin insufficiency, and exhibits gradual onset, long course, vomiting with faint low voice, small amount of vomitus, mild sour and foul-smelling odor, often accompanied with listlessness, lassitude, lack of strength and weak forceless pulse.

2. Differentiation of Vomitus

The differentiation is based on the color, texture and smell of the vomitus. If the vomitus is putrid sour, or undigested food, it mostly caused by food retention. If it is yellow water with bitter taste, it mostly pertains to liver qi invading the stomach. If it is clear water or phlegm-drool, it is mostly due to internal obstruction of phlegm and fluid retention. If there is no or little volume of vomitus, it is mostly caused by stomach yin insufficiency.

Syndrome Differentiation

1. Syndrome of External Pathogen Invading the Stomach

[Clinical Manifestations] Sudden vomiting, and epigastric and abdominal fullness and oppression. For wind-cold cases, the concurrent symptoms include fever, aversion to cold, headache, generalized aching pain, white thin tongue coating and float tight pulse. For wind-heat cases, the symptoms include aversion to wind, headache, generalized pain, sweating, red-tipped tongue with thin white or thin yellow tongue coating and float rapid pulse. For summerheat-dampness cases, the symptoms are chest and gastric stuffiness and oppression, generalized fever, heart vexation, thirst, red tongue with yellow slimy coating and soggy rapid pulse.

[Manifestations Analysis] External pathogen invading the stomach causes stomach qi failing to descend but ascend instead, leading to sudden vomiting as well as epigastric and abdominal fullness and oppression. Pathogen fettering the exterior triggers disharmony between the nutrient and defensive aspects, causing aversion to cold, fever, headache and generalized pain.

[Nursing Principle] Dispersing pathogen and releasing the exterior; harmonizing the stomach and descending adverse qi.

[Suggested Formula] Wind-cold: Huoxiang Zhengqi Powder; wind-heat: Yinqiao Powder; summerheat-dampness: Huanglian Xiangru Decoction.

2. Syndrome of Food Retention

[Clinical Manifestations] Large amount of sour putrid vomitus or undigested food, belching, anorexia, epigastric and abdominal fullness and distention aggravated after meal while alleviated after vomiting, constipation or loose stool with foul smell, thick slimy tongue coating, and slippery, replete and forceful pulse.

[Manifestations Analysis] Improper diet and stomach qi stagnation makes counterflow of turbid qi accompanied with food, resulting in sour putrid vomitus. Food stagnating in the middle energizer leads to disturbance of qi movement, causing belching, anorexia and epigastric and abdominal fullness and distention. Qi movement is disinhibited after vomiting, so epigastric and abdominal fullness and distention is alleviated. Disorder of qi movement in the middle energizer causes conveyance dysfunction of large intestine, leading to constipation or loose stool with foul smell. Thick slimy tongue coating and slippery, replete and forceful pulse are signs of food retention.

[Nursing Principle] Promoting digestion and resolving food retention; harmonizing the stomach and descending adverse qi.

[Suggested Formula] Baohe Pills.

3. Syndrome of Liver Qi Invading the Stomach

[Clinical Manifestations] Vomiting with acid regurgitation, or retching and upflowed nausea, distending pain in the epigastrium and rib-side, vexation and oppression, frequent belching, symptoms induced or aggravated by emotional frustration, tongue with red-margins and thin slimy or slightly yellow coating, and wiry pulse.

[Manifestations Analysis] Liver qi depression transversely invades the stomach and causes ascending of stomach qi, causing vomiting, acid regurgitation, and frequent belching. Liver meridian runs along both rib-sides, and the stomach locates in the upper abdomen. Liver qi transversely invades the stomach, so there is distending pain in the epigastrium and rib-side. Emotional frustration aggravates liver depression that transversely invades the stomach, so symptoms are induced or aggravated by emotional frustration. Tongue with red-margins and thin slimy or slightly yellow coating and wiry pulse are signs of liver qi depression and stagnation.

[Nursing Principle] Soothing the liver and harmonizing the stomach; descending adverse qi and arresting vomiting.

[Suggested Formula] Sini Powder and Banxia Houpo Decoction.

4. Syndrome of Internal Obstruction of Phlegm and Fluid-Retention

[Clinical Manifestations] Vomiting watery fluids, phlegm and saliva, or stomach filled with water, chest and gastric stuffiness and oppression, anorexia, dizziness, palpitation, or gradual emaciation, or vomiting with borborygmus, white, slippery and slimy tongue coating, and sunken, wiry and slippery pulse.

[Manifestations Analysis] Internal obstruction of phlegm and fluid-retention causes stomach qi counterflow, leading to vomiting watery fluids, phlegm and salivation, or stomach filled with water, chest and gastric stuffiness and oppression. Pathogenic fluid-retention invading upward leads to failure of clear yang to ascend and malnourishment of clear orifices, so dizziness and palpitation are felt. White, slippery and slimy tongue coating and sunken, wiry and slippery pulse are signs of internal obstruction of phlegm and fluid-retention.

[Nursing Principle] Warming and resolving phlegm and fluid retention; harmonizing the stomach and descending adverse qi.

[Suggested Formula] Xiao Banxia Decoction and Linggui Zhugan Decoction.

5. Syndrome of Deficiency-Cold of the Spleen and Stomach

[Clinical Manifestations] Intermittent vomiting easily triggered by little more intake of food, difficult digestion, chest and gastric stuffiness and oppression, poor appetite, bright white complexion, lassitude, lack of strength, cold limbs, thirst without desire to drink or preference for hot drinks, thin loose stool, pale tongue with white thin coating, and soggy weak or sunken pulse.

〔Manifestations Analysis〕 Dysfunction of the spleen in transportation and transformation due to its deficiency causes stomach qi ascending counterflow, causing intermittent vomiting easily triggered by little more intake of food. Devitalization of middle yang makes yang qi fail to reach the four extremities, leading to bright white complexion, lassitude, lack of strength, and cold limbs. Dysfunction of the spleen in transportation and transformation due to its deficiency also causes thin loose stool. Pale tongue with white thin coating and soggy weak or sunken pulse are manifestations of deficiency-cold of the spleen and stomach.

〔Nursing Principle〕 Warming the middle and invigorating the spleen; harmonizing the stomach and descending adverse qi.

〔Suggested Formula〕 Lizhong Pills.

6. Syndrome of Stomach Yin Insufficiency

〔Clinical Manifestations〕 Recurrent vomiting, or frequent retching, nausea, gastric upset, feeling like hunger but without desire to eat, dry mouth and throat, red tongue with scanty fluids and coating, and thready rapid pulse.

〔Manifestations Analysis〕 Stomach yin insufficiency cannot moisten the stomach and descend stomach qi, leading to recurrent vomiting or frequent retching. Stomach yin insufficiency also causes failure of the stomach to govern reception and decomposition, resulting in gastric upset and feeling like hunger but without desire to eat. Stomach yin insufficiency causes failure to convey fluids upward to the mouth, so dry mouth and throat are felt. Red tongue with scanty fluids and coating and thready rapid pulse are signs of yin deficiency with heat.

〔Nursing Principle〕 Nourishing stomach yin, descending adverse qi and arresting vomiting.

〔Suggested Formula〕 Maimendong Decoction.

Nursing Measures

For cases with vomiting, nurses should observe the frequency, severity, and duration of vomiting; the amount, color, texture and smell of vomitus; the location, severity, duration and inducing factors of abdominal distention; the location, severity, nature, frequency, duration and inducing factors of abdominal pain; and the presence or absence of nausea, belching, acid regurgitation, chocking cough and intestine-shaped mass in the abdomen. They should also check the consciousness, complexion, sensation of cold or heat, sweating, blood pressure, tongue and pulse, and inquire the patients about their appetite, urination, defecation, alcohol intake history and the emotional state. If there is coffee-colored or bloody vomitus, or dripping cold sweating, pale complexion, dysphoria and headache, or cyanosis, it is advisable to report to the doctors immediately.

Syndrome-Based Nursing Measures

1. Syndrome of External Pathogen Invading the Stomach

（1）Daily life nursing. The ward should be away from wind. The patients should rest in bed, and rinse the mouth with warm water after vomiting. Keep the epigastric region and abdomen warm to prevent re-infection with external pathogens, and massage the epigastric region from top to bottom with the palm. For patients with exogenous cold, keep warm and apply hot compress on the epigastric region and abdomen.

（2）Diet nursing. For patients with wind cold, drink zisuye（perilla leaf）tea, or shengjiang（fresh ginger）brown sugar water; eat foods that warm the middle and dissipate cold, such as baihujiao（white pepper）, leaf mustard, xiaohuixiang（fennel）and congbai（scallion white）; avoid cold-natured foods, such as duck meat, crabs and bananas. For patients with wind heat, drink jinyinhua（honeysuckle）tea, juhua（chrysanthemum）tea; eat foods that disperse wind and clear heat, such as bailuobo（white radish）and bohe（Peppermint）. For patients with summerheat-dampness, eat foods that clear summerheat and resolve dampness, such as watermelons, heye（lotus leaf）, chixiaodou（adzuki bean）, lüdou（mung bean）and baibiandou（white hyacinth bean）; avoid pungent, spicy, fatty and too-sweet foods.

（3）Emotion nursing. Nurses may use emotional transference and dispositional change therapy to encourage the patients to close their eyes to nourish the spirit, or listen to light music to distract their attention.

（4）Medication nursing. Decoction should be prepared fast with strong fire and taken hot after meals, multiple times in small portions. Slight perspiration after taking medicine is preferred. Drip some shengjiang（fresh ginger）juice on the root of tongue before taking medicine to arrest vomiting.

（5）Manipulation techniques. ① Paste application therapy: select Zhongwan（CV 12）and Neiguan（PC 6）; grind into powder biba（long pepper fruit）and chuanjiao（pricklyash peel）; blend the powder with shengjiang（fresh ginger）juice to make pastes, and apply them on the acupoints, 12 hours each time, and once per day. It is suitable for patients with wind cold. ② Acupressure therapy: select Neiguan（PC 6）, Zhongwan（CV 12）, Weishu（BL 21）, Zusanli（ST 36）, Waiguan（TE 5）and Dazhui（GV 14）; apply thumb kneading, rubbing and one-finger pushing manipulations on each of the acupoints until the area turns hot or the patient has the feelings of soreness, numbness, distension and heaviness in the area; once per day. And it is contraindicated in pregnancy.

2. Syndrome of Food Retention

（1）Daily life nursing. The ward should be warm, dry and full of fresh air, and avoid strong and convective wind. Keep the respiratory track clean, and take a lateral decubitus position with the head slightly raised. Encourage the patients to vomit, pat on their back, and use suction apparatus if necessary. Rinse the mouth with warm water after vomiting, clean the vomitus in time, and change the contaminated clothes and coverings. The patients may do moderate exercise to keep a normal bowel movement.

（2）Diet nursing. Patients are fasted for 12~24 hours if necessary. Offer the patients semi-liquid foods after the vomiting stops, with a light diet in small frequent meals, and gradual increase of meat. Shanzha maiya (Chinese hawthorn fruit and germinated barley) tea and shengjiang jiaomi (fresh ginger and scorch-fried rice) tea are recommended. Eat foods that promote digestion and remove food stagnation, such as chenpi (aged tangerine peel), white radish, rice vinegar, kumquat, white radish leaf and ji'neijin (chicken gizzard lining). Greasy and roasted foods should be avoided, such as fat meat, roast meat and deep-fried dough sticks.

(3) Emotion nursing. Because the symptoms are severe, nurses may encourage patients' family members to accompany and comfort them to ensure their safety without being worried or anxious.

(4) Medication nursing. Decoction should be concentrated and taken warm after meals.

(5) Manipulation techniques. ① Paste application therapy: select Zhongwan (CV 12) and Neiguan (PC 6); use shengjiang (fresh ginger) juice to stir-fry huangliang (coptis rhizome), zisuye (perilla leaf), baikouren (round cardamon kernel) and shenqu (medicated leaven); grind the above medicinals into fine powder and blend with shengjiang (fresh ginger) juice to make pastes, and apply the mixture on the acupoints, 12 hours each time, once per day. ② Inducing vomiting therapy: irritate the pharynx with a tongue depressor or a feather, or drink warm dilute saline and use a finger to irritate the pharynx, to induce vomiting of food retention. It is suitable for patients who desire but fail to vomit. ③ Purgation therapy: follow the doctor's advice to swallow shengdahuang (raw rhubarb root and rhizome) power 3 ~ 6 g. It is suitable for patients with constipation, and contraindicated in pregnancy. ④ Acupressure therapy: select Neiguan (PC 6), Zhongwan (CV 12), Weishu (BL 21), Zusanli (ST 36), Liangmen (ST 21) and Tianshu (ST 25); apply thumb kneading, rubbing and one-finger pushing manipulations on each of the acupoints until the area turns hot or the patient has the feelings of soreness, numbness, distension and heaviness in the area; once per day. And it is contraindicated in pregnancy.

3. Syndrome of Liver Qi Invading the Stomach

(1) Daily life nursing. The ward should be cool, quiet, and full of fresh air. The patients should rest in bed and have adequate sleep.

(2) Diet nursing. For patients with severe vomiting, fast for 4 ~ 6 hours if necessary. When the vomiting stops, the patients should have liquid diet, then semi-liquid, soft diet, and finally general diet, in small frequent meals. Meiguihua (rose flower) tea and xianlugen (fresh reed rhizome) juice are recommended. Eat foods that sooth the liver and regulate qi, such as kumquat, orange, foshou (finger citron fruit) and white radish. The patients should refrain from cigarettes and alcohol as well as foods that are greasy, pungent, spicy, and flatulent, such as sweet potatoes.

(3) Emotion nursing. Because emotional frustration often causes the disease to occur or aggravate, it is important for the patients to stay calm. Nurses may use emotional transference and dispositional change therapy to distract the patients' attention. Nurses should find out the causes of patients' irritation, anger and depression, encourage their family members to accompany them, and lead communications among wardmates to create a stress-free atmosphere.

(4) Medication nursing. Decoction should be concentrated and taken warm after meals, multiple

times in small portions.

（5）Manipulation techniques. ① Paste application therapy: select Zhongwan（CV 12）, Zusanli（ST 36）and Shenque（CV 8）, mix finely ground wuzhuyu（medicinal evodia fruit）3 g with shengjiang（fresh ginger）juice to make pastes, and apply them on the acupoints, once per day; or select Yongquan（KI 1）, spread white sugar on some clean fresh dilong（earth worms）to make them mushy, and blend with wheat flour to apply on the acupoints. ② Acupoint-pressing therapy: select Neiguan（PC 6）; apply forceful finger-pressing manipulation on it for one minute. It is suitable for patients with severe vomiting. ③ Water acupuncture therapy: select a unilateral Zusanli（ST 36）; inject Vitamin B$_6$ injection into the acupoint. It is suitable for patients with severe belching. ④ Acupressure therapy: select Neiguan（PC 6）, Zhongwan（CV 12）, Weishu（BL 21）, Zusanli（ST 36）, Taichong（LR 3）and Qimen（LR 14）; apply thumb kneading, rubbing and one-finger pushing manipulations on each of the acupoints until the area turns hot or the patient has the feelings of soreness, numbness, distension and heaviness in the area; once per day. And it is contraindicated in pregnancy.

4. Syndrome of Internal Obstruction of Phlegm and Fluid-Retention

（1）Daily life nursing. The ward should be warm, dry and full of fresh air, and avoid strong and convective wind. The patients should rest in bed with a sitting or semi-supine position, keep the abdomen warm, and turn the head aside during vomiting.

（2）Diet nursing. Take shengjiang（fresh ginger）juice 10~15 mL with rice soup frequently to arrest vomiting. Eat foods that invigorate the spleen and remove dampness, such as sharen（villous amomum fruit）, red bean, heye（lotus leaf）and yiyiren（coix seed）. The patients should refrain from alcohol, and foods that are cold, raw and greasy.

（3）Emotion nursing. Due to a long course of disease and severe symptoms, nurses may use verbal enlightenment therapy and patiently answer the patients' questions to eliminate their anxiety.

（4）Medication nursing. Decoction should be concentrated and taken warm after meals.

（5）Manipulation techniques. ① Paste application therapy: select Zhongwan（CV 12）, Neiguan（PC 6）and Shenque（CV 8）; mix qingbanxia（prepared pinelliae rhizome）powder with shengjiang（fresh ginger）juice to make pastes, and apply them on the acupoints, 12 hours each time, once per day. And it is contraindicated in pregnancy. ② Acupressure therapy: select Neiguan（PC 6）, Zhongwan（CV 12）, Weishu（BL 21）, Zusanli（ST 36）, Fenglong（ST 40）and Gongsun（SP 4）; apply thumb kneading, rubbing and one-finger pushing manipulations on each of the acupoints until the area turns hot or the patient has the feelings of soreness, numbness, distension and heaviness in the area; once per day. And it is contraindicated in pregnancy.

5. Syndrome of Deficiency-Cold of the Spleen and Stomach

（1）Daily life nursing. The ward should be warm, dry, quiet, comfortable and full of bright light and fresh air, and avoid strong and convective wind. The patients should rest in bed, keep the abdomen warm, and pay attention to skin care. Nurses should assist the patients in turning over every two hours to prevent pressure sores.

(2) Diet nursing. The foods should be warm and diversified with nice color, smell and taste. The patients should have small frequent meals. Shengjiang hongtang chenpi (fresh ginger, aged tangerine peel, and brown sugar) tea is recommended. Eat foods that dissipate cold and harmonize the stomach, such as lianzi (lotus seed), qianshi (euryale seed), fuling (poria), shanyao (common yam rhizome) and yiyiren (coix seed). Food therapy: pig stomach porridge, dingxiang jiang (clove flower and fresh ginger) sugar. The patients should refrain from liquor, Chinese chives, chili, and coffee and foods that are raw, cold and hard.

(3) Emotion nursing. Because the patients are weak with a long course of disease, nurses may use verbal enlightenment therapy, submission therapy and music therapy to impart them knowledge about the disease, care for them, invite them to listen to soothing music to make them comfortable and avoid pessimism and depression.

(4) Medication nursing. The decoction should be concentrated and taken hot before meals, multiple times in small portions. Several drops of shengjiang (fresh ginger) juice could be supplemented while taking medicine. Stroke on the patients' back gently when they are taking medicine. The patients may take some rest in bed after taking medicine.

(5) Manipulation techniques. ① Medicated ironing therapy: select the epigastric region; follow the doctor's advice to grind and stir-fry the medicinals that warm the middle, invigorate the spleen, harmonize the stomach and descend adverse qi, and put them into a cloth bag for medicated ironing at a temperature of 60~70℃, 20 minutes each time, once per day. And it is contraindicated in pregnancy. ② Moxibustion therapy: select Yinbai (SP 1) and Pishu (BL 20); place the moxa stick 2 ~ 3 centimeters away from the skin to perform mild moxibustion on each of the acupoints until the area turns red and the patient feels warm and comfortable without the sensation of burning pain, once per day. ③ Acupressure therapy: select Neiguan (PC 6), Zhongwan (CV 12), Weishu (BL 21), Zusanli (ST 36), Pishu (BL 20) and Gongsun (SP 4); apply thumb kneading, rubbing and one-finger pushing manipulations on each of the acupoints until the area turns hot or the patient has the feelings of soreness, numbness, distension and heaviness in the area; once per day. And it is contraindicated in pregnancy.

6. Syndrome of Stomach Yin Insufficiency

(1) Daily life nursing. The ward should be cool and comfortable. The patients should rest in bed to ensure adequate sleep, and reduce the frequency of turning over. Follow the doctor's advice to keep the vomitus for further test. Pay attention to oral hygiene, rinse the mouth with dilute saline or jinyinhua gancao (honeysuckle flower and licorice root) liquid. The patients should avoid watching thrilling books, journals or TV shows.

(2) Diet nursing. The diet should be light, soft and juicy. The patients may drink xiangjiang (clove flower and fresh ginger) milk, ganzhe shengjiang (sugarcane and fresh ginger) juice, or sheep milk. Herbal tea made of xianlugen (fresh reed rhizome) 30 g, tiepishihu (dendrobium officinale) 10 g and maidong (dwarf lilyturf tuber) 10 g is recommended. Eat foods that replenish the stomach and nourish yin, such as biqi (waternut), wild jujube, lianzi (lotus seed), baihe (lily bulb), sangshen (mulberry)

and oujie (lotus rhizome node). Food therapy: wumei fengmi (smoked plum and honey) extract. For patients with constipation, more fresh vegetables rich in fiber are recommended to relieve constipation, and avoid purgatives. The patients should refrain from cigarettes, alcohol, scallion, Chinese chives and garlic, and foods that are fatty, too-sweet, pungent, spicy, aromatic and dry-natured.

(3) Emotion nursing. Because the patients have deficiency fire with a long course of disease, nurses may use verbal enlightenment therapy as well as emotional transference and dispositional change therapy to impart patients the disease condition to eliminate their fear and anxiety, and distract their attention to help them stay calm.

(4) Medication nursing. Decoction should be concentrated slowly and taken warm slowly before meals, multiple times in small portions. Before taking medicine, eat a little digestible food, or drip some shengjiang (fresh ginger) juice into the decoction, or chew some shengjiang (fresh ginger). After taking medicine, the patients should rest in bed.

(5) Manipulation techniques. ① Acupressure therapy: select Neiguan (PC 6), Zhongwan (CV 12), Weishu (BL 21), Zusanli (ST 36), Pishu (BL 20) and Sanyinjiao (SP 6); apply thumb kneading, rubbing and one-finger pushing manipulations on each of the acupoints until the area turns hot or the patient has the feelings of soreness, numbness, distension and heaviness in the area; once per day. And it is contraindicated in pregnancy. ② Healthcare massage therapy: select the epigastric region; apply clockwise rubbing manipulation with the palm until the area turns hot, ten minutes each time. The preferred time for massage is before and after meals.

Patient Education

The room should be quiet and full of fresh air, and avoid wind, strong light and loud noise. The patients should live a regular life, balance work and rest, do moderate exercise, and keep the stomach warm to prevent colds.

The diet should be light, nutritious and digestible. The patients should follow a moderate diet, have small frequent meals at low speed, avoid being too hungry or too full, and pay attention to food hygiene. For patients who are intolerant to cold fruit, immerse the fruit in warm water before eating. The patients should refrain from cigarettes, alcohol, strong tea, coffee and foods that are raw, cold, fatty, greasy, too-sweet, sticky, pungent, spicy, and flatulent.

The patients should regulate their emotions and keep themselves comfortable.

For patients with frequent vomiting, find out the cause in time.

第九节　胃　脘　痛

胃脘痛,是指因寒热侵扰,或因饮食失调,阴阳气血不足,气滞血瘀而引起的,以自觉剑突下的上腹部疼痛,或切按则痛为临床特征的病证。西医的急性胃炎、慢性胃炎、消化性溃疡、胃癌,以及部分肝、胆、胰疾病,以上腹部疼痛为主要表现的,可参照本节进行护理。

一、病因病机

胃脘痛的病因包括六淫外袭、情志所伤、饮食失调、起居失宜、瘀血停滞、脾胃虚弱。六淫外袭皮毛,内传胃脘,或经口鼻内客胃脘,与饮食相抟结,停于中焦,阻滞气机,不通则痛,可发为胃脘痛。病人思虑伤脾、脾气郁结,或郁郁寡欢、肝郁乘脾,或暴怒急躁、肝气横逆犯脾,或过悲伤肺、子病及母,可致脾胃升降失常,气机阻滞。病人暴饮暴食,饥饱无常,宿食停滞,过食生冷、粗糙、辛辣、炙煿,过饮烈酒,或年老久病,脾虚难化,可生痰化热,耗伤胃阴,阻滞气机,发为胃脘痛。病人久坐湿地,冒雨涉水,或暑季贪凉,寒湿困脾,气机逆乱,血行不畅,可发为胃脘痛。气滞日久,或脾虚失运,均可导致瘀血阻络,发为胃脘痛。病人素体脾胃虚寒,或劳倦太过,失血久病,致胃脘脉络失于温养,亦可发为胃脘痛。

胃脘痛的病机为胃气郁滞,不通则痛,或脾胃虚弱,不荣则痛。病位在胃,与肝、脾有关。胃脘痛初期多为实证,后期往往虚实夹杂。

二、常见证型

（一）辨证要点

1. 辨急性与慢性　根据发病速度、病程长短、疼痛程度等来辨别。若发病急,病程短,疼痛剧烈,持续半小时以上不得缓解,多为急性。若起病缓,病程长,疼痛可耐受,服药后即可缓解或消失,反复发作,则多为慢性。

2. 辨虚实　根据体质特点、疼痛性质、大便情况、脉象等来辨别。若其人体壮,起病急,疼痛剧烈,持续无休,位置固定不移,拒按,食后痛甚,大便闭结不通,脉盛,则多为实证。若其人年老、久病、体弱,疼痛徐缓,反复发作,位置不固定,得食痛减,或劳倦后加重,休息后减轻,喜按,大便无闭结,脉虚,则多为虚证。

3. 辨寒热　根据病因、疼痛性质、缓解因素、舌脉等来辨别。若因受寒或过食生冷而起,胃脘绞痛,得温痛减,遇寒加重,苔白,脉紧,多为寒证。若胃脘灼痛,得冷痛减,遇热加重,苔黄,脉数,则多为热证。

4. 辨在气在血　根据诱因、疼痛性质等来辨别。若疼痛与情志因素相关,胀痛,连及两胁,嗳气频频,多为气滞。若痛如针刺或刀割,痛有定处,入夜尤甚,或兼吐血、黑便,舌质紫暗或有瘀斑,脉涩,则多为血瘀。

（二）证候分型

1. 寒邪客胃证

［主要证候］胃痛暴作,恶寒喜暖,得温痛减,遇寒加重,口淡不渴,或喜热饮;舌淡,苔薄白,脉弦紧。

［证候分析］寒邪凝胃,气机阻滞,故胃痛暴作;寒邪得温则自散,得寒则增其邪势,故恶寒喜暖,得温痛减,遇寒加重;中寒内盛,阳气被遏,运化不健,和降失司,故口淡不渴,或喜热饮;舌淡,苔薄白,脉弦紧,均为寒邪客胃之象。

［护治原则］温胃散寒,理气止痛。

［常用方剂］良附丸合香苏饮。

2. 肝气犯胃证

［主要证候］胃脘胀痛,痛连两胁,遇烦恼则痛作或痛甚,嗳气、矢气则痛舒,胸闷嗳气,喜长叹息,大便不畅;舌苔薄白,脉弦。

［证候分析］肝气郁滞,胃失和降,故胃脘胀痛;胁为肝络之分野,故痛连两胁;滞气上行,故胸闷嗳气;恼怒会加重气机不畅,故遇烦恼则痛作或痛甚;气郁于胸,故喜长叹息;舌苔薄白,脉弦,均为肝气犯胃之象。

［护治原则］疏肝理气,和胃止痛。

［常用方剂］柴胡疏肝散。

3. 痰饮停胃证

［主要证候］胃脘痞痛,胸腹堵闷;呕吐痰涎,口黏不爽,肢体沉重,口淡不饥;苔白厚腻,脉弦滑。

［证候分析］痰饮中阻,胃失和降,故胃脘痞痛,胸腹堵闷;痰湿困脾,脾失健运,故呕吐痰涎,口黏不爽,肢体沉重,口淡不饥;苔白厚腻,脉弦滑,均为痰浊中阻之象。

［护治原则］温化痰饮,理气和胃。

［常用方剂］苓桂术甘汤合二陈汤。

4. 饮食积滞证

［主要证候］胃脘疼痛,胀满拒按,嗳腐吞酸,或呕吐不消化食物,其味腐臭,吐后痛减,不思饮食,大便不爽,得矢气及便后则稍舒;舌苔厚腻,脉滑。

［证候分析］饮食积滞,阻碍气机,故胃脘疼痛,胀满拒按;胃气不降,浊气上逆,故嗳腐吞酸,或呕吐不消化食物,其味腐臭;吐出食物后,气机得畅,故吐后痛减;食积下迫,大肠传导失司,故大便不爽,得矢气及便后则稍舒;舌苔厚腻,脉滑,均为食积内阻之象。

［护治原则］消食导滞,理气和胃。

［常用方剂］保和丸。

5. 湿热蕴胃证

［主要证候］胃脘疼痛,痛势急迫,脘闷灼热,口干口苦,口渴而不欲饮,纳呆恶心,小便色黄,大便不畅;舌红,苔黄腻,脉滑数。

［证候分析］湿热内蕴,阻滞中焦,故胃脘疼痛,痛势急迫,脘闷灼热;湿热上犯于口,故口干、口苦、口渴;水津不布,故渴不欲饮;湿热熏蒸于胃脘,故纳呆恶心;湿热下侵膀胱,故小便色黄;湿热阻滞肠道,故大便不畅;舌红,苔黄腻,脉滑数,均为湿热蕴胃之象。

［护治原则］清化湿热,理气和胃。

［常用方剂］清中汤。

6. 瘀血阻络证

［主要证候］胃脘刺痛,痛有定处,按之痛甚,食后加剧,入夜尤甚,或见吐血、黑便;舌质紫暗或有瘀斑,脉涩。

［证候分析］瘀血阻络,气机壅滞,故胃脘刺痛;瘀血有形,故痛有定处,按之痛甚;瘀血为阴邪,故入夜尤甚;瘀血停胃,胃失和降,故食后加剧;瘀血损伤络脉,血不循经,故吐血、黑便;舌质紫暗或有瘀斑,脉涩,均为瘀血内阻之象。

［护治原则］活血化瘀,理气和胃。

［常用方剂］丹参饮合失笑散。

7. 胃阴亏虚证

［主要证候］胃脘隐隐灼痛,似饥而不欲食,口燥咽干,五心烦热,消瘦乏力,口渴思饮,大便干结;舌红少津,脉细数。

［证候分析］胃阴不足,络脉失养,故胃脘隐隐灼痛;气津不足,纳食不化,故似饥而不欲食;胃失濡养,气机不畅,上不布津,故口燥咽干,口渴思饮;阴液不足,无以下溉,肠道失润,故大便干结;五心烦热,消瘦乏力,舌红少津,脉细数,均为阴虚内热之象。

［护治原则］养阴生津,益胃止痛。

［常用方剂］益胃汤合芍药甘草汤。

8. 脾胃虚寒证

［主要证候］胃凉隐痛,绵绵不休,喜按喜温,遇冷痛重,空腹痛甚,得食痛减;劳累或受凉后发作或加重,泛吐清水,神疲纳呆,四肢倦怠,手足不温,大便溏薄;舌淡苔白,脉虚弱或迟缓。

［证候分析］脾阳亏虚,寒自内生,故胃凉隐痛,喜按喜温;寒得温而散,得冷则凝,故遇冷痛重,得食痛减;脾虚中寒,水不运化而上逆,故泛吐清水;脾虚水谷受纳失常,故纳呆;脾虚生湿下渗,故便溏;舌淡苔白,脉虚弱或迟缓,均为脾胃虚寒之象。

［护治原则］温中健脾,和胃止痛。

［常用方剂］黄芪健中汤。

三、护理措施

对于胃脘痛的病人,应观察疼痛的性质、程度、发生时间、持续时间、次数、诱发因素、缓解因素;腹胀的部位、性质、程度、发生时间、诱发因素;嗳气、反酸、呕吐的频率和程度;呕吐物和大便的颜色、性状,是否带血。注意观察胃口、食量、舌脉。若病人出现吐血、黑便,伴面色苍白,冷汗时出,四肢厥冷,烦躁不安,血压下降;或突然出现胃痛加剧,伴恶心呕吐,全腹硬满,疼痛拒按,应立即报告医生,并配合抢救。

（一）辨证施护

1. 寒邪客胃证

（1）生活起居护理　居室温暖避风。卧床休息，注意保暖。

（2）饮食护理　饮食宜温热、易消化。可饮生姜大枣茶。宜食散寒止痛的食物，如葱白、大蒜、小茴香。食疗方：丁香肉桂红糖煎、白胡椒猪肚汤。不宜食生冷、肥甘的食物。

（3）情志护理　护士可运用语言开导疗法，多与病人沟通，帮助病人保持乐观的情绪。

（4）用药护理　中药汤剂宜饭后热服。服药后加盖衣被，用热水袋热敷胃脘部。

（5）操作技术　① 敷贴疗法：取中脘、上脘、胃俞、脾俞、足三里，将吴茱萸、小茴香、细辛、冰片打粉，与生姜汁调成糊状敷贴，每次 2 小时，每日 1 次；孕妇禁用。② 灸法：取中脘、足三里、脾俞、胃俞，用温和灸，艾条燃着端悬于施灸部位上，距离皮肤 2~3 厘米，灸至病人有温热舒适无灼痛的感觉，皮肤稍有红晕，每日 1 次。③ 穴位按摩法：取中脘、内关、足三里，用拇指揉法、摩法、一指禅推法，按摩至局部发热或有酸麻重胀感，每日 1 次；孕妇禁用。

2. 肝气犯胃证

（1）生活起居护理　居室安静整洁，可设置花、草、盆景。衣裤宽松。做好口腔护理，发生嗳腐吞酸时随时漱口。若疼痛剧烈，应卧床休息。当疼痛缓解时，可适量锻炼。饭后取直立位，从饭后 1 小时开始，散步 30 分钟，以身体发热或微汗、不疲劳为宜。睡前不进食，晚餐与入睡的间隔时间不少于 3 小时，睡眠时将床头抬高 30°。

（2）饮食护理　饮食宜清淡，少食多餐，减少饮食摄入量和饮水量，郁怒、悲伤时避免进食。可喝陈佛饮、茉莉花茶。宜食疏肝理气的食物，如金橘、白萝卜、玫瑰花。食疗方：胡萝卜炒陈皮瘦肉丝。不宜食生冷、油腻、辛辣、坚硬、过甜、过烫、易产气的食物，如红薯。

（3）情志护理　护士可运用语言开导疗法，帮助病人消除忧虑。或采用移情易性疗法，转移病人的注意力，消除恼怒的情绪。或运用暗示解惑疗法，消除病人的心理压力。为病人营造轻松愉悦的就餐环境，使肝气条达。

（4）用药护理　中药汤剂应饭后温服，少量频服。

（5）操作技术　① 敷贴疗法：取中脘或神厥，用槟榔、莱菔子、枳实、厚朴、木香、大腹皮、香附等份研粉，与茶油搅拌成膏外敷，每次 2~8 小时，每日 1 次；孕妇禁用。② 穴位按摩法：取中脘、内关、足三里、阳陵泉、太冲、行间、章门、期门、肝俞，用拇指揉法、摩法、一指禅推法，按摩至局部发热或有酸麻重胀感，每日 1 次；孕妇禁用。③ 耳压疗法：取交感、神门、肝、胃等耳穴，用耳穴压丸贴片贴压，每日按揉 4~5 次，以局部发热泛红为度，留置 2~4 日；孕妇禁用。

3. 痰饮停胃证

（1）生活起居护理　居室温暖干燥，空气新鲜。卧床休息，可做少量轻缓的运动，如散步、打太极拳，不可过劳。

（2）饮食护理　少食多餐，减少饮食摄入量。宜食健脾除湿的食物，如薏苡仁、山药。食疗方：赤小豆鲫鱼羹。不宜食生冷、油腻、辛辣、坚硬、易产气的食物，如红薯。

（3）情志护理　护士可运用语言开导疗法，多安慰病人，消除病人忧虑，从而使其增强脾胃功能。

（4）用药护理　中药汤剂宜饭后温服，少量频服。

（5）操作技术 ① 灸法：取中脘、神阙、气海、关元，用温和灸，艾条燃着端悬于施灸部位上，距离皮肤2~3厘米，灸至病人有温热舒适无灼痛的感觉，皮肤稍有红晕，每日1次；孕妇腹部禁用。② 穴位按摩法：取中脘、天枢、关元、脾俞、胃俞、足三里，用拇指揉法、摩法、一指禅推法，按摩至局部发热或有酸麻重胀感，每日1次；孕妇禁用。

4. 饮食积滞证

（1）生活起居护理 居室安静避风，光线柔和，空气新鲜。进食后取半仰卧位，改变体位时动作要慢。做好口腔护理，经常用温水漱口。

（2）饮食护理 疼痛剧烈时暂时禁食。病情缓解后，从流食、半流食、软食转到普食。饮食有节，不暴饮暴食。宜食消食化积的食物，如白萝卜、柠檬、麦芽、陈皮。食疗方：神曲山楂粥。鸡莱散：莱菔子9g，鸡内金5g，炒黄，研磨成粉，分3次用温开水调服。不宜食生冷、肥甘、甜黏的食物。

（3）情志护理 病人症状虽重，但属于新病，病位浅，预后好。护士可鼓励家属多陪伴病人，鼓励病友间多交流疾病的防治经验，以增强病人对于治疗的信心。

（4）用药护理 中药汤剂宜饭后温服，少量频服。服药前可含姜片或山楂片。中药丸剂可用温水溶化后服用。

（5）操作技术 ① 点穴疗法：取神门、内关，用拇指按压对侧腧穴，当有酸胀感时，再继续按压半分钟。② 涌吐法：以压舌板或羽毛刺激咽部，或饮温盐水后用手指探吐；适用于欲吐不得吐者。

5. 湿热蕴胃证

（1）生活起居护理 居室宜凉爽，空气新鲜。衣物轻薄宽松。做好口腔护理，饭后用金银花甘草液漱口。保持肛周皮肤清洁干燥。保持大便通畅，排便时不可久蹲或过于用力。

（2）饮食护理 饮食宜清淡。可饮荷叶茶、绿茶。宜食清热祛湿的食物，如香椿、薏苡仁、茯苓、苦瓜、绿豆、豆腐、小白菜。不宜食辛辣、助湿生热的食物。

（3）情志护理 病人为实热证，症状较重，护士可运用移情易性疗法，转移其注意力，消除烦躁的情绪。

（4）用药护理 中药汤剂宜饭后温服或偏凉服。

（5）操作技术 ① 敷贴疗法：取中脘、上脘、胃俞、脾俞、足三里，用黄连、黄芩、乳香、没药、冰片打成粉，与凡士林调成糊状敷贴，每次8小时，每日1次，孕妇禁用；或用仙人掌，不拘多少，捣烂，敷于痛处。② 拔罐疗法：取脾俞、胃俞，留罐10分钟；或取足太阳膀胱经、督脉，循经走罐；隔日1次；孕妇禁用。

6. 瘀血阻络证

（1）生活起居护理 居室温暖避风，安静舒适，空气新鲜。卧床休息，注意腹部保暖。若出现吐血、黑便，应绝对卧床。若发生吐血，应去枕平卧，头偏向一侧，及时清除呕吐物，保持呼吸道通畅。吐血后用淡盐水漱口。待吐血和黑便停止后，方可下床活动。

（2）饮食护理 吐血时应禁食，待病情稳定后，由流食逐渐过渡到普食。可饮红花茶。宜食理气活血的食物，如山楂、陈皮、香菇、丝瓜、茄子。食疗方：木须肉片黄花菜、大枣赤豆莲藕粥。不宜食生冷、粗糙、硬固、煎炸、厚味、易产气的食物，如红薯。

（3）情志护理 护士可运用语言开导疗法，关心体贴病人，宣传关于疾病的知识，解释检查结果，以消除病人的恐癌心理。或运用顺意疗法，当病人出现紧张、恐惧、忧思情绪时，允许病人合理表达。或运用移情易性疗法,指导病人放松,如缓慢地深呼吸、阅读娱乐性读物、打太极拳等,以减轻心理压力。

（4）用药护理　中药汤剂宜饭后温服,少量频服。

（5）操作技术　① 敷贴疗法:取中脘、神阙、关元、天枢,用细辛、川芎、白芷、皂角刺、茜草、红花打成粉,与芝麻油调成膏状,选择1~3个腧穴敷贴,每次4~6小时,每日1次。② 足浴疗法:用当归、细辛、川芎、木瓜、红花、甘草,煎煮后待水温降至37~42℃时洗按足部,每次20分钟,每日1次;血压过低者慎用。③ 水针疗法:取单侧足三里,用丹参注射液或复方当归注射液进行穴位注射。④ 穴位按摩法:取中脘、内关、胃俞、肝俞、太冲、期门、血海、膈俞,用拇指揉法、摩法、一指禅推法,按摩至局部发热或有酸麻重胀感,每日1次;孕妇禁用。

7. 胃阴亏虚证

（1）生活起居护理　居室凉爽湿润,安静舒适。多卧床休息。胃脘痛发作时,可饮温开水或少量进食,以缓解不适。病情缓解后,可适量运动,以保持大便通畅。

（2）饮食护理　少食多餐。可饮铁皮石斛茶、麦冬茶。宜食益胃生津的食物,如甘蔗、百合、莲子、银耳、鳖肉、藕、大白菜、桑椹、雪梨、葡萄、山药、鱼胶、蜂蜜。食疗方:木瓜生姜煲米醋。忌酒类、浓茶、咖啡,不宜食生冷、油腻、辛辣、质地粗糙的食物。

（3）情志护理　病人身体虚弱且病程较长,护士可运用语言开导疗法,向病人讲解饮食营养对于健康的重要性。

（4）用药护理　中药汤剂宜文火久煎,饭前温服,少量频服。

（5）操作技术　① 穴位按摩法:取胃俞、脾俞、血海、中脘、内关、足三里、三阴交、太溪,用拇指揉法、摩法、一指禅推法,按摩至局部发热或有酸麻重胀感,每日1次;孕妇禁用。② 耳压疗法:取胃、脾、交感、神门、皮质下等耳穴,用耳穴压丸贴片贴压,每日按揉4~5次,以局部发热泛红为度,留置2~4日;孕妇禁用。③ 保健按摩疗法:病人取仰卧位,双腿屈曲,用掌心在腹部做顺时针按摩,也可从上腹往下腹缓缓按摩,每次5~10分钟,每日3~4次。

8. 脾胃虚寒证

（1）生活起居护理　居室向阳,温暖干燥,安静舒适,光线明亮,不可有强风、对流风。衣被宜厚。多卧床休息,尤其饭后宜卧床休息片刻。睡眠充足,注意胃脘部保暖。定时翻身,预防压疮。症状缓解后,可适量运动。运动时注意安全,不可过劳,以防止跌仆。

（2）饮食护理　饮食宜温热,少食多餐。宜食温中健脾的食物,如猪肚、龙眼肉、大枣、黄鱼、鳝鱼、羊肉,可用生姜、小葱、白胡椒调味。食疗方:杞精炖鹌鹑、桂花莲子羹。不宜食生冷、寒凉、肥腻、甜黏、炙煿的食物。

（3）情志护理　病人体虚久病,护士可运用语言开导疗法,向病人讲解胃脘痛的病因和诱因,告诉病人应避免受凉、生气、饮食不节。注意了解病人的心理状态,帮助其保持乐观的情绪,避免悲观、消沉。

（4）用药护理　中药汤剂宜文火久煎,饭前热服。

（5）操作技术　① 热敷疗法:用盐炒麸皮,装入布袋中,制成温度为60~70℃的布包,放在痛处热敷20分钟,每日1次;孕妇禁用。② 灸法:取中脘、足三里、神阙、气海、关元,用温和灸,艾条燃着端悬于施灸部位上,距离皮肤2~3厘米,灸至病人有温热舒适无灼痛的感觉,皮肤稍有红晕,每日1

次;孕妇腹部禁用。③ 足浴疗法:用花椒、黄芪各 30 g,姜黄、延胡索、红花、制附子片各 15 g,煎煮后待水温降至 37~42℃时洗按足部,每次 20 分钟,每日睡前 1 次;血压过低者慎用。④ 水针疗法:取足三里,用黄芪注射液或生脉注射液进行穴位注射。⑤ 穴位按摩法:取足三里、血海、关元、天枢、内庭、脾俞、章门,用拇指揉法、摩法、一指禅推法,按摩至局部发热或有酸麻重胀感,每日 1 次;孕妇禁用。

（二）健康教育

起居有常,劳逸适度,睡眠充足,慎避风寒暑湿之邪。进行适量的体育锻炼,不可过劳。饭后休息半小时,不宜马上运动,亦不宜平躺。

饮食宜清淡、营养、易消化。食物宜温,进食宜慢。少食多餐,定时定量。注意饮食卫生。烹调以蒸、煮、炒、煲为主,不宜煎炸、烟熏、腊腌、生拌。忌烟酒、浓茶、咖啡,不宜食辛辣、肥腻、甜黏、炙煿、粗糙、硬固、易产气的食物。

保持情绪平和,心情舒畅,避免抑郁、焦虑、忧思、恼怒。学会放松,可通过下棋、看报、听音乐进行自我调节,以保持心情愉快,增强抗病能力。

若胃脘痛反复发作,迁延不愈,应定期到门诊复查,遵医嘱进行相关检查,筛查危险因素,进行针对性干预,以防止恶变。

Section 9　Epigastric Pain

Epigastric pain is a disease characterized by pain or tenderness in the upper abdomen below the xiphoid process. It is caused by invasion of cold or heat, improper diet, insufficiency of yin, yang, qi and blood, qi stagnation and blood stasis. This section can be referred to for the nursing of some diseases with epigastric pain as the main manifestation, such as acute gastritis, chronic gastritis, peptic ulcer, gastric cancer, as well as some diseases of the liver, gallbladder and pancrea in Western medicine.

ETIOLOGY AND PATHOGENESIS

The etiology includes external invasion of six excesses, emotional damage, improper diet, irregular daily life, blood stasis and constitutional deficiency of the spleen and stomach. Six excesses invade the skin and hair externally and transmit to the epigastric region internally or enter the epigastric region via mouth and nose, then they intermingle with food, and subsequently stagnate in the middle energizer and hinder qi movement to cause pain. Contemplation damaging the spleen causes spleen qi depression, liver depression overwhelms the spleen, violent rage triggers liver qi transversely invading the spleen, or excessive sorrow damaging the lung induces disorder of the child-organ (the lung) affecting the mother-organ (the spleen), all these may lead to abnormal ascending and descending of spleen qi and stomach qi as well as hinderance of qi movement, and consequently bring about epigastric pain. Improper diet, such as irregular eating, food retention, excessive consumption of raw, cold, coarse, pungent, spicy and fried foods, and over-drinking of alcohol, or being aged with prolonged disease and spleen deficiency that causes dysfunction of the spleen in transportation and transformation, all these may generate phlegm that transforms into heat to consume stomach yin and block qi movement, and consequently bring about epigastric pain. Sitting on the wetland for a long time, wading in rain, or desire for coolness in the summer, may cause cold-dampness encumbering the spleen that induces disorder of qi movement and inhibition of blood flow, and consequently bring about epigastric pain. Prolonged qi stagnation or dysfunction of the spleen in transportation and transformation due to its deficiency may induce blood stasis blocking meridians and collaterals, and consequently bring about epigastric pain. Constitutional deficiency-cold of the spleen and stomach, excessive overstrain, excessive loss of blood or prolonged disease, all may cause lack of warmth and nourishment for meridians and collaterals of epigastric region, and consequently bring about epigastric pain.

The pathogenesis is depression and stagnation of stomach qi or weakness of the spleen and stomach. The disease is located in the stomach but connected to the liver and spleen. The initial phrase of epigastric pain mainly belongs to excess syndrome while later to deficiency-excess in complexity.

COMMON SYNDROMES

Key Points in Syndrome Differentiation

1. Differentiation of Being Acute from Chronic

The differentiation is based on the onset speed, course of disease and severity of pain. Acute syndrome is characterized by sudden onset, short course, and severe pain lasting more than half an hour without relief. On the contrary, chronic syndrome is characterized by gradual onset, long course, tolerable pain relieved or disappearing after medication, and recurrent attacks.

2. Differentiation of Deficiency from Excess Syndrome

The differentiation is based on the constitutional characteristics, the nature of pain, stool and pulse manifestation. Excess syndrome occurs mostly in patients with a strong physique, and shows sudden onset, constant severe pain with fixed location and aggravation after eating, constipation, and strong pulse. Deficiency syndrome occurs mostly in patients at an old age, or have prolonged illness or weak constitution, and exhibits mild recurrent pain with unfixed location and relief after eating or aggravation with exertion and relief after rest, preference for pressure, no constipation, and feeble pulse.

3. Differentiation of Cold from Heat Syndrome

The differentiation is based on the cause, nature and relieving factors of the pain, and the manifestations of tongue and pulse. Cold syndrome is caused by cold or excessive consumption of raw or cold foods, showing epigastric colicky pain that decreases with warmth and worsens with cold, white tongue coating and tight pulse. Heat syndrome shows epigastric burning pain that decreases with cold and worsens with heat, yellow tongue coating and rapid pulse.

4. Differentiation of Qi Aspect from Blood Aspect

The differentiation is based on the cause and nature of the pain. If the pain is associated with emotional factors, accompanied with distending pain at both rib-sides and frequent belching, it is identified as syndrome of qi stagnation. If it shows stabbing pain with fixed location, aggravating at night, or concurrent symptoms of hematemesis and tarry stool, dark purple tongue with possible ecchymoses and unsmooth pulse, it is identified as syndrome of blood stasis.

Syndrome Differentiation

1. Syndrome of Cold Pathogen Attacking the Stomach

[Clinical Manifestations] Sudden stomachache, aversion to cold, preference for warmth, the pain relieved with warmth and aggravated with cold, bland taste in mouth without desire to drink, or preference for hot drinks, pale tongue with thin white coating, and wiry tight pulse.

[Manifestations Analysis] Cold pathogen congealing in the stomach hinders qi movement, so there is sudden stomachache. The cold pathogen dissipates with warmth and worsens with cold, leading to aversion to cold, preference for warmth, and pain relieved with warmth and aggravated with cold. Cold exuberance in the middle energizer constrains yang qi and causes dysfunction of the spleen in transportation and transformation as well as failure of the stomach to harmonize and descend, causing bland taste in the mouth without desire to drink or preference for hot drinks. Pale tongue with thin white coating and wiry tight pulse are signs of cold pathogen attacking the stomach.

[Nursing Principle] Warming the stomach and dissipating cold; regulating qi and relieving pain.

[Suggested Formula] Liangfu Pills and Xiangsu Decoction.

2. Syndrome of Liver Qi Invading the Stomach

[Clinical Manifestations] Epigastric distending pain radiating to both rib-sides, induced or aggravated with vexation and relieved after belching and flatus, chest oppression, belching, frequent long sigh, inhibited defecation, thin white tongue coating, and wiry pulse.

[Manifestations Analysis] Liver qi depression and stagnation causes failure of the stomach to harmonize and descend, causing epigastric distending pain. The branch of the liver meridian runs through the rib-sides, so there is pain radiating to both rib-sides. Depressed qi flowing upward leads to chest oppression and belching. Vexation worsens the obstruction of qi movement, so the pain is induced or aggravated with vexation. Qi stagnates in the chest, so there is frequent long sigh. Thin white tongue coating and wiry pulse are signs of liver qi invading the stomach.

[Nursing Principle] Soothing the liver and regulating qi; harmonizing the stomach and relieving pain.

[Suggested Formula] Chaihu Shugan Powder.

3. Syndrome of Phlegm and Fluid-Retention Stagnating in the Stomach

[Clinical Manifestations] Epigastric stuffiness and pain, chest and abdominal oppression, vomiting of phlegm and saliva, sticky and slimy sensation in the mouth, heavy limbs, bland taste in the mouth without hunger, white, thick and slimy tongue coating, and wiry slippery pulse.

[Manifestations Analysis] Phlegm and fluid retention obstructs the middle energizer and causes failure of the stomach to harmonize and descend, leading to epigastric stuffiness and pain, and chest and abdominal oppression. Phlegm-dampness encumbering the spleen triggers dysfunction of the spleen in transportation and transformation, causing vomiting of phlegm and saliva, sticky and slimy sensation in the mouth, heavy limbs, and bland taste in the mouth without hunger. White, thick and slimy tongue coating, and wiry slippery pulse all are signs of turbid phlegm obstructing the middle energizer.

[Nursing Principle] Warming and resolving phlegm and fluid retention; regulating qi and harmonizing the stomach.

[Suggested Formula] Linggui Zhugan Decoction and Erchen Decoction.

4. Syndrome of Food Retention

[Clinical Manifestations] Epigastric pain and significant tenderness with fullness and distention alleviated after vomiting, putrid belching and acid regurgitation, or vomiting of undigested putrid-smelling food, poor appetite, incomplete defecation alleviated after flatus or defecation, thick slimy tongue coating, and slippery pulse.

[Manifestations Analysis] Food retention obstructs qi movement, causing unpalpable epigastric pain with fullness and distention. Stomach qi fails to descend and turbid qi flows upward, leading to putrid belching and acid regurgitation, or vomiting of undigested putrid-smelling food. After vomiting, qi movement becomes smooth, so the pain is alleviated. Food retention causes conveyance dysfunction of the large intestine, resulting in incomplete defecation alleviated after flatus or defecation. Thick slimy tongue coating and slippery pulse are signs of internal obstruction of food retention.

[Nursing Principle] Promoting digestion and removing food stagnation; regulating qi and harmonizing the stomach.

[Suggested Formula] Baohe Pills.

5. Syndrome of Dampness-Heat Accumulating in Stomach

[Clinical Manifestations] Acute epigastric pain with oppression and scorching sensation, dry mouth with bitter taste, thirst without desire to drink, anorexia, nausea, dark urine, inhibited defecation, red tongue with yellow slimy coating, and slippery rapid pulse.

[Manifestations Analysis] Internal accumulation of dampness-heat obstructs qi movement in the middle energizer, causing acute epigastric pain with oppression and scorching sensation. Dampness-heat upward invades the mouth, resulting in dry mouth with bitter and thirst. Failure of fluids to be distributed brings on thirst without desire to drink. Dampness-heat fuming and steaming the stomach causes anorexia and nausea. Dampness-heat pouring down in the bladder explains dark urine. Dampness-heat obstructing the intestines is responsible for inhibited defecation. Red tongue with yellow slimy coating and slippery rapid pulse are signs of dampness-heat accumulating in the stomach.

[Nursing Principle] Clearing heat and resolving dampness; regulating qi and harmonizing the stomach.

[Suggested Formula] Qingzhong Decoction.

6. Syndrome of Blood Stasis Obstructing Collaterals

[Clinical Manifestations] Stabbing epigastric pain with fixed location aggravated with pressure, after diet, and especially at night, or hematemesis and tarry stool, dark purple tongue with possible ecchymoses, and unsmooth pulse.

[Manifestations Analysis] Blood stasis obstructs collaterals and hinders qi movement, causing stabbing epigastric pain. Blood stasis is tangible, leading to epigastric pain with fixed location aggravated with pressure. Blood stasis is yin pathogen, so the pain aggravates especially at night. Blood stasis accumulating in the stomach causes failure of the stomach to harmonize and descend, so the pain aggravates after diet. Blood stasis damaging collaterals makes blood fail to stay in the meridians, so there are hematemesis and tarry stool. Dark purple tongue with possible ecchymoses and unsmooth pulse are signs of internal obstruction of blood stasis.

[Nursing Principle] Activating blood and resolving stasis; regulating qi and harmonizing the stomach.

[Suggested Formula] Danshen Decoction and Shixiao Powder.

7. Syndrome of Stomach Yin Deficiency

[Clinical Manifestations] Dull epigastric pain with scorching sensation, feeling like hunger but without desire to eat, dry mouth and throat, vexing heat in the chest, palms and soles, emaciation, lack of strength, thirst with desire to drink, dry stool, red tongue with scanty fluids, and thready rapid pulse.

[Manifestations Analysis] Stomach yin insufficiency deprives collaterals of nourishment, so there is dull epigastric pain with scorching sensation. Qi and fluid insufficiency as well as undigested food contributes to feeling like hunger but without desire to eat. Stomach being deprived of nourishment triggers qi movement inhibition and failure of fluids to be distributed upward, resulting in dry mouth and throat, and thirst with desire to drink. Insufficient yin fluid cannot distribute downward to moisten the intestines, so there is dry stool. Vexing heat in the chest, palms and soles, emaciation, lack of strength, red tongue with scanty fluids, and thready rapid pulse, all are manifestations of yin deficiency with internal heat.

[Nursing Principle] Nourishing yin and promoting fluid production; replenishing the stomach and relieving pain.

[Suggested Formula] Yiwei Decoction and Shaoyao Gancao Decoction.

8. Syndrome of Deficiency-Cold in the Spleen and Stomach

[Clinical Manifestations] Persistent dull epigastric pain with cool sensation, preference for pressure and warmth, pain induced with overstrain or cold, aggravated with cold, hunger or overstrain and alleviated after diet, vomiting watery fluids, mental and physical fatigue, anorexia, cold limbs, thin loose stool, pale tongue with white coating, and weak or slow moderate pulse.

[Manifestations Analysis] Deficiency of spleen yang causes internal generation of cold, so there is dull epigastric pain with cool sensation, and preference for pressure and warmth. The cold dissipates with warmth and congeals with cold, thus the pain is aggravated with cold and alleviated after diet. Spleen deficiency and cold in the middle energizer triggers ascending of watery fluids, leading to vomiting of watery fluids. Spleen deficiency fails to transport and transform food, so anorexia is felt. Spleen deficiency generates dampness that descends, so there is loose stool. Pale tongue with white coating and weak or slow moderate pulse are signs of deficiency-cold in the spleen and stomach.

[Nursing Principle] Warming the middle and invigorating the spleen; harmonizing the stomach and relieving pain.

[Suggested Formula] Huangqi Jianzhong Decoction.

NURSING MEASURES

For patients with epigastric pain, nurses should observe the nature, degree, onset time, duration, frequency and inducing and alleviating factors of pain; the location, nature, degree, onset time, and inducing factors of abdominal distention; the frequency and degree of belching, acid regurgitation and vomiting; the color, property and form of vomitus and stool; and the presence or abscence of blood in vomitus and stool. They should also check the appetite, amount of food intake, tongue and pulse of the patients. For patients with hematemesis and tarry stool, accompanied with pale complexion, frequent cold sweat, cold limbs, dysphoria and decrease of blood pressure; or those with suddenly aggravated epigastric pain, accompanied with nausea, vomiting, hardness and fullness of the whole abdomen and unpalpable abdominal pain, it is advisable to report to the doctor immediately and assist in emergency treatment.

Syndrome-Based Nursing Measures

1. Syndrome of Cold Pathogen Attacking the Stomach

(1) Daily life nursing. The ward should be warm and away from wind. The patients should rest in bed and keep warm.

(2) Diet nursing. The diet should be warm and digestible. Shengjiang dazao (fresh ginger and Chinese date) tea is recommended. Eat foods that dissipate cold and relieve pain, such as congbai (scallion white), garlic, and xiaohuixiang (fennel). Food therapy: dingxiang rougui hongtang (clove flower, cinnamon bark, and brown sugar) decoction, and baihujiao zhudu (white pepper and pig stomach) soup. Raw, cold, fatty and sweet foods should be avoided.

(3) Emotion nursing. Nurses may use verbal enlightenment therapy to communicate with the patients as much as possible to help them maintain an optimistic mood.

(4) Medication nursing. Decoction should be taken hot after meals. After taking medicine, put on more clothes, tuck in quilts, and put a bag full of hot water on the epigastric region.

(5) Manipulation techniques. ① Paste application therapy: select Zhongwan (CV 12), Shangwan (CV 13), Weishu (BL 21), Pishu (BL 20) and Zusanli (ST 36); grind into powder wuzhuyu (medicinal evodia fruit), xiaohuixiang (fennel), xixin (Manchurian wild ginger) and bingpian (borneol); blend the powder with shengjiang (fresh ginger) juice to make pastes, and apply them on the acupoints, two hours each time, once per day. And it is contraindicated in pregnancy. ② Moxibustion therapy: select Zhongwan (CV 12), Zusanli (ST 36), Pishu (BL 20) and Weishu (BL 21); place the moxa stick 2 ~ 3 centimeters away from the skin to perform mild moxibustion on each of the acupoints until the area turns red and the patient feels warm and comfortable without the sensation of burning pain, once per day. ③ Acupressure therapy: select Zhongwan (CV 12), Neiguan (PC 6) and Zusanli (ST 36); apply thumb kneading, rubbing and one-finger pushing manipulations on each of the acupoints until the area turns hot or the patient has the feelings of soreness, numbness, distension and heaviness in the area. And it is contraindicated in pregnancy.

2. Syndrome of Liver Qi Invading the Stomach

(1) Daily life nursing. The ward should be quiet, tidy, and decorated with flowers, plants and bonsai. The patients should wear loose clothes. Pay attention to oral hygiene, rinse the mouth after meals, or rinse the mouth immediately after putrid belching and acid regurgitation. Patients with severe pain should rest in bed. When the pain eases, the patients should do moderate exercise. They should take an upright position after meals, take a walk for 30 minutes one hour after the meals until they feel warm

or perspire slightly but without fatigue. Eating before sleep should be prohibited. The time gap between supper and sleep should be more than three hours. Raise the head of the bed up to 30°.

（2）Diet nursing. The diet should be light. The patients should have small frequent meals with reduced food and water intake, and avoid eating in the mood of depression, anger or grief. Chenfo（aged tangerine peel and finger citron fruit）drink and jasmine tea are recommended. Eat foods that sooth the liver and regulate qi, such as kumquat, white radish and meiguihua（rose flower）. Food therapy：carrot stir-fried with chenpi shourousi（aged tangerine peel and sliced pork）. Raw, cold, greasy, pungent, spicy, hard, too-sweet, too-hot and flatulent foods should be avoided, such as sweet potatoes.

（3）Emotion nursing. Nurses may use verbal enlightenment therapy to help the patients to get over worries, use emotional transference and dispositional change therapy to distract their attention and eliminate their angry feelings, or use suggestive and doubts-dispelling therapy to eliminate their psychological stress. Moreover, nurses should create an easy and happy dining environment, so that the patients' liver qi can act freely.

（4）Medication nursing. Decoction should be taken warm after meals, multiple times in small portions.

（5）Manipulation techniques. ① Paste application therapy：select Zhongwan（CV 12）and Shenque（CV 8）；grind into powder equal parts of binlang（betel nut）, laifuzi（radish seed）, zhishi（immature bitter orange）, houpo（magnolia bark）, muxiang（common aucklandia root）, dafupi（areca husk）and xiangfu（cyperus）；blend the powder with tea-seed oil to make pastes, and apply them on the acupoints, eight hours each time, once per day. And it is contraindicated in pregnancy. ② Acupressure therapy：select Zhongwan（CV 12）, Neiguan（PC 6）, Zusanli（ST 36）, Yanglingquan（GB 34）, Taichong（LR 3）, Xingjian（LR 2）, Zhangmen（LR 13）, Qimen（LR 13）and Ganshu（BL 18）；apply thumb kneading, rubbing and one-finger pushing manipulations on each of the acupoints until the area turns hot or the patient has the feelings of soreness, numbness, distension and heaviness in the area；once per day. And it is contraindicated in pregnancy. ③ Auricular pressure therapy：select the auricular points of sympathetic（AH6a）, shenmen（TF4）, liver（CO12）and stomach（CO4）；apply specialized pasters on the points, press on each of them till the area feels hot and turns red, 4~5 times per day, and keep the pasters for 2~4 days. And it is contraindicated in pregnancy.

3. Syndrome of Phlegm and Fluid-Retention Stagnating in the Stomach

（1）Daily life nursing. The ward should be warm, dry, and full of fresh air. The patients should rest in bed, do moderate exercise such as slow walking or Taiji, and avoid being exhausted.

（2）Diet nursing. The patients should have small frequent meals, reduce the food intake, and eat foods that invigorate the spleen and dispel dampness, such as yiyiren（coix seed）and shanyao（common yam rhizome）. Food therapy：chixiaodou jiyu（adzuki bean and crucian）thick soup. The patient should not eat raw, cold, greasy, pungent, spicy, hard and flatulent foods, such as sweet potatoes.

（3）Emotion nursing. Nurses may use verbal enlightenment therapy to constantly comfort the patients to remove their anxiety and invigorate the function of their spleen and stomach.

（4）Medication nursing. Decoction should be taken warm after meals, multiple times in small portions.

（5）Manipulation techniques. ① Moxibustion therapy: select Zhongwan（CV 12）, Shenque（CV 8）, Qihai（CV 6）and Guanyuan（CV 4）; place the moxa stick 2~3 centimeters away from the skin to perform mild moxibustion on each of the acupoints until the area turns red and the patient feels warm and comfortable without the sensation of burning pain, once per day. And it cannot be applied on the abdomen of pregnant women. ② Acupressure therapy: select Zhongwan（CV 12）, Tianshu（ST 25）, Guanyuan（CV 4）, Pishu（BL 20）, Weishu（BL 21）and Zusanli（ST 36）; apply thumb kneading, rubbing and one-finger pushing manipulations on each of the acupoints until the area turns hot or the patient has the feelings of soreness, numbness, distension and heaviness in the area; once per day. And it is contraindicated in pregnancy.

4. Syndrome of Food Retention

（1）Daily life nursing. The ward should be quiet, full of gentle light and fresh air, and away from wind. The patients should take a semi-supine position after meals, move slowly to change the body positions, pay attention to oral hygiene, and often rinse the mouth with warm water.

（2）Diet nursing. Temporary fasting is recommended for patients with severe pain. When the condition is stabilized, the patients should have liquid diet, then semi-liquid, soft diet, and finally general diet. They should follow a moderate diet without being too hungry or too full, and eat foods that promote digestion and resolve accumulation, such as white radish, lemon, maiya（germinated barley）and chenpi（aged tangerine peel）. Food therapy: shenqu shanzha（medicated leaven and Chinese hawthorn fruit）porridge. Jilai（chicken gizzard lining and radish seed）powder is recommended: stir-fry laifuzi（radish seed）9 g and ji'neijin（chicken gizzard lining）5 g until they turn yellow, grind them into powder, divide the powder into three equal parts, and take each portion with warm water, three times per day. Raw, cold, greasy, too-sweet and sticky foods should be avoided.

（3）Emotion nursing. Although the symptoms are severe, it is new onset with shallow disease location and good prognosis. Nurses may encourage patients' family members to often accompany the patients, encourage them to communicate with other patients about the prevention and treatment measures of the disease to build up confidence.

（4）Medication nursing. Decoction should be taken warm after meals, multiple times in small portions. Before taking medicine, eat a slice of shengjiang（fresh ginger）or shanzha（Chinese hawthorn fruit）. Pills could be dissolved in warm water.

（5）Manipulation techniques. ① Acupoint-pressing therapy: select Shenmen（HT 7）and Neiguan（PC 6）; apply pressing manipulation with one thumb on the acupoints of the other hand, keep pressing for extra half a minute after the patient has feeling of pain and distention. ② Inducing vomiting therapy: irritate the pharynx with a tongue depressor or a feather, or drink warm dilute saline and use a finger to irritate the pharynx to induce vomiting. It is suitable for patients who desire but fail to vomit.

5. Syndrome of Dampness-Heat Accumulating in the Stomach

（1）Daily life nursing. The ward should be cool and full of fresh air. The clothes should be thin and baggy. Pay attention to oral hygiene, and rinse the mouth with jinyinhua gancao (honeysuckle flower and licorice root) liquid after meals. Keep the perianal skin clean and dry. Keep a normal bowel movement, and avoid overexertion and long-time squatting in defecation.

（2）Diet nursing. Eat light diet. Heye (lotus leaf) tea and green tea are recommended. Eat foods that clear heat and remove dampness, such as tender leaves of Chinese toon, yiyiren (coix seed), fuling (poria), balsam pear, lüdou (mung bean), bean curd and pakchoi. Pungent, spicy, dampness- and heat-generated foods should be avoided.

（3）Emotion nursing. Because the patients have excess heat syndrome with severe symptoms, nurses may use emotional transference and dispositional change therapy to distract their attention and eliminate dysphoria.

（4）Medication nursing. Decoction should be taken warm or slightly cool after meals.

（5）Manipulation techniques. ① Paste application therapy: select Zhongwan (CV 12), Shangwan (CV 13), Weishu (BL 21), Pishu (BL 20) and Zusanli (ST 36); grind into powder huanglian (coptis rhizome), huangqin (scutellaria root), ruxiang (frankincense), moyao (myrrh) and bingpian (borneol); blend the powder with vaseline to make pastes, and apply them on the acupoints, eight hours each time, once per day. And it is contraindicated in pregnancy. Or take some cactuses, smash, and apply the pulp on the affected region. ② Cupping therapy: select Pishu (BL 20) and Weishu (BL 21), and retain the cup on them for ten minutes; or select the area along the bladder meridian of foot-taiyang and governor vessel for sliding cupping, once every other day. It is contraindicated in pregnancy.

6. Syndrome of Blood Stasis Obstructing Collateral

（1）Daily life nursing. The ward should be warm, quiet, comfortable, full of fresh air, and away from wind. The patients should rest in bed, and keep the abdomen warm. For patients with hematemesis and tarry stool, take absolute bed rest. For patients with hematemesis, remove the pillow, turn the head aside, and clear vomitus in time to keep the respiratory track clean. Rinse the mouth with dilute saline after hematemesis. When the hematemesis and tarry stool are resolved, the patients could do some out-of-bed activities.

（2）Diet nursing. Patients with hematemesis are fasted. When the condition is stabilized, take liquid diet, and gradually change it to general diet. Honghua (safflower) tea is recommended. Eat foods that regulate qi and activate blood, such as shanzha (Chinese hawthorn fruit), chenpi (aged tangerine peel), xianggu (lentinus edodes), luffa, and eggplants. Food therapy: muxu roupian huanghuacai (sliced pork, black fungus, egg and day lily), dazao chidou lian'ou (Chinese date, adzuki bean, and lotus root) porridge. Raw, cold, coarse, hard, fried, rich and flatulent foods should be avoided, such as sweet potatoes.

（3）Emotion nursing. Nurses may use verbal enlightenment therapy to care for the patients, impart them disease-related knowledge and explain the test results to eliminate their fear of cancer. Nurses may use submission therapy to allow the patients to express fear, fright and worry reasonably. Nurses may use emotional transference and dispositional change therapy to help the patients to relax and alleviate their psychological pressure, such as taking a deep breath, reading entertainment books, or practising Taiji.

(4) Medication nursing. Decoction should be taken warm after meals, multiple times in small portions.

(5) Manipulation techniques. ① Paste application therapy: select Zhongwan (CV 12), Shenque (CV 8), Guanyuan (CV 4) and Tianshu (ST 25); grind into powder xixin (Manchurian wild ginger), chuanxiong (Sichuan lovage root), baizhi (angelica root), zaojiaoci (Chinese honeylocust spine), qiancao (Indian madder root) and honghua (safflower); blend the powder with sesame oil to make pastes, and apply them on the acupoints, 1~3 acupoint(s) each time, 4~6 hours each time, once per day. ② Foot bath therapy: decoct danggui (Chinese angelica), xixin (Manchurian wild ginger), chuanxiong (Sichuan lovage root), mugua (Chinese quince fruit), honghua (safflower) and gancao (licorice root); wash the feet with the decoction at a temperature of 37~42℃ and massage, 20 minutes each time, once per day. And it should be used with caution for patients with hypotension. ③ Water acupuncture therapy: select unilateral Zusanli (ST 36); inject danshen (danshen root) injection or compound danggui (Chinese angelica) injection into the acupoint. ④ Acupressure therapy: select Zhongwan (CV 12), Neiguan (PC 6), Weishu (BL 21), Ganshu (BL 18), Taichong (LR 3), Qimen (LR 14), Xuehai (SP 10) and Geshu (BL 17); apply thumb kneading, rubbing and one-finger pushing manipulations on each of the acupoints until the area turns hot or the patient has the feelings of soreness, numbness, distension and heaviness in the area; once per day. And it is contraindicated in pregnancy.

7. Syndrome of Stomach Yin Deficiency

(1) Daily life nursing. The ward should be cool, moist, quiet and comfortable. The patients should take more rest in bed. During the onset stage of epigastric pain, drink warm boil water or eat a little food to alleviate the pain. When the condition is stabilized, the patients may do moderate exercise to keep a normal bowel movement.

(2) Diet nursing. The patients should have small frequent meals. Tiepishihu (dendrobium officinale) tea or maidong (dwarf lilyturf tuber) tea is recommended. Eat foods that benefit the stomach and generate fluid, such as sugarcane, baihe (lily bulb), lianzi (lotus seed), yin'er (tremella), meat of soft-shelled turtles, lotus root, Chinese cabbage, sangshen (mulberry), snow pear, grapes, shanyao (common yam rhizome), fish gelatin, and honey. Food therapy: mugua shengjiang (Chinese quince fruit and fresh ginger) stewed with rice vinegar. The patients should refrain from alcohol, coffee, strong tea, and foods that are raw, cold, greasy, pungent, spicy and coarse.

(3) Emotion nursing. Because the patients are weak with a long course of disease, nurses may use verbal enlightenment therapy to explain the importance of diet nutrition for health maintenance.

(4) Medication nursing. Decoction should be prepared slowly over low heat and taken warm before meals, multiple times in small portions.

（5）Manipulation techniques. ① Acupressure therapy: select Weishu（BL 21）, Pishu（BL 20）, Xuehai（SP 10）, Zhongwan（CV 12）, Neiguan（PC 6）, Zusanli（ST 36）, Sanyinjiao（SP 6）and Taixi（KI 3）; apply thumb kneading, rubbing and one-finger pushing manipulations on each of the acupoints until the area turns hot or the patient has the feelings of soreness, numbness, distension and heaviness in the area; once per day. And it is contraindicated in pregnancy. ② Auricular pressure therapy: select the auricular points of stomach（CO4）, spleen（CO13）, sympathetic（AH6a）, shenmen（TF4）and subcortex（AT4）; apply specialized pasters on the points, knead each of them till the area turns hot and red, 4~5 times per day, and keep the pasters for 2~4 days. And it is contraindicated in pregnancy. ③ Healthcare massage therapy: the patients should take a supine position, bend two legs, and apply rubbing manipulation clockwise on the abdomen with the center of the palm, or slow rubbing from the upper abdomen to the lower abdomen, 3~4 times a day, and 5~10 minutes every time.

8. Syndrome of Deficiency-Cold in the Spleen and Stomach

（1）Daily life nursing. The ward should be sunward, warm, dry, quiet, comfortable and full of bright light, and avoid strong and convective wind. The patients should rest in bed with thick coverings, and keep the epigastric region warm. They should have adequate sleep, take some rest in bed after meals, and turn over regularly to prevent pressure sores. When the symptoms are alleviated, the patients may do moderate exercise but be cautious to avoid overstrain and falling while doing exercise.

（2）Diet nursing. The food should be warm. The patients should have small frequent meals, and foods that warm the middle and invigorate the spleen, such as pig stomach, longyanrou（longan）, dazao（Chinese date）, yellow croaker, ricefield eel and mutton, which may be seasoned with shengjiang（fresh ginger）, spring onion and baihujiao（white pepper）. Food therapy: qijing（Chinese wolfberry fruit and rhizoma polygonati）stewed with quail, and guihua lianzi（sweet-scented Osmanthus and lotus seed）thick soup. Raw, cold, cold-natured, greasy, sweet, sticky and roasted foods should be avoided.

（3）Emotion nursing. Because the patients are weak with a long course of disease, nurses may use verbal enlightenment therapy to explain the causes and inducing factors of epigastric pain to the patients and tell them to avoid cold, anger and improper diet in daily life. Nurses should know about the psychological state of the patients and help them to stay happy and avoid pessimism and depression.

（4）Medication nursing. Decoction should be prepared slowly over low heat and taken hot before meals.

（5）Manipulation techniques. ① Hot compress therapy: stir-fry salt with bran, and put it into a cloth bag for hot compress at a temperature of 60~70℃; 20 minutes each time, once per day. And it is contraindicated in pregnancy. ② Moxibustion therapy: select Zhongwan（CV 12）, Zusanli（ST 36）, Shenque（CV 8）, Qihai（CV 6）and Guanyuan（CV 4）; place the moxa stick 2~3 centimeters away from the skin to perform mild moxibustion on each of the acupoints until the area turns red and the patient feels warm and comfortable without the sensation of burning pain, once per day. And it cannot be applied on the abdomen of pregnant women. ③ Foot bath therapy: decoct huajiao（pricklyash peel）

30 g, huangqi (astragalus root) 30 g, jianghuang (turmeric root tuber) 15 g, yanhusuo (corydalis rhizome) 15 g, honghua (safflower) 15 g and sliced zhifuzi (prepared aconite root) 15 g; wash the feet with the decoction at a temperature is 37~42℃ before sleep, 20 minutes each time, once per day. And it should be used with caution for patients with hypotension. ④ Water acupuncture therapy: select Zusanli (ST 36); inject huangqi (astragalus root) injection or Shengmai Injection to the acupoint. ⑤ Acupressure therapy: select Zusanli (ST 36), Xuehai (SP 10), Guanyuan (CV 4), Tianshu (ST 25), Neiting (ST 44), Pishu (BL 20) and Zhangmen (LR 13); apply thumb kneading, rubbing and one-finger pushing manipulations on each of the acupoints until the area turns hot or the patient has the feelings of soreness, numbness, distension and heaviness in the area; once per day. And it is contraindicated in pregnancy.

Patient Education

The patients should live a regular life, balance work and rest, take adequate sleep, and avoid exogenous pathogenic factors, such as wind, cold, summer-heat and dampness. They should do moderate exercise without overstrain, and rest for half an hour after meals, avoiding lying flat or doing exercise immediately after meals.

The diet should be light, nutritious and digestible. The foods should be warm. The patients should have small frequent meals of proper quantity, at fixed time and slow speed, and pay attention to food hygiene. In cooking, steaming, boiling and stir-frying are prefered to deep-frying, smoking, pickling, curing, or raw mixing. The patients should refrain from cigarettes, alcohol, strong tea, coffee, and foods that are pungent, spicy, greasy, sweet, sticky, fried, roasted, coarse, hard and flatulent.

The patients should stay calm, enjoy a happy mood, and avoid depression, anxiety, worry and anger. They should also learn to get relaxed and regulate emotions by playing chess, reading newspaper or listening to music for the purpose of making themselves cheerful and improving the resistence to disease.

For patients with chronic recurrent epigastric pain, regular outpatient examination is recommended. They should follow the doctor's advice to have relevant tests to screen the risk factors and receive targeted intervention to prevent deterioration.

第十节 泄 泻 病

泄泻病，是指因外感风寒湿热之邪，或因饮食所伤，情志失调，或因久病，脾肾阳气亏虚而引起的，以大便次数增多，粪质稀薄，或完谷不化，甚至泻下水样便为临床特征的脾系病。西医的肠结核、炎症性肠病、功能性胃肠病，以腹泻为主要表现的，可参照本节进行护理。

一、病因病机

泄泻病的病因包括感受外邪、饮食不节、情志不调、脏腑虚衰。病人淋雨涉水，久坐湿地，寒湿困遏脾阳，或外感湿热、暑湿之邪，湿热壅遏脾胃，下迫大肠，可致脾胃气机失调，肠道功能失常，发为泄泻。病人饮食不节，或饮食饮酒过量，或偏嗜肥甘、辛辣、生冷，可致脾胃受损，肠道功能失常，发为泄泻。病人抑郁愤怒，焦虑紧张，导致肝郁乘脾，或思虑过度，土虚木乘，可致脾胃气机失调，肠道功能失常，发为泄泻。病人先天脾虚，年老体虚，久病劳倦，可使脾失健运，或年老久病，肾阳不足，不能温煦脾土，运化失常，湿滞内停，阻碍气机，水谷混杂，下走大肠，均可发为泄泻。

泄泻病的病机为脾虚湿盛，脾失健运，水湿不化，肠道清浊不分，传化失司。病位在脾、胃、大肠、小肠，与肝、肾有关。急性暴泻多为实证，慢性久泻多为虚证或虚实夹杂之证。

二、常见证型

（一）辨证要点

1. **辨暴泻与久泻**　根据病因、起病速度、发作频率、病程长短等来辨别。若因外邪或饮食而起，突然起病，症状剧烈，腹泻如倾，次频量多，泻下多水，或伴津伤气脱，病程在3周以内，多为暴泻。若因情志、饮食、劳倦而起，起病缓慢，间歇发作，伴倦怠乏力，病程超过3周，则多为久泻。

2. **辨寒热**　根据大便的量、色、质、气味等来辨别。若粪质清稀如水，完谷不化，伴腹痛，畏寒喜温，则多为寒。若粪便色黄褐而臭秽，伴肛门灼热，泻下急迫，小便短赤，口渴喜冷饮，则多为热。

3. **辨虚实**　根据起病速度、病程长短，以及大便的量、色、质等来辨别。若起病急，病程较短，次数频多，伴腹痛拒按，泻后痛减，多为实证。若起病缓慢，病程较长，反复发作，次数较少，伴腹痛不甚，喜温喜按，神疲肢冷，则多为虚证。

4. **辨泻下物**　根据大便的量、色、质、气味等来辨别邪气的种类。若大便清稀，或如水样，味秽腥，多为寒湿。若大便稀溏，色黄褐而臭，伴肛门灼热，多为湿热。若大便溏垢，臭如败卵，夹有不消化的食物残渣，则多为食积。

（二）证候分型

1. 暴泻

（1）寒湿内盛证

［主要证候］泻下清稀,甚至如水样;伴腹痛肠鸣,脘闷食少,或见恶寒发热,鼻塞头痛,肢体酸痛;舌苔薄白或白腻,脉濡缓。

［证候分析］寒湿侵袭,脾失健运,清浊不分,肠腑传导失司,故泻下清稀,甚至如水样;肠道气机受阻,寒主收引,故腹痛肠鸣;寒湿困脾,脾失健运,故脘闷食少;风寒湿邪束于肌表,故恶寒发热,鼻塞头痛,肢体酸痛;舌苔薄白或白腻,脉濡缓,均为寒湿内盛之象。

［护治原则］芳香化湿,解表散寒。

［常用方剂］藿香正气散。

（2）湿热中阻证

［主要证候］泄泻腹痛,泻下急迫,或泻而不爽,粪色黄褐臭秽,肛门灼热,烦热口渴,小便短黄;舌质红,苔黄腻,脉滑数或濡数。

［证候分析］湿热侵袭,肠道气机不畅,传化失常,故泻下急迫;热在肠中,湿热互结,腑气不扬,故泻而不爽,伴腹痛;湿热下迫,故大便色黄褐臭秽,肛门灼热,小便短黄;湿热蕴蒸,故烦热口渴;舌质红,苔黄腻,脉滑数或濡数,均为湿热内盛之象。

［护治原则］清热燥湿,分消止泻。

［常用方剂］葛根芩连汤。

（3）食滞肠胃证

［主要证候］腹痛肠鸣,泻下粪便臭如败卵,泻后痛减,脘腹胀满,嗳腐酸臭,不思饮食;舌苔垢浊或厚腻,脉滑。

［证候分析］宿食内停,肠胃传化失司,故腹痛肠鸣,泻下粪便臭如败卵;泻后腐浊之邪得以外出,故泻后痛减;脾胃不和,纳少化迟,故脘腹胀满,不思饮食;宿食不化,浊气上逆,故嗳腐酸臭;舌苔垢浊或厚腻,脉滑,均为饮食内停之象。

［护治原则］消食导滞,和中止泻。

［常用方剂］保和丸。

2. 久泻

（1）肝气乘脾证

［主要证候］平时心情抑郁,或急躁易怒,每因抑郁恼怒,或情绪紧张而发生泄泻,伴有胸胁胀闷,嗳气食少,腹痛攻窜,肠鸣矢气;舌淡红,脉弦。

［证候分析］情志不畅,肝失条达,横逆乘脾,脾运无权,故每因抑郁恼怒,或情绪紧张而发生泄泻;肝气郁结,气机郁闭,故平时心情抑郁,或急躁易怒,伴有胸胁胀闷;肝失疏泄,脾虚不运,故嗳气食少,腹痛攻窜,肠鸣矢气;舌淡红,脉弦,均为肝气郁结之象。

［护治原则］抑肝扶脾,调中止泻。

［常用方剂］痛泻要方。

（2）脾胃虚弱证

［主要证候］大便时溏时泻,迁延反复,稍进油腻食物,则大便溏稀,次数增加,或完谷不化,伴

食少纳呆,脘闷不舒,面色萎黄,倦怠乏力;舌质淡,苔白,脉细弱。

[证候分析]脾胃虚弱,运化无权,故大便时溏时泻,迁延反复,稍进油腻食物,则大便溏稀,次数增加,或完谷不化;脾阳不振,运化失司,故食少纳呆,脘闷不舒;久泻伤脾,气血化源不足,故面色萎黄,倦怠乏力;舌质淡,苔白,脉细弱,均为脾气虚弱之象。

[护治原则]健脾益气,化湿止泻。

[常用方剂]参苓白术散。

(3)肾阳虚衰证

[主要证候]黎明前腹部作痛,肠鸣即泻,泻后痛减,完谷不化,腹部喜暖喜按,形寒肢冷,腰膝酸软;舌淡苔白,脉沉细。

[证候分析]肾阳虚衰,火不暖土,脾失健运,黎明之前阴寒较盛,故黎明前腹部作痛,肠鸣即泻,又称"五更泻";泻后腑气通利,故泻后痛减;命门火衰,不能助脾腐熟水谷,故完谷不化;阳虚失于温煦,故形寒肢冷;腰为肾之府,肾主骨,肾阳衰惫,故腰膝酸软;舌淡苔白,脉沉细,均为肾阳不足之象。

[护治原则]温肾健脾,固涩止泻。

[常用方剂]四神丸。

三、护理措施

对于泄泻病的病人,应该观察排便的时间、次数,大便的量、色、质、气味;腹痛的性质、部位,以及腹痛的发生时间与泄泻之间的关系。注意观察神志、体温、口渴和饮水情况、尿量、腹胀、舌脉和皮肤弹性。如果病人出现眼窝凹陷,口干舌燥,皮肤弹性下降;或腹泻骤止,伴呼吸深长,烦躁不安,恶心呕吐,四肢厥冷,少尿或无尿,均应立即报告医生。

(一)辨证施护

1. 寒湿内盛证

(1)生活起居护理　居室宜向阳,温暖避风,空气新鲜。卧床休息,注意腹部保暖。若发热,不可冷敷。

(2)饮食护理　泄泻发作期间,吃流食或半流食。多饮水,可饮生姜大枣茶。宜食散寒化湿的食物,如白胡椒、肉桂、红糖。食疗方:姜橘椒鱼羹。不宜食生冷、油腻、辛辣的食物。

(3)情志护理　护士可运用语言开导疗法,宣教关于疾病的知识,帮助病人正确对待疾病,避免焦虑、紧张。

(4)用药护理　中药汤剂宜饭后热服,服后覆被静卧并微微汗出。

(5)操作技术　① 热敷疗法:用大葱100 g,与食盐炒热,装入布袋中,制成温度为60~70℃的中药热罨包,在腹部热敷20分钟,每日1次;女性月经期或妊娠期禁用。② 敷贴疗法:用生姜20 g,附子15 g,大葱2根,捣烂敷于涌泉;或用大蒜1头,白胡椒20粒,艾叶3 g,捣烂后与白酒调成糊状,敷于神阙;孕妇禁用。③ 穴位按摩法:取天枢、神阙、大肠俞、上巨虚、三阴交、脾俞、阴陵泉,用拇指揉法、摩法、一指禅推法,按摩至局部发热或有酸麻重胀感,每日1次;孕妇禁用。

2. 湿热中阻证

（1）生活起居护理　居室宜凉爽,空气新鲜。卧床休息。注意口腔护理,饭后用金银花甘草液漱口。勤换内裤,内裤应棉质、宽松、柔软。保持肛周清洁干燥,便后用柔软的厕纸擦拭。用温水清洁肛门,或用马齿苋 60 g 煎水坐浴,坐浴后在肛周涂青黛膏。

（2）饮食护理　泄泻发作期间,吃流食或半流食。饮食宜清淡。多饮水,可饮荷叶茶、雪梨汁、荸荠汁、藕汁。宜食清热化湿的食物,如薏苡仁、黄瓜叶、赤小豆、马齿苋。食疗方：小麦麸饼。不宜食油腻、生冷、硬固、辛辣的食物。

（3）情志护理　护士可运用语言开导疗法,关心和安慰病人,保持其情绪稳定,避免烦躁、恐惧。

（4）用药护理　中药汤剂宜饭后温服或偏凉服。

（5）操作技术　① 穴位按摩疗法：取天枢、神阙、大肠俞、上巨虚、三阴交、合谷、下巨虚,用拇指揉法、摩法、一指禅推法,按摩至局部发热或有酸麻重胀感,每日 1 次;孕妇禁用。② 涂药法：用九华膏或三黄膏;用棉签蘸药物涂抹于肛周,每日 2 次;适用于因便次频多而发生肛门糜烂、出血者。③ 浸洗疗法：用苍术、花椒煎水坐浴;适用于肛门灼热者,女性月经期或妊娠期禁用。

3. 食滞肠胃证

（1）生活起居护理　居室温暖干燥,空气新鲜,必要时可燃线香。卧床休息。

（2）饮食护理　泄泻发作期间,可禁食数小时至 1 天。待宿食泻尽后,逐渐从流食、半流食过渡到普食。食物宜清淡、细软,少食多餐。可饮酸梅汤、麦芽茶、谷芽茶、白萝卜汁或神曲茶。宜食消食化积的食物,如山楂、鸡内金、荞麦苗。食疗方：焦米粥。忌浓茶、咖啡,不宜食生冷、肥甘、厚味、甜腻的食物。

（3）情志护理　护士可运用语言开导疗法,告诉病人要注意饮食卫生,饭前便后要洗手,冰箱里的食物不宜存放过久,勿食用霉烂变质的食物。

（4）用药护理　中药汤剂宜温服,少量频服。若病人发生呕吐,可在服药前用生姜擦舌面,或用少许生姜汁滴舌。

（5）操作技术　① 穴位按摩法：取天枢、神阙、大肠俞、上巨虚、三阴交、中脘、建里,用拇指揉法、摩法、一指禅推法,按摩至局部发热或有酸麻重胀感,每日 1 次;孕妇禁用。② 保健按摩疗法：病人睡前取仰卧位,双膝屈曲,自行用双手叠于腹部左侧,顺时针按摩 20~30 次;或将单掌放于中脘,掌根发力,按摩 20 次。③ 耳压疗法：取大肠、小肠、脾、胃、交感、神门,用耳穴压豆胶布贴压,每日按揉 4~5 次,以局部发热泛红为度,留置 2~4 日;孕妇禁用。

4. 肝气乘脾证

（1）生活起居护理　居室安静舒适,空气新鲜。卧床休息,不可过劳。

（2）饮食护理　增进食欲,经常更换饮食品种,提高菜品的色、香、味。可饮玫瑰花茶、茉莉花茶。宜食疏肝健脾的食物,如金橘、陈皮、柚子、芡实、薏苡仁。食疗方：山楂荞麦饼。不宜食易产气的食物,如红薯。

（3）情志护理　护士可运用语言开导疗法、移情易性疗法、顺意疗法,经常与病人交流,了解导致其泄泻的心理因素,调节病人的情绪,避免忧虑、抑郁、恼怒。

（4）用药护理　中药汤剂宜饭后温服,少量频服。

（5）操作技术　①拔罐疗法：取天枢、中脘，留罐10分钟，隔日1次。②穴位按摩法：取天枢、神阙、大肠俞、上巨虚、三阴交、期门、太冲，用拇指揉法、摩法、一指禅推法，按摩至局部发热或有酸麻重胀感，每日1次；孕妇禁用。

5. 脾胃虚弱证

（1）生活起居护理　居室温暖干燥，安静避风。卧床休息，衣被宜厚，注意腹部保暖。起居有常，劳逸适度，不可久行、久站、进行重体力劳动或剧烈运动。排便时不可久蹲或过于用力。保持肛周清洁干燥，便后用温水清洗。经常做提肛运动。若发生脱肛，用温水坐浴后取侧卧位，涂黄连软膏，用灭菌纱布将脱出物推回肛内，再用丁字带压迫固定，卧床休息。若病情平稳，可进行少量的体育运动，如散步、打太极拳，以不疲劳为度。

（2）饮食护理　饮食宜清淡少油，温热软烂，少食多餐。宜食健脾止泻的食物，如莲子、芡实、百合、鲫鱼、猪肚、小米。食疗方：山药炖羊肉、茯苓饼、参枣米饭、姜汁牛肉饭。不宜食辛辣、肥甘、生冷、油腻、多渣、易产气的食物。

（3）情志护理　病人体虚久病，护士可运用语言开导疗法，态度和蔼，耐心讲解疾病的相关知识，使其积极配合治疗，避免紧张、忧虑。

（4）用药护理　中药汤剂宜文火久煎，饭前温服，少量频服。

（5）操作技术　①灸法：取天枢、大肠俞、上巨虚、三阴交、脾俞、足三里，或取足外踝高点直下，赤白肉际处，用温和灸，艾条燃着端悬于施灸部位上，距离皮肤2～3厘米，灸至病人有温热舒适无灼痛的感觉，皮肤稍有红晕，每日1次；孕妇腹部及腰骶部禁用。②保健按摩疗法：病人睡前取仰卧位，双膝屈曲，自行用双手叠于腹部，逆时针按摩20～30次。③热敷疗法：在腹部，用60～70℃的热水袋进行热敷，每次20分钟，每日1次；女性月经期或妊娠期禁用。④敷脐疗法：取神阙，用肉桂、川椒各0.5 g，研磨成粉后与芝麻油调匀，纳入脐中，每次2～8小时，每日1次；孕妇禁用。

6. 肾阳虚衰证

（1）生活起居护理　居室宜向阳，温暖避风，空气新鲜。卧床休息，衣被宜厚，注意腹部保暖。凌晨如厕时注意保暖。注意皮肤护理，定时翻身，预防压疮。若病情平稳，可进行少量的体育运动，如散步、打太极拳，注意安全，防止跌仆，不可过劳。

（2）饮食护理　饮食宜清淡、细软。可饮乌梅茶。宜食温阳止泻的食物，如芡实、鹿肉、麻雀肉、羊乳，常用肉桂、高良姜、荜茇、白胡椒调味。食疗方：四神腰花、椒姜羊肉汤、羊肾苁蓉羹。不宜食肥甘、生冷的食物。

（3）情志护理　病人体虚久病，护士可运用顺意疗法，多与病人交谈，鼓励其表达情绪。

（4）用药护理　中药汤剂宜文火久煎，饭前温服，少量频服。

（5）操作技术　①药熨疗法：取胃脘部，用肉桂、小茴香等量，研磨盐炒，装入布袋中，制成温度为60～70℃的中药热罨包，药熨20分钟，每日1次；孕妇禁用。②灸法：取天枢、神阙、大肠俞、上巨虚、三阴交、肾俞、命门、关元，隔附子饼灸。将附子研磨成粉，与黄酒调成直径2～3厘米、厚0.5～0.8厘米的薄饼，中间以针刺数孔，放置于施灸处，每处5～7壮，灸至皮肤稍有红晕，每日2次；孕妇禁用。③敷脐疗法：取神阙，用五倍子10 g，研磨成粉后与醋调为糊状敷贴，每次2～8小时，每日1次，连用3次；孕妇禁用。④足浴疗法：用生黄芪、酒大黄、当归、党参、鸡血藤各30 g，煎煮后待水温降至37～42℃时洗按足部，每次20分钟，每日1次；血压过低者慎用。

（二）健康教育

起居有常，注意腹部保暖。慎避外邪，勿贪凉露宿、冒雨涉水。进行适量的体育锻炼。

饮食宜清淡、营养、易消化。食物宜温热，进食速度宜慢，少食多餐，不可过饥、过饱。注意饮食卫生。宜食健脾益胃的食物。不宜食生冷、辛辣、油腻、肥甘的食物。

调畅情志，保持情绪稳定，避免精神刺激。

Section 10　Diarrhea

Diarrhea is a spleen disease characterized by increased bowel movements with thin loose stool or undigested food in stool or even watery stool. It is caused by external contraction of wind-cold and dampness-heat, dietary damage, emotional disorder, or yang deficiency of the spleen and kidney due to prolonged disease. This section can be referred to for the nursing of some diseases with diarrhea as the main manifestation such as intestinal tuberculosis, inflammatory bowel disease, and functional gastrointestinal diseases in Western medicine.

ETIOLOGY AND PATHOGENESIS

The etiology includes invasion of external pathogens, improper diet, emotional disorder and debilitation of zang-fu organs. Specifically speaking, getting soaked in the rain, wading into the water or keeping sedentary on the damp places causes cold-dampness encumbering spleen yang, or external invasion of pathogenic dampness-heat and summerheat-dampness leads to dampness-heat obstructing the spleen and stomach and pouring downward into the large intestine, all these may lead to qi movement disorder of the spleen and stomach as well as dysfunction of the intestine, thus resulting in diarrhea. Improper diet, over drinking or eating, predilection for fatty, too-sweet, pungent, spicy, raw and cold foods, all these could damage the spleen and stomach and cause dysfunction of the intestine, so diarrhea occurs. Depression, anger, anxiety and nervousness causes liver depression overwhelming the spleen, or excessive contemplation triggers over-restriction of the earth by the wood, all could cause qi movement disorder of the spleen and stomach and dysfunction of the intestine, leading to diarrhea. Congenital spleen deficiency, old age with weak constitution, or overstrain due to prolonged disease, all may lead to dysfunction of the spleen in transformation and transportation, causing diarrhea. Old age with prolonged disease, or insufficiency of kidney yang that fails to warm the spleen, all may induce dysfunction of the spleen in transportation and transformation as well as internal dampness stagnation, which blocks qi movement and makes water and food pour downward into the large intestine, leading to diarrhea.

The pathogenesis is spleen deficiency and dampness exuberance as well as dysfunction of the spleen in transportation and transformation, which causes non-transformation of water-dampness and failure of intestines to separate the clear from the turbid and to convey the waste of food. The disease is located in the spleen, stomach, large intestine and small intestines, and involves the liver and kidney. Acute fulminant diarrhea often pertains to excess syndrome whereas chronic diarrhea often to deficiency syndrome or deficiency-excess in complexity.

COMMON SYNDROMES

Key Points in Syndrome Differentiation

1. Differentiation of Fulminant from Chronic Diarrhea

The differentiation is based on the cause, developing speed, frequency and course of the disease. If it is caused by external pathogen or diet, with sudden onset, severe symptoms, frequent pouring and watery diarrhea in large volume, possibly accompanied by fluid damage and qi collapse, and the course is within three weeks, it is identified as fulminant diarrhea. If it is induced by emotional factors, diet and overstrain, with slow onset, intermittent attack, accompanied by lassitude and lack of strength, and the course is more than three weeks, it is identified as chronic diarrhea.

2. Differentiation of Cold from Heat Syndrome

The differentiation is based on the color, texture, volume and smell of the stool. Cold syndrome shows thin and clear stool, undigested food in stool, accompanied by abdominal pain, aversion to cold and preference for warmth. Heat syndrome exhibits brown foul-smelling stool, accompanied by urgency of bowel movement with scorching sensation in the anus, scanty dark urine, and thirst with desire for cold drinks.

3. Differentiation of Deficiency from Excess Syndrome

The differentiation is based on the developing speed, course of the disease and the color, texture and volume of the stool. Excess syndrome shows acute onset, frequent occurrence, short disease course, thin and clear stool, accompanied by unpalpable abdominal pain relieved after diarrhea. However, deficiency syndrome exhibits slow onset, less times, long disease course, disease recurrence, accompanied by mild abdominal pain, preference for warmth and pressure, lassitude and cold limbs.

4. Differentiation of the Stool

The differentiation is based on the color, texture, volume and smell of the stool. Clear thin or watery stool with fishy foul-smell indicates cold-dampness. Loose foul-smelling stool with brown color, and accompanied by scorching sensation in the anus means dampness-heat. Loose filthy and putrid foul-smelling stool with undigested food suggests food accumulation.

Syndrome Differentiation

1. Fulminant Diarrhea

(1) Syndrome of Internal Exuberance of Cold-Dampness

〔Clinical Manifestations〕 Clear thin or even watery stool, accompanied by abdominal pain, borborygmus, epigastric fullness, reduced appetite, or possible aversion to cold, fever, nasal congestion, headache, aching pain in the limbs, white thin or white slimy tongue coating, and soggy moderate pulse.

〔Manifestations Analysis〕 Invasion of cold-dampness and dysfunction of the spleen in transportation and transformation lead to failure of intestines to separate the clear from the turbid and to convey the waste of food, resulting in clear thin or even watery stool. The obstruction of qi movement in intestines and cold causing contracture and tension explain abdominal pain and borborygmus. Cold-dampness encumbering the spleen and dysfunction of the spleen in transportation and transformation contribute to epigastric fullness and reduced appetite. Wind-cold and dampness fetters the exterior, causing aversion to cold, fever, nasal congestion, headache and aching pain in the limbs. White thin or white slimy tongue coating and soggy moderate pulse pertain to internal exuberance of cold-dampness.

〔Nursing Principle〕Resolving dampness with aromatics; releasing exterior and dissipating cold.

〔Suggested Formula〕Huoxiang Zhengqi Powder.

（2）Syndrome of Dampness-Heat Obstruction in the Middle

〔Clinical Manifestations〕Diarrhea with abdominal pain, urgent or unsmooth bowel movement, brown foul-smelling stool, scorching sensation in the anus, heat vexation, thirst, scanty dark urine, red tongue with yellow slimy coating, and slippery rapid or soggy rapid pulse.

〔Manifestations Analysis〕Invasion of dampness-heat and disinhibition of qi movement in intestines cause dysfunction of the spleen in transportation and transformation, lending to urgent bowel movement. Heat in the intestines intermingling with dampness causes failure of fu-organ qi to ascend, so there is unsmooth bowel movement and abdominal pain. Dampness-heat pours downward, causing brown foul-smelling stool, scorching sensation in the anus, heat vexation, thirst, and scanty dark urine. Dampness-heat brews and steams, resulting in heat vexation and thirst. Red tongue with yellow slimy coating, slippery rapid or soggy rapid pulse pertains to internal dampness-heat exuberance.

〔Nursing Principle〕Clearing heat and dry dampness; separating dispersion and checking diarrhea.

〔Suggested Formula〕Gegen Qinlian Decoction.

（3）Syndrome of Food Stagnation in the Stomach and Intestine

〔Clinical Manifestations〕Abdominal pain, borborygmus, putrid foul-smelling stool, abdominal pain relieved after diarrhea, epigastric and abdominal distension and fullness, belching of putrid sour qi, poor appetite, dirty turbid or thick slimy tongue coating, and slippery pulse.

〔Manifestations Analysis〕Food stagnation causes dysfunction of the stomach and intestine in conveyance, so there are abdominal pain, borborygmus and putrid foul-smelling stool. Putrid and turbid pathogens are expelled out with diarrhea, so the pain decreases. Disharmony between the spleen and stomach causes reduced appetite, so there are epigastric and abdominal distension and fullness, and poor appetite. Food accumulation causes turbid qi ascending upward, so there is belching of putrid sour qi. Dirty turbid or thick slimy tongue coating and slippery pulse mean food stagnation in the stomach and intestine.

〔Nursing Principle〕Promoting digestion and removing food stagnation; harmonizing the middle and checking diarrhea.

〔Suggested Formula〕Baohe Pills.

2. Chronic Diarrhea

（1）Syndrome of Liver Qi Overwhelming the Spleen

［Clinical Manifestations］Emotional depression in normal times, irritability, occurrence of diarrhea always induced by depression, anger or nervousness, accompanied by distending oppression in the chest and hypochondrium, belching, reduced appetite, scurrying abdominal pain, borborygmus and flatus, pale red tongue, and wiry pulse.

［Manifestations Analysis］Emotional depression and failure of the liver to act freely cause transverse invasion of liver qi to overwhelm the spleen, which causes dysfunction of the spleen in transportation and transformation, so diarrhea is always induced by depression, anger or nervousness.

［Nursing Principle］Repressing the liver and supporting the spleen; harmonizing the middle and checking diarrhea.

［Suggested Formula］Tongxie Yaofang Formula.

（2）Syndrome of Spleen-Stomach Weakness

［Clinical Manifestations］Recurrent alternating loose stool and diarrhea, thin loose stool and increase of bowel movement after eating greasy food, or undigested food in stool, accompanied by anorexia, epigastric oppression and discomfort, sallow complexion, lassitude, pale tongue with white coating, and thready weak pulse.

［Manifestations Analysis］Weakness of the spleen and stomach causes failure in transportation and transformation, leading to recurrent alternating loose stool and diarrhea, thin loose stool and increase of bowel movement after eating greasy food, or undigested food in stool. Spleen yang devitalization causes failure in transportation and transformation, so there are anorexia, epigastric oppression and discomfort. Chronic diarrhea damages the spleen that cannot provide sufficient source for the generation and transformation of qi and blood, so the patients show sallow complexion and lassitude. Pale tongue with white coating and thready weak pulse suggests weakness of spleen qi.

［Nursing Principle］Invigorating the spleen and replenishing qi; resolving dampness and checking diarrhea.

［Suggested Formula］Shenling Baizhu Powder.

（3）Syndrome of Kidney Yang Debilitation

［Clinical Manifestations］Diarrhea usually at dawn upon abdominal pain and borborygmus, abdominal pain relieved after diarrhea, undigested food in stool, preference for warmth and pressure in abdomen, cold body and limbs, soreness and weakness in the waist and knees, pale tongue with white coating, and sunken thready pulse.

［Manifestations Analysis］Debilitation of kidney yang and fire failing to warm earth lead to failure of the spleen in transportation and transformation. Yin cold is exuberant at dawn, so diarrhea usually occurs at dawn upon abdominal pain and borborygmus. That is why it is also called "*wugengxie* (daybreak diarrhea)". Disinhibition of qi movement in fu-organ after diarrhea relieves the pain. Debilitation of life gate fire fails to assist the spleen to decompose foodstuff, so there is undigested food in stool. Yang debilitation fails to warm the body, so cold body and limbs are felt. Lumbus is the house of the kidney that governs the bones, so when kidney yang is in debilitation, there is soreness and weakness in the waist and knees. Pale tongue with white coating and sunken thready pulse suggest debilitation of kidney yang.

[Nursing Principle] Warming the kidney and invigorating the spleen; checking diarrhea with astringents.

[Suggested Formula] Sishen Pills.

NURSING MEASURES

For cases with diarrhea, nurses should observe the time and frequency of defecation; the quantity, color, consistency, odor of the stool; the nature and location of abdominal pain; the interrelationship between the onset time of abdominal pain and diarrhea. Nurses should also monitor the spirit, body temperature, thirst, drinking of water, urine output, abdominal distension, tongue, pulse as well as skin elasticity. For cases with sunken eye socket, dry mouth and tongue, decreased skin elasticity, or sudden stoppage of diarrhea accompanied by deep and long breathing, restlessness, nausea, vomiting, cold limbs, little or no urine, it should be immediately reported to doctors.

Syndrome-Based Nursing Measures

1. Syndrome of Internal Exuberance of Cold-Dampness

(1) Daily life nursing. The ward should be sunward, warm, full of fresh air, and away from wind. The patients should rest in bed and keep the abdomen warm. For patients with fever, cold compress is forbidden.

(2) Diet nursing. During the onset period of diarrhea, liquid or semi-liquid diet is recommended. The patients should drink more water, may drink shengjiang dazao (fresh ginger and Chinese date) tea, and eat cold-dissipating and dampness-resolving foods, such as baihujiao (white pepper), rougui (cinnamon bark) and brown sugar. Food therapy: jiangju jiaoyu (fresh ginger, tangerine pericarp, pricklyash peel and crucian) thick soup. Raw, cold, greasy, pungent and spicy foods should be avoided.

(3) Emotion nursing. Nurses may use verbal enlightenment therapy to impart patients the knowledge of the disease to help them better understand the disease and prevent anxiety and nervousness.

(4) Medication nursing. The decoction should be taken hot after meals. After taking medicine, the patients should take some rest in bed and put on more clothes and quilt to perspire slightly.

(5) Manipulation techniques. ① Hot compress therapy: stir-fry 100 g of scallion with salt, and put it into a cloth bag for hot compress at a temperature of 60~70℃; 20 minutes each time, once per day. And it is contraindicated in women during menstruation or pregnancy. ② Paste application therapy: mash 15 g of fuzi (monkshood), 20 g of shengjiang (fresh ginger), and two stalks of scallion, and apply the pastes on Yongquan (KI 1); or mash one whole grain of dasuan (garlic bulb), 20 grains of baihujiao (white pepper), and 3 g of mugwort leaves, add in proper amount of liquor and apply the pastes on

Shenque (CV 8). And it is contraindicated in pregnancy. ③ Acupressure therapy: select Tianshu (ST 25), Shenque (CV 8), Dachangshu (BL 25), Shangjuxu (ST 37), Sanyinjiao (SP 6), Pishu (BL 20), and Yinlingquan (SP 9); apply thumb kneading, rubbing and one-finger pushing manipulations on each of the acupoints until the area turns hot or the patient has the feelings of soreness, numbness, distension and heaviness in the area; once per day. And it is contraindicated in pregnancy.

2. Syndrome of Dampness-Heat Obstruction in the Middle

(1) Daily life nursing. The ward should be cool and full of fresh air. The patients should rest in bed, maintain oral hygiene by rinsing with jinyinhua gancao (honeysuckle flower and licorice root) liquid, and wear cotton, loose, soft underwear and change it frequently. Keep the perianal region dry and clean with soft toilet paper to wipe it after defecation; clean the anus with warm water, or have a hip bath with decoction made by 60 g of machixian (purslane) and then apply Qingdai Paste on the anus.

(2) Diet nursing. During the onset period of diarrhea, the patients should have light liquid or semi-liquid diet. They should drink more water, may drink heye (lotus leaf) tea, snow pear juice, biqi (waternut) juice and lotus root juice, and eat foods that clear heat and resolve dampness, such as yiyiren (coix seeds), cucumber leaves, chixiaodou (adzuki beans) and machixian (purslane). Food therapy: wheat bran pancake. Greasy, raw, cold, hard, pungent and spicy foods should be avoided.

(3) Emotion nursing. Nurses may use the verbal enlightenment therapy to care about and console the patients to keep their mood stable and alleviate vexation or fear.

(4) Medication nursing. Decoction should be taken warm or slightly cool after meals.

(5) Manipulation techniques. ① Acupressure therapy: select Tianshu (ST 25), Shenque (CV 8), Dachangshu (BL 25), Shangjuxu (ST 37), Sanyinjiao (SP 6), Hegu (LI 4), and Xiajuxu (ST 39); apply thumb kneading, rubbing and one-finger pushing manipulations on each of the acupoints until the area turns hot or the patient has the feelings of soreness, numbness, distension and heaviness in the area; once per day. And it is contraindicated in pregnant women. ② Application therapy: apply Jiuhua Paste or Sanhuang Paste; use cotton swabs dipped in the paste to apply it on the perianal area, twice per day; and it is suitable for patients with erosion and bleeding for frequent defecation. ③ Steeping and washing therapy: have hip baths with decoction prepared with cangzhu (atractylodes rhizome) and huajiao (pricklyash peel); this is effective for patients with a burning sensation of the anus. And it is contraindicated in females during menstruation or pregnancy.

3. Syndrome of Food Stagnation in the Stomach and Intestine

(1) Daily life nursing. The ward should be warm, dry, and full of fresh air. Joss sticks could be burned if necessary. The patients should rest in bed.

(2) Diet nursing. During the onset period of diarrhea, the patients could fast for several hours to one day. After the retained food is eliminated from the body, they could shift the diet gradually from liquid or semi-liquid one to general one. The diet should be light, soft, and taken multiple times in small portions. Plum syrup, maiya (germinated barley) tea, guya (grain sprout) tea, white radish juice or shenqu (medicated leaven) tea are recommended. It is advisable to eat foods that promote digestion and

resolve accumulation, such as shanzha (Chinese hawthorn fruit), ji'neijin (chicken gizzard lining) and buckwheat sprout. Food therapy: scorch-fried-rice porridge. Coffee, strong tea, as well as raw, cold, fatty, sweet, rich and greasy foods should be avoided.

(3) Emotion nursing. Nurses may use verbal enlightenment therapy to inform patients that they should pay attention to food hygiene and safety, wash hands before meals and after using the bathroom, and avoid storing food in refrigerators for an extended period of time or eating rotten and spoiled food.

(4) Medication nursing. Decoction should be taken warm, multiple times in small portions. For patients with vomiting, rub shengjiang (fresh ginger) slice on the surface of the tongue or have a few drops of shengjiang (fresh ginger) juice on the tongue before taking the medicine.

(5) Manipulation techniques. ① Acupressure therapy: select Tianshu (ST 25), Shenque (CV 8), Dachangshu (BL 25), Shangjuxu (ST 37), Sanyinjiao (SP 6), Zhongwan (CV 12), and Jianli (CV 11); apply thumb kneading, rubbing and one-finger pushing manipulations on each of the acupoints until the area turns hot or the patient has the feelings of soreness, numbness, distension and heaviness in the area; once per day. And it is contraindicated in pregnancy. ② Health massage therapy: before sleep, patients should take a supine position, bend knees, put their hands on the left side of the abdomen and massage the area clockwise 20~30 cycles; or place one palm on Zhongwan (CV 12), massage the acupoint with the base of the palm for 20 cycles. ③ Auricular pressure therapy: select the auricular points of large intestine (CO7), small intestine (CO6), spleen (CO13), stomach (CO4), sympathetic (AH6a), and shenmen (TF4); apply specialized pasters on the points, knead each of them till the area turns hot and red, 4~5 times per day, and keep the pasters for 2~4 days. And it is contraindicated in pregnant women.

4. Syndrome of Liver Qi Overwhelming the Spleen

(1) Daily life nursing. The ward should be quiet, comfortable, and full of fresh air. The patients should rest in bed and avoid overstrain.

(2) Diet nursing. The patients should try to build their appetite by diversifying the food and improving the taste, fragrance and appearance of the dishes. Meiguihua (rose flower) tea and jasmine tea are recommended. Foods that soothe the liver and invigorate the spleen, such as kumquat, chenpi (aged tangerine peel), pomelo, qianshi (euryale seeds), and yiyiren (coix seeds), are preferred. Food therapy: shanzha qiaomai (hawthorn and buckwheat) pancake. Foods that may lead to flatulence, such as sweet potatoes, should be avoided.

(3) Emotion nursing. Nurses may use verbal enlightenment therapy, emotional transference and dispositional change therapy as well as submission therapy to communicate with the patients, discover the psychological causes for their diarrhea, and regulate their moods to prevent distress, depression and annoyance.

(4) Medication nursing. Decoction should be taken warm after meals, multiple times in small portions.

(5) Manipulation techniques. ① Cupping therapy: select Tianshu (ST 25) and Zhongwan (CV

12); retain the cup on them for ten minutes, once every other day. ② Acupressure therapy: select Tianshu (ST 25), Shenque (CV 8), Dachangshu (BL 25), Shangjuxu (ST 37), Sanyinjiao (SP 6), Qimen (LR 14), and Taichong (LR 3); apply thumb kneading, rubbing, and one-finger pushing manipulations on each of the acupoints until the area turns hot or the patient has the feelings of soreness, numbness, distension and heaviness in the area; once per day. And it is contraindicated in pregnant women.

5. Syndrome of Spleen-Stomach Weakness

(1) Daily life nursing. The ward should be warm, dry, quiet and away from wind. The patients should rest in bed, wear thick clothes, get under thick covers, and keep the abdomen warm. They should live a regular life, balance work and rest, and avoid prolonged period of sitting or standing as well as heavy labor or strenuous activity. They should also keep the perianal region clean and dry, use warm water to clean the area after defecation, practise anus-contraction exercise constantly, and avoid long squatting or overexertion in defecation. In case of anal prolapse, the patients, after a warm hip bath, could lie on the side, apply Huanglian Paste, use sterilized gauze to push back the prolapse, fix it with a T-shape-bandage and rest in bed. When the condition is stabilized, take moderate exercise without overexertion, such as walking and Taiji.

(2) Diet nursing. The diet should be light, warm (hot), tender and well-cooked with minimal oil. The patients should have small frequent meals and foods that invigorate the spleen and check diarrhea, such as lianzi (lotus seed), qianshi (euryale seed), baihe (lily bulb), crucian, pig stomach and millet. Food therapy: mutton stewed with shanyao (common yam rhizome), fuling (poria) pancake, shenzao (ginseng and Chinese date) rice, and jiangzhi niurou (fresh ginger juice and beef) rice. Pungent, spicy, fatty, sweet, raw, cold, greasy, coarse-fiber and flatulent foods should be avoided.

(3) Emotion nursing. For weak patients with a long course of disease, nurses may use verbal enlightenment therapy to inform them patiently and warmly about the disease to make them cooperate with the treatment and relieve their tension and distress.

(4) Medication nursing. Decoction should be prepared slowly over low heat, and taken warm before meals, multiple times in small portions.

(5) Manipulation techniques. ① Moxibustion therapy: select Tianshu (ST 25), Dachangshu (BL 25), Shangjuxu (ST 37), Sanyinjiao (SP 6), Pishu (BL 20), and Zusanli (ST 36), or select the border between the red and white flesh vertically below the external malleolus; place the moxa stick 2~3 centimeters away from the skin to perform mild moxibustion on each of the points until the area turns red and the patient feels warm and comfortable without the sensation of burning pain, once per day. And it cannot be applied on the abdomen and lumbosacral region of pregnant women. ② Healthcare massage therapy: before sleep, the patients should take a supine position, bend their knees, fold their hands on the abdomen and massage the area counterclockwise 20~30 times. ③ Hot compress therapy: put a hot-water bag on the abdomen at a temperature of 60~70℃, 20 minutes each time, once per day. And it is contraindicated in females during menstruation or pregnancy. ④ Umbilical compress therapy: grind into

powder 0.5 g of rougui (cinnamon bark) and 0.5 g of chuanjiao (Sichuan pricklyash peel), blend the powder with sesame oil to make a paste, and apply the paste on the navel, 2~8 hours each time, once per day. And it is contraindicated in pregnancy.

6. Syndrome of Kidney Yang Debilitation

(1) Daily life nursing. The ward should be sunward, warm, full of fresh air, and away from wind. The patients should rest in bed, wear thick clothes, get under thick covers, and keep the abdomen warm. They should also keep warm when using the bathroom before dawn, and turn over regularly to prevent pressure sores. If the condition becomes stable, some exercise, such as walking and Taiji, could be taken. Moreover, they should take extra care to prevent traumatic impairment and avoid falls and overexertion.

(2) Diet nursing. Wumei (smoked plum) tea is preferred. The patients should have light and tender diet as well as foods that warm yang and check diarrhea, such as qianshi (euryale seeds), venison, sparrow meat, and sheep milk, which are often seasoned with rougui (cinnamon bark), gaoliangjiang (galangal), biba (long pepper fruit), and baihujiao (white pepper). Food therapy: sishen pig kidneys, jiaojiang yangrou (pricklyash peel, fresh ginger and mutton) soup, yangshen congrong (sheep kidneys and desert cistanche) thick soup. Fatty, sweet, raw and cold foods should be avoided.

(3) Emotion nursing. For weak patients with a long course of disease, nurses may use verbal enlightenment therapy to talk with the patients as much as possible to encourage them to express their emotions.

(4) Medication nursing. Decoction should be slowly prepared over low heat, and taken warm before meals, multiple times in small portions.

(5) Manipulation techniques. ① Medicated ironing therapy: grind into powder rougui (cinnamon bark) and xiaohuixiang (fennel) and stir-fry the powder with salt; put it into a cloth bag for medicated ironing at a temperature of 60~70℃; 20 minutes each time, once per day. And it is contraindicated in pregnancy. ② Moxibustion therapy: select Tianshu (ST 25), Shenque (CV 8), Dachangshu (BL 25), Shangjuxu (ST 37), Sanyinjiao (SP 6), Shenshu (BL 23), Mingmen (GV 4), and Guanyuan (CV 4); apply monkshood-cake-partitioned moxibustion on them. The procedure is to mix finely ground fuzi (monkshood) powder with yellow wine to make thin medicated cakes with a diameter of 2~3 centimeters and thickness of 0.5~0.8 centimeters, pierce several holes through the cakes with sharp needle, and place the cakes on the acupoints, 5~7 moxa-cones on every acupoint until the area turns red, twice every day. And it is contraindicated in pregnancy. ③ Umbilical compress therapy: select Shenque (CV 8); grind into powder 10 g of wubeizi (gallnut of Chinese sumac), blend the powder with vinegar to make a paste, and apply the paste on the navel, 2~8 hours each time, once per day, for three consecutive times. And it is contraindicated in pregnant women. ④ Foot bath therapy: decoct 30 g of shenghuangqi (raw astragalus root), 30 g of jiudahuang (yellow wine prepared rhubarb root and rhizome), 30 g of danggui (Chinese angelica), 30 g of dangshen (codonopsis root), and 30 g of jixueteng (suberect spatholobus stem); wash the feet with the decoction at a temperature of 37~42℃

and massage, 20 minutes each time, once per day. And it should be used with caution for patients with hypotension.

Patient Education

The patients should live a regular life, keep the abdomen warm, and take moderate exercise. They should also cautiously avoid pathogenic factors, braving rain or wading in water.

The diet should be light, nutritious and digestible. Food should be taken warm and slowly. The patients should have multiple small meals, pay attention to food hygiene, eat foods that invigorate the spleen and benefit the stomach and avoid foods that are raw, cold, pungent, spicy, greasy, fatty and sweet.

Patients should regulate their emotions, keep their mood stable and prevent mental disturbance.

第十一节 黄 疸

　　黄疸,泛指因外感湿热疫毒,酒客湿热内蕴,或因寒湿困脾,结石、肿块梗阻,导致气滞血瘀,迫使胆汁外溢,以面目发黄、身黄、小便黄为临床特征的一类疾病。西医的病毒性肝炎、自身免疫性肝病、药物性肝病、肝硬化、肝外胆系结石及炎症、胆道系统肿瘤,以黄疸为主要表现的,可参照本节进行护理。

一、病因病机

　　黄疸的病因包括感受外邪、饮食不节、脾胃虚寒、他病所致等。病人外感湿热、寒湿或时气疫毒,内蕴中焦,交蒸于肝胆,胆液不循常道,可发为黄疸。过食肥甘,或嗜酒无度,或饮食不节,脾胃受损,生湿化热,熏蒸肝胆,胆汁不循常道,可发为黄疸。病人恣食生冷,或饥饱失常,脾虚生湿,困遏中焦,肝失疏泄,胆汁外溢,可发为黄疸。素体脾虚,或劳倦太过,或久病伤脾,使运化失司,寒湿阻滞中焦,胆汁外溢,可发为黄疸。砂石、虫体或瘀血阻滞胆道,胆汁外溢,亦可发为黄疸。

　　黄疸的病机为湿邪困遏脾胃,壅塞肝胆,疏泄失常,胆汁泛溢肌肤。病位在脾胃、肝胆,与心、肾有关。外感或急性发作的黄疸,多为实证。内伤或慢性发作的黄疸,多为虚实夹杂之证。

二、常见证型

（一）辨证要点

1. 辨阳黄与阴黄　根据起病速度、病程长短、黄疸的颜色等来辨别。若起病快,病程短,黄色鲜明,舌红,脉弦数,多属热证、实证,为阳黄。若起病急骤,黄色如金,病情急转直下,舌绛,多为急黄。若起病缓,病程长,黄色晦暗,舌淡,脉迟或弱,多属寒证、虚证,为阴黄。

2. 辨热重与湿重　根据发热程度等来辨别。若发热重,口干而苦,口渴,大便秘结,苔黄腻,多为热重于湿。若发热轻,头身困重,胸脘痞满,大便溏垢,苔微黄腻,多为湿重于热。

（二）证候分型

1. 急黄

疫毒炽盛证

［主要证候］发病急骤,黄疸迅速加深,其色如金;皮肤瘙痒,高热口渴,胁痛腹满,神昏谵语,烦躁抽搐,或见衄血、便血,或肌肤瘀斑;舌质红绛,苔黄而燥,脉弦滑或数。

［证候分析］疫毒热炽,内扰于胆,胆汁浸淫肌肤,故发病急骤,黄疸迅速加深,其色如金,皮肤瘙痒;邪热耗损气阴,故高热口渴;脾胃肝胆气机壅滞,故胁痛腹满;邪陷厥阴,故神昏谵语,烦躁抽

搐;邪热迫血妄行,故衄血、便血、肌肤瘀斑;舌质红绛,苔黄而燥,脉弦滑或数,均为邪毒炽盛之象。

[护治原则]清热解毒,凉血开窍。

[常用方剂]犀角散。

2.阳黄

(1)热重于湿证

[主要证候]身目俱黄,黄色鲜明;发热口渴,或见心中懊恼,腹部胀闷,口干而苦,恶心呕吐,小便短少黄赤,大便秘结;舌苔黄腻,脉弦数。

[证候分析]湿热熏蒸肝胆,胆汁外溢肌肤,故身目俱黄;热重于湿,故黄色鲜明;湿热蕴阻中焦,故腹部胀闷,恶心呕吐;热结胃腑伤津,故发热口渴,心中懊恼,口干而苦,大便秘结;湿热下注膀胱,故小便短少黄赤;舌苔黄腻,脉弦数,均为湿热内盛之象。

[护治原则]清热通腑,利湿退黄。

[常用方剂]茵陈蒿汤。

(2)湿重于热证

[主要证候]身目俱黄,黄色不及前者鲜明;头重身困,胸脘痞满,食欲减退,恶心呕吐,腹胀或大便溏垢;舌苔厚腻微黄,脉濡数或濡缓。

[证候分析]湿热熏蒸肝胆,胆汁排泄不畅,故身目俱黄;湿重热轻,故黄色不甚鲜明;湿困肌表,故头重身困;湿热蕴阻中焦,故胸脘痞满,食欲减退,恶心呕吐,腹胀;湿热夹滞,阻于肠道,故大便溏垢;舌苔厚腻微黄,脉濡数或濡缓,均为湿热内蕴之象。

[护治原则]利湿化浊运脾,佐以清热。

[常用方剂]茵陈五苓散合甘露消毒丹。

(3)胆腑郁热证

[主要证候]身目发黄,黄色鲜明;上腹、右胁胀闷疼痛,牵引肩背,身热不退,或寒热往来,口苦咽干,呕吐呃逆,尿黄赤,大便秘结;舌红,苔黄,脉弦滑数。

[证候分析]虫石阻塞胆道,胆汁溢于肌肤,故身目发黄;胆热瘀结,肝气壅滞,故上腹、右胁胀闷疼痛,牵引肩背;胆热瘀阻,胃气上逆,故口苦咽干,呕吐呃逆;脾胃运化升降失常,故大便秘结;郁热侵袭少阳,故寒热往来;郁热流注下焦,故尿黄赤;舌红,苔黄,脉弦滑数,均为胆腑郁热之象。

[护治原则]疏肝泄热,利胆退黄。

[常用方剂]大柴胡汤。

3.阴黄

(1)寒湿阻遏证

[主要证候]身目俱黄,黄色晦暗,或如烟熏;脘腹痞胀,纳食减少,大便不实,神疲畏寒,口淡不渴;舌淡苔腻,脉濡缓或沉迟。

[证候分析]寒湿困脾,阳气受遏,胆汁外溢肌肤,故身目俱黄;寒湿为阴邪,故黄色晦暗,或如烟熏;寒湿困脾,故脘腹痞胀,纳食减少,大便不实;寒湿为阴邪,阳气不能温煦肢体,故神疲畏寒,口淡不渴;舌淡苔腻,脉濡缓或沉迟,均为寒湿阻遏之象。

[护治原则]温中化湿,健脾和胃。

[常用方剂]茵陈术附汤。

（2）脾虚血亏证

［主要证候］面目及肌肤淡黄,甚则晦暗不泽;肢软乏力,心悸气短,腹胀纳少,大便溏薄;舌质淡,苔薄,脉濡或细弱。

［证候分析］黄疸日久,脾虚失健,气血亏败,湿滞残留,故面目及肌肤淡黄,甚则晦暗不泽;气血不足,心脾失养,故见肢软乏力,心悸气短;脾虚不健,则腹胀纳少,大便溏薄;舌质淡,苔薄,脉濡或细弱,均为血虚之象。

［护治原则］健脾养血,祛湿退黄。

［常用方剂］黄芪建中汤。

三、护理措施

对于黄疸的病人,应观察黄疸的部位、色泽、程度、消长情况;大小便的量、色、质、次数;呕吐物的量、色、质、气味。注意观察神志、面色、体温、脉搏、呼吸、血压、食欲、舌脉,以及是否有腹胀、腹痛、皮肤瘙痒。若有发热,每4小时测1次体温和脉搏。若有出血,观察出血的量、颜色、部位。若病人出现黄疸加深,伴神昏谵语,烦躁抽搐,瘀斑出血,尿少色赤;或病人出现右胁下或上腹部疼痛剧烈,伴高热寒战,均应立即报告医生。

（一）辨证施护

1. 疫毒炽盛证

（1）生活起居护理 居室安静整洁,光线柔和,床褥平整干燥。最好安排单人房间,进行消化道隔离、血液隔离、空气消毒。绝对卧床,减少探视。每2小时翻身1次,经常用金银花甘草液漱口。若衄血,应及时清除口、鼻部的血块。若呕吐,取半仰卧位,头偏向一侧,轻拍其背部,或在胃脘部自上而下缓慢摩推。若皮肤瘙痒,嘱病人不要搔抓,可涂冰硼水止痒。若持续高热,可用温水擦浴。若神昏烦躁,可加床栏,必要时由专人看护。准备好床旁抢救设备。

（2）饮食护理 若恶心、呕吐频发,可暂时禁食。若神志昏愦,不能进食,可鼻饲清淡流食,严格限制蛋白质的摄入。宜食流食,少食多餐。待病情好转后,过渡到半流食。多饮水,可饮藕汁、果汁、鲜芦根茶。多吃新鲜的水果和蔬菜,如黄瓜、冬瓜、白菜、荠菜。宜食薏苡仁、赤小豆。遵医嘱使用食疗方:茵陈黄花菜汤。不宜食生冷、辛辣、油腻、甜黏、硬固的食物。

（3）情志护理 病人病情重,预后较差,思想负担较重,护士可运用语言开导疗法,解答病人的疑问,鼓励病人,使其积极配合治疗。

（4）用药护理 中药汤剂应浓煎,少量多次频服。服药前可用生姜汁滴舌,服药后静卧休息。必要时鼻饲或保留灌肠。

（5）操作技术 ①穴位按摩法:取足三里、至阳、胆俞、大椎、太冲、阴陵泉、蠡沟、肝俞,用拇指揉法,揉按力度宜大,按摩至局部发热或有酸麻重胀感,每日1次;孕妇禁用。②刺血疗法:取少商,皮肤消毒后揉按局部使其充血,用三棱针的3毫米针尖,快速刺入并出针,放出1.0 mL以下的血液,用无菌干棉球擦拭或按压;适用于高热不退者。③敷脐疗法:取神阙,用麝香1 g,田螺、大葱适量,捣烂外敷2~8小时;适用于尿闭腹胀者,孕妇禁用。④热敷疗法:用食盐1 kg,装入布袋中,制成温度为60~70℃的中药热罨包,在腹部热敷20分钟,每日1次;适用于尿闭腹胀者,孕妇禁用。

⑤ 点穴疗法：取内关、合谷、中脘、足三里,每处各点按 1 分钟,适用于剧烈呕吐时。

2. 热重于湿证

（1）生活起居护理　居室凉爽安静。衣物宽大、棉质、柔软。卧床休息,不可过劳。做好口腔护理,饭后漱口。做好皮肤护理。若皮肤瘙痒,可外涂炉甘石洗剂,剪短指甲,不可抓挠,每日用温水擦洗皮肤,水温不可过高。保持大便通畅。

（2）饮食护理　多饮水,可饮五汁饮、鲜白茅根茶。多吃高纤维的食物,以保持大便通畅。若频繁呕吐,可服少量生姜汁。宜食清热利湿的食物,如蚬肉、茯苓、赤小豆、薏苡仁、冬瓜、芹菜、绿豆。食疗方：泥鳅炖豆腐、藿香芦根粥。不宜食牛肉、羊肉。

（3）情志护理　病人为新病,护士可运用语言开导疗法,告知病人黄疸可随病情好转而减退或消失,以使病人情志舒畅,安心静养。

（4）用药护理　中药汤剂宜饭后温服或偏凉服,少量频服。

（5）操作技术　① 熏蒸疗法：用石菖蒲、丹皮各 15 g,白鲜皮、地肤子各 10 g,甘草 6 g;或用苦参 30 g;加水 1 000 mL 共煮,浓缩至 300 mL,倒入熏蒸锅中,加水至 2 000 mL,温度 50~70℃时熏蒸全身,微微出汗,每次 20 分钟,每日 1 次,熏蒸后休息 30 分钟方可外出。② 穴位按摩法：取肝俞、胆俞、阴陵泉、内庭、足三里、太冲,用拇指揉法,按摩至局部发热或有酸麻重胀感,每日 1 次;孕妇禁用。③ 敷贴疗法：取生姜、茵陈各 250 g,捣烂后敷于前胸和四肢,并用它时时揉擦全身。④ 灌肠疗法：用茵陈、栀子、大黄、甘草煎汤,进行保留灌肠;适用于高热便结者,高血压病人慎用。

3. 湿重于热证

（1）生活起居护理　居室安静避风。卧床休息,睡眠充足。黄疸期间不宜洗澡。黄疸消退 10 天后,可适量运动,以保持大便通畅。避免受凉,不可过劳。

（2）饮食护理　进食清淡、营养、易消化的软食或半流食,温热细软,少食多餐。可饮玉米须茶、李子茶。宜食利湿清热的食物,如蚬肉、茯苓、赤小豆、白扁豆、陈皮、山楂。食疗方：薏苡仁冬瓜猪瘦肉汤、黄花菜粥。待黄疸消退后,可食肉、鱼、蛋、奶。忌酒,不宜食生冷、油腻、辛辣、硬固的食物。

（3）情志护理　护士可运用顺意疗法,鼓励病人表达对于疾病的疑问,满足病人的合理要求,避免因多虑忧思伤脾而导致病程延长。

（4）用药护理　中药汤剂宜饭后温服,少量频服。

（5）操作技术　① 穴位按摩法：取胆俞、阴陵泉、内庭、太冲、阳陵泉、建里,用拇指揉法,按摩至局部发热或有酸麻重胀感,每日 1 次;孕妇禁用。② 熏洗疗法：取地骨皮 120 g,煎汤熏洗全身后,用生姜、茵陈各等份捣烂,用布包好,揉擦全身,每日 1~2 次。③ 灌肠疗法：用大承气汤加减,保留灌肠。

4. 胆腑郁热证

（1）生活起居护理　居室凉爽舒适。卧床休息。保持皮肤清洁,每日用温水擦洗,勿用手搔抓。注意口腔清洁,饭后漱口。养成定时排便的习惯。病情平稳后,适量运动,以保持大便通畅。

（2）饮食护理　饮食宜清淡。多饮水,可饮蒲公英茶。多吃新鲜的水果和蔬菜,如芹菜、菠菜、苋菜、香蕉。宜食疏肝清热的食物,如金橘、佛手。食疗方：鲤鱼赤豆陈皮汤、炒猪肝萝卜。忌烟酒、牛肉、羊肉,不宜食辛辣、油腻、甜腻、易产气的食物。

（3）情志护理　护士可运用语言开导疗法,告诉病人及家属情志舒畅有助于疾病痊愈,为病人营造良好的环境,避免急躁易怒。

（4）用药护理　中药汤剂宜饭后温服,少量频服。若呕吐频繁,可用生姜汁滴舌。

（5）操作技术　① 熏洗疗法:用苍术、川椒、艾叶、蛇床子、茵陈、苦参,合而煮沸,水温50~70℃时熏蒸皮肤瘙痒处,水温降至37~40℃时浸泡、淋洗,每次20分钟,每日1次;女性月经期或妊娠期不可坐浴及外阴部熏洗。② 穴位按摩法:取合谷、内关、足三里、阳陵泉、胆囊、肝俞、胆俞,用拇指揉法,按摩至局部发热或有酸麻重胀感,每日1次;孕妇禁用。③ 耳压疗法:取胰胆、肝、脾、胃、耳中、大肠、直肠等耳穴,用耳穴压丸贴片贴压,每日按揉4~5次,以局部发热泛红为度,留置2~4日;孕妇禁用。④ 灌肠疗法:用大黄乌梅汤,保留灌肠;适用于便秘者。

5. 寒湿阻遏证

（1）生活起居护理　居室温暖干燥,安静避风,光线明亮。卧床休息,注意保暖。病情稳定时,适量运动,但要避免剧烈运动和重体力劳动。

（2）饮食护理　饮食宜温热,少食多餐。饮水量不宜过大,可饮少量生姜红糖水。可食肉、鱼、蛋、奶,以加强营养。宜食温中化湿的食物,如山药、芡实、莲子、茯苓、橘皮。忌烟酒、发物,不宜食生冷、甜腻、厚味的食物。

（3）情志护理　病人的病程迁延反复,护士可运用移情易性疗法,转移病人的注意力,为病人安排娱乐活动,如听音乐、聊天、练习气功等,以使病人保持乐观的情绪,避免忧思、焦虑。

（4）用药护理　中药汤剂宜饭后温服,少量频服。服药后可食薏苡仁粥以和胃气。

（5）操作技术　① 灸法:取神阙,用隔姜灸,把生姜切成直径2~3厘米、厚0.4~0.6厘米的薄片,中间以针刺数孔,放置于施灸处,每处5壮,每日2次;孕妇禁用。② 热敷疗法:将大葱装入布袋中,制成温度为60~70℃的中药热罨包,热敷腹部20分钟,每日1次;孕妇禁用。③ 熏洗疗法:取连翘、赤小豆、防风、白鲜皮、地肤子、金钱草、虎杖各30 g,麻黄、鸡内金各20 g,薄荷10 g,合而煮沸,水温50~70℃时熏蒸皮肤黄染处,水温降至37~40℃时浸泡、淋洗,每次20分钟,每日1次;女性月经期或妊娠期不可坐浴及外阴部熏洗。④ 灌肠疗法:用真武汤加减,保留灌肠。⑤ 穴位按摩法:取至阳、脾俞、胆俞、中脘、三阴交、肾俞、足三里、肝俞,用拇指揉法、一指禅推法,按摩至局部发热或有酸麻重胀感,每日1次;孕妇禁用。

6. 脾虚血亏证

（1）生活起居护理　居室温暖避风,安静舒适,光线柔和。起居有常,注意腹部和下肢保暖。劳逸适度,适量运动,不可过劳。保持肛周干燥清洁,便后用温水清洗。若心悸,应卧床休息。

（2）饮食护理　饮食有节,少食多餐,食物宜清淡少渣、温热软烂。宜食健脾养血的食物,如芡实、山药、莲子、薏苡仁、茯苓、羊肉。多吃鱼、肉、蛋,佐以生姜、小茴香、小葱、韭菜。食疗方:枸杞猪肉汤。若腹胀,可食白萝卜、金橘、焦米茶。不宜食发物和生冷、辛辣、油腻的食物。

（3）情志护理　病人体虚,病程迁延反复,护士可运用顺意疗法,鼓励病人表达自己的想法,认同其感受,解答病人提出的问题,介绍治疗效果较好的病例,以增强病人战胜疾病的信心。

（4）用药护理　中药汤剂宜文火久煎,饭前温服,少量频服。

（5）操作技术　① 穴位按摩法:取足三里、至阳、脾俞、胆俞、中脘、三阴交,用拇指揉法、一指禅推法,按摩至局部发热或有酸麻重胀感,每日1次;孕妇禁用。② 水针疗法:取胆俞、肝俞、期门、阳陵泉、阴陵泉、至阳,每次选择 2~3 个腧穴,用复方丹参注射液进行穴位注射。③ 耳压疗法:取胰胆、肝、脾、胃、耳中等耳穴,用耳穴压丸贴片贴压,每日按揉 4~5 次,以局部发热泛红为度,留置 2~4 日;孕妇禁用。

（二）健康教育

起居有常,顺应四时,劳逸适度。慎避外邪,不可过劳。

食物宜清淡、营养、易消化。多吃新鲜的蔬菜、豆类、粗粮,以及高蛋白、低脂的食物,如猪瘦肉、豆腐。饮食有节,注意饮食卫生。戒烟限酒,不可暴饮暴食、饮食偏嗜,不宜食发物和生冷、油腻、辛辣、甜腻、硬固的食物。

对于有传染性的病人,从发病之日起至少隔离 30~45 天,消毒措施必须严格、彻底。

治愈出院后,休息 3 个月,1 年内不进行重体力劳动。定期门诊复查,积极治疗原发病。坚持遵医嘱服药,不可滥用药物。

Section 11　Jaundice

Jaundice is a disease clinically characterized by yellow face and eyes, yellow body skin, and dark urine. It is caused by qi stagnation and blood stasis forcing bile to flow outward which is induced by either external invasion of epidemic dampness-heat toxin, internal accumulation of dampness-heat in alcoholist, cold-dampness encumbering the spleen, or obstruction of calculi and lumps. This section can be referred to for the nursing of some diseases with jaundice as the main manifestation, such as viral hepatitis, autoimmune liver disease, drug-induced liver disease, cirrhosis, extrahepatic biliary calculi and inflammation, biliary system tumor in Western medicine.

ETIOLOGY AND PATHOGENESIS

The etiology includes invasion of external pathogen, improper diet, deficiency-cold of the spleen and stomach and other diseases. External dampness-heat, cold-dampness or seasonal epidemic toxin accumulates in the middle energizer, steams the liver and gallbladder, and forces bile to flow outward, and subsequently, jaundice occurs. Excessive consumption of fatty and too-sweet foods, excessive drinking, or improper diet may damage the spleen and stomach as well as produce dampness-heat that steams the liver and gallbladder, and forces bile to flow outward, and subsequently, jaundice forms. Excessive consumption of raw and cold foods or dietary irregularities may induce spleen deficiency and generate dampness. The dampness encumbering the middle makes failure of the liver to act freely, and forces bile to flow outward, and subsequently, jaundice occurs. Spleen deficiency constitution, overstrain, or spleen damage due to chronic disease may cause dysfunction of the spleen in transportation and transformation as well as obstruction of cold-dampness in the middle energizer, and forces bile to flow outward, and subsequently, jaundice develops. Calculi, parasites or blood stasis obstructs biliary tract and forces bile to flow outward, and subsequently, jaundice occurs.

The pathogenesis is that pathogenic dampness encumbers the spleen and stomach as well as congests the liver and gallbladder, which consequently causes failure of the liver to govern free flow of qi and outward flow of bile. The disease is located in the spleen, stomach, liver and gallbladder but connected to the heart and kidney. Jaundice caused by external invasion or acute jaundice mostly belongs to excess syndrome. However, jaundice triggered by internal damage or chronic jaundice mostly belongs to deficiency-excess in complexity.

COMMON SYNDROMES

Key Points in Syndrome Differentiation

1. Differentiation of Yang Jaundice from Yin Jaundice

The differentiation is based on the onset speed, disease course and skin color. Yang jaundice of heat syndrome and excess syndrome shows sudden onset, short course, bright yellow color, and red tongue with wiry rapid pulse. Acute jaundice displays sudden onset, golden yellow color, rapid deterioration, and crimson tongue. Yin jaundice of cold syndrome and deficiency syndrome exhibits gradual onset, long course, dim yellow color, and pale tongue with slow or weak pulse.

2. Differentiation of Heat Preponderance from Dampness Preponderance

The differentiation is based on the severity of fever. Severe fever, dry and bitter mouth, thirst, constipation and slimy yellow coating indicate preponderance of heat over dampness. Mild fever, heaviness of the head, drowsiness, chest and gastric stuffiness and fullness, grimy loose stool and slimy yellowish coating suggests preponderance of dampness over heat.

Syndrome Differentiation

1. Acute Jaundice

Syndrome of Epidemic Toxin Exuberance

[Clinical Manifestations] Sudden onset, rapidly darkening gold-like jaundice, skin itching, high fever, thirst, hypochondriac pain, abdominal fullness, coma, delirious speech, restlessness, convulsion, or epistaxis, blood in stool, or skin ecchymosis, crimson tongue with yellow dry coating, and wiry slippery or rapid pulse.

[Manifestations Analysis] Exuberant epidemic toxin disturbing the gallbladder internally causes bile spreading outward to the skin, leading to sudden onset, rapid darkening gold-like jaundice, and skin itching. Pathogenic heat consumes qi and yin, thus high fever and thirst occur. Congested qi movement of the spleen, stomach, liver and gallbladder induces hypochondriac pain and abdominal fullness. Pathogen invades jueyin meridian, resulting in coma, delirious speech, restlessness, and convulsion. Pathogenic heat causes frenetic movement of blood, causing epistaxis, blood in stool, and skin ecchymosis. Crimson tongue with yellow dry coating and wiry slippery or rapid pulse are signs of exuberant pathogenic toxin.

[Nursing Principle] Clearing heat and removing toxin; cooling blood and opening orifice.

[Suggested Formula] Xijiao Powder.

2. Yang Jaundice

(1) Syndrome of Preponderance of Heat Over Dampness

[Clinical Manifestations] Yellow body skin and eyes, bright yellow color, high fever, thirst, or anguish, abdominal distension and oppression, dry mouth with bitter taste, nausea, vomiting, scanty dark urine, constipation, slimy yellow tongue coating, and wiry rapid pulse.

[Manifestations Analysis] Dampness-heat fuming and steaming the liver and gallbladder causes outward flow of bile to the skin, resulting in yellow body skin and eyes. Preponderance of heat over dampness explains bright yellow color. Dampness-heat encumbers the middle energizer, then abdominal distension and oppression, nausea and vomiting are felt. Heat accumulation in the stomach damages fluids, causing fever, thirst, anguish, dry mouth with bitter taste, and constipation. Dampness-heat pouring down into the bladder contributes to scanty dark urine. Slimy yellow tongue coating and wiry rapid pulse are signs of internal exuberance of dampness-heat.

[Nursing Principle] Clearing heat and dredging fu-organs; draining dampness and abating jaundice.

[Suggested Formula] Yinchenhao Decoction.

(2) Syndrome of Preponderance of Dampness Over Heat

[Clinical Manifestations] Yellow body skin and eyes (yellow is not as bright as the previous syndrome), heaviness of the head, drowsiness, chest and gastric stuffiness and fullness, reduced appetite, nausea, vomiting, abdominal distention or grimy loose stool, thick slimy tongue coating with yellowish color, and soggy rapid pulse or soggy moderate pulse.

[Manifestations Analysis] Dampness-heat fuming and steaming the liver and gallbladder causes inhibited excretion of bile, resulting in yellow body skin and eyes. Preponderance of dampness over heat explains the color of yellow not as bright as the previous syndrome. Dampness encumbers the muscles and skin, then heaviness of the head and drowsiness are felt. Dampness-heat encumbers the middle energizer, then there exhibit chest and gastric stuffiness and fullness, reduced appetite, nausea, vomiting, and abdominal distention. Dampness-heat obstructs the intestinal tract, then grimy loose stool occurs. Thick slimy tongue coating with yellowish color and soggy rapid pulse or soggy moderate pulse are signs of internal accumulation of dampness-heat.

[Nursing Principle] Draining dampness and resolving the turbid; activating spleen yang and clearing heat.

[Suggested Formula] Yinchen Wuling Powder and Ganlu Xiaodu Pellets.

(3) Syndrome of Heat Stagnation in Gallbladder

[Clinical Manifestations] Yellow body skin and eyes, bright yellow color, distending and dull pain in upper abdomen and right hypochondrium that radiates to the shoulder and back, unabating fever, or alternating chills and fever, dry throat and bitter taste in the mouth, vomiting, hiccup, dark urine, constipation, red tongue with yellow coating, and wiry, slippery and rapid pulse.

[Manifestations Analysis] Calculi and parasites obstructing biliary tract causes outward flow of bile to the skin, resulting in yellow body skin and eyes. Stagnation of gallbladder heat leads to congestion of liver qi, causing distending and dull pain in upper abdomen and right hypochondrium that radiates to the shoulder and back. Stagnation of gallbladder heat causes stomach qi ascending counterflow, leading to dry throat and bitter taste in the mouth, vomiting, and hiccup. Dysfunction of the spleen and stomach in transportation and transformation as well as ascending and descending leads to constipation. Stagnated heat invading shaoyang meridian induces alternating chills and fever. Stagnated heat pouring into lower energizer, and dark urine appears. Red tongue with yellow coating and wiry, slippery and rapid pulse are signs of heat stagnation in the gallbladder.

[Nursing Principle] Soothing the liver and discharging heat; promoting function of the gallbladder and abating jaundice.

[Suggested Formula] Da Chaihu Decoction.

3. Yin Jaundice

(1) Syndrome of Cold-Dampness Obstruction

[Clinical Manifestations] Yellow body skin and eyes, dim yellow or smoked color, abdominal and gastric stuffiness and distension, reduced appetite, loose stool, mental fatigue, fear of cold, bland taste in the mouth, absence of thirst, pale tongue with slimy coating, and soggy moderate pulse or sunken slow pulse.

[Manifestations Analysis] Cold-dampness encumbering the spleen causes constraint of yang qi and outward flow of bile to the skin, resulting in yellow body skin and eyes. Cold-dampness belongs to yin pathogen and leads to dim yellow or smoked color. Cold-dampness encumbering the spleen causes abdominal and gastric stuffiness and distension, reduced appetite and unsolid stool. Cold-dampness belongs to yin pathogen and yang qi cannot warm the body and limbs, causing mental fatigue, fear of cold, bland taste in the mouth, and absence of thirst. Pale tongue with slimy coating and soggy moderate pulse or sunken slow pulse indicate cold-dampness obstruction.

[Nursing Principle] Warming the middle and resolving dampness; invigorating the spleen and harmonizing stomach.

[Suggested Formula] Yinchen Zhufu Decoction.

(2) Syndrome of Spleen Deficiency and Blood Depletion

[Clinical Manifestations] Yellowish, or even dim yellow and lusterless face, eyes and skin, weak limbs and lack of strength, palpitation, shortness of breath, abdominal distension, reduced appetite, thin loose stool, pale tongue with thin coating, and soggy pulse or thready weak pulse.

[Manifestations Analysis] Chronic jaundice causes spleen deficiency, qi-blood depletion and lingering dampness, resulting in yellowish, or even dim yellow and lusterless face, eyes and skin. Qi-blood depletion cannot nourish the heart or spleen, so exhibit weak limbs and lack of strength, palpitation, and shortness of breath. Spleen deficiency triggers abdominal distension, reduced appetite, and thin loose stool. Pale tongue with thin coating and soggy pulse or thready weak pulse are signs of blood deficiency.

[Nursing Principle] Invigorating the spleen and nourishing blood; removing dampness and abating jaundice.

[Suggested Formula] Huangqi Jianzhong Decoction.

NURSING MEASURES

For patients with jaundice, nurses should observe the location, color, severity, and exuberance or debilitation of jaundice; the volume, color, quality, and frequency of urine and stool, as well as the volume, color, quality and smell of the vomitus. The nurses should also observe the patients' changes in consciousness, complexion, body temperature, pulse, respiration, blood pressure, appetite, and manifestations of tongue and pulse; the presence or abscence of abdominal distension and pain, and skin itching. For those with fever, the nurses should take body temperature and pulse every four hours. For patients with bleeding, the nurses should observe the amount, color and location of bleeding. If the patient has worsening jaundice accompanied with unconsciousness, delirious speech, restlessness, convulsion, skin ecchymosis, bleeding, scanty and dark urine, or severe pain in the right rib-side and upper abdomen, accompanied with high fever, and chill, it is advisable to report to the doctor immediately.

Syndrome-Based Nursing Measures

1. Syndrome of Epidemic Toxin Exuberance

(1) Daily life nursing. The ward should be quiet, tidy, air-disinfected, and full of gentle light. The bedding should be smooth and dry. Patients should be arranged respectively in a single ward for digestive tract and blood isolation. The patients should take absolute bed rest, keep visits minimal, turn over every two hours, and rinse the mouth with jinyinhua gancao (honeysuckle flower and licorice root) liquid frequently. For patients with episaxis, clean the blood clot in the mouth and nose. For vomiting patients, take a semi-supine position with the head tilted to one side while the nurses pat them on the back or gently rub their stomach from top to bottom. For patients with skin itching, ask them not to scratch, and apply Bingpeng Lotion to relieve itching. For those with persistent high fever, have a warm sponge bath. For unconscious and agitated patients, add guardrails to their beds, and if necessary, they should have an assigned caretaker. First-aid equipment should be readily available at the bedside.

(2) Diet nursing. In case of frequent nausea and vomiting, patients could fast temporarily. For unconscious patients, give light liquid foods by nasal feeding, with strict restriction of protein intake. It is advisable for patients to have liquid foods and multiple small meals. After conditions are improved, they could eat semi-liquid foods. They should drink more water, may drink lotus root juice, fruit juice, and xianlugen (fresh reed rhizome) tea, and eat more fresh vegetables and fruit, such as cucumber, Chinese waxgourd, Chinese cabbage and shepherd's purse. Yiyiren (coix seed) and chixiaodou (adzuki bean) are recommended. Follow the doctor's advice to adopt food therapy: yinchen huanghuacai (virgate wormwood herb and day lily) soup. Raw, cold, pungent, spicy, greasy, sweet, sticky and hard foods should be avoided.

(3) Emotion nursing. Because of the serious condition and poor prognosis, patients may have heavy mental stress. Nurses may use verbal enlightenment therapy to answer the patients' questions and encourage them to actively comply with treatment.

(4) Medication nursing. Decoction should be concentrated and taken multiple times in small portions. Drip some shengjiang (fresh ginger) juice on the tongue before taking medicine. And take some rest in bed after taking medicine. If necessary, nasal feeding or retention enema therapy could be used.

(5) Manipulation techniques. ① Acupressure therapy: select Zusanli (ST 36), Zhiyang (GV 9), Danshu (BL19), Dazhui (GV 14), Taichong (LR 3), Yinlingquan (SP 9), Ligou (LR 5) and Ganshu (BL 18); apply thumb kneading manipulation on each of the acupoints until the area turns hot or the patient has the feelings of soreness, numbness, distension and heaviness in the area, once per day. And it is contraindicated in pregnancy. ② Blood-letting therapy: select Shaoshang (LU 11); after the skin is disinfected, rub the local area to make it hyperemic, use a three-edged needle to quickly pierce the skin at a depth of 3 millimeters, remove the needle to release blood less than 1.0 mL, and wipe or press the pierced point with a sterile dry cotton ball. It is suitable for patients with unabating high fever. ③ Umbilical compress therapy: select Shenque (CV 8); mash 1 g of musk with proper amounts of field snails and scallion to make a paste, and apply the paste on the navel, 2~8 hours each time. It is suitable for patients with uroschesis and abdominal distention, and contraindicated in pregnant women. ④ Hot compress therapy: heat one kilogram of salt, and put it into a cloth bag for hot compress on the abdomen at 60~70℃; 20 minutes each time, once per day. It is appropriate for patients with uroschesis and abdominal distention, and contraindicated in pregnant women. ⑤ Acupoint-pressing therapy: select Neiguan (PC 6), Hegu (LI 4), Zhongwan (CV 12), and Zusanli (ST 36), and press on them, one minute for each acupoint. And it is suitable for severe vomiting.

2. Syndrome of Preponderance of Heat Over Dampness

(1) Daily life nursing. The ward should be cool and quiet. Patients should wear loose, cotton and soft clothes, rest in bed, avoid overstrain, pay attention to oral hygiene, rinse the mouth after meals, and keep a normal bowel movement. They should also take good care of their skin. If the skin itches, calamine lotion could be applied, and the patients' nails should be trimmed to avoid scratching. Besides, they should wash the skin every day with warm water at moderate temperature.

(2) Diet nursing. The patients should drink more water, may drink Wuzhi Juice, biqi (waternut) juice or xianbaimaogen (fresh woolly grass) tea, and take high-fiber foods to keep bowel movement normal. Patients with frequent vomiting could take a few drops of shengjiang (fresh ginger) juice. Foods that clear heat and remove dampness are recommended, such as clam meat, fuling (poria), chixiaodou (adzuki bean), yiyiren (coix seed), Chinese waxgourd, celery, and lüdou (mung bean). Food therapy: bean curd stewed with loach, and huoxiang lugen (agastache and reed rhizome) porridge. Avoid eating beef or mutton.

(3) Emotion nursing. As the disease just develops, nurses may use verbal enlightenment therapy to inform the patients that jaundice would subside or disappear as their conditions improve to make them relaxed and free from anxiety.

(4) Medication nursing. Decoction should be taken warm or slightly cool after meals, multiple times in small portions.

(5) Manipulation techniques. ① Fumigating and steaming therapy: take shichangpu (grassleaf sweetflag rhizome) 15 g, danpi (tree peony bark) 15 g, baixianpi (dictamnus root bark) 10 g, difuzi (belvedere fruit) 10 g, and gancao (licorice root) 6 g; or kushen (light yellow sophora root) 30 g;

then, decoct the ingredients above with 1 000 mL of water to get 300 mL of concentrated decoction; pour the decoction into the fumigation pot and add water to get 2 000 mL of liquid to fumigate and steam the whole body at 50 ~ 70℃ until sweating slightly, 20 minutes each time, once per day. After fumigating, the patients need to take a rest for 30 minutes before leaving. ② Acupressure therapy: select Ganshu (BL 18), Danshu (BL19), Yinlingquan (SP 9), Neiting (ST 44), Zusanli (ST 36), and Taichong (LR 3); apply thumb kneading manipulation on each of the acupoints until the area turns hot the patient has the feelings of soreness, numbness, distension and heaviness in the area, once per day. And it is contraindicated in pregnant women. ③ Paste application therapy: mash shengjiang (fresh ginger) 250 g and yinchen (virgate wormwood herb) 250 g to make pastes; apply the pastes on the chest and limbs, and use them to rub the whole body constantly. ④ Enema therapy: decoct yinchen (virgate wormwood herb), zhizi (gardenia), dahuang (rhubarb root and rhizome), and gancao (licorice root) for retention enema. It is suitable for patients with high fever and dry stool. And it should be used with caution for patients with high blood pressure.

3. Syndrome of Preponderance of Dampness Over Heat

(1) Daily life nursing. The ward should be quiet and away from wind. The patients should rest in bed as much as possible to get adequate sleep. They should not bathe during the disease but may do moderate exercise to keep a normal bowel movement after the jaundice subsides for more than ten days. Besides, they should also avoid catching cold and overstrain.

(2) Diet nursing. The diet should be light, nutritious and digestible. The patients should take soft or semi-liquid warm foods, and have small frequent meals. They may drink yumixu (cornsilk) tea or plum tea, and eat foods that clear heat and remove dampness, such as clam meat, fuling (poria), chixiaodou (adzuki bean), baibiandou (white hyacinth bean), chenpi (aged tangerine peel) and shanzha (Chinese hawthorn fruit). Food therapy: yiyiren donggua zhushourou (coix seed, Chinese waxgourd, and lean pork) soup, and day lily porridge. Meat, fish, egg and milk are allowed when jaundice subsides. Don't drink liquor, or eat raw, cold, greasy, pungent, spicy and hard foods.

(3) Emotion nursing. Nurses may use submission therapy to encourage patients to ask questions about the disease and meet their reasonable requirements to prevent excessive worry that damages the spleen and prolongs the disease course.

(4) Medication nursing. Decoction should be taken warm after meals, multiple times in small portions.

(5) Manipulation techniques. ① Acupressure therapy: select Danshu (BL19), Yinlingquan (SP 9), Neiting (ST 44), Taichong (LR 3), Yanglingquan (SP 9), and Jianli (CV 11); apply thumb kneading manipulation on each of the acupoints until the area turns hot or the patient has the feelings of soreness, numbness, distension and heaviness in the area; once per day. And it is contraindicated in pregnancy. ② Fumigating and washing therapy: decoct digupi (Chinese wolfberry root-bark) 120 g and use the decoction to fumigate and wash the whole body; then, mash equal amount of shengjiang (fresh ginger) and yinchen (virgate wormwood herb), and pack it with a cloth bag to rub the whole body,

once to twice per day. ③ Enema therapy: use modified Dachengqi Decoction for retention enema.

4. Syndrome of Heat Stagnation in the Gallbladder

(1) Daily life nursing. The ward should be cool and comfortable. The patients should rest in bed as much as possible, keep skin hygiene by washing the skin everyday with warm water and without scratching it, pay attention to oral hygiene by rinsing the mouth after meals, and develop the habit of regular defecation. After the condition is stabilized, the patients may exercise moderately to keep a normal bowel movement.

(2) Diet nursing. The patients should have a light diet and drink more water, may drink pugongying (dandelion) tea, eat more fresh vegetables and fruit, such as celery, spinach, amaranth and bananas, and take foods that soothe the liver and clear heat, such as kumquat and foshou (finger citron fruit). Food therapy: liyu chidou chenpi (carp, adzuki bean, and aged tangerine peel) soup, and pig liver stir-fried with white radish. The patients should also refrain from cigarette, alcohol, beef, mutton and foods that are pungent, spicy, greasy, sweet and flatulent.

(3) Emotion nursing. To provide a good environment for patients and prevent their impetuousness and irritability, nurses may use verbal enlightenment therapy to inform patients and their families that good mood is beneficial to their recovery.

(4) Medication nursing. Decoction should be taken warm after meals, multiple times in small portions. For patients with severe vomiting, drip some shengjiang (fresh ginger) juice on the tongue.

(5) Manipulation techniques. ① Fumigating and washing therapy: prepare cangzhu (atractylodes rhizome), Sichuan pricklyash peel, aiye (mugwort leaf), shechuangzi (cnidium fruit), yinchen (virgate wormwood herb) and kushen (light yellow sophora root); decoct the above ingredients for fumigating the itching skin at a temperature of $50 \sim 70 \text{℃}$, and for washing the itching skin at a temperature of $37 \sim 40 \text{℃}$, 20 minutes each time, once per day. And it is contraindicated for females to apply hip bath and vulva fumigating and washing during menstruation or pregnancy. ② Acupressure therapy: select Hegu (LI 14), Neiguan (PC 6), Zusanli (ST 36), Yanglingquan (SP 9), Dannang (EX－LE 6), Ganshu (BL 18), and Danshu (BL 19); apply thumb kneading manipulation on each of the acupoints until the area turns hot or the patient has the feelings of soreness, numbness, distension and heaviness in the area; once per day. And it is contraindicated in pregnancy. ③ Auricular pressure therapy: select the auricular points of pancreas and gallbladder (CO11), liver (CO12), spleen (CO13), stomach (CO4), ear center (HX1), large intestine (CO7), and rectum (HX2); apply specialized pasters on the points, knead each of them till the area turns hot and red, $4 \sim 5$ times per day, and keep the pasters for $2 \sim 4$ days. And it is contraindicated in pregnancy. ④ Enema therapy: use Dahuang Wumei Decoction for retention enema. It is suitable for patients with constipation.

5. Syndrome of Cold-Dampness Obstruction

(1) Daily life nursing. The ward should be warm, dry, quiet, full of light, and away from wind. The patients should rest in bed and keep themselves warm. When the condition is stabilized, they may exercise moderately, avoiding strenuous exercise and heavy physical labor.

（2）Diet nursing. The patients should take warm foods, have small frequent meals, and reduce the water intake. They can drink a little shengjiang hongtang (fresh ginger and brown sugar) tea, eat meat, fish, egg and milk for more nutrition, and take foods that warm the middle and resolve dampness, such as shanyao (common yam rhizome), qianshi (euryale seed), lianzi (lotus seed), fuling (poria) and jupi (tangerine pericarp). They should also refrain from cigarette, alcohol, foods that induce or aggravate disease, and foods that are raw, cold, sweet, greasy and rich.

（3）Emotion nursing. As the disease is prolonged and recurrent, nurses may use emotional transference and dispositional change therapy to shift the patients' attention and arrange some recreational activities for them, such as listening to music, chatting and practising Qigong, so they can be optimistic and have no worry or anxiety.

（4）Medication nursing. Decoction should be taken warm after meals, multiple times in small portions. After taking medicine, the patients can take yiyiren (coix seed) porridge to harmonize stomach qi.

（5）Manipulation techniques. ① Moxibustion therapy：select Shenque (CV 8) and perform ginger-partitioned moxibustion. The procedure is to slice shengjiang (fresh ginger) into thin pieces with a diameter of 2～3 centimeters and thickness of 0.4～0.6 centimeters, pierce several holes through the ginger slice with a sharp needle, and place the ginger slice on the acupoint, five moxa-cones on the acupoint until the area turns red, and twice every day. And it is contraindicated in pregnancy. ② Hot compress therapy：put scallions into a cloth bag for hot compress on the abdomen at 60～70℃, 20 minutes each time, once per day. And it is contraindicated in pregnant women. ③ Fumigating and washing therapy：take lianqiao (weeping forsythia capsule), chixiaodou (adzuki bean), fangfeng (siler), baixianpi (dictamnus root bark), difuzi (belvedere fruit), jinqiancao (lysimachia), and huzhang (giant knotweed rhizome) 30 g respectively, mahuang (ephedra) 20 g, ji'neijin (chicken gizzard lining) 20 g, and bohe (field mint) 10 g; decoct the above ingredients for fumigating the yellowed skin at a temperature of 50～70℃, and for washing the yellowed skin at a temperature of 37～40℃, 20 minutes each time, once per day. And it is contraindicated for females to apply hip bath and vulva fumigating and washing during menstruation or pregnancy. ④ Enema therapy：use modified Zhenwu Decoction for retention enema. ⑤ Acupressure therapy：select Zhiyang (GV 9), Pishu (BL 20), Danshu (BL 19), Zhongwan (CV 12), Sanyinjiao (SP 6), Shenshu (BL 23), Zusanli (ST 36), and Ganshu (BL 18); apply thumb kneading and one-finger pushing manipulations on each of the acupoints until the area turns hot or the patient has the feelings of soreness, numbness, distension and heaviness in the area; once per day. And it is contraindicated in pregnancy.

6. Syndrome of Spleen Deficiency and Blood Depletion

（1）Daily life nursing. The ward should be warm, quiet, comfortable, full of gentle light, and away from wind. The patients should live a regular life, keep the abdomen and lower limbs warm, balance work and rest, do moderate physical exercise, keep the perianal region dry and clean, and wash it with warm water after defecation. Patients with palpitation should rest in bed.

（2）Diet nursing. The patients should have a moderate diet and small frequent meals. The foods should be light, warm and soft with little dregs. Foods that invigorate the spleen and nourish blood are recommended, such as qianshi (euryale seed), shanyao (common yam rhizome), lianzi (lotus seed), yiyiren (coix seed), fuling (poria) and mutton. They may eat more fish, meat and eggs, seasoned with shengjiang (fresh ginger), xiaohuixiang (fennel), spring onion, and Chinese chives. Food therapy: gouqi zhurou (Chinese wolfberry fruit and pork) soup. For patients with abdominal distention, they can eat white radish and kumquat, or drink scorch-fried-rice tea. Don't eat raw, cold, pungent, spicy, and greasy foods, or foods that induce or aggravate disease.

（3）Emotion nursing. Because of the patients' weak constitution and extended repetitive course of disease, nurses may use submission therapy to encourage the patients to express their feelings for recognition, answer their questions, and introduce patients with better curative effect to enhance their confidence in fighting the disease.

（4）Medication nursing. Decoction should be prepared slowly over low heat and taken warm before meals, multiple times in small portions.

（5）Manipulation techniques. ① Acupressure therapy: select Zusanli (ST 36), Zhiyang (GV 9), Pishu (BL 20), Danshu (BL 19), Zhongwan (CV 12), and Sanyinjiao (SP 6); apply thumb kneading and one-finger pushing manipulations on each of the acupoints until the area turns hot or the patient has the feelings of soreness, numbness, distension and heaviness in the area; once per day. And it is contraindicated in pregnancy. ② Water acupuncture therapy: select Danshu (BL 19), Ganshu (BL 18), Qimen (LR 14), Yanglingquan (GB 34), Yinlingquan (SP 9), and Zhiyang (GV 9); inject compound danshen (danshen root) injection to the acupoints, 2~3 acupoints each time. ③ Auricular pressure therapy: select the auricular points of pancreas and gallbladder (CO11), liver (CO12), spleen (CO13), stomach (CO4), and ear center (HX1); apply specialized pasters on the points, knead each of them till the area turns hot and red, 4~5 times per day, and keep the pasters for 2~4 days. And it is contraindicated in pregnancy.

Patient Education

The patients should live a regular life, comply with seasonal changes, balance work and rest, stay away from external pathogens and avoid overstain.

The diet should be light, nutritious and digestible. More fresh vegetables, beans, whole grains and foods with high protein and low fat should be supplemented, such as lean pork and bean curd. The patients should have a moderate diet, pay attention to food hygiene, refrain from cigarette, alcohol, gluttony, diet preference, and foods that are raw, cold, greasy, pungent, spicy, sweet and hard.

For infectious patients, quarantine should last at least 30~45 days from the date of onset, and the disinfection measures must be strictly carried out.

Patients should rest for three months after clinical recovery and discharge. Don't take heavy physical labor within one year. They should have regular outpatient examination, actively treat the primary disease, and strictly follow the doctor's advice in medication.

第十二节　水　　肿

水肿，泛指因外邪侵袭，劳倦内伤，饮食失调，导致气化不利，水液潴留，泛滥肌肤，以眼睑、头面、四肢、全身浮肿，或按之凹陷为临床特征的一类疾病。西医的原发性肾小球疾病、继发性肾病、甲状腺功能减退症、原发性醛固酮增多症，以水肿为主要表现的，可参照本节进行护理。

一、病因病机

水肿的病因包括风邪袭表、疮毒内陷、水湿内侵、饮食不节、情志失调、劳欲过度、他病所致。病人外感风寒或风热之邪，肺气失宣，风水相搏，溢于肌肤，可发为水肿。痈疡疮毒未解，损伤脾肺，导致水液代谢障碍，溢于肌肤，发为水肿。病人久居湿地，或冒雨涉水，脾为湿困，不能制水，溢于肌肤，可发为水肿。过饥伤脾，或过食肥甘、生冷，脾虚生湿，溢于肌肤，可发为水肿。病人抑郁伤肝，疏泄失常，三焦气机不畅，水道不利；或忧思伤脾，脾虚失运，水湿泛于肌肤，均可发为水肿。过劳伤脾，或房劳多产伤肾，水液代谢失司，可发为水肿。病人久病，损伤肺脾肾三脏，水液代谢不畅，或病久入络，瘀血阻滞三焦，水道壅塞，亦可发为水肿。

水肿的病机为肺失通调，脾失运化，肾失开阖，三焦气化不利，水液潴留，泛溢肌肤。病位在肺、脾、肾。水肿多为本虚标实之证，阳水以标实为主，阴水以本虚为主。

二、常见证型

（一）辨证要点

1. 辨阳水与阴水　根据病因、起病速度、病程长短、水肿部位等来辨别。若因外邪而起，发病急，病程短，水肿由上而下，水肿处皮肤光亮，按之即起，多为阳水。若因内伤而起，发病缓，病程长，反复发作，水肿由下而上，按之凹陷不易恢复，伴神疲乏力，则多为阴水。

2. 辨病位　根据水肿部位等来辨别。若先眼睑浮肿，继而四肢皆肿，伴恶寒发热，多病位在肺。若全身水肿，伴肢体困重，脘闷食少，多病位在脾。若全身水肿，腰以下为甚，伴腰膝酸软，多病位在肾。

3. 辨外感与内伤　根据病程长短等来辨别。若起病急，病程短，伴恶寒，发热，头疼身痛，脉浮，多为外感。若起病缓，病程长，反复发作，伴内脏亏虚，正气不足之象，则多为内伤。

（二）证候分型

1. 阳水

（1）风水相搏证

[主要证候] 初起眼睑浮肿，迅即四肢及全身皆肿；且兼恶风发热，肢节酸楚，小便不利；偏于风

寒者,恶寒,咳喘,舌苔薄白,脉浮滑或紧;偏于风热者,咽喉红肿疼痛,舌质红,脉浮滑数。

　　[证候分析]外邪袭肺,肺失宣降,不能通调水道、下输膀胱,水液代谢失常,故水肿,小便不利;风性轻扬,善行数变,风助水势,故初起眼睑浮肿,迅即四肢及全身皆肿;邪在肌表,卫阳受遏,故恶风发热,肢节酸楚;若风邪兼寒,则恶寒,咳喘,舌苔薄白,脉浮滑或紧;若风邪兼热,则咽喉红肿疼痛,舌质红,脉浮滑数。

　　[护治原则]疏风清热,宣肺行水。

　　[常用方剂]越婢加术汤。

　　(2)湿毒浸淫证

　　[主要证候]眼睑浮肿,延及全身,皮肤光亮,尿少色赤,身发疮痍,甚则溃烂,恶风发热;舌质红,苔薄黄,脉浮数或滑数。

　　[证候分析]湿毒未清,累及肺脾,肺失通调水道,脾失运化水湿,故尿少,水肿;湿毒未解,故身发疮痍,甚则溃烂;湿毒夹风,营卫失和,故眼睑浮肿,延及全身,恶风发热;舌质红,苔薄黄,脉浮数或滑数,均为湿毒内蕴之象。

　　[护治原则]宣肺解毒,利湿消肿。

　　[常用方剂]麻黄连翘赤小豆汤合五味消毒饮。

　　(3)水湿浸渍证

　　[主要证候]全身水肿,下肢明显,按之没指,小便短少,身体困重,胸闷,纳呆,泛恶,起病缓慢,病程较长;苔白腻,脉沉缓。

　　[证候分析]脾虚水湿泛溢,精微不敛,久则元气虚衰,气化失常,故小便短少;水湿之邪下趋,故全身水肿,下肢明显,按之没指;湿性黏腻,故起病缓慢,病程较长;脾为湿困,阳气不得舒展,故身体困重,胸闷,纳呆,泛恶;苔白腻,脉沉缓,均为湿盛之象。

　　[护治原则]运脾化湿,通阳利水。

　　[常用方剂]五皮饮合胃苓汤。

　　(4)湿热壅盛证

　　[主要证候]遍体浮肿,皮肤绷急光亮,胸脘痞闷,烦热口渴,小便短赤,大便干结;舌红,苔黄腻,脉沉数或濡数。

　　[证候分析]水湿化热,壅滞三焦,故遍体浮肿,皮肤绷急光亮;热耗津液,气机失常,故胸脘痞闷;热盛消耗津液,故烦热口渴,小便短赤,大便干结;舌红,苔黄腻,脉沉数或濡数,均为湿热之象。

　　[护治原则]分利湿热。

　　[常用方剂]疏凿饮子。

　　2.阴水

　　(1)脾阳虚衰证

　　[主要证候]身肿日久,腰以下为甚,按之凹陷不易恢复,脘腹胀闷,纳减便溏,面色不华,神疲乏力,四肢倦怠,小便短少;舌质淡,苔白腻或白滑,脉沉缓或沉弱。

　　[证候分析]脾阳虚衰,气不化水,故身肿日久,腰以下为甚;脾虚运化失司,故脘腹胀闷,纳减便溏;脾虚气血生化乏源,故面色不华;阳虚失于温煦,故神疲乏力,四肢倦怠;阳虚失于气化,故小便短少;舌质淡,苔白腻或白滑,脉沉缓或沉弱,均为脾阳虚衰之象。

［护治原则］健脾温阳利水。

［常用方剂］实脾饮。

（2）肾阳衰微证

［主要证候］水肿反复消长不已,面浮身肿,腰以下为甚,按之凹陷不起,尿量减少或反多,腰酸冷痛,四肢厥冷,怯寒神疲,面色苍白,心悸胸闷,喘促难卧,腹大胀满;舌质淡胖,苔白,脉沉细或沉迟无力。

［证候分析］阳虚气化失司,水湿难去,故水肿反复消长不已;阳虚膀胱开阖不利,故尿量减少或反多;腰为肾之府,阳虚则腰酸冷痛;阳虚失于温煦,故四肢厥冷;肾阳不足,心阳亦亏,水气上凌心肺,故心悸胸闷,喘促难卧;舌质淡胖,苔白,脉沉细或沉迟无力,均为肾阳衰微之象。

［护治原则］温肾助阳,化气行水。

［常用方剂］真武汤。

（3）瘀水互结证

［主要证候］水肿延久不退,肿势轻重不一,四肢或全身浮肿,以下肢为主,或有皮肤瘀斑,腰部刺痛,或伴血尿;舌紫暗,苔白,脉沉细涩。

［证候分析］久病入络,络脉瘀阻,水道不通,水渗肌肤,故水肿延久不退,肿势轻重不一,四肢或全身浮肿,以下肢为主;血水同源,水液久蓄脉道,脉络胀滞,故皮肤瘀斑,腰部刺痛,或伴血尿;舌紫暗,苔白,脉沉细涩,均为瘀血内停之象。

［护治原则］活血祛瘀,化气行水。

［常用方剂］桃红四物汤合五苓散。

三、护理措施

对于水肿的病人,应观察水肿的部位、程度、消长规律;小便的量、色、质、次数;大便的颜色、次数。注意观察神志、面色、呼吸、血压、心率、体温,以及用药后的反应。询问有无胸闷、腰痛、呕吐、出血、泡沫尿。记录24小时液体出入量。定期测量腹围、体重,检查血常规、尿常规、肝功能、肾功能。若病人出现小便不通、呕吐,伴头痛,口有尿味,应立即报告医生,并配合抢救。

（一）辨证施护

1. 风水相搏证

（1）生活起居护理　居室向阳避风。卧床休息,抬高头部,定时翻身。待症状缓解后,可适当活动,不可过于劳累。出汗后及时用干毛巾擦拭。若咽喉肿痛,可用锡类散或双料喉风散喷喉,喷药后20分钟内不要饮水及进食。急性期不可洗澡。

（2）饮食护理　限盐,不可过饱,控制饮水量。根据水肿程度不同,予低盐或无盐饮食。若发热,可适当增加饮水量。玉米须30 g,加水煮沸30分钟至300 mL,代茶饮。宜食疏风利水的食物,如薏苡仁、冬瓜、茯苓、赤小豆。不宜食辛辣、厚腻、肥甘的食物。

（3）情志护理　病人起病急,可能产生恐惧、忧虑、急躁的情绪,护士可运用语言开导疗法,经常巡视,主动关心病人,进行跟疾病相关的知识指导,使病人情绪稳定。

（4）用药护理　石膏先煎,车前子包煎。中药汤剂应武火快煎,饭后热服,服药后食少许热饮或热粥,盖被安卧,微微汗出。

（5）操作技术　①药浴疗法：用紫苏叶、防风、土茯苓、丹参,煎煮后兑水浸洗全身,药液温度38~40℃,每次20分钟,隔日1次;适用于水肿明显,或经休息、限盐、利尿后,水肿消退不理想的病人;女性月经期或妊娠期禁用。②穴位按摩法：取水道、三焦俞、委中、阴陵泉、肺俞、列缺、合谷,用拇指揉法,按摩至局部发热或有酸麻重胀感,每日1次;孕妇禁用。③熏蒸疗法：用浮萍煮水,对头面部进行熏蒸,每次20分钟;适用于头面部严重水肿者。④耳压疗法：取脾、肾、内分泌等耳穴,用耳穴压丸贴片贴压,每日按揉4~5次,以局部发热泛红为度,留置2~4日;孕妇禁用,耳部水肿者禁用。

2.湿毒浸淫证

（1）生活起居护理　居室凉爽避风,空气新鲜。床单衣物平整、柔软、清洁、干燥。卧床休息,抬高头部。定时翻身,每日用温水擦洗,协助病人修剪指甲,避免搔抓皮肤。保持口腔清洁,饭前、饭后、睡前用黄芩水漱口。注射拔针后,按压的时间要长,以不渗液为宜。水肿部位不宜进行针法和推拿疗法。

（2）饮食护理　限盐。高热者予流食或半流食。宜食健脾利湿的食物,如绿豆、冬瓜、白萝卜、白扁豆、赤小豆、丝瓜、苦瓜、山药。食疗方：薏苡仁煲瘦肉。不宜食辛辣、油腻、生冷的食物。

（3）情志护理　病人起病急,病情重,护士可运用语言开导疗法,鼓励病人积极配合治疗,认真实施护理措施,以增加病人的安全感,避免恐惧、忧虑、急躁、悲观。

（4）用药护理　赤小豆打碎煎。中药汤剂宜浓煎,饭后温服,少量频服。

（5）操作技术　①敷贴疗法：用新鲜蒲公英、马齿苋、野菊花各等量,洗净捣烂外敷;适用于皮肤溃烂处。②熏蒸疗法：用葛根、桂枝、白芍、紫苏叶、荆芥、防风、香薷、紫菀、生姜,煮水成500 mL,温度37~42℃,熏蒸水肿部位,每次20分钟,熏蒸后休息30分钟方可外出,隔日1次;适用于高度水肿无汗者,禁用于严重高血压者。③药浴疗法：用制苍术、白术、茯苓、泽泻、猪苓、车前子(包煎)、姜半夏、陈皮各10 g,煎煮后兑水浸洗全身,药液温度38~40℃,每次20分钟,隔日1次;女性月经期或妊娠期禁用。

3.水湿浸渍证

（1）生活起居护理　居室温暖干燥,安静避风,空气新鲜。卧床休息。若胸闷,取半仰卧位。若下肢水肿严重,适当抬高下肢。注意皮肤护理,定时翻身。输液时,严格控制滴速。若发生呕吐,应协助取坐位或侧卧位,头转向一边,吐后用温水漱口,及时清理呕吐物,保持床单清洁。

（2）饮食护理　限盐。增加菜肴的色、香、味,食物温度宜温,进食速度宜慢,少食多餐。限制饮水量。可用玉米须30 g,大枣10 g,煮水至300 mL,代茶饮。若泛恶,可含生姜片。宜食健脾利水的食物,如冬瓜、瓠瓜、白萝卜、丝瓜、莲子、荠菜、芹菜、茯苓、木瓜、荸荠、紫菜、藕。食疗方：薏苡仁粥、赤小豆炖鲤鱼。不宜食辛辣、油腻、生冷、酸涩的食物,如柚子、枇杷。

（3）情志护理　病人起病缓,病程长,护士可运用语言开导疗法,多鼓励病人,指导家属温暖、支持病人。或用顺意疗法,疏导病人的不良情绪,避免抑郁、焦虑。

（4）用药护理　中药汤剂宜浓煎,饭后温服,少量频服。服药后食少许热饮或热粥,以助药力。若泛恶,可在服药前用生姜片擦舌。

（5）操作技术　①点穴疗法：取内关、合谷,点按3分钟;适用于泛恶时。②水针疗法：取足三里、三阴交、阴陵泉,用维生素 B_1 注射液进行穴位注射。③ 灌肠疗法:用苍术、藿香、煅牡蛎、土茯苓、生大黄,保留灌肠。④ 敷贴疗法:取肾俞、天枢、足三里,用生黄芪、丹参、酒大黄、紫苏叶、川芎、积雪草、淫羊藿、白芷、丁香、吴茱萸、厚朴、木香,研磨成粉后与黄酒调成糊状敷贴;孕妇禁用。⑤ 敷脐疗法:取神阙,用田螺、大蒜、车前子各等份,捣碎纳入脐中,用胶布固定后用热水袋加温,每次 2~8 小时,每日 1 次;孕妇禁用。

4. 湿热壅盛证

(1) 生活起居护理　居室凉爽安静。卧床休息,取半仰卧位。保持皮肤清洁干燥,加强口腔护理。保持会阴部清洁,阴囊水肿者可垫起局部。经常顺时针按摩腹部,以保持大便通畅。排便时不可久蹲或过于用力。

(2) 饮食护理　若高度浮肿,予无盐饮食。控制饮水量,可少量饮绿豆汤、西瓜汁。宜食清热利湿的食物,如冬瓜、瓠瓜、菊花、白萝卜、莲子、赤小豆、丝瓜、绿豆芽、苦瓜。食疗方:薏苡仁煲鲫鱼、鲜芦根粥。不宜食辛辣、油腻、生冷的食物。

(3) 情志护理　病人症状较重,可能会有生命受威胁感,护士可运用移情易性疗法,如听音乐、练气功,帮助病人放松,避免紧张、焦虑、恐惧。

(4) 用药护理　赤小豆打碎煎。中药汤剂宜浓煎,晨起空腹少量频服。服药后记录二便的量及次数,中病即止。

(5) 操作技术　① 水针疗法:取肾俞、足三里,用鱼腥草注射液进行穴位注射。② 药浴疗法:用龙胆草、柴胡、泽泻、车前子、通草、生地、当归、炒栀子、炒黄芩、甘草,煎煮后兑水浸洗全身,药液温度 38~40℃,每次 20 分钟,隔日 1 次。③ 敷脐疗法:取神阙,用甘遂、京大戟、芫花各等量,共研细末,以 1~3 g 置脐内,外加纱布覆盖,胶布固定;每次 2~8 小时,每日 1 次;女性月经期或妊娠期禁用。④ 足浴疗法:用羌活、槟榔、大腹皮、茯苓皮、通草、泽泻、赤小豆各 30 g,煎煮后待水温降至 37~42℃时洗按足部,每次 20 分钟,每日 1 次;血压过低者慎用。⑤ 灌肠疗法:用大黄 60 g,牡蛎 30 g,煮水至 100~200 mL,保留灌肠。⑥ 敷贴疗法:用芒硝,捣成粉末,装入敷药袋内敷贴水肿处,每次 8~10 小时,每日 1 次。

5. 脾阳虚衰证

(1) 生活起居护理　居室温暖向阳,安静避风。床单干燥平整,衣物宽松柔软。卧床休息,注意保暖,适当抬高下肢,定时改变体位,经常活动脚踝。水肿减轻后,可适量运动,不可过劳,防止跌仆。

(2) 饮食护理　食物温度宜温,进食速度宜慢。增加菜肴的色、香、味,少食多餐。宜食温阳健脾的食物,如茯苓、木瓜、白胡椒、芡实、甘栗、大枣、山药、鹌鹑。若肾功能不全,只宜进食少量的高蛋白食物。若肾功能正常,可多吃肉、鱼、蛋、奶。食疗方:黄芪炖乳鸽、赤小豆鲤鱼汤。忌烈酒,不宜食辛辣、油腻、生冷、易产气的食物,如红薯。

(3) 情志护理　病人体虚久病,可能会对治疗信心不足,护士可运用语言开导疗法和移情易性疗法,鼓励和劝导病人,消除其不良情绪,指导病人培养兴趣爱好,参加力所能及的家庭或社交娱乐活动,如种植花草、下棋。

(4) 用药护理　中药汤剂宜饭前温服,少量频服。

(5) 操作技术　① 灸法:取肺俞、脾俞、肾俞、三阴交、足三里、关元,用温和灸,艾条燃着端悬于施灸部位上,距离皮肤2~3厘米,灸至病人有温热舒适无灼痛的感觉,皮肤稍有红晕,每日1次;孕妇腹部及腰骶部禁用。② 足浴疗法:用党参、生黄芪、生白术、茯苓、薏苡仁、杜仲、牛膝、泽泻、甘草,煎煮后待水温降至37~42℃时洗按足部,每次20分钟,每日1次;血压过低者慎用。③ 敷贴疗法:取肾俞、复溜、足三里、脾俞、气海,用温阳益气的药物,研磨成粉后与生姜汁调成糊状,选择2~3个腧穴敷贴,每次2~6小时,每日1次。

6. 肾阳衰微证

(1)生活起居护理　居室温暖向阳,安静舒适。床单平整干燥,衣物宽松柔软。绝对卧床,取半仰卧位,吸氧,注意保暖。保持皮肤清洁,定时翻身。注意口腔卫生,饭后用温水漱口。若口中有氨味,可用柠檬水漱口。病情平稳时,可适量运动,动作宜缓,以不疲劳为度。

(2)饮食护理　无盐、低蛋白饮食。食用优质蛋白,如肉、蛋、奶。宜食温阳利水的食物,如肉桂、韭菜、泥鳅、鸡肉、黑芝麻、黑豆。食疗方:赤小豆冬瓜炖鲫鱼。不宜食辛辣、生冷、油腻的食物。

(3)情志护理　病人体虚久病,护士可运用语言开导疗法和顺意疗法,了解病人的心理状况,鼓励病人说出焦虑、恐惧的原因,进行有效的心理疏导,避免病人由于焦虑紧张而乱投医、乱服药,导致病情加重。

(4)用药护理　中药汤剂宜文火久煎,饭前温服。

(5)操作技术　① 灸法:取气海、关元、阴陵泉、三阴交、足三里、太溪、肾俞、脾俞,用温和灸,艾条燃着端悬于施灸部位上,距离皮肤2~3厘米,灸至病人有温热舒适无灼痛的感觉,皮肤稍有红晕,每日1次;孕妇腹部及腰骶部禁用。② 药熨疗法:取腰部,用吴茱萸250 g,粗盐50 g,炒热后装入布袋中,制成温度为60~70℃的中药热罨包,药熨20分钟,每日1次;孕妇禁用。③ 敷贴疗法:取关元,用附子、肉桂、细辛,打粉与生姜汁调成饼状;或用附子、干姜、川续断、大葱,捣泥外敷,每次2~4小时,每日1~2次。④ 灌肠疗法:用附子、肉苁蓉、煅牡蛎、生大黄煎汤,保留灌肠,每周2次。⑤ 水针疗法:取肾俞、关元、足三里,用参附注射液进行穴位注射。⑥ 保健按摩疗法:取足三里、肾俞,经常用拇指揉法进行自我按摩。

7. 瘀水互结证

(1)生活起居护理　居室温暖避风,安静舒适。卧床休息,定时翻身,注意保暖。若发生血尿,应绝对卧床。当病情平稳时,可适量运动,以不疲劳为度。注意皮肤和口腔清洁,操作时动作轻柔,避免出血。

(2)饮食护理　宜食活血化瘀的食物,如乌鸡、黑鱼、山楂、香菇、黑木耳、洋葱、紫菜、黑豆、葡萄、桃子。不宜食辛辣、油腻、生冷的食物。

(3)情志护理　病人病程较长,或伴出血,可能会恐惧、焦虑、抑郁,护士可运用语言开导疗法,多与病人沟通,说明积极治疗可以缓解病情,以及本病与情志的关系,使病人保持情绪稳定,积极配合治疗。

(4)用药护理　中药汤剂宜饭后温服。

(5)操作技术　① 灌肠疗法:用炒杜仲、肉苁蓉、煅牡蛎、生大黄、红花、丹参;或用柴胡、当归、生地、川芎、赤芍、牛膝、桔梗、枳壳、甘草、桃仁、红花;保留灌肠。② 水针疗法:取太溪、太冲、血海,用灯盏细辛注射液或参附注射液进行穴位注射。③ 足浴疗法:用红花、牛膝、刘寄奴,煎煮后待水温降至37~42℃时洗按足部,每次20分钟,每日1次;血压过低者慎用。④ 穴位按摩法:取三阴交、阳陵泉、脾俞、太溪,用拇指揉法,按摩至局部发热或有酸麻重胀感,每日1次;孕妇禁用。

（二）健康教育

居室安静避风,光线充足,空气新鲜。多卧床休息,睡眠充足。注意个人卫生,勤漱口。保持皮肤清洁,定时翻身。病情平稳时,适量运动。预防感冒,不可冒雨涉水。不可过劳,节制性行为。

饮食宜清淡、营养、易消化,少食多餐。宜食高热量、高维生素、低脂、低嘌呤的食物。进食少量的优质动物蛋白,多吃新鲜蔬菜。依据水肿程度,予低盐或无盐饮食。控制饮水量和蛋白质的摄入量。忌烟酒、发物、腌制品、致敏食物,不宜食生冷、辛辣的食物。

保持情绪稳定。正确认识疾病,学会自我调节,放慢行为节奏,消除心理压力,避免焦虑、紧张、抑郁、恐惧、愤怒。

遵医嘱用药。谨慎使用抗生素和镇痛药。忌用肾毒性药物,如马兜铃、关木通、木防己、青木香、益母草。

定期复诊,检查尿常规、肝功能、肾功能等。积极治疗原发病,及时治疗反复感染的病灶。

Section 12　Edema

Edema is a disease clinically characterized by swelling of the eyelids, face, four limbs and whole body, or concavities on the skin after pressure. It is caused by disturbance of qi transformation and water retention due to either external pathogen, overstrain and internal damage, or improper diet. This section can be referred to for the nursing of some diseases with edema as the main manifestation, such as primary glomerular disease, secondary nephropathy, hypothyroidism, and primary aldosteronism in Western medicine.

ETIOLOGY AND PATHOGENESIS

The etiology includes pathogenic wind attacking the exterior, inward sinking of sore-toxin, internal invasion of water-dampness, improper diet, emotional disorders, overstrain and sexual indulgence, and other diseases. External invasion of wind-cold or wind-heat induces failure of lung qi to disperse and descend. The wind and water combine with each other, and subsequently edema occurs. Residual toxin of abscess and ulcer damages the spleen and lung, which leads to disturbance of water metabolism, and subsequently edema occurs. Long-term residence in damp place, braving rain or wading in water causes internal retention of water-dampness that encumbers the spleen and triggers dysfunction of the spleen to restrain water, and subsequently edema develops. Improper diet, such as excessive hunger, or over intake of fatty, too-sweet, raw and cold foods, causes spleen deficiency and dampness, and subsequently edema takes place. Depression damaging the liver triggers failure of the liver to act freely, which leads to inhibited qi movement of the triple energizer and impeded water passage; or anxiety and contemplation damaging the spleen induces failure of the spleen in transportation and transformation; both may subsequently generate edema. Overstrain damaging the spleen, or sexual indulgence and multiparity damaging the kidney, may bring about disturbance of water metabolism, and subsequently edema happens. Chronic illness damaging the lung, spleen and kidney gives rise to inhibited water metabolism; or chronic illness entering collaterals makes blood stasis obstruct triple energizer and congestion of water passage; both may subsequently result in edema.

The pathogenesis is failure of the lung to dredge and regulate water passage, dysfunction of the spleen in transportation and transformation, and failure of the kidney to govern opening and closing, which all cause inhibited qi movement of the triple energizer and water retention, and consequently edema. The disease is located in the lung, spleen and kidney. Edema mostly belongs to the syndrome of root deficiency and tip excess. Yang edema is primarily tip excess while yin edema root deficiency.

COMMON SYNDROMES

Key Points in Syndrome Differentiation

1. Differentiation of Yang Edema from Yin Edema

The differentiation is based on the causes, onset speed, course and location of edema. Generally, yang edema is caused by external pathogen with acute onset, short course, development from top to bottom, bright swollen skin, spontaneous restoration of concavities on the skin after pressure. On the contrary, the edema caused by internal damage with gradual onset, long course, repeated occurrence, development from bottom to top, difficult restoration of concavities on the skin after pressure, accompanied with mental and physical fatigue, mostly belongs to yin edema.

2. Differentiation of Disease Location

The differentiation is based on the location of edema. If edema starts from eyelids, and then spreads to four limbs, and accompanied with aversion to cold and fever, the location is in the lung. If edema spreads to the whole body, and accompanied with heavy sensation of extremities, gastric stuffiness and reduced appetite, the location is in the spleen. If edema spreads to the whole body with severe swelling below the waist, and accompanied with soreness and weakness of waist and knees, the location is in the kidney.

3. Differentiation of External Invasion from Internal Damage

The differentiation is based on the course of disease. Edema caused by external invasion exhibits acute onset, short course, and accompanied with aversion to cold, fever, headache, body pain and floating pulse. However, edema induced by internal damage demonstrates gradual onset, repeated occurrence, long course, and accompanied with depletion of viscera and deficiency of healthy qi.

Syndrome Differentiation

1. Yang Edema

（1）Syndrome of Mutual Wind-Water Contention

［Clinical Manifestations］Edema starting from the eyelids and then spreading to the four limbs and all over the body rapidly, accompanied with aversion to cold, fever, soreness of joints and inhibited urination. For wind-heat syndrome: red, swollen and sore throat, red tongue and floating, slippery and rapid pulse. For wind-cold syndrome: aversion to cold, cough and asthma, thin white tongue coating, and floating, slippery or tight pulse.

［Manifestations Analysis］Exterior pathogen attacking the lung leads to failure of the lung to disperse and descend as well as to dredge and regulate water passage, which consequently gives rise to abnormal water metabolism, resulting in edema and inhibited urination. Pathogenic wind is apt to migrate and change, and tends to aid water pathogens, so edema starts from the eyelids, and then spreads to the four limbs and all over the body rapidly. Pathogen invades the exterior and constrain defensive yang, so exhibits aversion to cold, fever, and soreness of joints. Pathogenic wind carrying heat is the reason for red, swollen and sore throat, red tongue, and floating, slippery and rapid pulse. Pathogenic wind carrying cold contributes to aversion to cold, cough, asthma, thin white tongue coating, and floating, slippery or tight pulse.

〔Nursing Principle〕Dispersing wind and clearing heat; ventilating the lung and moving water.

〔Suggested Formula〕Yuebi Jiazhu Decoction.

（2）Dampness Toxin Spreading Syndrome

〔Clinical Manifestations〕Edema starting from the eyelids, and then spreading to the whole body, bright color skin, scanty dark urine, sores on the body or even ulcerations, aversion to wind, fever, red tongue with thin yellow coating, and floating rapid or slippery rapid pulse.

〔Manifestations Analysis〕Residue dampness toxin involving the spleen and lung leads to failure of the lung to govern dredging and regulating of water passage as well as dysfunction of the spleen in transportation and transformation, so scanty urine and edema occur. Residual dampness toxin contributes to sores on the body or even ulcerations. Dampness toxin carrying wind brings about disharmony of nutrient and defensive aspects, causing edema starting from the eyelids and then spreading to the whole body, aversion to wind and fever. Red tongue with thin yellow coating and floating rapid or slippery rapid pulse are the signs of internal accumulation of dampness toxin.

〔Nursing Principle〕Ventilating the lung and clearing toxin; removing dampness and relieving swelling.

〔Suggested Formula〕Mahuang Lianqiao Chixiaodou Decoction and Wuwei Xiaodu Decoction.

（3）Water-Dampness Retention and Diffusion Syndrome

〔Clinical Manifestations〕General edema especially in lower limbs, difficult restoration of concavities on the skin after pressure, scanty urine, heavy sensation of the body, chest oppression, anorexia, upflow nausea, gradual onset, long course, white slimy tongue coating, and sunken moderate pulse.

〔Manifestations Analysis〕Spleen deficiency causes effusion of water-dampness and fails to constrain nutritious essence, which gradually and subsequently causes debilitation of primordial qi and abnormal qi transformation, so scanty urine occurs. Pathogenic dampness tends to move downwards, causing general edema especially in lower limbs, and difficult restoration of concavities on the skin after pressure. Dampness is viscous and slimy, resulting in edema with gradual onset and long course. Spleen is encumbered by dampness and yang qi cannot spread to the whole body, leading to heavy sensation of the body, chest oppression, anorexia, and upflow nausea. White slimy tongue coating and sunken moderate pulse are signs of exuberant dampness.

〔Nursing Principle〕Activating spleen yang and resolving dampness; unblocking yang and promoting urination.

〔Suggested Formula〕Wupi Drink and Weiling Decoction.

（4）Exuberant Dampness-Heat Congestion Syndrome

〔Clinical Manifestations〕General edema, tight bright color skin, chest and gastric stuffiness and oppression, vexation, thirst, scanty dark urine, dry stool, red tongue with yellow slimy coating, and sunken rapid or soggy rapid pulse.

[Manifestations Analysis] Water-dampness transforms to heat and obstructs the triple energizer, so there are general edema, and tight bright color skin. Heat consuming fluids causes abnormal qi movement, so there is chest and gastric stuffiness and oppression. Exuberant heat consumes fluids, so the patients show vexation, thirst, scanty dark urine, and dry stool. Red tongue with yellow slimy coating and sunken rapid or soggy rapid pulse means dampness-heat.

[Nursing Principle] Separating and removing dampness-heat.

[Suggested Formula] Shuzao Yinzi Decoction.

2. Yin Edema

(1) Syndrome of Spleen-Yang Debilitation

[Clinical Manifestations] General edema for long time especially below the waist, difficult restoration of concavities on the skin after pressure, gastric and abdominal distension and stuffiness, reduced appetite, loose stool, lusterless complexion, mental and physical fatigue, lassitude, scanty urine, pale tongue with white slimy or white slippery coating, and sunken moderate or sunken weak pulse.

[Manifestations Analysis] Debilitation of spleen yang causes failure of qi to promote water transformation, so shows general edema for long time especially below the waist. Dysfunction of the spleen in transportation and transformation contributes to gastric and abdominal distension and stuffiness, reduced appetite, and loose stool. Deficient spleen fails to generate enough qi and blood, so the complexion is lusterless. Deficiency yang cannot warm the body, leading to mental and physical fatigue and lassitude. Yang deficiency triggers failure of qi transformation, resulting in scanty urine. Pale tongue with white slimy or white slippery coating and sunken moderate pulse or sunken weak pulse suggest debilitation of spleen yang.

[Nursing Principle] Invigorating the spleen, warming yang and draining water.

[Suggested Formula] Shipi Drink.

(2) Debilitation of Kidney Yang Syndrome

[Clinical Manifestations] Persistent and recurrent edema, facial puffiness and general edema especially below the waist, difficult restoration of indent after pressure, reduced or adversely increased urine amount, lumbar soreness and cold pain, reversal cold of four limbs, fear of cold, mental fatigue, pale complexion, palpitation, chest oppression, hasty panting with inability to lie flat, abdominal distension and fullness, pale enlarged tongue with white coating, and sunken thready pulse or sunken, slow and forceless pulse.

[Manifestations Analysis] Yang deficiency causes failure of qi transformation and retention of water-dampness, causing persistent and recurrent edema. Yang deficiency leads to inhibited opening and closing of the bladder, resulting in reduced or adversely increased urine amount. Lumbus is the house of the kidney, therefore, yang deficiency causes lumbar soreness and cold pain. Yang deficiency cannot warm the body, so reversal cold of four limbs is felt. Debilitation of kidney yang induces deficiency of heart yang, therefore, water pathogen intimidates the heart and lung, then there exhibit palpitation, chest oppression, and hasty panting with inability to lie flat. Pale enlarged tongue with white coating and sunken thready pulse or sunken, slow and forceless pulse are signs of debilitation of kidney yang.

[Nursing Principle] Warming the kidney and assisting yang; transforming qi and moving water.

[Suggested Formula] Zhenwu Decoction.

(3) Syndrome of Mutual Binding of Stasis and Water

[Clinical Manifestations] Persistent edema with varying severity, dropsy in extremities or all over the body, especially in the lower limbs, or possible skin ecchymosis, stabbing pain of lumbus, or accompanied with bloody urine, dark purple tongue with white coating, and sunken thready and unsmooth pulse.

[Manifestations Analysis] Chronic illness entering the collaterals causes obstruction of collateral vessels and water passage, which subsequently induces effusion of water to the skin. Therefore, there is persistent edema with varying severity, and dropsy in extremities or all over the body, especially in the lower limbs. Blood and water share the same origin and long-time water retention in the vessels causes distention and stagnation of collateral vessels. Therefore, there are possible skin ecchymosis, stabbing pain of lumbus, or accompanied with bloody urine. Dark purple tongue with white coating and sunken thready and unsmooth pulse are signs of internal stagnation of blood stasis.

[Nursing Principle] Activating blood and removing stasis; transforming qi and moving water.

[Suggested Formula] Taohong Siwu Decoction and Wuling Powder.

NURSING MEASURES

For patients with edema, nurses should observe the location, severity as well as exuberance or debilitation of edema; the volume, color, quality and frequency of urine; and the color and frequency of stool. They should also observe the patients' consciousness, complexion, respiration, blood pressure, heart rate, temperature and reaction to medication. Nurses should inquire the presence or abscence of chest oppression, lumbus pain, vomiting, bleeding, or foaming urine, record the 24-hour intake and output, regularly measure abdominal circumference and body weight, and take routine blood test, routine urine test, liver function test and kidney function test. If the patient has urinary obstruction, vomiting, accompanied with headache, and urinary smell in the mouth, it is advisable to report to doctor immediately and assist in emergency treatment.

Syndrome-Based Nursing Measures

1. Syndrome of Mutual Wind-Water Contention

(1) Daily life nursing. The ward should be sunward, dry, quiet, and away from wind. The patients should rest in bed with the head slightly raised and turn over regularly. When the symptoms are relieved, they can do moderate activities but should avoid overexertion. Wipe the sweat with a dry towel

immediately after perspiration. For patients with swollen and sore throat, Xilei Powder or Shuangliao Houfeng Powder could be used to spray the throat and don't drink or eat within 20 minutes after spraying medicine. Don't bathe in the acute phase of disease.

(2) Diet nursing. The patients should limit salt intake, avoid overeating, and drink less water. A low-salt or salt-free diet is given to the patients according to the different severities of edema. For cases with high fever, water intake could be increased and yumixu (cornsilk) tea could be used for drinking (i.e. decoct 30 g of cornsilk with water for 30 minutes to get 300 mL decoction for drinking). The patients may eat foods that disperse wind and excrete water, such as yiyiren (coix seed), Chinese waxgourd, fuling (poria), and chixiaodou (adzuki bean). Don't eat pungent, spicy, rich, greasy, fatty and sweet foods.

(3) Emotion nursing. Due to acute onset, the patients may feel fear, anxiety, and impatience. Nurses may use verbal enlightenment therapy to care for the patients initiatively and impart them the knowledge of the disease to keep them calm.

(4) Medication nursing. Shigao (gypsum) should be decocted first and cheqianzi (plantago seed) should be wrap-boiled. Decoction should be brewed fast with strong fire and taken hot after meals. After taking the medicine, the patients should take hot drinks or porridge and covered with a quilt to perspire slightly.

(5) Manipulation techniques. ① Medicated bath therapy: prepare zisuye (perilla leaf), fangfeng (siler), tufuling (poria) and danshen (danshen root); first decoct the above medicinals, and then add water into the decoction to steep and wash the whole body at a temperature of $38 \sim 40\ ℃$, 20 minutes each time, once every other day. It is appropriate for the patients with apparent edema, or those with unsatisfactory effect after rest, salt-limiting and diuresis. And it is contraindicated in females during menstruation or pregnancy. ② Acupressure therapy: select Shuidao (ST 28), Yinlingquan (SP 94), Feishu (BL 13), Lieque (LU 7) and Hegu (LI 4); apply thumb kneading manipulation on each of the points until the area turns hot or the patient has the feelings of soreness, numbness, distension and heaviness in the area, once per day. And it is contraindicated in pregnant women. ③ Fumigating and steaming therapy: decoct fuping (duckweed) with water to fume and steam the head and face, 20 minutes each time. It is appropriate for the patients with severe swelling of head and face. ④ Auricular pressure therapy: select spleen (CO13), kidney (CO10) and endocrine (CO18); apply specialized pasters on the points, press on each of them until the area turns hot and red, $4 \sim 5$ times per day, and keep the pasters for $2 \sim 4$ days. And it is contraindicated in pregnant women and patients with ear edema.

2. Dampness Toxin Spreading Syndrome

(1) Daily life nursing. The ward should be cool, dry, quiet, full of fresh air and away from wind. Sheets and clothing should be tidy, soft, clean and dry. The nurses should assist patients to trim the fingernails to prevent them from scratching the skin. The patients should rest in bed with the head slightly raised, turn over regularly, scrub the body with warm water every day, and keep oral hygiene by gargling the mouth with huangqin (scutellaria root) liquid before and after meals as well as before sleep.

After injection, press the needle hole for a long time to avoid seepage. The edema area should not be acupunctured and massaged.

(2) Diet nursing. The patients should limit salt intake. For patients with high fever, eat liquid or semi-liquid foods. The patients may eat foods that invigorate the spleen and drain dampness, such as lüdou (mung bean), Chinese waxgourd, white radish, baibiandou (white hyacinth bean), chixiaodou (adzuki bean), luffa, bitter gourd and shanyao (common yam rhizome). Food therapy: lean meat stewed with yiyiren (coix seed). Don't eat pungent, spicy, greasy, raw and cold foods.

(3) Emotion nursing. Due to the acute onset and severe condition, nurses may use verbal enlightenment therapy to encourage the patients to comply with the treatment and properly implement nursing measures to enhance their sense of security and prevent fear, anxiety, impatience and pessimism.

(4) Medication nursing. Chixiaodou (adzuki bean) should be crushed. Decoction should be concentrated and taken warm after meals, multiple times in small portions.

(5) Manipulation techniques. ① Paste application therapy: clean and mash equal amount of fresh pugongying (dandelion), machixian (purslane) and yejuhua (wild chrysanthemum flower), and apply it on the skin. It is appropriate for the patients with skin ulceration. ② Fumigating and steaming therapy: prepare gegen (kudzuvine root), guizhi (cinnamon twig), baishao (white peony root), zisuye (perilla leaf), jingjie (schizonepeta), fangfeng (siler), xiangru (aromatic madder), ziyuan (tatarian aster root), and shengjiang (fresh ginger); decoct the above ingredients to get 500 mL of concentrated decoction, and use it to fumigate the swollen area at 37~42℃, 20 minutes each time, once every other day. After fumigating, the patients need to take a rest for 30 minutes before leaving. It is appropriate for the patients with serious edema and without sweating, and contraindicated in patients with severe hypertension. ③ Medicated bath therapy: prepare zhicangzhu (prepared atractylodes rhizome), baizhu (white atractylodes rhizome), fuling (poria), zexie (water plantain rhizome), zhuling (polyporus), cheqianzi (plantago seed) (wrap-boiled), jiangbanxia (pinellia rhizome prepared with fresh ginger juice), and chenpi (aged tangerine peel) 10 g respectively; first decoct the above medicinals, and then add water into the decoction to steep and wash the whole body at a temperature of 38~40℃, 20 minutes each time, once every other day. And it is contraindicated in females during menstruation or pregnancy.

3. Water-Dampness Retention and Diffusion Syndrome

(1) Daily life nursing. The ward should be warm, dry, quiet, full of fresh air, and away from wind. Patients should rest in bed as much as possible. If chest oppression occurs, patients should stay in semi-supine position. If severe edema presents in lower limbs, patients should raise their legs properly. They should pay attention to skin care and turn over regularly. Nurses should strictly control the dripping rate of transfusion. For patients with vomiting, the nurses should assist them to take a sitting or lateral decubitus position with the head turning to one side, gargle with warm water after vomiting, clean the vomitus in time, and keep the sheets clean.

(2) Diet nursing. The patients should limit salt intake, have multiple small meals at slow speed, and drink less water. The color, aroma, taste of dishes could be enhanced and food should be warm.

Herbal tea is recommended：decoct yumixu（cornsilk）30 g, dazao（Chinese date）10 g and water to get 300 mL of liquid for drinking. For patients with nausea, keep shengjiang（fresh ginger）slice in the mouth. The patients may eat foods that invigorate the spleen and drain water, such as Chinese waxgourd, bottle gourd, white radish, luffa, lianzi（lotus seed）, shepherd's purse, celery, fuling（poria）, mugua（Chinese quince fruit）, biqi（waternut）, laver and lotus root. Food therapy：yiyiren（coix seed）porridge, carp stewed with chixiaodou（adzuki bean）. Don't eat pungent, spicy, greasy, raw, cold, sour and astringent foods, such as grapefruit and loquat.

（3）Emotion nursing. Due to slow onset and long course of disease, nurses may use verbal enlightenment therapy to encourage patients as much as possible and guide their families to give them support. Nurses may also use submission therapy to ease patients' bad emotions and prevent their depression and anxiety.

（4）Medication nursing. Decoction should be concentrated and taken warm after meals, multiple times in small portions. After taking the medicine, the patients could drink a few hot drinks or porridge to enhance the efficacy of medication. For patients with nausea, wipe the tongue with shengjiang（fresh ginger）slice before taking medicine.

（5）Manipulation techniques. ① Acupoint-pressing therapy：select Neiguan（PC 6）and Hegu（LI 4）; press on them for three minutes. It is appropriate for patients with nausea. ② Water acupuncture therapy：select Zusanli（ST 36）, Sanyinjiao（SP 6）, and Yinlingquan（SP 9）; inject Vitamin B_1 injection to the acupoints. ③ Enema therapy：decoct cangzhu（atractylodes rhizome）, huoxiang（agastache）, duanmuli（calcined oyster shell）, tufuling（glabrous greenbrier rhizome）, and shengdahuang（raw rhubarb root and rhizome）; use the decoction for retention enema. ④ Paste application therapy：select Shenshu（BL 23）, Tianshu（ST 25）, and Zusanli（ST 36）; grind into powder shenghuangqi（astragalus root）, danshen（danshen root）, jiudahuang（yellow wine prepared rhubarb root and rhizome）, zisuye（perilla leaf）, chuanxiong（Sichuan lovage root）, jixuecao（asiatic pennywort）, yinyanghuo（aerial part of epimedium）, baizhi（angelica root）, dingxiang（clove flower）, wuzhuyu（medicinal evodia fruit）, houpo（magnolia bark）, and muxiang（common aucklandia root）; blend the powder with yellow wine to make pastes, and apply the pastes on the acupoints. And it is contraindicated in pregnant women. ⑤ Umbilical compress therapy：select Shenque（CV 8）; mash equal proportions of river snails, dasuan（garlic bulb）and cheqianzi（plantago seed）, apply the paste on the navel, fix it with adhesive tape, and warm it with hot water bag, 2~8 hours each time, once per day. And it is contraindicated in pregnancy.

4. Exuberant Dampness-Heat Congestion Syndrome

（1）Daily life nursing. The ward should be cool, dry, quiet and comfortable. The patients should rest in bed, stay in semi-supine position, keep the skin clean and dry, pay attention to oral hygiene, and keep the perineal region clean. Scrotum edema can be locally padded. The patients should also often massage abdomen clockwise to keep a normal bowel movement and avoid extended periods of squatting and overexertion in defecation.

（2）Diet nursing. Patients with severe edema should have salt-free diet and reduce water intake. A moderate amount of lüdou（mung bean）soup and watermelon juice is recommended. They may eat foods that clear heat and drain dampness, such as Chinese waxgourd, bottle gourd, juhua（chrysanthemum flower）, white radish, lianzi（lotus seed）, chixiaodou（adzuki bean）, luffa, and mung bean sprouts. Food therapy: crucian stewed with yiyiren（coix seed）, and xianlugen（fresh reed rhizome）porridge. Don't eat pungent, spicy, greasy, raw and cold foods.

（3）Emotion nursing. Due to serious symptoms, the patients may have life-threatening feeling. Nurses may use emotional transference and dispositional change therapy, such as listening to music, practising Qigong, to help patients relax and prevent tension, anxiety and fear.

（4）Medication nursing. Chixiaodou（adzuki bean）should be crushed. Decoction should be concentrated and taken on an empty stomach in the morning, multiple times in small portions. After taking the medicine, the quantity of urine and stool and frequency of urination and defecation should be recorded, and medication should be discontinued immediately after recovery.

（5）Manipulation techniques. ① Water acupuncture therapy: select Shenshu（BL 23）and Zusanli （ST 36）; inject yuxingcao（heartleaf houttuynia）injection to the acupoints. ② Medicated bath therapy: prepare longdan cao（Chinese gentian）, chaihu（bupleurum）, zexie（water plantain rhizome）, cheqianzi（plantago seed）, tongcao（rice paper plant pith）, shengdi（rehmannia root）, danggui （Chinese angelica）, chaozhizi（stir-fried gardenia）, chaohuangqin（stir-fried scutellaria root）, and gancao（licorice root）; first decoct the above medicinals, and then add water into the decoction to steep and wash the whole body at a temperature of $38 \sim 40\,℃$, 20 minutes each time, once every other day. ③ Umbilical compress therapy: select Shenque（CV 8）; grind into powder equal amount of gansui （gansui root）, jingdaji（Peking euphorbia root）, and yuanhua（lilac daphne flower bud）; put $1 \sim 3$ g of the powder into the umbilicus and then fix it with gauze and bondage, $2 \sim 8$ hours each time, once per day. And it is contraindicated in females during menstruation or pregnancy. ④ Foot bath therapy: decoct qianghuo（notoptetygium root）, binglang（betel nut）, dafupi（areca husk）, fulingpi（poria peel）, tongcao（rice paper plant pith）, zexie（water plantain rhizome）, and chixiaodou（adzuki bean）; wash the feet with the decoction at $37 \sim 42\,℃$ and massage, 20 minutes each time, once per day. And it should be used with caution for patients with hypotension. ⑤ Enema therapy: decoct dahuang（rhubarb root and rhizome）60 g, and duanmuli（calcined oyster shell）30 g, and use $100 \sim 200$ mL of the decoction for retention enema. ⑥ Paste application therapy: crush mangxiao（sodium sulphate）into powder, put it into a cloth bag, and apply the bag to the edema area, $8 \sim 10$ hours each time, once per day.

5. Syndrome of Spleen-Yang Debilitation

（1）Daily life nursing. The ward should be warm, sunward, quiet and away from wind. The sheet should be dry and tidy while the clothing is loose and soft. The patients should rest in bed, keep themselves warm, raise the lower limbs slightly, change postures regularly, and do dorsiflexion and extension of feet frequently. After the edema is relieved, the patients may do moderate exercise but should avoid falls and overexertion.

（2）Diet nursing. The color, aroma and taste of dishes could be enhanced and food should be warm. The patients should have multiple small meals at slow speed and foods that warm yang and invigorate the spleen, such as fuling (poria), mugua (Chinese quince fruit), baihujiao (white pepper), qianshi (euryale seed), chestnuts, dazao (chinese date), shanyao (common yam rhizome), and quails. For patients with renal insufficiency, eat a little foods with high protein. For patients with normal kidney function, take more meat, fish, eggs and milk. Food therapy: huangqi (astragalus root) stewed with squab, and chixiaodou liyu (adzuki bean and carp) soup. Don't drink liquor and eat foods that are pungent, spicy, greasy, raw, cold and flatulent, such as sweet potatoes.

（3）Emotion nursing. Due to weakness and long course of disease, the patients may have insufficient confidence in treatment. Nurses may use verbal enlightenment therapy to encourage and persuade the patients to eliminate their bad emotions. Nurses may also use emotional transference and dispositional change therapy to guide the patients to develop hobbies and take part in family or social recreational activities, such as planting flowers and playing chess.

（4）Medication nursing. Decoction should be taken warm before meals, multiple times in small portions.

（5）Manipulation techniques. ① Moxibustion therapy: select Feishu (BL 13), Pishu (BL 20), Shenshu (BL 23), Sanyinjiao (SP 6), Zusanli (ST 36), and Guanyuan (CV 4); place the moxa stick 2~3 centimeters away from the skin to perform mild moxibustion on each of the acupoints until the area turns red and the patient feels warm and comfortable without the sensation of burning pain, once per day. And it is contraindicated on the abdomen and lumbosacral region for pregnant women. ② Foot bath therapy: decoct dangshen (codonopsis root), shenghuangqi (raw astragalus root), shengbaizhu (raw white atractylodes rhizome), fuling (poria), yiyiren (coix seed), duzhong (eucommia bark), niuxi (two-toothed achyranthes root), zexie (water plantain rhizome), and gancao (Licorice root); wash the feet with the decoction at 37~42℃ and massage, 20 minutes each time, once per day. And it should be used with caution for patients with hypotension. ③ Paste application therapy: select Shenshu (BL 23), Fuliu (KI 7), Zusanli (ST 36), Pishu (BL 20), and Qihai (CV 6); grind into powder the herbs that warm yang and replenish qi, blend the powder with shengjiang (fresh ginger) juice to make pastes, and apply the pastes on the acupoints for 2~6 hours, 2~3 acupoints each time, once per day.

6. Debilitation of Kidney Yang Syndrome

（1）Daily life nursing. The ward should be warm, sunward, quiet and comfortable. The sheet should be dry and tidy whereas the clothing should be loose and soft. The patients should rest in bed absolutely, stay in semi-supine position, have oxygen inhalation and keep themselves warm. They should also keep the skin clean, turn over regularly, pay attention to oral hygiene and gargle with warm water after meals. If smell of ammonia presents in the mouth, the patients should gargle with lemon water. When the condition is stabilized, do moderate physical exercise gently.

（2）Diet nursing. The patients should keep a salt-free and low protein diet and consume high-quality protein, such as milk, egg and lean meat. They may eat foods that warm yang and drain water, such as rougui（cinnamon bark）, Chinese chives, loach, chicken, heizhima（black sesame）, and heidou（black soybean）. Food therapy: chixiaodou donggua jiyu（adzuki bean, Chinese waxgourd, and crucian）soup. Don't eat pungent, spicy, raw, cold and greasy foods.

（3）Emotion nursing. Due to weakness and long course of disease, nurses may use verbal enlightenment therapy and submission therapy to know about patients' psychological conditions, encourage them to speak out the causes of anxiety and fear, and give thom effective psychological counselling to prevent them from seeking medical treatment and taking medicines randomly out of anxiety and tension, which could aggravate the condition.

（4）Medication nursing. Decoction should be brewed slowly over low heat and taken warm before meals.

（5）Manipulation techniques. ① Moxibustion therapy: select Qihai（CV 6）, Guanyuan（CV 4）, Yinlingquan（SP 9）, Sanyinjiao（SP 6）, Zusanli（ST 36）, Taixi（KI 3）, Shenshu（BL 23）and Pishu（BL 20）; place the moxa stick 2~3 centimeters away from the skin to perform mild moxibustion on each of them until the area turns red and the patient feels warm and comfortable without the sensation of burning pain, once per day. And it is contraindicated on the abdomen and lumbosacral region for pregnant women. ② Medicated ironing therapy: stir-fry wuzhuyu（medicinal evodia fruit）250 g and crude salt 50 g, and put them into a cloth bag to iron the lumbar region at a temperature of 60~70℃, 20 minutes each time, once per day. And it is contraindicated in pregnant women. ③ Paste application therapy: select Guanyuan（CV 4）; grind into powder fuzi（monkshood）, rougui（cinnamon bark）, and xixin（manchurian wild ginger）, blend the powder with shengjiang（fresh ginger）juice to make a paste, and apply it on the acupoint; or mash fuzi（monkshood）, ganjiang（dried ginger rhizome）, chuanxuduan（Himalayan teasel root）and scallions, and apply it on the acupoint; 2~4 hours each time, once or twice per day. ④ Enema therapy: decoct fuzi（monkshood）, roucongrong（desert cistanche）, duanmuli（calcined oyster shell）, and shengdahuang（raw rhubarb root and rhizome）, and apply the decoction for retention enema, twice per week. ⑤ Water acupuncture therapy: select Shenshu（BL 23）, Guanyuan（CV 4）, and Zusanli（ST 36）; inject Shenfu Injection to the acupoints. ⑥ Healthcare massage therapy: select Zusanli（ST 36）and Shenshu（BL 23）; apply thumb kneading manipulation for healthcare massage by the patients' themselves.

7. Syndrome of Mutual Binding of Stasis and Water

（1）Daily life nursing. The ward should be warm, quiet and comfortable, and away from wind. The patients should rest in bed, turn over regularly, and keep themselves warm. In case of blood urine, the patients must absolutely stay in bed. When the condition is stabilized, patients could take moderate exercise without overexertion. They should also maintain skin and oral hygiene with gentle actions to prevent bleeding.

（2）Diet nursing. The patients may eat foods that activate blood and remove stasis, such as black chicken, black fish, shanzha（Chinese hawthorn fruit）, xianggu（lentinus edodes）, heimuer（black fungus）, onion, laver, heidou（black soybean）, grapes, and peaches. Don't eat pungent, spicy, greasy, raw and cold foods.

(3) Emotion nursing. Due to the long course of disease or accompanying bleeding, the patients may have fear, anxiety and depression. Nurses may use verbal enlightenment therapy to inform patients that active treatment could ease their condition and explain the relationship between the disease and emotions, so that they maintain emotional stability and actively comply with treatment.

(4) Medication nursing. Decoction should be taken warm after meals.

(5) Manipulation techniques. ① Enema therapy: decoct chaoduzhong (stir-fried eucommia bark), roncongrong (desert cistanche), duanmuli (calcined oyster shell), shengdahuang (raw rhubarb root and rhizome), honghua (safflower), and danshen (danshen root); or decoct chaihu (bupleurum), danggui (Chinese angelica), shengdi (rehmannia root), chuanxiong (Sichuan lovage root), chishao (red peony root), niuxi (two-toothed achyranthes root), jiegen (platycodon root), zhiqiao (bitter orange), gancao (licorice root), and taoren (peach kernel); use the decoction for retention enema. ② Water acupuncture therapy: select Taixi (KI 3), Taichong (LR 3) and Xuehai (SP 10); inject Dengzhanxixin (fleabane) Injection or Shenfu Injection into the acupoints. ③ Foot bath therapy: decoct honghua (safflower), niuxi (two-toothed achyranthes root) and liujinu (artemisia); wash the feet with the decoction at a temperature of 37~42℃ and massage, 20 minutes each time, once per day. And it should be used with caution for patients with hypotension. ④ Acupressure therapy: select Sanyinjiao (SP 6), Yanglingquan (GB 34), Pishu (BL 20) and Taixi (KI 3); apply thumb kneading manipulation on each of them until the area turns hot or the patient has the feelings of soreness, numbness, distension and heaviness in the area, once per day. And it is contraindicated in pregnant women.

Patient Education

The room should be quiet, full of light and fresh air, and away from wind. The patients should rest in bed to get adequate sleep, pay attention to personal hygiene, often gargle the mouth, keep the skin clean and turn over regularly. When the condition is stabilized, patients could take moderate exercise without overexertion. They should prevent colds, avoid braving rain or wading in water, and value sexual abstinence.

The diet should be light, nutritious and digestible. The patients should have small frequent meals, and foods with high calories, high vitamin, low fat, and low purine. They may eat moderate amounts of high-quality animal protein and more fresh vegetables, take a low-salt or salt-free diet according to the severity of the edema, control water and protein intake, refrain from cigarette, alcohol, pickles, allergenic foods, foods that aggravate or induce diseases, and foods that are raw, cold, pungent and spicy. Patients should maintain emotional stability, understand the disease correctly, learn to self-regulate, slow down the pace of behaviors, eliminate psychological pressure, and avoid negative emotions such as anxiety, tension, depression, fear, and anger.

Patients should follow the doctor's advice in medication, be cautious to use antibiotics and analgesics, and avoid using nephrotoxic drugs, such as madouling (birthwort fruit), guanmutong (manchurian dutchmans pipe stem), mufangji (Southern fangji root), qingmuxiang (slender dutchmanspipe root) and yimucao (motherwort).

Patients should be checked regularly for routine urine test, liver function test and kidney function test. The primary disease should be treated actively, and repeatedly infected lesions should be treated timely.

第十三节　消　　渴

消渴，泛指因恣食肥甘，情志过极，房事不节，温热邪伤，滥服金石药物，导致胃热液涸，或因肺热化燥，心火偏盛，肾阴受灼，导致气化失常，津液精微不约而下泄，以多饮、多食、多尿为临床特征的一类疾病。西医的糖尿病等疾病可参照本节进行护理。

一、病因病机

消渴的病因包括饮食不节、禀赋不足、情志失调、房劳过度、过服温燥。病人嗜食醇酒与肥甘辛辣，积热伤津，脏腑经络失于濡养。先天不足，肾精亏虚，燥热内生。病人长期抑郁，焦虑紧张，劳心竭虑，营谋强思，郁火伤阴。或房室不节，肾精亏损，虚火内生。病人长期大量服用温燥壮阳药物，或久病误服温燥的药物，燥热内生，阴津亏损。以上病因皆可导致消渴。

消渴的病机为阴津亏损，燥热偏盛。病位在肺、胃（脾）、肾，以肾为本。消渴以阴虚为本，燥热为标，属于本虚标实、虚实夹杂之病。

二、常见证型

（一）辨证要点

1. **辨预后**　根据发病年龄、病程长短等来辨别。若发病年龄小，起病急，发展快，病情重，症状典型，多预后较差。若中年之后发病，起病缓，则病程长，症状不典型，则常有痈疽、肺痨，以及心、脑、肾、眼等处的并发症。

2. **辨标本虚实**　本病初起以燥热为主，继则燥热与阴虚并见，后期以阴虚或阴阳两虚为主。本病之虚，以阴虚为主，可兼见气虚、阳虚。本病之实，除燥热外，尚可见湿热、痰、瘀等。

3. **辨本症与并发症**　除"三多一少（多饮、多食、多尿和消瘦）"的本症外，消渴的并发症也很重要。多数病人先有本症，随病情发展再出现并发症。而少数中老年病人，本症不明显，却因并发症，如痈疽、眼疾、心脑血管疾病等前来就诊，从而发现消渴。

4. **辨病位**　根据症状特点等来辨别。若以多饮为主，为肺燥，多为上消。若以多食为主，为胃热，多为中消。若以多尿为主，为肾虚，多为下消。此三种情况往往相互并见。

（二）证候分型

1. 上消

肺热津伤证

[主要证候]口渴多饮，口舌干燥，尿频量多；烦热多汗；舌边尖红，苔薄黄，脉洪数。

[证候分析]肺为燥热所伤，无力敷布津液，津液直行膀胱排泄而出，故尿频量多；津液不能上

承,故口渴多饮,口舌干燥;壮火食气,燥热伤津耗气,故烦热多汗;烦热,舌边尖红,苔薄黄,脉洪数,均为燥热之象。

[护治原则] 清热润肺,生津止渴。

[常用方剂] 消渴方。

2. 中消

(1) 胃热炽盛证

[主要证候] 多食易饥,口渴,尿多,形体消瘦;大便干燥;苔黄,脉滑实有力。

[证候分析] 阳明热盛,津液被伤,故口渴;饮水虽多,但燥热伤肺,肺失治节,不能统摄敷布水液,津液自趋下泄,故尿多;胃热过盛,所食之物随火而化,故多食易饥;水谷精微损耗过多,故形体消瘦;热灼津液,故大便干燥;苔黄,脉滑实有力,均为内热之象。

[护治原则] 清胃泻火,养阴增液。

[常用方剂] 玉女煎。

(2) 气阴亏虚证

[主要证候] 口渴引饮,能食与便溏并见,或饮食减少,精神不振,四肢乏力,体瘦;舌质淡红,苔白而干,脉弱。

[证候分析] 消渴未止,脾胃反伤,燥热之邪未祛,故能食;脾失健运,谷气下泄,从大便出,故便溏;津液不能上输,故口渴引饮;脾胃失于健运,水谷不化精微,不得布散于周身,故精神不振,四肢乏力,体瘦;舌质淡红,苔白而干,脉弱,均为气阴亏虚之象。

[护治原则] 益气健脾,生津止渴。

[常用方剂] 七味白术散。

3. 下消

(1) 肾阴亏虚证

[主要证候] 尿频量多,混浊如脂膏,或尿甜,腰膝酸软;乏力,头晕耳鸣,口干唇燥,皮肤干燥,瘙痒;舌红苔少,脉细数。

[证候分析] 肾失固摄,水谷精微直趋膀胱,故尿频量多,混浊如脂膏,或尿甜;腰为肾之府,肾虚则腰膝酸软;精血亏虚,不能濡润清窍,故头晕耳鸣;津液不能上承,故口干唇燥;水谷精微不能濡养肌肤,故皮肤干燥,瘙痒;舌红苔少,脉细数均为阴虚之象。

[护治原则] 滋阴固肾。

[常用方剂] 六味地黄丸。

(2) 阴阳两虚证

[主要证候] 小便频数,混浊如膏,甚至饮一溲一;面容憔悴,耳轮干枯,腰膝酸软,四肢欠温,畏寒肢冷,阳痿或月经不调;舌苔淡白而干,脉沉细无力。

[证候分析] 阴损及阳,肾阳失于气化,精微与水液下注,故小便频数,混浊如膏,饮一溲一;肾开窍于耳,腰为肾之府,阴虚则面容憔悴,耳轮干枯,腰膝酸软;阳虚无力温煦,故四肢欠温,畏寒肢冷,阳痿或月经不调;舌苔淡白而干,脉沉细无力,均为阴阳两虚之象。

[护治原则] 滋阴温阳,补肾固涩。

[常用方剂] 金匮肾气丸。

三、护理措施

对于消渴的病人，应观察排尿次数、尿量、尿色的变化。注意观察基础生命体征、神志、体重、饮水量、食量、皮肤、大便和舌脉。定期测量并记录血糖、尿糖、尿酮体、视力等。若病人出现心慌头晕，汗出过多，脸色苍白，饥饿，软弱无力，视力模糊，应立即口服糖水或果汁。若病人出现烦躁不安，头痛头昏，恶心呕吐，甚至呼气有烂苹果味；或病人出现神志昏愦，四肢冰凉，血压下降，脉微欲绝，应立即报告医生，并配合抢救。

（一）辨证施护

1. 肺热津伤证

（1）生活起居护理　居室凉爽安静。起居有常，不可熬夜。适量运动，如打太极拳、气功锻炼，从饭后 1 小时开始，持续半小时，以不疲劳为度。

（2）饮食护理　控制饮水量，可饮生白萝卜汁、鲜芦根茶、鲜藕汁、荸荠汁、乌梅茶或铁皮石斛茶。宜食清热生津的食物，如燕窝、鸽肉、黄瓜、苦瓜、菠菜、西葫芦、番茄、枸杞子、百合、兔肉、葛根。食疗方：萝卜煲鲍鱼。多吃新鲜蔬菜，以保持大便通畅。戒烟限酒，不宜食辛辣的食物。

（3）情志护理　护士可运用语言开导疗法，向病人宣传关于消渴的知识，消除其忧虑、恐惧的情绪，使病人积极配合治疗。

（4）用药护理　中药汤剂宜饭后温服，中西药之间间隔30分钟以上。

（5）操作技术　① 穴位按摩法：取肺俞、肾俞、肝俞、三阴交、足三里，用拇指揉法，按摩至局部发热或有酸麻重胀感，每日 1 次；孕妇禁用。② 耳压疗法：取皮质下、内分泌、脾、胰胆、三焦等耳穴，用耳穴压丸贴片贴压，每日按揉 4~5 次，以局部发热泛红为度，留置 2~4 日；孕妇禁用。

2. 胃热炽盛证

（1）生活起居护理　居室凉爽安静。起居有常，不可熬夜。鞋袜不宜过紧。做好口腔护理，饭前、饭后、睡前用黄芩水漱口。保持皮肤清洁，定期洗头、洗澡。保持会阴部清洁，若会阴部搔痒，可用苦参煎汤外洗。保持大便通畅。适量运动，如打太极拳、练习气功，以不疲劳为度。

（2）饮食护理　少食多餐，多吃蔬菜，防止暴饮暴食。控制主食量，每日 250~400 g，可食南瓜、燕麦、荞麦、玉米。可饮山药汁、铁皮石斛茶。可用黄瓜、番茄代替水果。宜食清胃养阴的食物，如白萝卜、猪胰、茭白、洋葱、苦瓜、鸡毛菜、白菜、山药、冬瓜、豆类、菠菜。可多吃牛奶、鸡蛋、兔肉、鱼、鸡肉、牛肉。食疗方：芡实莲子瘦肉汤。戒烟限酒，不宜食含糖多的食物，如蜂蜜、藕粉、过甜的水果。不宜食辛辣、油腻、易产气的食物，如红薯。

（3）情志护理　若病人过早出现饥饿，护士可运用移情易性疗法，转移病人的注意力，同时可配合食用少量蔬菜。

（4）用药护理　中药汤剂宜饭后温服。

（5）操作技术　① 穴位按摩法：取肺俞、脾俞、胃脘下俞、膈俞、中脘、足三里、鱼际、太渊、心俞，用拇指揉法，按摩至局部发热或有酸麻重胀感，每日 1 次；孕妇禁用。② 耳压疗法：取皮质下、内分泌、胰胆、脾、交感，用耳穴压丸贴片贴压，每日按揉 4~5 次，以局部发热泛红为度，留置 2~4 日；孕妇禁用。③ 吹药疗法：用锡类散吹至局部；适用于口腔糜烂者。

3. 气阴两虚证

（1）生活起居护理 居室安静舒适，空气新鲜，光线柔和，避免阳光直射。睡眠充足，衣着宽松，注意肢端保暖，避免被热水袋烫伤。进餐1小时后开始适量运动，如散步、做家务，以保证大便通畅。保持皮肤和会阴部的清洁，每日检查双脚的皮肤。定期检查视力和眼底，避免用眼过度。不可熬夜、过劳、食后即卧、终日久坐。

（2）饮食护理 可饮黄精茶、大枣乌梅汤。宜食益气养阴的食物，如枸杞子、茯苓、酸枣、黑木耳、银耳、蛋类、鱼、乌鸡、鸽肉。食疗方：兔肉煲山药、蘑菇瘦肉汤。不宜食辛辣、生冷、油腻的食物。

（3）情志护理 病人体虚久病，护士可组织病人互相交流，请治疗效果较好的病人介绍经验，以提高病人对于治疗的信心。

（4）用药护理 石膏先煎。中药汤剂宜饭后温服，少量频服。

（5）操作技术 ① 敷贴疗法：取肾俞、天枢、足三里，用生黄芪、丹参、酒大黄、紫苏叶、川芎、积雪草、淫羊藿、白芷，研磨成粉后与醋调成糊状敷贴。② 穴位按摩法：取肺俞、脾俞、胃脘下俞、膈俞、足三里、内庭、三阴交、胃俞、中脘，用拇指揉法、一指禅推法，按摩至局部发热或有酸麻重胀感，每日1次；孕妇禁用。

4. 肾阴亏虚证

（1）生活起居护理 居室安静整洁，光线柔和，避免阳光直射与强风直吹。卧床休息，床单干燥柔软，注意肢端保暖。每日检查口腔和全身皮肤，定时翻身。饭后用金银花甘草液漱口。每日用温水清洁会阴部。勤剪指甲，不可搔抓损伤皮肤。病人应常闭目养神，定期检查视力和眼底。进餐1小时后适量运动，如散步。保持大便通畅，排便时不可过于用力。节制性行为，不可熬夜与过劳。

（2）饮食护理 不可随意加餐或吃零食，睡前少饮水。宜食滋阴降火的食物，如猪脊髓、猪肾、桑椹、黑芝麻、鳖肉、鸭肉、百合、银耳、茼蒿。食疗方：枸杞蒸鸡、山药莲子粥。不宜食辛辣、燥烈的食物。

（3）情志护理 病人体虚久病，容易出现急躁、悲观的情绪，护士可运用语言开导疗法，关心和理解病人，使病人感到温暖和愉快。若病人情绪郁怒，可运用以情胜情疗法，调节病人的情绪。

（4）用药护理 石膏先煎，中药汤剂宜饭后温服，少量频服。

（5）操作技术 ① 穴位按摩法：取肺俞、脾俞、胃脘下俞、膈俞、足三里、内庭、三阴交、胃俞、中脘、气海、关元、涌泉，用拇指揉法、一指禅推法，按摩至局部发热或有酸麻重胀感，每日1次；孕妇禁用。② 耳压疗法：取皮质下、内分泌、肾、胰胆等耳穴，用耳穴压豆胶布贴压，每日按揉4~5次，以局部发热泛红为度，留置2~4日；孕妇禁用。③ 敷贴疗法：取涌泉，用吴茱萸、肉桂，研磨成粉后与米醋调成糊状敷贴，每晚1次，次日早晨取下；适用于失眠者。

5. 阴阳两虚证

（1）生活起居护理 居室温暖安静，整洁避风。卧床休息，睡眠充足。注意肢端保暖，衣物鞋袜应宽大。做好皮肤护理，保持床铺清洁干燥，定时帮病人翻身，每日用红花乙醇溶液按摩受压部位，检查双脚皮肤。保持会阴部清洁，勤换内裤。保持口腔清洁，选用软毛牙刷，刷牙动作要轻，饭后用金银花甘草液漱口。进餐1小时后适量运动，如散步，以保持大便通畅。防止跌仆，节制性行为，不可过劳。

（2）饮食护理 宜食滋阴温阳的食物，如猪胰、山药、芡实、生姜、羊肉、狗肉、羊肉、鹿肉、牛肉、猪肾、黑豆、黑芝麻。食疗方:韭菜炒虾仁、清炖枸杞鸽、香菇木耳汤。不宜食辛辣、生冷、油腻的食物。

(3)情志护理　护士可用移情易性疗法,指导病人培养兴趣爱好,如听音乐、听相声、练书法、养鸟、栽培花草,以保持心情愉快,情绪稳定。或用语言开导疗法,告诉病人本病需长期坚持治疗,遇事勿恼怒烦忧,可闭目静坐,全身放松,平静呼吸。或用顺意疗法,鼓励病人表达心中疾苦,耐心倾听,对病人进行心理疏导。

(4)用药护理　附子、龟甲先煎。中药汤剂宜文火久煎、浓煎,饭后温服。

(5)操作技术　①足浴疗法:用温补肾阳的中药煎汤,待水温降至37~42℃时洗按足部,每次20分钟,每日1次;适用于肢冷者,禁用于皮肤破溃者,血压过低者慎用。②穴位按摩法:取肺俞、脾俞、胃脘下俞、膈俞、足三里、太溪、太冲、肝俞、肾俞、关元、太阳、睛明、四白、丝竹空,用拇指揉法,按摩至局部发热或有酸麻重胀感,每日1次;孕妇禁用。③气功锻炼:练习八段锦中的"两手攀足固肾腰"。

(二)健康教育

终身遵医嘱用药。定期到内分泌科、眼科、心脑血管科、营养科等科室复查。护士应向病人及家属介绍血糖、尿糖的自测方法。

起居有常,劳逸适度。鞋袜柔软、宽大、透气。注意肢端保暖。保护视力。保持皮肤清洁干燥,注意口腔、足部的卫生。根据个人情况选择适合的运动,如八段锦、易筋经、五禽戏。运动时以周身发热、微微出汗为宜,不可大汗淋漓或剧烈运动。外出时随身携带急救信息卡、糖果、饼干。节制性行为,不可熬夜及过劳。

饮食有节,少食多餐,定时定量。控制饮水量和进食量,避免过饥、过饱。清淡饮食,以高维生素、低糖、低盐、低脂、低胆固醇为原则,主食为全谷杂粮,副食为蛋、奶、豆制品、含糖少的蔬菜,肉类为乌鸡、鳖肉、兔肉等。戒烟限酒,少吃面食,不宜食含糖高的水果、饮料,以及辛辣、油腻、煎炸、肥甘的食物。

心情舒畅,安心静养,勿恼怒、忧思、抑郁、惊恐。

Section 13　Wasting-Thirst

Wasting-thirst is a disease clinically characterized by polydipsia, polyphagia and polyuria. It is caused by stomach heat and fluid dry-up due to excessive consumption of fatty sweet foods, emotional disturbance, sexual indulgence, pathogenic warm-heat injury, or abuse of metallic or mineral medicine, and by failure of qi transformation and downward flowing of fluids and nutritious essence due to lung-heat transforming into dryness, heart-fire exuberance or heat scorching kidney yin. This section can be referred to for the nursing of diabetes mellitus in Western medicine.

ETIOLOGY AND PATHOGENESIS

The etiology includes improper diet, constitutional insufficiency, emotional disorders, sexual strain and excessive intake of warm or dry-natured foods or medicines. Predilection for alcohol and fatty, too-sweet, pungent and spicy foods leading to accumulation of heat and damages fluids, and consequently makes zang-fu organs and meridians deprived of nourishment. Congenital insufficiency with kidney essence depletion produces internal dryness-heat. Long-term depression, anxiety and nervousness, and over-contemplation generates depressed fire that damages yin. Sexual indulgence consumes kidney essence and causes internal deficiency fire. Long-term overdose of medicines that invigorate yang or misusing warm or dry-natured medicines for chronic illness generates internal dryness-heat that consumes yin fluids. All above causes may lead to wasting-thirst.

The pathogenesis is depletion of yin fluids and exuberance of dryness-heat. The disease is located in the lung, stomach (spleen) and kidney, of which the kidney is primary location. For wasting-thirst, yin deficiency is the root while dryness-heat is the tip. It belongs to the syndrome of root deficiency and tip excess, and is a disease of deficiency-excess in complexity.

COMMON SYNDROMES

Key Points in Syndrome Differentiation

1. Differentiation of Prognosis

The differentiation is based on the age of onset and course of disease. Young patients with urgent onset, rapid development, serious condition and typical symptoms have worse prognosis. Middle-aged and elderly patients with slow onset, long course and atypical symptoms often have carbuncle, lung abscess, and complications of the heart, brain, kidney and eyes.

2. Differentiation of Root from Tip as well as Deficiency from Excess

At the initial stage of the disease, the primary clinical manifestation is dryness-heat, and then is coexistence of both dryness-heat and yin deficiency. However, at the late stage, the clinical manifestations is mostly yin deficiency or dual deficiency of yin and yang. Deficiency nature of wasting-thirst mainly refers to yin deficiency, though possibly accompanied with qi deficiency and yang deficiency. On the other hand, excess nature of the disease is probably dampness-heat, phlegm and blood stasis, besides dryness-heat.

3. Differentiation of Fundamental Symptoms and Complications

Except the fundamental symptoms of polydipsia, polyphagia, polyuria and emaciation, the complications of wasting-thirst also deserve special attention. For most patients, the fundamental symptoms first appear and complications follow with the development of the disease. However, for a few middle-aged and elderly patients without obvious fundamental symptoms, they are diagnosed with the disease when they come to see a doctor for complications, such as carbuncle, eye disease, and cardiovascular and cerebrovascular diseases.

4. Differentiation of Disease Location

The differentiation is based on symptom characteristics. Upper wasting-thirst is mainly characterized by lung dryness with polydipsia; middle one, stomach heat with polyphagia; and lower one, kidney deficiency with polyuria. These three conditions usually exist together.

Syndrome Differentiation

1. Upper Wasting-Thirst

Lung Heat Damaging Fluids Syndrome

[Clinical Manifestations] Thirst, polydipsia, dry mouth and tongue, polyuria, vexing heat, profuse sweating, red tip and margins of the tongue, thin yellow tongue coating, and surging rapid pulse.

[Manifestations Analysis] The lung damaged by dryness-heat can't transmit fluids, which subsequently induces downward flowing of fluids to the bladder, so there is polyuria. The fluids fail to be distributed upwards, so thirst, polydipsia, and dry mouth and tongue are felt. Vigorous fire consumes qi and dryness-heat damages both fluids and qi, so vexing heat and profuse sweating occur. Vexing heat, red tip and margins of the tongue, thin yellow coating and surging rapid pulse are signs of dryness-heat.

[Nursing Principle] Clearing heat and moistening the lung; promoting fluid production to quench thirst.

[Suggested Formula] Xiaoke Formula.

2. Middle Wasting-Thirst

（1）Stomach Heat Exuberance Syndrome

[Clinical Manifestations] Polyphagia with easy hunger, thirst, polyuria, emaciation, dry stool, yellow tongue coating, and slippery, replete and forceful pulse.

[Manifestations Analysis] Heat exuberance in yangming meridian damages fluids, so thirst is felt.

In spite of polyphagia, dryness-heat damaging the lung makes failure of the lung to govern management and regulation, which subsequently induces downward flowing of fluids, then polyuria occurs. Effulgent stomach fire digests the foodstuff quickly, causing polyphagia with easy hunger. Excessive consumption of essence of grain and water causes emaciation. Heat scorching fluids leads to dry stool. Yellow tongue coating and slippery, replete and forceful pulse are signs of internal heat.

[Nursing Principle] Clearing the stomach and reducing fire; nourishing yin and supplementing fluid.

[Suggested Formula] Yunü Decoction.

(2) Deficiency of Qi and Yin Syndrome

[Clinical Manifestations] Thirst with taking of fluids, coexistence of polyphagia and loose stool, or reduced appetite, dispiritedness, lack of strength of extremities, emaciation, pale red tongue with white dry coating, and weak pulse.

[Manifestations Analysis] Persistent wasting-thirst, spleen-stomach damage and lingering dryness-heat work together to cause polyphagia. Dysfunction of the spleen in transportation and transformation causes downward of food qi and loose stool. Failure of fluids to be distributed upwards causes thirst with taking of fluids. The spleen and stomach cannot transform water and grain into nutrient essence and distribute it to the whole body, leading to dispiritedness, lack of strength of extremities and emaciation. Pale red tongue with white dry coating and weak pulse are signs of deficiency of qi and yin.

[Nursing Principle] Replenishing qi and invigorating the spleen; promoting fluid production to quench thirst.

[Suggested Formula] Qiwei Baizhu Power.

3. Lower Wasting-Thirst

(1) Kidney Yin Deficiency Syndrome

[Clinical Manifestations] Polyuria, turbid paste-like urine or sweet urine, soreness and weakness of waist and knees, lack of strength, dizziness, tinnitus, dry mouth and lips, dry itching skin, red tongue with sparse coating, and thready rapid pulse.

[Manifestations Analysis] Failure of the kidney in securing and containing causes nutritious essence of water and grain to directly reach the bladder, resulting in polyuria and turbid paste-like urine or sweet urine. Lumbus is the house of the kidney, therefore, kidney deficiency may cause soreness and weakness of waist and knees. Deficiency of essence and blood can't nourish clear orifices, so dizziness and tinnitus are felt. Failure of fluids to be distributed upwards causes dry mouth and lips. Nutritious essence of water and grain cannot nourish the skin, causing dry itching skin. Red tongue with sparse coating and thready rapid pulse suggest yin deficiency.

[Nursing Principle] Nourishing yin and securing the kidney.

[Suggested Formula] Liuwei Dihuang Pills.

(2) Syndrome of Dual Deficiency of Yin and Yang

[Clinical Manifestations] Polyuria, turbid paste-like urine with profuse volume, haggard look, withering ear helices, soreness and weakness of waist and knees, cold extremities, aversion to cold, impotence or irregular menstruation, dry pale-white tongue coating, and sunken, thready and forceless pulse.

〔Manifestations Analysis〕Yin impairment affecting yang causes dysfunction of kidney yang in qi transformation and downward flow of nutritious essence and fluids, causing polyuria, turbid paste-like urine with profuse volume. Kidney opens into ears and lumbus is the house of the kidney, therefore, yin deficiency induces haggard look, withering ear helices as well as soreness and weakness of waist and knees. Yang deficiency cannot warm the body, leading to cold extremities, aversion to cold, impotence or irregular menstruation. Dry pale-white tongue coating and sunken, thready and forceless pulse demonstrate dual deficiency of yin and yang.

〔Nursing Principle〕Nourishing yin and warming yang; tonifying the kidney and consolidating essence.

〔Suggested Formula〕Jingui Shenqi Pills.

NURSING MEASURES

For patients with wasting-thirst, nurses should observe the urination frequency, the volume and color of urine, basic vital signs, consciousness, weight, water intake, food intake, skin, stool, tongue and pulse. The nurses should also regularly measure and record blood sugar, urine sugar, urine ketone body, vision, etc. If the patient has flusteredness, dizziness, excessive sweating, pale complexion, hunger, weakness, blurred vision, drink sugar water or fruit juice immediately. If the patient has fidgetiness, headache, dizziness, nausea and vomiting, and even breath with rotten apple smell; or coma, cold limbs, decreased blood pressure and faint pulse verging on expiry, it is advisable to report to the doctor immediately and assist in emergency treatment.

Syndrome-Based Nursing Measures

1. Lung Heat Damaging Fluids Syndrome

（1）Daily life nursing. The ward should be cool and quiet. The patients should live a regular life without staying up late, and take moderate half-an-hour exercise one hour after meals, such as Taiji and Qigong.

（2）Diet nursing. The patients should control water intake, and can take raw white radish juice, xianlugen（fresh reed rhizome）tea, fresh lotus root juice, biqi（waternut）juice, wumei（smoked plum）tea or tiepishihu（dendrobium officinale）tea. They may eat foods that clear heat and promote fluid production, such as yanwo（edible bird's nest）, pigeon meat, cucumber, bitter gourd, spinach, zucchini, tomato, gouqizi（Chinese wolfberry fruit）, baihe（lily bulb）, rabbit meat, and gegen（kudzuvine root）. Food therapy: luobo stewed with baoyu（white radish stewed with abalone）. The patients should eat more fresh vegetables to keep a normal bowel movement, and refrain from cigarette, alcohol, and foods that are pungent and spicy.

（3）Emotion nursing. Nurses may use verbal enlightenment therapy to inform patients about wasting-thirst to remove their worries and fears and encourage them to actively comply with treatment.

（4）Medication nursing. Decoction should be taken warm after meals. The interval between taking Chinese and Western medicine should exceed 30 minutes.

（5）Manipulation techniques. ① Acupressure therapy：select Feishu（BL 13）, Shenshu（BL 23）, Ganshu（BL 18）, Sanyinjiao（SP 6）and Zushanli（ST 36）; apply thumb kneading manipulation on each of the acupoints until the area turns hot or the patient has the feelings of soreness, numbness, distension and heaviness in the area; once per day. And it is contraindicated in pregnant women. ② Auricular pressure therapy：select subcortex（AT4）, endocrine（CO18）, spleen（CO13）, pancreas and gallbladder（CO11）, and triple energizer（CO17）; apply specialized pasters on the points, press on each of them till the area turns hot and red, 4~5 times per day, and keep the pasters for 2~4 days. And it is contraindicated in pregnancy.

2. Stomach Heat Exuberance Syndrome

（1）Daily life nursing. The ward should be cool and quiet. The patients should live a regular life without staying up late, wear loose shoes and socks, pay attention to oral care, and gargle with huangqin（scutellaria root）liquid before and after meals as well as before sleep. They should also keep the skin clean, wash the hair and take shower regularly, and keep the perineal region clean. If the perineal region itches, kushen（light yellow sophora root）decoction can be used to wash the area externally. The patients should take moderate exercise to keep a normal bowel movement, such as Taiji and Qigong.

（2）Diet nursing. The patients should have small frequent meals without craputence, take more vegetables, and limit the daily staple foods to 300~400 g, like pumpkin, oats, buckwheat, and corn. Shanyao（common yam rhizome）juice and tiepishihu（dendrobium officinale）tea are recommended. Cucumbers and tomatoes could be consumed instead of fruit. They may have more milk, eggs, rabbit meat, fish, chicken, beef and foods that clear stomach heat and nourish yin, such as white radish, tomatoes, pig pancreas, water bamboo, onion, bitter gourd, Chinese little greens, Chinese cabbage, shanyao（common yam rhizome）, Chinese waxgourd, beans and spinach. Food therapy：qianshi lianzi shourou（euryale seed, lotus seed, and lean pork）soup. The patients should refrain from cigarette, alcohol, sugary foods（such as honey, lotus root powder, and sweet fruit）as well as pungent, spicy, greasy and flatulent foods, such as sweet potatoes.

（3）Emotion nursing. For patients with early hunger pangs, nurses may use emotional transference and dispositional change therapy to divert their attention and let them eat some vegetables.

（4）Medication nursing. Decoction should be taken warm after meals.

（5）Manipulation techniques. ① Acupressure therapy：select Feishu（BL 13）, Pishu（BL 20）, Weiwanxiashu（EX－B3）, Geshu（BL 18）, Zhongwan（CV 12）, Zushanli（ST 36）, Yuji（LU 10）, Taiyuan（LU 9）and Xinshu（BL 15）; apply thumb kneading manipulation on each of the acupoints until the area turns hot or the patient has the feelings of soreness, numbness, distension and heaviness in the area; once per day. And it is contraindicated in pregnancy. ② Auricular pressure therapy：select subcortex（AT4）, endocrine（CO18）, pancreas and gallbladder（CO11）, spleen（CO13）and sympathetic（AH6a）; apply specialized pasters on the points, press on each of them till the area turns hot and red, 4~5 times per day, and keep the pasters for 2~4 days. And it is contraindicated in pregnant women. ③ Insufflation therapy: insufflate Xilei Powder into the affected area; it is appropriate for patients with oral erosion.

3. Deficiency of Qi and Yin Syndrome

（1）Daily life nursing. The ward should be warm, quiet, full of fresh air and gentle light. The patients should get adequate sleep, wear loose clothes, keep extremities warm without being burnt by hot-water bag, and take moderate half-an-hour exercise one hour after meals, such as walking and doing housework to keep a normal bowel movement. They should also keep the skin and perineal region clean, check foot skin every day, and have regular eyesight and ocular fundus examinations. Moreover, they should avoid over-use of eyes, staying up late, overstrain, lying down immediately after eating or sitting still all day long.

（2）Diet nursing. Huangjing（rhizoma polygonati）tea, or dazao wumei（Chinese date and smoked plum）soup is recommended. The patients may eat foods that replenish qi and nourish yin, such as gouqizi（Chinese wolfberry fruit）, fuling（poria）, wild jujube, heimuer（black fungus）, yin'er（tremella）, eggs, fish, black chicken and pigeon meat. Food therapy: rabbit meat stewed with shanyao（common yam rhizome）, and lean meat soup with mushroom. Don't eat pungent, spicy, raw, cold and greasy foods.

（3）Emotion nursing. Given patients' weak constitution and long course of disease, nurses may organize patients to communicate with each other, and ask those who have good curative effect to share experience to boost others' confidence in treatment.

（4）Medication nursing. Shigao（gypsum）should be decocted first. Decoction should be taken warm after meals, multiple times in small portions.

（5）Manipulation techniques. ① Paste application therapy: select Shenshu（BL 23）, Tianshu（ST 25）, and Zusanli（ST 36）; grind into powder shenghuangqi（raw astragalus root）, danshen（danshen root）, jiudahuang（yellow wine prepared rhubarb root and rhizome）, zisuye（perilla leaf）, chuanxiong（Sichuan lovage root）, jixuecao（asiatic pennywort）, yinyanghuo（aerial part of epimedium）, and baizhi（angelica root）; blend the powder with vinegar to make pastes, and apply the pastes on the acupoints. ② Acupressure therapy: select Feishu（BL 13）, Pishu（BL 20）, Weiwanxiashu（EX - B3）, Geshu（BL 18）, Zushanli（ST 36）, Neiting（ST 44）, Sanyinjiao（SP 6）, Weishu（BL 21）and Zhongwan（CV 12）; apply thumb kneading and one-finger pushing manipulations on each of the acupoints until the area turns hot or the patient has the feelings of soreness, numbness, distension and heaviness in the area, once per day. And it is contraindicated in pregnant women.

4. Kidney Yin Deficiency Syndrome

（1）Daily life nursing. The ward should be quiet, tidy, full of gentle light, and without direct sunlight or strong wind. The sheet should be dry and soft. The patients should rest in bed, keep extremities warm, check oral cavity and body skin every day, turn over regularly, and rinse the mouth with jinyinhua gancao (honeysuckle flower and licorice root) liquid after meals. Patients should also clean the perineal region with warm water everyday, trim the nails frequently to avoid scratching the skin, close their eyes often to refresh themselves, and have regular eyesight and ocular fundus examinations. Moreover, they should take moderate exercise one hour after meals, such as walking, to keep a normal bowel movement, and avoid sexual indulgence, staying up late and overstain.

(2) Diet nursing. The patients should not eat extra meals or snacks, drink less water before sleep, and may eat foods that nourish yin and reduce fire, such as pig bone marrow, pig kidneys, sangshen (mulberry), heizhima (black sesame), meat of soft-shelled turtles, duck meat, baihe (lily bulb), yin'er (tremella) and garland chrysanthemum. Food therapy: chicken steamed with gouqi (Chinese wolfberry fruit), shanyao lianzi (common yam rhizome and lotus seed) porridge. Don't eat pungent, spicy, and dry-natured foods.

(3) Emotion nursing. Due to patients' weak constitution and long course of disease, they are prone to irritability and pessimism. Nurses may use verbal enlightenment therapy to care for and appreciate the patients. For patients with depression and anger, nurses may use the therapy of emotion predominating over emotion to adjusted their mood.

(4) Medication nursing. Shigao (gypsum) should be decocted first. Decoction should be taken warm before meals, multiple times in small portions.

(5) Manipulation techniques. ① Acupressure therapy: select Feishu (BL 13), Pishu (BL 20), Weiwanxiashu (EX−B3), Geshu (BL 18), Zushanli (ST 36), Neiting (ST 44), Sanyinjiao (SP 6), Weishu (BL 21), Zhongwan (CV 12), Qihai (CV 6), Guanyuan (CV 4) and Yongquan (KI 1); apply thumb kneading and one-finger pushing manipulations on each of the acupoints until the area turns hot or the patient has the feelings of soreness, numbness, distension and heaviness in the area; once per day. And it is contraindicated in pregnant women. ② Auricular pressure therapy: select subcortex (AT4), endocrine (CO18), kidney (CO10), and pancreas and gallbladder (CO11); apply specialized pasters on the points, press on each of them till the area turns hot and red, 4~5 times per day, and keep the pasters for 2~4 days. And it is contraindicated in pregnant women. ③ Paste application therapy: select Yongquan (KI 1); grind into powder wuzhuyu (medicinal evodia fruit) and rougui (cinnamon bark); blend the powder with rice vinegar to make pastes, and apply the pastes on the acupoint, once every night, and remove it on the next morning. It is suitable for patients with insomnia.

5. Syndrome of Dual Deficiency of Yin and Yang

(1) Daily life nursing. The ward should be warm, quiet, tidy, and away from wind. Nurses should keep the sheet clean and dry, take care of patients's skin, help them to turn over regularly, massage the compressed area with honghua (safflower) ethanol solution daily, and examine the skin of the feet. The patients should rest in bed to get adequate sleep, keep extremities warm, wear loose-fitting clother, shoes and socks. They should keep the perineal region clean, change underwear frequently, maintain oral hygiene, use a soft-bristled toothbrush to brush teeth gently, and rinse the mouth with jinyinhua gancao

（honeysuckle flower and licorice root）liquid after meals. They should also take moderate exercise one hour after meals, such as walking, to keep a normal bowel movement, value sexual abstinence, and avoid falls and overstrain.

（2）Diet nursing. The patients may eat foods that nourish yin and warm yang, such as pig pancreas, shanyao（common yam rhizome）, qianshi（euryale seed）, shengjiang（fresh ginger）, mutton, dog meat, vension, beef, pig kidneys, heidou（black soybean）and heizhima（black sesame）. Food therapy: Chinese chives fried with shelled shrimps, pigeon stewed with gouqi（Chinese wolfberry fruit）, xianggu muer（lentinus edodes and wood ear）soup. Don't eat pungent, spicy, raw, cold and greasy foods.

（3）Emotion nursing. Nurses may use emotional transference and dispositional change therapy to guide patients to cultivate hobbies such as listening to music or crosstalk, practising calligraphy, raising birds, planting flowers and plants, in order to stay cheerful. Nurses may also use verbal enlightenment therapy to inform patients that their disease needs long-term treatment, and that when something troublesome comes, they may sit quietly with their eyes closed, relax their whole body, and breathe calmly rather than get angry or upset. Still, nurses may use submission therapy to encourage patients to express their sufferings, listen to them patiently and provide psychological counseling for them.

（4）Medication nursing. Fuzi（monkshood）and guijia（tortoise shell）should be decocted first. Decoction should be concentrated slowly over low heat and taken warm before meals.

（5）Manipulation techniques. ① Foot bath therapy: decoct herbs that warm yang and tonify the kidney; wash the feet with the decoction at a temperature of $37 \sim 42℃$, 20 minutes each time, once per day. It is appropriate for patients with cold extremities and is contraindicated for patients with skin ulceration. And it should be used with caution for patients with hypotension. ② Acupressure therapy: select Feishu（BL 13）, Pishu（BL 20）, Weiwanxiashu（EX－B 3）, Geshu（BL 18）, Zushanli（ST 36）, Taixi（KI 3）, Taichong（LR 3）, Ganshu（BL 18）, Shenshu（BL 23）, Guanyuan（CV 4）, Taiyang（EX－HN5）, Jingming（BL 1）, Sibai（ST 2）, Sizhukong（TE 23）; apply thumb kneading manipulation on each of the acupoints until the area turns hot or the patient has the feelings of soreness, numbness, distension and heaviness in the area, once per day. And it is contraindicated in pregnant women. ③ Qigong therapy: practise the exercise of "moving the hands down and touching the feet to strengthen the kidney and waist" in Baduanjin.

Patient Education

Patients should follow the doctor's advice in medication for life, regularly recheck themselves in endocrinology, ophthalmology, cardiovascular and cerebrovascular, and nutrition departments. Nurses should inform the patients and their family about methods of testing blood sugar and urine sugar by themselves.

The patients should follow a regular daily routine, balance work and rest, wear soft, loose, and air-permeable shoes and socks. They should also keep extremities warm, protect their eyesight, keep the skin clean and dry, pay attention to the hygiene of the mouth and feet, and choose the appropriate exercise according to individual constitution, such as Baduanjin (eight-sectioned exercise), Yijinjing (muscle-bone strengthening exercise) and Wuqinxi (five-animal exercise). When exercising, perspire slightly with mild warm sensation of the whole body rather than sweat profusely or exercise vigorously. When going out, carry first-aid information card, candy and biscuits with themselves. Moreover, they should value sexual abstinence and avoid staying up late and overstrain.

The diet should be light, with high vitamins, low sugar, low salt, low fat, and low cholesterol as the norm, whole grain cereals as the staple food, eggs, milk, soy products, and vegetables with less sugar as the non-staple food, and black chicken, meat of soft-shelled turtles, and rabbit meat as the meat food. The patients should have a moderate diet in multiple small meals and regular dietary schedule and amount, and control the intake amount of water and food. They should eat less cooked wheaten food, and refrain from cigarette, alcohol, fruit and drinks high in sugar, or foods that are pungent, spicy, greasy, fried, fatty and sweet.

The patients should stay in a peaceful state of mind and set aside their anger, distress, depression or panic to have a rest cure.

第二章
外科病证的中医护理

据《周礼》记载,在周代时出现了主治肿疡、溃疡、金创和折疡的外科医生:疡医。《五十二病方》记载了痔瘘、皮肤病等外科疾病。在《黄帝内经》中,有针砭、按摩等多种外科疗法和猪膏等外用药物。东汉末年,华佗发明麻沸散,进行全身麻醉剂和开腹手术。《刘涓子鬼遗方》(公元499年)是我国现存第一部中医外科学专著。隋代《诸病源候论》记载了外科手术疗法和40多种皮肤病。唐代,孙思邈著《备急千金要方》,首创葱管导尿术。后世,中医外科学发展壮大,形成了不同的学术流派。

现代中医外科学的范围包括疮疡、瘿、瘤、岩、皮肤、乳房、肛肠、男性前阴、周围血管及其他外伤性疾病,还包括内痈、急腹症、疝、泌尿生殖疾病和性传播疾病等。外科疾病一般根据其发病部位、病因、形态、颜色、疾病特征等进行命名。

外科疾病的常见病因有六淫邪气、特殊之毒、外来伤害、情志失调、饮食不节、劳伤虚损和痰饮、瘀血、脓毒。在六淫中,风邪走注甚速,多发于人体上部。寒邪易侵袭筋骨关节,患处皮色紫、青、暗,痛有定处。暑邪致病,患处焮红肿胀。湿邪侵袭皮肤,可发为丘疹、水疱,破后滋水淋漓不尽,瘙痒。燥邪致病,患处干燥、枯槁、皲裂脱屑。火邪来势猛急,患处焮红灼热,肿痛剧烈,易化脓腐烂。虫毒、蛇毒、狂犬毒、漆毒、药毒、食物毒和疫疠之毒侵袭人体,可因禀赋不耐或机体不胜克防而发病。意外跌仆、沸水、火焰、寒冷,均可使局部气血凝滞而发为外科疾病。情志内伤,常发为肝胆经络循行处的乳房、胸胁、颈两侧的疾病。饮食太过,内伤脾胃,生湿化热;饮食不及,脾胃损伤,气血流行不畅,均可导致外科疾病。房劳伤肾,外邪趁虚而入;劳倦伤脾,气血不足,血行不畅,均易导致外科疾病。痰饮、瘀血、脓毒等病理产物致病范围广,病种多,症状较为复杂。

外科疾病的诊断方法包括望、闻、问、切。在望诊中,常用望形态、舌象,以及望局部的四种基本颜色,即红、白、黑、紫。红色多为阳证、热证,白色多为阴证、寒证,黑色多为死肌,青紫色多为瘀血。在闻诊中,常嗅脓和病变部位的气味。在问诊中,要问发病日期、治疗经过和现在症状。在脉诊中,主要体会脉象是有余还是不足。在触诊中,需注意患处的大小、肿痛、硬度、冷热和深浅。

外科疾病的辨证以八纲辨证、六经辨证、脏腑辨证和卫气营血辨证为主。

外科疾病,若疾患轻浅,单用外治即可;若为重证,往往采取内外合治。外科疾病的外治法有消、腐、收三个法则。外治方法包括药物疗法、手术疗法和其他疗法。药物疗法,是运用膏药、油膏、箍围药、掺药、酊剂、草药等各种药物直接施治于病变部位,使药效直达病所来治疗疾病的方法。手术疗法,是运用各种器械和手法操作,如切开法、烙法、砭镰法、挂线法、结扎法等来治疗疾病的方法。其他疗法,包括引流法、垫棉法、药筒拔法、灸法、熏法、熨法、浸渍法、热烘疗法、滚刺疗法、洗涤法等方法。外科疾病的内治法有消、托、补三个法则。消法,包括疏表、通里、清火、消痰、除湿、温经、舒肝、活血等方法,可使很多肿疡消散于无形,或使疮疡由重变轻,适用于尚未化脓的肿疡初期,为内治三大法则之首。托法,可托毒外出,使毒邪由深出浅,易化脓成熟,防止邪毒内攻入里或邪毒内陷,适用于肿疡和疮疡开始化脓者。补法,可加快生肌收口,常用于疮疡溃后脓血过多或久不收口者。

Chapter 2
Nursing of External Diseases

According to the *Rites of Zhou*, external disease doctors (traumato-orthopedic surgeons) treating swollen sores, ulcers, incised wounds and fractures emerged in the Zhou Dynasty. In *Prescriptions for Fifty-two Diseases*, hemorrhoid and fistula, and skin diseases were recorded. In *Huangdi's Internal Classic*, there were various external disease therapies such as stone needle therapy and tuina, and external medicines such as pig lard. At the end of the Eastern Han Dynasty, Hua Tuo invented Mafei Powder for general anesthesia and laparotomy. *Liu Juan-zi's Ghost-Bequeathed Prescriptions* (499 A.D.) is the first extant monograph on external medicine of TCM in China. *Treatise on the Pathogenesis and Manifestations of All Diseases* in the Sui Dynasty recorded surgical treatments and more than 40 skin diseases. *Essential Prescriptions Worth A Thousand Gold for Emergencies* written by Sun Simiao in the Tang Dynasty described his original catheterization with green onion tube. Later, external medicine of TCM developed and different academic schools emerged.

In modern times, the scope of external medicine of TCM includes not only sores and ulcers, goiters, tumors, cancers, skin diseases, breast diseases, anorectal diseases, male external genitalia diseases, peripheral vascular diseases and other traumatic diseases, but also internal carbuncles, acute abdominal disease, hernia, urogenital diseases and sexually transmitted diseases. External medicine diseases are generally named according to their locations, causes, shapes, colors, and other characteristics.

The etiology of external medicine diseases is six excesses, special toxicity, external trauma, emotional damage, improper diet, overstrain and taxation damage, phlegm-fluid retention, blood stasis and purulent toxin. Among the six excesses, wind pathogen is prone to being mobile and changeable, and usually attacks the upper parts of the body. Cold pathogen is prone to attacking the bones and joints, with purple, green-blue and dark skin color and fixed painful location. When summer-heat pathogen causes disease, the affected area shows redness, swelling and distention. When dampness pathogen attacks the skin, papules and blisters can occur, with itching and profuse effusion after diabrosis. When dryness pathogen induces diseases, the affected area is dry or withered, with rhagadia and desquamation. Disease triggered by fire pathogen has a sudden onset and severe condition, and the affected area experiences scorching redness, burning sensation, severe swelling pain, and possibility to be purulent and putrid. When special toxin, such as insect toxin, snake toxin, rabies toxin, lacquer toxin, medicinal toxin, food toxin and epidemic pestilence, attacks the human body, patients' intolerable constitution or weak constitution may result in diseases. Accidental falls, boiling water, fire and cold all can induce external medicine diseases via localized stagnation of qi and blood. Internal emotional damage usually leads to the disease in breast, chest and hypochondrium, and both sides of neck where the liver meridian and gallbladder meridian run through. Overeating damages the spleen and stomach internally and induces dampness-heat. Inadequate eating attacks the spleen and stomach and inhibits qi-blood circulation. Both of the causes may lead to external medicine diseases. Sexual taxation damaging the kidney makes it possible for pathogenic qi to enter the body and cause external medicine diseases. Overstrain damaging the spleen leads to deficiency of qi-blood and inhibition of blood circulation, and subsequently external medicine diseases occur. Phlegm-fluid retention, blood stasis, purulent toxin and other pathological products trigger a wide range of diseases, with more complicated symptoms.

The diagnostic methods of external medicine diseases include inspection, listening and smelling, inquiry, as well as pulse taking and palpation. Inspecting physique, posture, tongue manifestation, and four basic colors (red, white, black and purple) of localized areas are common diagnostic methods of inspection. Generally speaking, red belongs to yang syndrome and heat syndrome; white, yin syndrome and cold syndrome; black mainly is the sign of necrotic muscles and purple, blood stasis. The doctors need to smell the odors of pus and lesions. The doctors should also ask the onset date, treatment and present symptoms of the patients. In the pulse taking, the doctors should feel the patients' pulse and judge its surplus or insufficiency. In the palpation, the doctors should pay attention to the size, swelling, pain, hardness, cold and heat, and depth of the affected area.

The differentiation of external medicine diseases depends mainly on eight-principle syndrome differentiation, six-meridian syndrome differentiation, visceral syndrome differentiation and defense-qi-nutrient-blood syndrome differentiation.

For external medicine diseases, if the disease is mild, external treatment alone would be enough; for severe syndromes, combined internal with external treatment are often used. External therapeutic principles of external medicine diseases include resolving, corroding and wound-closing. External therapies include medicine therapy, operative therapy and other therapies. Medicine therapy directly applies plaster, ointment, encircling medicinal, medicinal powder, tincture and herbs on the affected areas. Operative therapy employs a variety of apparatus and manipulations, such as incision, cauterization, stone needle therapy, threaded ligation, and ligation to treat disease. Other therapies include drainage therapy, cotton-padding drainage therapy, medicated bamboo cupping, moxibustion therapy, fumigation therapy, medicated ironing therapy, maceration therapy, baking therapy, needling roller therapy, and rinsing and compressing therapy. Internal therapeutic principles include resolving, promoting and tonifying. Resolving includes relieving exterior, purgative method, reducing fire, dispersing phlegm, removing dampness, warming meridians, soothing the liver and activating blood. It can dissipate swollen sores or reduce the severity of sores and ulcers, so it is suitable for swollen sores at early stages before pus forms and it is the first choice among three approaches. Promoting can expel toxin from the depth in the body to the surface and enable it to suppurate, thereby preventing the internal invasion or internal sinking of pathogenic toxin. It is suitable for swollen sores and ulcers that just begin to fester. Tonifying can promote tissue regeneration and wound healing. It is suitable for sores and ulcers with profuse pus and blood or persistently unhealing wounds.

第一节 丹　　毒

丹毒,是指因皮肤、黏膜破损,火毒与血热抟结,蕴阻肌肤,不得外泄而引起的,以患部皮肤突然鲜红成片,色如涂丹,灼热肿胀,迅速蔓延,可伴见寒战、高热为临床特征的皮肤疾病。丹毒好发于下肢及颜面。发于头面的称"抱头火丹";发于下肢者称"流火";新生儿则多发于臀部,常为游走性,称"赤游丹"。西医的丹毒可参照本节进行护理。

一、病因病机

丹毒的病因多为血热和火毒。病人素有血热,加之外感火毒之邪,可因热毒蕴结于血分,发为丹毒。病人肌肤擦伤,或脚癣糜烂,或遇毒虫咬伤,皆可因毒邪趁隙而入,发为丹毒。

丹毒的病机为风湿热邪化火成毒,蕴结于皮肤。病位在皮肤。丹毒的病性多为实热证。

二、常见证型

(一)辨证要点

辨风热与湿热　根据皮损部位和脉象等来辨别。若发于头面部,伴恶寒,发热,头疼,脉浮,多为风热。若发于下肢,伴胃纳不香,脉滑,则多为湿热。

(二)证候分型

1. 风热蕴毒证

[主要证候]发于头面部,皮肤焮红灼热、肿胀疼痛、水疱,眼胞肿胀难睁;恶寒,发热,头疼;舌质红,舌苔薄黄,脉浮数。

[证候分析]风热化火上行,热郁皮肤,故皮肤焮红灼热、水疱;热阻经络,气血不畅,故皮肤肿胀疼痛,眼胞肿胀难睁,头疼;风火相煽,抟结于头面,正邪交争,故恶寒,发热;舌质红,舌苔薄黄,脉浮数,均为风热之象。

[护治原则]疏风清热解毒。

[常用方剂]普济消毒饮。

2. 肝脾湿火证

[主要证候]发于胸腹腰胯部,皮肤红肿蔓延,肿胀疼痛,触之灼手;伴口苦,口干;舌质红,舌苔黄腻,脉弦滑数。

[证候分析]肝郁化火乘脾,脾失健运,痰湿内生,湿与火相互抟结,氤氲于肌肉皮肤之间,故皮肤红肿蔓延,肿胀疼痛,触之灼手;舌质红,舌苔黄腻,脉弦滑数均为肝脾湿火之象。

[护治原则]清肝泻火利湿。

［常用方剂］龙胆泻肝汤。

3. 湿热蕴毒证

［主要证候］发于下肢,皮肤红赤肿胀、灼热疼痛,或见水疱、紫斑,甚至结毒化脓或皮肤坏死,或反复发作,可形成大脚风;伴发热,胃纳不香;舌质红,舌苔黄腻,脉滑数。

［证候分析］湿热下注,蕴蒸肌肤,阻塞经络,故下肢皮肤红赤肿胀、灼热疼痛;热毒蕴肤,故见水疱、紫斑,甚至结毒化脓或皮肤坏死;湿性黏滞且趋下,故疾病在下肢反复发作,形成大脚风;湿邪困脾,故胃纳不香;舌质红,舌苔黄腻,脉滑数,均为湿热之象。

［护治原则］清热利湿解毒。

［常用方剂］萆薢渗湿汤。

4. 胎火蕴毒证

［主要证候］发生于新生儿,多见于臀部,局部红肿灼热,可呈游走性,并有壮热烦躁,甚则神昏谵语,恶心呕吐。

［证候分析］新生儿胎火蕴毒,结于臀部,故臀部皮肤红肿灼热;火毒入于心包,心神受扰,故壮热烦躁,甚则神昏谵语;热邪犯脾,胃失和降,故恶心呕吐。

［护治原则］清热凉血解毒。

［常用方剂］犀角地黄汤。

三、护理措施

对于丹毒的病人,应观察皮损的颜色、形态、分布和肿胀程度;疼痛的部位、性质、程度和持续时间;有无水疱。每日定时,在固定的地点,用软尺测量患肢的肿胀部位的周长。监测体温。对于皮损由头面或由四肢向胸腹扩大的病人,应观察神志情况;若病人出现神昏谵语,头痛高热,恶心呕吐,应立即报告医生。

(一) 辨证施护

1. 风热蕴毒证

(1) 生活起居护理　居室安静凉爽,光线柔和,空气新鲜。取半仰卧位,多休息。可进行轻缓的锻炼,如太极拳。注意个人卫生,修剪指甲,保持口腔、眼部、鼻及外耳道的清洁。皮损处不可搔抓挤压、风吹日晒或用热水烫洗,不可掏耳朵和挖鼻孔。若皮损在眼眶周围,应在涂药时做好包扎固定。若皮损在唇颊部,应少说话。

(2) 饮食护理　若皮损在唇颊部,应予软食或半流食,减少咀嚼。多饮水,可饮金银花茶、菊花茶。宜食清热散风的食物,如藕、绿豆、甘蔗、冬瓜、苦瓜。赤小豆薏苡仁汤:赤小豆、薏苡仁各100 g;浸泡半天,加水500 mL,文火煮烂。不宜食辛辣、油腻、助热生火的食物。忌发物,如羊肉、虾、蟹、辣椒、香椿。

(3) 情志护理　病人突发头疼且眼胞肿胀难睁,护士可运用语言开导疗法和移情易性疗法,加强疾病常识宣教,多与病人及家属沟通,营造良好的环境,使病人保持心情舒畅,避免抑郁、烦躁、紧张、焦虑。

(4) 用药护理　中药汤剂宜武火快煎,饭后温服。服药后观察皮损红肿的消退情况。

（5）操作技术　① 药膏疗法：用金黄膏、玉露膏、青黛膏或芩柏膏敷贴于皮损处，涂抹厚度为1~2毫米，敷药面积超过红肿边缘1~2厘米，每次4~6小时，每日1次，适用于皮损无破溃者；或用黄连膏，适用于皮损破溃者；若用药期间出现红疹、瘙痒，应立即停用。② 湿泥疗法：用鲜蒲公英、鲜紫花地丁或鲜马齿苋，择一洗净后捣烂为泥，用适量芝麻油调成糊状，敷布于皮损处；待湿泥干燥后调换，或以冷开水时时湿润，每日2次，每次4~6小时，温度以24~31℃为宜。③ 穴位按摩法：取合谷、太阳、印堂、百会，用拇指揉法，按摩至局部发热或有酸麻重胀感，每日1次；孕妇禁用。

2. 肝脾湿火证

（1）生活起居护理　居室凉爽湿润，安静舒适，空气新鲜。衣物宽松、柔软、棉质。卧床休息，经常改变体位，以防皮损受压。保持皮肤清洁，勤换衣，擦洗动作宜轻，不可搔抓。若水疱直径超过3厘米，遵医嘱抽吸疱液。保持口腔清洁，饭后含漱金银花甘草液。减少探视，病情稳定后可适量锻炼。

（2）饮食护理　多饮水，可饮芦根茶。多吃高蛋白、富含维生素和烟酸的食物。多吃新鲜的水果和蔬菜，以保持大便通畅。宜食清热利湿的食物，如薏苡仁、马齿苋、猕猴桃。不宜食发物和辛辣的食物。

（3）情志护理　病人为实热证，容易有焦虑、烦躁的情绪，护士可运用移情易性疗法，如组织病友活动，以转移病人的注意力，使其保持情绪稳定。

（4）用药护理　中药汤剂宜饭后温服或偏凉服。服药后观察局部皮损情况。

（5）操作技术　① 湿敷疗法：用黄柏、白鲜皮；或黄连、白头翁、金银花、马齿苋、土槿皮、红花；煎煮后，用5~6层纱布浸透4~15℃的药液敷于患处，每次20分钟，每日1次。② 穴位按摩法：取大椎、合谷、曲池，用拇指揉法，力度宜大，频率宜快，按摩至局部发热或有酸麻重胀感，每日1次；孕妇禁用。③ 耳压疗法：取皮质下、神门、内分泌、三焦等耳穴，用耳穴压豆胶布贴压，每日按揉4~5次，以局部发热泛红为度，留置2~4日；孕妇禁用。

3. 湿热蕴毒证

（1）生活起居护理　居室安静凉爽，光线柔和，空气新鲜，床单整洁干燥。衣裤和袜子棉质、宽松。卧床休息，将患肢抬高30°~40°。保持足部清洁，积极治疗皮肤破损及足癣。指导病人进行轻缓的体育锻炼，如打太极拳，以保持大便通畅。避免使用刺激性强的皮肤清洁用品，不可搔抓、摩擦或用热水烫洗皮肤。避免劳累及长久站立。

（2）饮食护理　清淡饮食。多饮水，可饮绿豆汤、鲜芦根茶。多吃新鲜的水果和蔬菜。宜食清热利湿的食物，如冬瓜、苦瓜、西瓜、赤小豆。茯苓红花粥：茯苓、薏苡仁各30 g，红花5 g；茯苓与红花熬汁去渣，加入薏苡仁及少许大米，用文火煮成粥，每日早晚服用。戒烟限酒，不宜食辛辣、油腻、助热生火的食物。不宜食发物，如羊肉、牛肉、猪头肉、辣椒。

（3）情志护理　疾病反复发作，病程较长，病人有发怒倾向，护士可运用语言开导疗法，加强疾病常识宣教，多与病人及家属沟通。或运用移情易性疗法，组织形式多样、寓教于乐的病友活动和同伴支持教育，介绍成功案例，鼓励病友之间交流防治经验，使病人保持心情舒畅，避免烦躁、焦虑。或运用顺意疗法，理解和同情病人，以避免情志刺激。

（4）用药护理　中药汤剂宜饭后温服或偏凉服。服药后观察皮损红肿的消退情况。

（5）操作技术　① 电离子导入疗法：用乳香、没药、川芎、川乌、威灵仙、蒲公英；煎煮后用药物离子透入仪导入，每次 20 分钟，每日 1 次；孕妇、婴儿禁用。②耳压疗法：取神门、交感、肾上腺、皮质下等耳穴，用耳穴压豆胶布贴压，每日按揉 4~5 次，以局部发热泛红为度，留置 2~4 日；孕妇禁用。③足部熏洗疗法：大蒜 500 g，煮水半桶，水温 50~70℃时熏蒸患肢（外盖棉被），水温降至 37~40℃时浸泡、淋洗患肢，每晚 1 次，每次 20 分钟；适用于大脚风，可配合使用医用弹力护套。

4. 胎火蕴毒证

（1）生活起居护理　居室安静凉爽，光线柔和，空气新鲜。床单整洁干燥。衣被宜薄。衣裤宽松，避免患处皮肤受压及摩擦。保护皮损，修剪患儿指甲以防搔抓挤压，避免阳光直射或用热水烫洗，患侧肢体严禁静脉输液。对于高热者，遵医嘱采取退热措施，以防止高热惊厥。

（2）饮食护理　饮食宜细软、易消化，少食多餐。多饮水，可饮绿豆汤、雪梨汁。宜食新鲜的水果和蔬菜，以及清热利湿的食物。忌发物，如羊肉、虾、蟹、辣椒、香椿，不宜食辛辣、油腻、助热生火的食物。

（3）情志护理　患儿壮热烦躁，护士可鼓励家属多陪伴和照顾患儿，多怀抱、安抚患儿，提供安全感，让患儿感到舒适。

（4）用药护理　中药汤剂宜饭后温服或偏凉服。服药后观察皮损红肿消退情况。

（5）操作技术　①敷贴疗法：将金黄散与鲜丝瓜叶汁调成糊状，敷贴于皮损处，涂抹厚度为 1~2 毫米，面积超过红肿边缘 1~2 厘米，每次 4~6 小时，每日 1 次，适用于皮损无破溃的患儿；若皮肤出现红疹、瘙痒，应立即停用。②湿泥疗法：用鲜荷叶、鲜马齿苋或绿豆芽，择一洗净后捣烂为泥，与适量芝麻油调成糊状，敷于皮损处；待湿泥干燥后调换，或以冷开水时时湿润，湿泥的温度以 24~31℃为宜，每次 4~6 小时，每日 2 次。

（二）健康教育

加强锻炼，调畅情志，注意休息。穿棉质、宽松的衣裤。注意与他人隔离，洁具专用。注意个人卫生，每日用温水洗脚。洗澡时轻轻擦洗，水温不宜过高，避免使用刺激性强的皮肤清洁用品。

多饮温开水，多吃新鲜的水果和蔬菜，如冬瓜、猕猴桃、番茄。薏苡仁 30 g，水煎，日服 1 剂，以预防复发。戒烟限酒，不宜食发物和辛辣、肥腻的食物，如羊肉、虾、蟹、大葱、大蒜、辣椒、香椿。

更换外用药时，应使用液体石蜡或植物油擦去原药迹，不可用水洗或用酒精擦拭。不宜过早停药。症状改善后，遵医嘱继续用药，以巩固治疗，防止复发。

保持局部皮肤清洁，每日用碘伏清洗创面。暴露水肿部位，避免翻身时擦伤、挤压而造成皮损剥脱或炎症扩散。患侧肢体严禁静脉输液。积极治疗皮肤黏膜的破损，以预防复发。

Section 1　Erysipelas

Erysipelas is a skin disease clinically characterized by sudden rapidly-spreading red skin with scorching heat and swelling, or possible chill and high fever. It is caused by skin and mucous membrane damage with fire and blood heat blocked in the skin. It is usually found on the lower limbs and the face. Erysipelas in the lower limbs is called "flowing fire (shank erysipelas)"; that in the head and face, "head erysipelas"; that in the newborns' buttocks often with wandering characteristic, "red wandering erysipelas". This section can be referred to for the nursing of erysipelas in Western medicine.

ETIOLOGY AND PATHOGENESIS

The etiology includes blood-heat and fire-toxin. Blood-heat constitution and external contraction of fire-toxin causes heat-toxin constrained in the blood level, developing as erysipelas. Skin abrasions, foot fungus eruptions, or poisonous insect bites would likely develop as erysipelas due to the toxin entering into blood level.

The pathogenesis is transformation of wind, dampness and heat pathogens into fire and toxin that accumulates within the skin. The disease is located in the skin. The disease nature is mostly excess heat syndrome.

COMMON SYNDROMES

Key Points in Syndrome Differentiation

Differentiation of Wind-Heat from Dampness-Heat

The differentiation is based on the location of lesion, accompanying symptoms and pulse manifestation. Wind-heat syndrome exhibits erysipelas in the head or face with the symptoms of aversion to cold, fever, headache and floating pulse. Dampness-heat syndrome displays erysipelas on the lower limbs with the symptoms of poor appetite and slippery pulse.

Syndrome Differentiation

1. Wind-Heat Toxin Accumulation Syndrome

[Clinical Manifestations] Erysipelas in the head and face, red scorching skin with swelling painful sensation and blisters, swollen eyes with difficulty to open, aversion to cold, fever, headache, red tongue with thin yellow coating and floating rapid pulse.

[Manifestations Analysis] Wind-heat transforms into fire that flows upward and is depressed in the skin, causing red scorching skin with blisters. Heat obstruction in the channels and collaterals brings on qi and blood inhibition, so there are symptoms of swelling painful skin, swollen eyes with difficulty to open, and headache. Wind and fire intermingling in the head and face leads to aversion to cold with fever. Red tongue with thin yellow coating and floating rapid pulse are the manifestations of wind-heat.

[Nursing Principle] Dispersing wind, clearing heat and removing toxin.

[Suggested Formula] Puji Xiaodu Drink.

2. Liver and Spleen Dampness-Fire Syndrome

[Clinical Manifestations] Erysipelas in the chest, abdomen, waist and crotch area, spreading red skin with swelling painful and burning sensation, accompanied by bitter and dry mouth, red tongue with yellow slimy coating, and wiry, slippery rapid pulse.

[Manifestations Analysis] Liver depression transforming into fire and overwhelming the spleen triggers failure of the spleen to transport and transform as well as internal generation of phlegm-dampness, and pathogenic fire binds with dampness that remains between the muscle and the skin. Therefore, there is spreading red skin with swelling painful and burning sensation. Red tongue with yellow slimy coating, and wiry, slippery rapid pulse are the manifestations of dampness-fire in the liver and spleen.

[Nursing Principle] Clearing liver fire and draining dampness.

[Suggested Formula] Longdan Xiegan Decoction.

3. Dampness-Heat Toxin Accumulation Syndrome

[Clinical Manifestations] Erysipelas on the lower limbs, red scorching skin with swelling painful sensation, or with blisters, purple spots, or even toxic nodules with pus, or skin necrosis, or repeated attacks that may lead to big foot wind (elephantiasis of leg), accompanied with fever, poor appetite, red tongue with yellow slimy coating, and slippery rapid pulse.

[Manifestations Analysis] Dampness-heat pouring downward steams the skin and obstructs the channels and collaterals, causing red scorching skin with swelling painful sensation. Heat toxin accumulation in the skin leads to blisters, purple spots, or even toxic nodules with pus, or skin necrosis. Dampness is sticky, stagnant and following downward, so the disease repeatedly attacks on the lower limbs and develops into big foot wind (elephantiasis of leg). Dampness encumbering the spleen leads to poor appetite. Red tongue with yellow slimy coating and slippery rapid pulse are the manifestations of dampness-heat.

[Nursing Principle] Clearing heat, draining dampness and removing toxin.

[Suggested Formula] Bixie Shenshi Decoction.

4. Fetal Fire-Toxin Accumulation Syndrome

[Clinical Manifestations] Erysipelas in newborns, mostly on the buttocks, localized red scorching skin with swelling sensation and wandering characteristic, accompanied with high fever and dysphoria, or even coma, delirium, nausea and vomiting.

[Manifestations Analysis] Newborns' fetal fire with toxin accumulates in the buttocks, causing red scorching skin with swelling sensation. Fire-toxin penetrates into the pericardium and disturbs the heart spirit, leading to high fever and dysphoria, or even coma and delirium. Pathogenic heat invading the spleen leads to the dysfunction of stomach-qi to descend, so nausea and vomiting are developed.

［Nursing Principle］Clearing heat, cooling blood and removing toxin.

［Suggested Formula］Xijiao Dihuang Decoction.

NURSING MEASURES

For cases with erysipelas, nurses should observe the color, shape, distribution and swelling degree of the lesions; the location, nature, degree and duration of pain; and the presence or absence of blisters. Nurses should also monitor the patients' body temperature and measure the circumference of the same swollen area of the affected limb with a soft ruler at a fixed time every day. For patients with lesions expanding from the head to the chest or from the four limbs to the chest and abdomen, the patients' mental status should be observed. If the patient has coma and delirious speech, headache, high fever, nausea and vomiting, it is advisable to immediately report to the doctors.

Syndrome-Based Nursing Measures

1. Wind-Heat Toxin Accumulation Syndrome

(1) Daily life nursing. The ward should be quiet and cool with mild light and fresh air. The patients should take a semi-supine position, rest in bed, and do moderate exercise, such as Taiji. They should maintain personal hygiene, trim the nails, and keep clean the mouth, eyes, nose and external ear canals. The lesions should not be scratched, squeezed, scalded by hot water or exposed to the sun and wind, and the ears and nostrils should not be picked. If the lesions are around the eyes, they should be fixed with a bandage when applying medicine. If the lesions are on the lips and cheeks, it is better for the patients to talk less.

(2) Diet nursing. If the lesions are on the lips and cheeks, liquid or semi-liquid diet should be given to reduce chewing. The patients should drink more water, may frequently drink jinyinhua (honeysuckle flower) tea or juhua (chrysanthemum flower) tea and eat foods with functions of clearing heat and dispersing wind, such as lotus root, lüdou (mung bean), sugarcane, Chinese waxgourd and bitter gourd. Chixiaodou yiyiren (adzuki bean and coix seed) soup is also recommended: chixiaodou (adzuki bean) 100 g and yiyiren (coix seed) 100 g; soak them for half a day, then add water to 500 mL and cook them thoroughly on a gentle fire. Don't eat pungent, spicy, greasy, heat- and fire-generating foods, or foods that induce or aggravate disease, such as mutton, shrimp, crab, chili and tender leaves of Chinese toon.

(3) Emotion nursing. When the disease occurs suddenly, the patients have headache and swollen eye cells that are difficult to open. So nurses may use verbal enlightenment therapy as well as emotional transference and dispositional change therapy to impart them the knowledge about the disease and communicate with them and their family members as much as possible to offer a relaxing environment so that the patients can keep in a pleasant state of mind and prevent depression, dysphoria, tension and anxiety.

(4) Medication nursing. Decoction should be decocted quickly with strong flame and be taken warm after meals. The local skin lesions should be observed after medication.

(5) Manipulation techniques. ① Ointment application therapy: for those whose skin lesions are not broken, Jinhuang Ointment, Yulu Ointment, Qingdai Ointment, or Qinbai Ointment can be applied to the skin lesions with a thickness of 1~2 millimeter(s) and an area of 1~2 centimeter(s) beyond the edges of the redness and swelling, remaining for 4~6 hours each time, once a day. If there are broken skin lesions, Huanglian Ointment can be applied; if there are red rash and itching during the medication, stop using it immediately. ② Wet mud therapy: xianpugongying (fresh dandelion), xianzihuadiding (fresh tokyo violet) or xianmachixian (fresh purslane); choose one of them, wash clean and pound it into mud, mix the mud with some sesame oil, then apply it on the skin lesions; change it when the wet mud becomes dry or wet it with cold boiled water, 4~6 hours each time, twice per day. The temperature should be remained between 24~31℃. ③ Acupressure therapy: select Hegu (LI 4), Taiyang (GB 1), Yintang (EX－HN3), and Baihui (GV 20); applying thumb kneading manipulation on them till the local area turns hot or feels soreness, numbness and heaviness and distension, once a day. And it is contraindicated in pregnancy.

2. Liver and Spleen Dampness-Fire Syndrome

(1) Daily life nursing. The ward should be cool, moist, quiet, comfortable, and full of fresh air. The clothes should be loose, soft and cotton. The patients should rest in bed and change position frequently to prevent pressure on the skin lesions. They should maintain skin hygiene and regularly change the the clothes. The scrubbing action should be gentle and don't scratch. If there are blisters of more than three centimeters in diameter, follow the doctor's advice to aspirate the blister fluid. They should also keep the mouth clean by gargling with jinyinhua gancao (honeysuckle flower and licorice root) liquid after meals. The visits from family and friends should be reduced and there should be some appropriate activities after stabilization of the disease.

(2) Diet nursing. The patients should drink more water, may take lugen (reed rhizome) tea and eat more foods that are high in protein, rich in vitamins and niacin. Also, they can eat more fresh fruit and vegetables to maintain a normal bowel movement, and eat foods with functions of clearing heat and draining dampness such as yiyiren (coix seed), machixian (purslane) and kiwi fruit. Don't eat pungent and spicy foods or foods that induce or aggravate disease.

(3) Emotion nursing. Because of the excess heat syndrome, patients are prone to anxiety and dysphoria. The nurses should adopt emotional transference and dispositional change therapy such as organizing activities for patients to divert their attention and keep them emotionally stable.

(4) Medication nursing. Decoction should be taken warm or slightly cool after meals. And the local skin lesions should be observed after medication.

(5) Manipulation techniques. ① Wet compress therapy: huangbai (amur cork-tree bark) and baixianpi (dictamnus root bark); or huanglian (coptis rhizome), baitouweng (Chinese anemone root), jinyinhua (honeysuckle flower), machixian (purslane), tujinpi (cortex pseudolaricis), and honghua

(safflower); first, decoct the medicinals, then soak 5~6 layers of gauze into the decoction of 4~15℃, and apply the gauze to the affected area, 20 minutes each time, once per day. ② Acupressure therapy: select Dazhui (GV 14), Hegu (LI 4) and Quchi (LI 11); apply powerful and quick thumb kneading manipulation on each of them till the local area turns hot or feels soreness, numbness and heaviness and distension; once per day. And it is contraindicated in pregnancy. ③ Auricular pressure therapy: select subcortex (AT4), shenmen (TF4), endocrine (CO18), and triple energizer (CO17); apply specialized pasters on them, press and knead each of them till the area turns hot and red, 4~5 times per day, and keep the pasters for 2~4 days. And it is contraindicated in pregnancy.

3. Dampness-Heat Toxin Accumulation Syndrome

(1) Daily life nursing. The ward should be quiet and cool with soft light and fresh air. The bedding should be neat and dry. The patients should rest in bed with the affected limb elevated 30°~40°. They should wear loose and cotton clothing and socks, keep the feet clean, actively treat skin lesions and tinea pedis. Nurses should guide patients to do soothing physical exercise such as Taiji to maintain a normal bowel movement. The patients should avoid straining, prolonged standing, using irritating skin cleansing products, and scratching, rubbing or washing the skin with hot water.

(2) Diet nursing. The patients should eat light diet and drink more water, may take lüdou (mung bean) soup or xianlugen (fresh reed rhizome) tea, and eat more fresh fruit and vegetables as well as foods with the functions of clearing heat and draining dampness such as Chinese waxgourd, bitter gourd, watermelon and chixiaodou (adzuki bean). Fuling honghua (poria and safflower) gruel is also strongly recommended: prepare fuling (poria) 30 g, yiyiren (coix seed) 30 g and honghua (safflower) 5 g; then boil fuling (poria) and honghua (safflower) with water and remove the dregs, put in yiyiren (coix seed) and some rice, and then boil them with mild fire to make gruel; take the gruel daily in the morning and evening. The patients should avoid alcohol and cigarettes as well as foods that induce or aggravate disease such as mutton, beef, pork and chili, so do pungent, spicy, greasy and heat-generating foods.

(3) Emotion nursing. The patients are prone to anger due to the recurrent attacks and long duration of the disease, so nurses may use verbal enlightenment therapy to impart the knowledge about the disease and communicate with patients and their families as much as possible, or adopt emotional transference and dispositional change therapy to organize various forms of funny educational activities for patients, such as peer support education, successful case introduction, and encourage patients to exchange experiences of prevention and treatment to keep them in a pleasant state of mind and avoid dysphoria and anxiety. Nurses could also use submission therapy to understand and sympathize with the patients to avoid emotional stimulation.

(4) Medication nursing. Decoction should be taken warm or slightly cool after meals and local skin lesions should be observed after medication.

(5) Manipulation techniques. ① Electrical iontophoresis therapy: prepare ruxiang (frankincense), moyao (myrrh), chuanxiong (Sichuan lovage root), chuanwu (common monkshood mother root), weilingxian (Chinese clematis root) and pugongying (dandelion); decoct the above medicinals and then use medicinal iontophoresis apparatus to conduct the medicinal ions of the decoction into the skin lesions, 20 minutes each time, once per day. And it should be avoided for pregnant women and infants. ② Auricular pressure therapy: select shenmen (TF4), sympathetic (AH6a), adrenal gland (TG2p) and subcortex (AT4); apply specialized pasters on them, press and knead each of them till the area turns hot and red, 4~5 times per day, and keep the pasters for 2~4 days. And it is contraindicated in pregnancy. ③ Fumigating and washing therapy: first boil 500 g of dasuan (garlic bulb) with half a bucket of water, then fumigate the affected limb (covered with quilts) with the water at a temperature of 50~70℃ and wash with it at a temperature of 37~40℃, 20 minutes each time, once per night. This method is suitable for big foot wind (elephantiasis of leg). Additionally, it can also be wrapped with medical elastic sheath.

4. Fetal Fire-Toxin Accumulation Syndrome

(1) Daily life nursing. The ward should be quiet and cool with soft light and fresh air. The bedding should be neat and dry. The patients should wear loose clothes and get under the thin covers to avoid pressure and friction on the affected skin. To protect skin lesion, the patients' nails should be trimmed, the affected skin should not be scratched, squeezed, washed with hot water, or exposed into the direct sunlight. Moreover, the affected limb is strictly prohibited from intravenous infusion. For the cases with high fever, take antipyretic measures as prescribed by the doctor to prevent febrile convulsions.

(2) Diet nursing. The diet should be soft and digestible. The patients should have small frequent meals and drink more water, may take lüdou (mung bean) soup or snow pear juice, and eat fresh fruit and vegetables as well as foods that have the functions of clearing heat and draining dampness. They should avoid pungent, spicy, greasy, and heat-generating foods and foods that induce or aggravate disease such as mutton, shrimp, crab, chili and tender leaves of Chinese toon.

(3) Emotion nursing. As the children are agitated by the high fever, the nurses should encourage the family members to spend more time with and care for the child, embrace and soothe the children as much as possible to cultivate a sense of security and comfort.

(4) Medication nursing. Decoction should be taken warm or slightly cool after meals and local skin lesions should be observed after medication.

(5) Manipulation techniques. ① Paste application therapy: whisk fresh luffa leaf juice with Jinhuang Powder to make a paste and apply it on the skin lesions with a thickness of 1~2 millimeter(s) and an area of 1~2 centimeter(s) beyond the edges of the redness and swelling, 4~6 hours each time, once a day; and it is suitable for those whose skin lesions are not broken. If there are red rash and itching during the medication, stop using it immediately. ② Wet mud therapy: xianheye (fresh lotus leaf), xianmachixian (fresh purslane) or fresh mung bean sprout; choose one of them, wash clean and pound it into mud, mix the mud with certain amount of sesame oil, then apply it on the skin lesions; change it when the wet mud becomes dry or wet it with cold boiled water, 4~6 hours each time, twice a day. The temperature should be remained between 24~31℃.

Patient Education

The patients should take more physical exercise, adjust the mood, have adequate rest, and wear cotton loose clothing. They should also be seperated from others in using personal sanitary appliances and keep personal hygiene, such as washing feet with warm water every day. When bathing, water temperature and scrubbing force should be moderate and irritating skin-cleaning products should be avoided.

The patients should drink more warm water. Fresh fruit and vegetables should be supplemented, such as Chinese waxgourd, kiwi fruit and tomatoes. Drink herbal tea made of 30 g of yiyiren (coix seed) each day to prevent reoccurrence. The patients should refrain from cigarette, alcohol and foods that induce or aggravate disease, such as mutton, shrimp, crab, scallions, dasuan (garlic bulb), chili and tender leaves of Chinese toon, so do pungent, spicy, fishy and greasy foods.

When replacing the externally-applied medicinal, wipe off the original drug stains with liquid paraffin or vegetable oil, instead of water or alcohol. After the improvement of disease condition, it is advisable to continue the medication as prescribed by the doctor to consolidate the treatment and prevent recurrence.

The patients should keep the local skin clean, daily disinfect the wound surface with iodophor, and expose the edematous area to avoid abrasion, extrusion, peeling-off or inflammatory diffusion of the skin lesions during turning over. The affected limb is strictly prohibited from intravenous infusion. And the patients should also actively treat the breakage of skin mucosa to prevent recurrence.

第二节 湿 疮

湿疮,是指因禀性不耐,风湿热邪客于肌肤而引起的,临床以对称分布的多形性皮疹,渗出流滋,剧烈瘙痒,反复发作为特征的一类皮肤病。根据病程可分为急性、亚急性和慢性三类。急性者以丘疹、水疱、糜烂、渗出为主。慢性者以干燥脱屑、苔藓样变为主。亚急性者介于急性与慢性之间。西医的湿疹可参照本节进行护理。

一、病因病机

湿疮的病因多为脾虚、湿热和血虚。病人素体脾虚,禀赋不耐,或过食辛热,日久伤脾,均可致脾虚内生湿热,浸淫肌肤,发为湿疮。湿热蕴久,耗伤阴血,或脾虚失运,气血生化乏源,均可致血虚风燥,肌肤失养,发为湿疮。

湿疮的病机为湿热浸淫肌肤。病位在肌肤。急性者为实证,以湿热浸淫肌肤为主;亚急性者为虚实夹杂,与湿邪困脾,脾失健运有关;慢性者为虚证,系久病耗伤阴血,血虚风燥所致。

二、常见证型

（一）辨证要点

1. 辨虚实　根据起病速度,皮损的颜色、形态和渗液情况,以及舌脉来辨别。若起病急,皮损颜色潮红,渗液多,伴丘疹,舌红苔黄,脉滑数,多为实证。若起病缓,皮损色暗,渗液少,以鳞屑和苔藓样变为主,舌淡苔薄,脉弦细,则多为虚证。

2. 辨燥湿　根据皮损的颜色、边界、粗糙程度和渗液情况来辨别。若皮损色红,以丘疹为主,渗出较多,边界不清,多为湿证。若皮损色暗,表面粗糙,呈苔藓样变,渗出较少,边界清晰,则多为燥证。

（二）证候分型

1. 湿热浸淫证

［主要证候］以潮红、肿胀、糜烂、渗出为主,可见丘疹、丘疱疹、水疱,自觉灼热,瘙痒;舌红,苔黄或黄腻,脉滑数。

［证候分析］湿热浸淫,热重于湿,故起病急,皮损潮红、灼热;湿热蕴阻,气血相搏,泛于肌肤,故皮损肿胀、糜烂、渗出,可见丘疹、丘疱疹、水疱;舌红,苔黄或黄腻,脉滑数,均为湿热之象。

［护治原则］清热利湿,祛风止痒。

［常用方剂］龙胆泻肝汤合萆薢渗湿汤。

2. 脾虚湿蕴证

［主要证候］以淡红色红斑、丘疹、丘疱疹,少量渗液为主,可见皮肤肥厚,自觉瘙痒;可伴有食

少,腹胀便溏;舌淡胖,苔腻,脉濡或滑。

　　[证候分析]脾虚生湿,日久化热,蕴积肌肤,故起病较缓,以淡红色红斑、丘疹、丘疱疹为主,自觉瘙痒;湿热相搏,湿重于热,故有少量渗液;湿阻中焦,运化失司,故食少,腹胀便溏;舌淡胖,苔腻,脉濡或滑,均为脾虚湿蕴之象。

　　[护治原则]健脾利湿,祛风止痒。

　　[常用方剂]除湿胃苓汤合参苓白术散。

　　3. 血虚风燥证

　　[主要证候]以肥厚、鳞屑、苔藓样变为主,可见色素沉着,自觉阵发性瘙痒;舌淡红,苔薄,脉弦细。

　　[证候分析]久病耗伤阴血,或脾虚生化乏源,致血虚肌肤失养,故皮损以肥厚、鳞屑、苔藓样变为主,可见色素沉着;血虚生风化燥,故自觉阵发性瘙痒;舌淡红,苔薄,脉弦细,均为血虚风燥之象。

　　[护治原则]养血润燥,祛风止痒。

　　[常用方剂]四物消风饮和当归饮子。

三、护理措施

　　对于湿疮的病人,应观察皮损的色泽、形态、部位、瘙痒程度、糜烂和渗液的情况,以及舌脉。若皮损渗液较多,浸润成片,瘙痒剧烈,或体温在38.5℃以上并伴有恶寒,均应及时报告医生。

　　(一)辨证施护

　　1. 湿热浸淫证

　　(1)生活起居护理　居室凉爽安静,空气新鲜。床单和被套整洁干燥。若渗出较多,要及时更换。衣物宽松、柔软、棉质。起居有常,睡眠充足。保持皮肤清洁,禁止搔抓和摩擦,不可使用肥皂清洁或用热水烫洗。

　　(2)饮食护理　可饮鲜芦根茶、金银花茶。宜食清热利湿的食物,如赤小豆、马齿苋、绿豆。食疗方:冬瓜薏米汤。不宜食发物和辛辣、油腻的食物,如虾、鸡肉、鹅肉、牛肉、羊肉、香菜、韭菜、生姜、大葱、大蒜。

　　(3)情志护理　由于奇痒难忍,病人容易急躁、焦虑或悲观,护士可运用语言开导疗法,详细介绍湿疮的知识,做好解释工作,使病人保持平和的心态。或运用移情易性疗法,鼓励病人多参加社交活动,以分散注意力,避免过思伤脾而导致病情迁延或加重。

　　(4)用药护理　中药汤剂宜饭后偏凉服或温服。

　　(5)操作技术　①涂药法:取三黄洗剂;摇匀后,用棉签蘸药物涂于患处,每日1次;适用于初期仅有红斑、丘疹、少量水疱,并且无渗出者。②湿敷疗法:用黄柏、蒲公英、马齿苋、生地榆、野菊花各20 g;任选1~2种煎煮,用5~6层纱布浸透4~15℃的药液敷于皮损处,每次20分钟,每日1次;适合水疱、糜烂、渗出较多,或伴有疼痛者。③敷贴疗法:用青黛散与芝麻油调成糊状,敷贴于皮损处,厚度为1~2毫米,面积超过红肿边缘1~2厘米,每次4~6小时,每日1次;适用于疾病后期,皮损结痂,渗出减少时。

2. 脾虚湿蕴证

（1）生活起居护理　居室温暖安静。起居有常，睡眠充足。保持皮肤清洁，禁止搔抓和摩擦，不可使用肥皂清洁或用热水烫洗。避免过劳。

（2）饮食护理　宜食健脾利湿的食物，如山药、芡实、莲子。食疗方：茯苓炖龟。不宜食发物和生冷、肥甘的食物。

（3）情志护理　病人的病程迁延，护士可运用语言开导疗法，经常巡视病房，主动向病人讲解有关湿疮的知识，鼓励病人，使病人保持心情舒畅，增加对于治疗的信心，避免紧张、焦虑。

（4）用药护理　中药汤剂宜温服。

（5）操作技术　① 涂药法：取黄柏霜、青黛膏或 10% 地榆氧化锌油；用棉签蘸药物涂于患处，每日 2~3 次；适用于无渗出者。② 湿敷疗法：取苦参汤或三黄洗剂；用 5~6 层纱布浸透 38~41℃ 的药液敷于皮损处或以绷带包扎，每次 20 分钟，每日 1 次；适合渗出较少者。

3. 血虚风燥证

（1）生活起居护理　居室安静。起居有常，睡眠充足，避免过劳。保持皮肤清洁，禁止搔抓和摩擦，不可使用肥皂清洁或用热水烫洗。

（2）饮食护理　可饮黑豆饮。宜食养血祛风的食物，如乌梢蛇、大枣、银耳、蛤蜊肉。食疗方：桑椹百合汤。不宜食发物和辛辣燥火的食物。

（3）情志护理　病人的病程迁延，护士可运用语言开导疗法，主动向病人讲解有关本病的知识，鼓励病人，使病人保持心情舒畅，增加战胜疾病的信心，避免消沉、抑郁。

（4）用药护理　中药汤剂宜文火久煎，饭前温服。

（5）操作技术　① 涂药法合封包疗法：取青黛膏、5%硫磺软膏或黑豆馏油软膏；用棉签蘸药物涂抹于患处，厚度为 1 毫米，用保鲜膜包裹 1~3 小时，每日 2 次，不必洗去油渍；适用于皮损肥厚，且无溃疡、感染的病人。② 穴位按摩法：取三阴交、血海、足三里、神门，用拇指揉法，揉按宜轻缓，按摩至局部发热或有酸麻重胀感，每日 1 次；孕妇禁用。③ 耳压疗法：取肺、神门、肾上腺、皮质下、交感等耳穴，用耳穴压豆胶布贴压，每日按揉 4~5 次，以局部发热泛红为度，留置 2~4 日；孕妇禁用。

（二）健康教育

检测过敏原。避免搔抓、摩擦、碰撞皮损。避开冷热源刺激，洗澡时水温不宜过高。忌用盐水、花椒水、碱性的香皂和沐浴液清洗皮损。避免使用刺激性的化妆品，头部湿疮者避免使用美发产品。避免皮肤直接接触化学纤维和皮毛制品。急性湿疮或慢性湿疮急性发作期间，暂缓疫苗接种。

居室安静，床单整洁干燥，衣物干净、宽松、棉质。起居有常，睡眠充足。恢复期可正常开展工作和学习，适当进行户外活动。保持皮肤清洁，及时修剪指甲。若皮肤较干，可使用性质温和的保湿乳。

饮食宜清淡、营养、易消化，少食多餐。多吃高纤维的食物。可食蜂蜜和黑芝麻，以保持大便通畅。湿疮与饮食密切相关，不当饮食极易加重病情。婴儿湿疮者，乳母也应忌口。不宜食油炸、煎烤、炙煿、甜黏、辛辣、油腻的食物。不宜食发物，如辣椒、海鱼、虾蟹、鸡肉、鹅肉、牛肉、羊肉、香菜、韭菜、大葱、大蒜。

加强情志疏导。病人常因奇痒难忍，病情反复而有较大的心理压力，容易出现急躁、恼怒、悲观的情绪。护士应详细介绍湿疮的知识，认真做好解释工作，鼓励病人多参加社交活动，以分散注意力。病人应积极治疗,合理调护,树立战胜疾病的信心。瘙痒时可运用移情易性疗法,如钓鱼、看电视、聊天,避免因过思伤脾导致湿热内生而加重病情。

定期复查,坚持正确用药。若局部有药痂,应清除药痂后再涂药。若用药后出现红斑、瘙痒,应立即停药,并报告医生。出院后若新起皮疹且剧烈瘙痒,应及时就医。

Section 2　Eczema

Eczema is a skin disease clinically characterized by symmetrically-distributed pleomorphic rash with effusion, severe itching and repeated attacks, which is caused by body constitution irresistant to some pathogenic factors and pathogenic wind-dampness-heat attacking the skin. Eczema can be divided into three types according to the course of disease: acute, subacute and chronic ones. The main clinical manifestations of acute patients are papules, blisters, erosion and effusion. The main clinical manifestations of chronic patients are dry desquamation and lichenification. And the main clinical manifestations of subacute patients are between the acute and chronic ones. This section can be referred to for the nursing of eczema in Western medicine.

ETIOLOGY AND PATHOGENESIS

The etiology includes spleen deficiency, dampness-heat and blood deficiency. Spleen deficiency constitution, body constitution irresistant to some pathogenic factors, or excessive intake of pungent spicy foods longly damaging the spleen, all may induce spleen deficiency that causes internal generation of dampness-heat. Thus, dampness-heat spreads on the skin and eczema occurs. Dampness-heat accumulation for longtime consuming yin-blood, or spleen deficiency failing in transportation and transportation, all lead to blood deficiency and wind-dryness as well as malnutrition of the skin. Thus, eczema occurs.

The pathogenesis is dampness-heat spreading on the skin. The disease is located in the skin. Generally speaking, acute eczema belongs to excess syndrome, with dampness-heat spreading on the skin as its main clinical manifestation; subacute eczema belongs to deficiency-excess in complexity, related to dampness encumbering the spleen that causes the spleen to fail in transportation and transformation; chronic eczema belongs to deficiency syndrome induced by chronic illness consuming yin-blood, which causes blood deficiency and wind-dryness.

COMMON SYNDROMES

Key Points in Syndrome Differentiation

1. Differentiation of Deficiency from Excess Syndrome

The differentiation is based on the onset of illness, color, shape and effusion of skin lesion, tongue and pulse manifestations. Generally speaking, excess syndrome shows acute onset, red skin lesion with plenty of effusion, visible papules, red tongue with yellow coating, and slippery rapid pulse. Deficiency syndrome shows slow onset, dark skin lesion with scanty effusion, scales and lichenification as the main symptoms, pale tongue with thin coating, and wiry thready pulse.

2. Differentiation of Dryness from Dampness Syndrome

The differentiation is based on the color, margin, roughness and effusion of skin lesion. Generally speaking, dampness syndrome displays red skin lesion with obscure margins, more papules and plenty of effusion. And dryness syndrome exhibits dark skin lesion with clear margins, rough skin surface, lichenification and scanty effusion.

Syndrome Differentiation

1. Syndrome of Dampness-heat Spreading on the Skin

[Clinical Manifestations] Flushed skin, swelling, erosion and effusion as the main symptoms, visible papule, papulovesicle and blister, conscious scorching heat sensation, itching, red tongue with yellow coating or yellow slimy coating, and slippery rapid pulse.

[Manifestations Analysis] Dampness-heat spreading on the skin and preponderance of heat over dampness contribute to acute onset, flushed skin and scorching heat sensation. Dampness-heat accumulation and mutual contention of qi and blood lead to water diffusion in the skin, causing swelling, erosion and effusion, visible papule, papulovesicle and blister. Such symptoms as red tongue with yellow coating or yellow slimy coating and slippery rapid pulse, all are signs of dampness-heat.

[Nursing Principle] Clearing heat and draining dampness; dispelling wind and relieving itching.

[Suggested Formula] Longdan Xiegan Decoction and Bixie Shenshi Decoction.

2. Syndrome of Spleen Deficiency with Dampness Accumulation

[Clinical Manifestations] Light red erythema, papule, papulovesicle, and scanty effusion as the main symptoms, visible thickening skin; conscious itching, possibly accompanied by reduced appetite, abdominal distention, loose stool, pale enlarged tongue with slimy coating, and soggy or slippery pulse.

[Manifestations Analysis] Spleen deficiency constitution, body constitution irresistant to some pathogenic factors, or excessive intake of pungent spicy foods longly damaging the spleen, all may induce spleen deficiency and dampness that transforms into heat and accumulates in the skin, causing slow onset, light red erythema, papule, papulovesicle and conscious itching. Mutual contention of dampness and heat and preponderance of heat over dampness lead to scanty effusion. Dampness obstructing the middle energizer can cause malfunction of transportation and transformation, resulting in reduced appetite, abdominal distention and loose stool. Such symptoms as pale enlarged tongue with slimy coating, and soggy or slippery pulse, all are signs of spleen deficiency with dampness accumulation syndrome.

[Nursing Principle] Invigorating the spleen and draining dampness; dispelling wind and relieving itching.

[Suggested Formula] Chushi Weiling Decoction and Shenling Baizhu Powder.

3. Blood Deficiency and Wind-Dryness Syndrome

〔Clinical Manifestations〕Thickening skin, scales, lichenification as the main symptoms, visible pigmentation, paroxysmal conscious itching, light red tongue with thin coating, and wiry thready pulse.

〔Manifestations Analysis〕Chronic illness consuming yin blood or insufficiency of the source of generation and transformation can induce blood deficiency that causes malnutrition of the skin, with thickening skin, scales, and lichenification as the main symptoms, and possibly visible pigmentation. Blood deficiency produces wind and dryness, so paroxysmal conscious itching is felt. Such symptoms as light red tongue with thin coating, and wiry thready pulse, all are signs of blood deficiency and wind-dryness.

〔Nursing Principle〕Nourishing blood and moistening dryness; dispelling wind and relieving itching.

〔Suggested Formula〕Siwu Xiaofeng Drink and Danggui Yinzi Decoction.

NURSING MEASURES

For cases with eczema, nurses should observe the color, shape, location, erosion and effusion of the skin lesion; degree of itching; and tongue and pulse manifestations. If the patient has plenty of effusion of the skin lesion, large scale infiltration, severe itching or a body temperature over 38.5℃ with chills, it is advisable to report to the doctor immediately.

Syndrome-Based Nursing Measures

1. Syndrome of Dampness-Heat Spreading on the Skin

（1）Daily life nursing. The ward should be cool, quiet, and full of fresh air. The bedding should be clean and dry, or even changed immediately in the presence of profuse effusion. The clothes should be loose, soft and cotton. The patients should follow a regular routine and get adequate sleep. They should not scratch, rub, or clean with soap or hot water while keeping the skin clean.

（2）Diet nursing. The patients may drink lugen（reed rhizome）tea and jinyinhua（honeysuckle flower）tea and eat foods that clear heat and drain dampness, such as chixiaodou（adzuki bean）, machixian（purslane）and lüdou（mung bean）. Food therapy: donggua yiyiren（Chinese waxgourd and coix seed）soup. They should avoid pungent, spicy and greasy foods or foods that induce or aggravate disease, such as shrimp, chicken, goose, beef, mutton, coriander, Chinese chives, shengjiang（fresh ginger）, scallions and dasuan（garlic bulb）.

（3）Emotion nursing. The patients are prone to irritability, anxiety or pessimism because of unbearable itching. Therefore, the nurses may use verbal enlightenment therapy to impart the patients knowledge of eczema to keep them in a peaceful state of mind. The nurses may also use emotional transference and dispositional change therapy to encourage them to participate in social intercourses to divert attention and eliminate distress. Spleen impairment due to excessive contemplation should be avoided, which can prolong or aggravate illness.

（4）Medication nursing. Decoction should be taken slightly cool or warm after meals.

（5）Manipulation techniques. ① Unction therapy: after shaking Sanhuang Lotion, apply the medicine on the affected area with a cotton swab, once per day. It is suitable for those with erythema, papules and a few blisters without exudation in the early stage. ② Wet compress therapy: huangbai （amur cork-tree bark）20 g, pugongying （dandelion）20 g, machixian （purslane）20 g, shengdiyu （garden burnet root）20 g, and yejuhua （wild chrysanthemum flower）20 g; choose 1~2 kind（s）of medicinals from them to make a decoction; soak 5~6 layers of gauze into the cooling decoction at a temperature of 4~15℃; then apply the gauze on the skin; 20 minutes each time, once per day. It is suitable for cases with blisters, erosion, plenty of effusion or accompanying pain. ③ Paste application therapy: whisk qingdai （natural indigo）powder with sesame oil to make a paste, and apply it to the skin lesions with a thickness of 1~2 millimeter（s）and size of 1~2 centimeter（s）beyond the edge of the redness and swelling, 4~6 hours each time, once a day. It is suitable for illness at late stage when exudation is reduced and skin lesions form scab.

2. Syndrome of Spleen Deficiency with Dampness Accumulation

（1）Daily life nursing. The ward should be warm and quiet. The patients should follow a regular routine and get adequate sleep. They should not scratch, rub, or clean with soap or hot water while keeping the skin clean. They should also avoid overstrain.

（2）Diet nursing. The patients may eat foods that invigorate the spleen and drain dampness, such as shanyao （common yam rhizome）, qianshi （euryale seed）, and lianzi （lotus seed）. Food therapy: fuling （poria）stewed with tortoise. Don't eat raw, cold, fatty and sweet foods or foods that induce or aggravate disease.

（3）Emotion nursing. Due to the prolonged course of disease, the nurses should often make the rounds of the wards and encourage the patients as much as possible, and may use verbal enlightenment therapy to impart the patients knowledge of eczema to keep them in a peaceful state of mind, and build up their confidence in treatment to relieve nervousness and anxiety.

（4）Medication nursing. Decoction should be taken warm.

（5）Manipulation techniques. ① Unction therapy: use huangbai （amur cork-tree bark）cream, qingdai （natural indigo）ointment or 10% diyu （garden burnet root）zinc-oxide oil; apply the medicine to the affected area with cotton swabs, 2~3 times per day. It is suitable for skin lesions without effusion. ② Wet compress therapy: use kushen （light yellow sophora root）decoction or Sanhuang Lotion; soak 5~6 layers of gauze into the cooling decoction at a temperature of 38~41℃; then apply the gauze on the skin or wrap them tightly with bandage; 20 minutes each time, once per day. It is suitable for cases with a little effusion.

3. Blood Deficiency and Wind-dryness Syndrome

（1）Daily life nursing. The ward should be quiet. The patients should live a regular life and get adequate sleep. They should not scratch, rub, or clean with soap or hot water while keeping the skin clean. They should also avoid overstrain.

（2）Diet nursing. The patients may drink heidou（black soybean）drink and eat foods that nourish blood and dispel wind, such as wushaoshe（black-tail snake）, dazao（Chinese date）, yin'er（tremella）and clam meat. Food therapy: sangshen baihe（mulberry and lily bulb）soup. Don't eat pungent, spicy, dry-natured and fire-generating foods or foods that induce or aggravate disease.

（3）Emotion nursing. Due to the prolonged course of disease, the nurses should encourage the patients as much as possible, and may use verbal enlightenment therapy to impart the patients knowledge of eczema to keep them in a peaceful state of mind, and build up their confidence in treatment to prevent depression.

（4）Medication nursing. Decoction should be brewed slowly over low heat and taken warm before meals.

（5）Manipulation techniques. ① Unction therapy combined with wrapping therapy: use qingdai（natural indigo）ointment, 5% sulphur ointment or black soybean oil ointment; apply the medicine of one millimeter thickness to the affected area with cotton swabs, then cover it with plastic wrap, 1～3 hour（s）each time, twice per day. There is no need to wash out the oil stains and it is only suitable for thickening skin lesions without effusion and infection. ② Acupressure therapy: select Sanyinjiao（SP 6）, Xuehai（SP 10）, Zusanli（ST 36）, and Shenmen（HT 7）; apply soft and slow thumb kneading manipulation on each of them till the local area turns hot or feels soreness, numbness and heaviness and distension, once per day. And it is contraindicated in pregnancy. ③ Auricular pressure therapy: select lung（CO14）, shenmen（TF4）, adrenal gland（TG2p）, subcortex（AT4）, and sympathetic（AH6a）; apply specialized pasters on them, press and knead each of them till the area turns hot and red, 4～5 times per day, and keep the pasters for 2～4 days. And it is contraindicated in pregnancy.

Patient Education

Patients should have allergen testing. They should not scratch, rub or touch skin lesion. Cold and heat should be avoided and the temperature of bath water should not be high. They should also avoid washing or cleaning skin lesion with saline water, Sichuan pricklyash peel water, alkaline soap or bath liquid, using irritating cosmetics as well as contacting chemical fibers and fur products. Patients with eczema on the head should keep themselves away from hair care products. During the course of acute eczema or acute attacks of chronic eczema, vaccination should be postponed.

The room should be quiet. The patients' sheets should be clean and dry. The patients should wear baggy, soft and cotton clothes. They should live a regular life and get adequate sleep. During the convalescent period, the patients can work and study normally and engage in outdoor activities appropriately. Keep the skin clean, and trim the nails. In case of dry skin, patients can use mild moisturizer.

The diet should be light, nutritious and digestible. The patients should have small frequent meals and plenty of foods rich in fiber. Honey and sesame seeds are beneficial to maintain smooth bowel movement. Eczema and diet are closely related, improper diet may easily aggravate the disease. For infants with eczema, their lactating mothers should also follow dietary restrictions. Don't eat fried, roasted, sweet, pungent, spicy and greasy foods or foods that induce or aggravate disease, such as chili, sea fish, shrimp, crab, chicken, goose, beef, mutton, coriander, Chinese chives, scallions and dasuan (garlic bulb).

Nurses should give patients more psychological support. Because of unbearable itching and relapse of illness, the patients are prone to irritability, agitation or pessimism under considerable psychological stress. Nurses should adequately inform the patients about eczema and encourage them to participate in social intercourses in order to distract attention, and increase their confidence in overcoming illness through active treatment and proper nursing care. When itch occurs, emotional transference and dispositional change therapy can be used, such as fishing, watching TV and chatting. Spleen impairment due to excessive contemplation should be avoided because it generates internal dampness-heat and aggravates the condition.

The patients should go back to the hospital for regular checks, and persist in correct use of medicine. Local medicine scab should be removed before applying medicine. In the presence of erythema and itchiness after medication, stop using the medicine and inform the doctor immediately. After their discharge from hospital, patients should seek immediate medical care when new severe itchy rash emerges.

第三节　蛇　串　疮

蛇串疮，是指因肝脾湿热，或肝经火盛，循经蕴肤，导致湿热火毒蕴积肌肤，以成簇疱疹沿身体单侧呈带状分布，初起为红斑，随即为丘疹、水疱，累累如串珠，剧烈疼痛，灼痛或针刺样痛，或部分破溃，局部渗液，干燥结痂、脱落，可伴见臖核肿痛为临床特征的皮肤病。西医的带状疱疹可参照本节进行护理。

一、病因病机

蛇串疮的病因多为情志内伤、饮食不节和感染毒邪。病人情志不畅，肝郁化火，火毒夹风邪外溢肌肤，可发为蛇串疮。饮食不节，脾虚生湿，复感毒邪，湿热与毒邪阻滞经络，外溢肌肤，亦可发为蛇串疮。病人年老体虚，血虚肝旺，湿热毒蕴，壅滞经脉，以致疼痛剧烈，病程迁延。

蛇串疮的病机是湿热毒邪，阻滞经络，气滞血瘀，外溢肌肤。病位在皮肤，与肝、脾、肾有关。蛇串疮初期以湿热火毒为主，后期为正气虚弱，湿毒瘀滞。

二、常见证型

（一）辨证要点

1. 辨虚实　根据皮损的颜色、疼痛程度，大便情况，以及舌脉等来辨别。若皮损鲜红，刺痛，大便干结，舌红苔黄，脉弦滑数，多为实证。若皮损颜色较淡，疼痛不剧烈，大便时溏，舌淡苔白，脉沉缓或滑，则多为虚证。

2. 辨初期与后期　根据皮损的持续时间、颜色和疼痛程度等来辨别。若皮损新起，鲜红，刺痛，多为初期。若皮损色淡，疼痛不剧烈，或皮疹完全消退仅留神经痛，迁延数月难愈，则多为后期。

（二）证候分型

1. 肝经郁热证

［主要证候］皮损鲜红，疱壁紧张，灼热刺痛；口苦咽干，烦躁易怒，大便干或小便黄；舌质红，舌苔薄黄或黄厚，脉弦滑数。

［证候分析］肝郁化火，外溢肌肤，故皮损鲜红，疱壁紧张；火毒阻滞经络，气血不通，故灼热刺痛；肝火夹胆气上溢，故口苦；心藏神，肝藏魂，热扰神魂，故烦躁易怒；火热灼津，故咽干，大便干或小便黄；舌质红，舌苔薄黄或黄厚，脉弦滑数，均为火热之象。

［护治原则］清肝泻火，活血解毒。

［常用方剂］龙胆泻肝汤。

2. 脾虚湿蕴证

［主要证候］皮损颜色较淡，疱壁松弛；口不渴，食少腹胀，大便时溏；舌质淡，舌苔白或白腻，脉沉缓或滑。

［证候分析］脾虚生湿,阻滞经络,外溢肌肤,故皮肤出现水疱;湿盛于热,故皮损颜色较淡,疱壁松弛;湿阻中焦,脾失健运,故食少腹胀;脾虚失运,水湿下注,故大便时溏;湿为阴邪,津液未伤,故口不渴;舌质淡,舌苔白或白腻,脉沉缓或滑,均为内湿蕴结之象。

［护治原则］健脾化湿,清热解毒。

［常用方剂］除湿胃苓汤。

3. 气滞血瘀证

［主要证候］常见于本病的恢复期及后遗神经痛期,皮疹消退后局部疼痛不止;倦怠乏力,大便秘结;舌质暗,苔白,脉弦细。

［证候分析］湿热毒邪虽退,但正气未复,气血阻滞,故皮疹消退后局部疼痛不止;正气未复,无力推动,故倦怠乏力,大便秘结;舌质暗,苔白,脉弦细,均为气滞血瘀之象。

［护治原则］理气活血,化瘀通络。

［常用方剂］血府逐瘀汤合金铃子散。

三、护理措施

对于蛇串疮的病人,应观察皮损的部位;疼痛的部位、性质、程度、持续时间及诱发因素;水疱的大小、数目、疱液性状、疱壁紧张度,以及有无继发感染。若病人出现头痛、耳痛、眼痛、耳聋、面瘫、呕吐、惊厥、味觉障碍或运动感觉障碍,考虑为严重的并发症,应立即报告医生。

（一）辨证施护

1. 肝经郁热证

（1）生活起居护理 居室安静凉爽,光线柔和,空气新鲜。床单和衣被整洁干燥,衣物宽松、柔软、棉质。多卧床休息,取健侧卧位以防止压破水疱。勤洗手,经常修剪指甲,避免搔抓皮损,忌用热水烫洗皮损。

（2）饮食护理 清淡饮食。多饮水,可饮金银花茶、菊花茶。多吃新鲜的水果和蔬菜,以保持大便通畅。宜食清热解毒的食物,如荸荠、绿豆。马齿苋粥:马齿苋100~200 g,洗净后切成小段,加大米适量,煮成稀粥。忌发物,如虾、蟹、鸡肉、鹅肉、牛肉、羊肉。不宜食辛辣的食物,如辣椒、胡椒、大蒜。

（3）情志护理 病人情志内伤,皮损疼痛,容易出现焦虑、烦躁、易怒的情绪,护士可运用语言开导疗法,向病人讲解疾病的相关知识,多与病人沟通交流,使其心情愉快,避免顾虑、恐惧。或用移情易性疗法,如聊天、看电视,以转移注意力。应取得家属的积极配合,为病人营造宽松愉悦的环境,以使其保持情绪稳定,避免不良情志刺激。

（4）用药护理 中药汤剂宜饭后温服。不宜久服,以免损伤正气。若服药后病人出现食欲减退,恶心呕吐,腹痛便溏,应立即报告医生。

（5）操作技术 ① 湿敷疗法:用三黄洗剂,或用浓茶水调青黛散;以5~6层纱布浸湿药液后湿敷患处,每次20分钟,每日3次,操作时动作应尽量轻柔、迅速;适用于皮损初起者。② 邮票贴敷法:用板蓝根、银花叶、木贼、虎杖、野菊花、黄柏各30 g,煎水;将单层纱布剪裁成创面的形状,蘸取冷却的药液,贴敷于裸露渗出的创面上,每日3次;适用于脓疱清创后的创面。③ 穴位按摩法:取阳陵泉、行间、太冲、肝俞、三阴交,用拇指揉法,力度大、速度快,按摩至局部发热或有酸麻重胀感,每日1次;孕妇禁用。

2. 脾虚湿蕴证

（1）生活起居护理　居室安静干燥,整洁明亮,空气新鲜。床单和衣被整洁干燥,衣物宽松、柔软、棉质。多卧床休息,睡眠充足。适量进行轻缓的运动,如散步、打太极拳。

（2）饮食护理　可饮柠檬豆芽汤。宜食健脾利湿的食物,如山药、赤小豆。薏苡仁粥:薏苡仁30~60 g,洗净,加适量大米,煮成稀粥;薏苡仁性微寒,若脾虚不耐,可加少许生姜汁。不宜食生冷、油腻的食物。

（3）情志护理　病人的病程迁延,可能出现抑郁的情绪。护士可运用语言开导疗法和移情易性疗法,主动关心病人,消除病人的顾虑,转移其注意力,以保持情绪稳定,防止因过思伤脾而加重病情。

（4）用药护理　中药汤剂宜饭前温服。若病人胃肠不适,可在饭后服用。向病人讲解除湿胃苓汤有利尿作用,不必因尿多而紧张。

（5）操作技术　① 敷脐疗法:土茯苓20 g,艾叶、干姜、栀子、泽兰、白芷、草豆蔻、吴茱萸各10 g;合而研磨成粉后与蜂蜜调成糊状,纳入脐中,用胶布固定后用热水袋加温,温度以自觉温热舒适为度,每次1小时,每日2次,结束后用温水洗净脐部。② 穴位按摩法:取阴陵泉、足三里、内庭、三阴交,用拇指揉法,力度不宜过大,按摩至局部发热或有酸麻重胀感,每日1次;孕妇禁用。

3. 气滞血瘀证

（1）生活起居护理　居室安静温暖,光线柔和,空气新鲜。床单和衣被整洁干燥。衣物宽松、柔软、棉质。多卧床休息,睡眠充足。适量进行轻缓的运动,如散步、打太极拳。

（2）饮食护理　宜食行气活血的食物,如山楂、白萝卜、陈皮、木瓜。不宜食过甜、易产气的食物。

（3）情志护理　病人的病程迁延,可能会抑郁、消沉,护士可运用语言开导疗法,主动关心病人,为病人讲解疾病的知识,以消除病人的顾虑。或运用移情易性疗法,建议病人多参加社交活动,以行气活血,保持情绪稳定。

（4）用药护理　中药汤剂宜饭后温服。

（5）操作技术　① 涂药法:取黄连膏;用棉签蘸药物涂于患处,每日1次;次日用甘草油将药膏轻轻清除干净。② 穴位按摩法:取肝俞、天枢、三阴交、血海以及阿是穴（原皮损部位）,用拇指揉法,按摩至局部发热或有酸麻重胀感,每日1次;孕妇禁用。③ 耳压疗法:取肺、肝、神门、内分泌、皮质下、肾上腺等耳穴,用耳穴压丸贴片贴压,每日按揉4~5次,以局部发热泛红为度,留置2~4日;孕妇禁用。

（二）健康教育

保持皮损干燥清洁,预防感染。若水疱较大,可用消毒空针抽吸疱液,保留疱皮,进行创面清洁。对于水疱破溃已有感染者,可用纱条蘸取双黄连液敷贴。病人应修剪指甲,避免摩擦和搔抓皮损。当皮损累及眼部时,白天每2~3小时滴1次眼药水,平时应多眨眼,避免强光刺激。注意观察眼部病情变化及视力的变化,防止发生眼睑粘连及溃疡性角膜炎。当皮损位于头皮、腋下、会阴部时,应剪去局部毛发。忌用热水和肥皂烫洗皮损。

对于免疫力低下者、婴幼儿及老年病人,应进行保护性隔离。安排病床时,可住单间。不能住单间者,应保持病室空气清新,不要与免疫力低下的病人同住。

起居有常,劳逸适度。注意天气变化,避免感冒。保持大便通畅。

饮食宜清淡、营养、易消化。多饮水,多吃新鲜的水果和蔬菜。戒烟限酒,不宜食发物和甜黏、辛辣、油腻的食物,如生姜、大蒜、辣椒、公鸡肉、牛肉、羊肉、香菜。

保持心情舒畅,忌发怒、忧虑。护士可向病人及家属宣教情志因素对于疾病的影响,为病人讲解疾病的相关知识及治疗成功的经验,以帮助病人树立信心,更好地配合治疗。

Section 3   Herpes Zoster

Herpes zoster, a kind of skin disease, is clinically characterized by clusters of zonal-distributed blisters along one side of the body, initial presence of red spots followed by beads-stringed papules and blisters, severe scorching pain or stabbing pain, partial diabrosis and localized exudation, dry crust or decrustation, and possible swollen lymph nodes. It is caused by dampness-heat in the liver and spleen or exuberant fire in the liver meridian that transmits along the meridian or amasses in the skin. This section can be referred to for the nursing of herpes zoster in Western medicine.

ETIOLOGY AND PATHOGENESIS

The etiology includes emotional internal damage, improper diet and contraction of pathogenic toxin. Emotional depression causes liver depression transforming into fire that intermingles with wind pathogen to outthrust externally into the skin, so herpes zoster occurs. Improper diet causes spleen deficiency and dampness generation, with which pathogenic toxin obstruct meridian and collaterals and outthrust externally into the skin, so herpes zoster occurs. Old age with weak constitution, blood deficiency with liver fire effulgence, dampness-heat-toxin accumulation and congestion in the meridian are responsible for severe pain and prolonged course of disease.

The pathogenesis is dampness-heat-toxin accumulation and congestion in the meridian that causes qi stagnation and blood stasis, and outthrusts externally into the skin. The disease is located in the skin, but related to the liver, spleen and kidney. Herpes zoster in the early stage is mainly associated with dampness-heat and fire-toxin whereas in the later stage, healthy qi deficiency and dampness-toxin stagnation.

COMMON SYNDROMES

Key Points in Syndrome Differentiation

1. Differentiation of Deficiency from Excess Syndrome

The differentiation is based on the color of skin lesions, the degree of pain, the characteristics of stool, and the manifestations of tongue and pulse. Bright red skin lesions, stabbing pain, dry stool, red tongue with yellow coating, and wiry, slippery and rapid pulse indicate excess syndrome. And light-colored skin lesion, slight pain, frequent loose stool, pale tongue with white coating, and sunken, moderate or slippery pulse are manifestations of deficiency syndrome.

2. Differentiation of Initial from Final Stage

The differentiation is based on the duration, color and pain severity of skin lesions. Initial stage shows new skin lesions with bright red color and stabbing pain. And final stage displays light-colored skin lesion, slight pain, or only neuralgia after disappearance of herpes that may last for several months and is difficult to heal.

Syndrome Differentiation

1. Syndrome of Heat Depression in the Liver Meridian

[Clinical Manifestations] Bright red skin lesions, tight blister wall, burning stabbing pain, bitter mouth, dry throat, dysphoria, irascibility, dry stool or dark urine, red tongue with thin yellow or yellow thick coating, and wiry, slippery and rapid pulse.

[Manifestations Analysis] Emotional depression causes liver depression transforming into fire that outthrusts externally into the skin, resulting in bright red skin lesions and tight blister wall. Fire-heat and toxin pathogen obstructing meridian and collateral leads to blockage of qi and blood, causing burning stabbing pain. Liver is a firm-characterized zang organ. Heat is depressed in liver meridian and liver fire gathers with gallbladder qi to flow upwards, causing bitter taste in mouth. Heart stores spirit and liver stores soul, so heat harassing spirit and soul causes dysphoria and irascibility. Fire-heat scorching fluids leads to dry throat, dry stool or dark urine. Red tongue with thin yellow or yellow thick coating and wiry, slippery and rapid pulse, all are manifestations of heat.

[Nursing Principle] Clearing the liver and reducing fire; activating blood and removing toxin.

[Suggested Formula] Longdan Xiegan Decoction.

2. Spleen Deficiency and Dampness Accumulation Syndrome

[Clinical Manifestations] Light-colored skin lesion, loose blister wall, no thirst, reduced appetite, abdominal distention, frequent loose stool, pale tongue with white or slimy white coating, and sunken, moderate or slippery pulse.

[Manifestations Analysis] Improper diet causes spleen deficiency and dampness generation, with which pathogenic toxin obstruct meridian and collaterals and outthrust externally into the skin, causing blisters. Preponderance of dampness over heat explains light-colored skin lesion and loose blister wall. Pathogenic dampness obstructs in middle energizer causes dysfunction of the spleen in transportation and transformation, resulting in reduced appetite and abdominal distention. Dysfunction of the spleen in transportation and transformation makes it unable to separate the lucid from the turbid and causes water-dampness pouring down, resulting in loose stool. As yin pathogen, dampness causes no damage to fluids, so there is no thirst. Pale tongue with white or slimy white coating and sunken, moderate or slippery pulse, all are manifestations of dampness.

[Nursing Principle] Invigorating the spleen and resolving dampness; clearing heat and removing toxin.

[Suggested Formula] Chushi Weiling Decoction.

3. Qi Stagnation and Blood Stasis Syndrome

〔Clinical Manifestations〕It is common in the convalescence and sequelae neuralgia period of this disease. Persistent neuralgia after disappearance of herpes, fatigue, constipation, dark tongue with white coating, and wiry thready pulse.

〔Manifestations Analysis〕Although dampness-heat and toxin pathogen are removed, healthy qi has not been recovered and qi and blood are still obstructed, showing persistent neuralgia after disappearance of herpes. Unrecovered healthy qi is powerless to propel the movement of qi and blood, causing fatigue and constipation. Dark tongue with white coating, and wiry thready pulse, all are manifestations of qi stagnation and blood stasis.

〔Nursing Principle〕Regulating qi and activating blood; resolving stasis and dredging collateral.

〔Suggested Formula〕Xuefu Zhuyu Decoction and Jinlingzi Powder.

NURSING MEASURES

For patients with herpes zoster, nurses should observe the location of skin lesions; the location, nature, degree, duration and predisposing factors of pain; the size and number of blisters; the properties and form of blister fluid; the tension of blister wall; and the presence or absence of the secondary infection. If the patient has headache, earache, eye pain, deafness, facial paralysis, vomiting, convulsions, dysgeusia or dysmotility, which is considered as a serious complication, it is advisable to timely report to the doctor.

Syndrome-Based Nursing Measures

1. Syndrome of Heat Depression in the Liver Meridian

(1) Daily life nursing. The ward should be quiet and cool, with soft light and fresh air. The bedding should be dry and clean and the clothes should be baggy, soft and cotton. The patients should rest in bed and lie on the healthy side to prevent crushing the blisters, often wash hands, trim finger nails, and avoid scratching the skin lesions and washing the local skin with hot water.

(2) Diet nursing. The diet should be light. The patients should drink more water, may drink jinyinhua (honeysuckle) tea and juhua (chrysanthemum flower) tea and eat more fresh fruit and vegetables to keep a normal bowel movement. They may eat heat-clearing and toxin-removing foods, such as biqi (waternut) and lüdou (mung bean). Purslane porridge is recommended: prepare 100~200 g of purslane, wash and cut into small pieces, add in an appropriate amount of rice, and make them into thin porridge. Don't eat foods that induce or aggravate disease, such as shrimp, crab, chicken, goose, beef and lamb, or pungent and spicy foods such as chili, hujiao (pepper fruit) and dasuan (garlic bulb).

(3) Emotion nursing. Because of emotional internal damage and painful skin lesions, the patients are prone to anxiety, dysphoria and irritability. Nurses may use verbal enlightenment therapy to impart the disease-related knowledge to the patients and talk with them as much as possible to make them feel

happy and eliminate worries and fears. Nurses may also use emotional transference and dispositional change therapy, such as chatting and watching TV, to distract their attention. Nurses should try to gain the active cooperation of patients' family members to create a relaxed and pleasant environment for the patients to keep good moods and prevent unhealthy emotional stimulation.

(4) Medication nursing. Decoction should be taken warm after meals; however, it cannot be taken for a long term, so as not to damage the healthy qi of the body. If the patient experiences loss of appetite, nausea, vomiting, abdominal pain and loose stool during medication, nurses should report to the doctor in a timely manner.

(5) Manipulation techniques. ① Wet compress therapy: apply 5~6 layers of gauze to the affected area after soaking in Sanhuang Lotion, or with Qingdai Powder blended with strong tea, 20 minutes each time, three times a day, act as gently and fast as possible during manipulation. The therapy is suitable for patients with initial skin lesions. ② Stamp-like application therapy: Use banlan'gen (isatis root), yinhuaye (honeysuckle leaf), muzei (common scouring rush), huzhang (giant knotweed rhizome), yejuhua (wild chrysanthemum flower) and huangbai (amur cork-tree bark), 30 g each, boil with hot water; cut a single layer of gauze into the shape of the wound, dip in the cooled liquid medicine, and apply it to the exposed wound, three times per day. It is suitable for the wound surface after debridement of pustules. ③ Acupressure therapy: Select Yinlingquan (SP 9), Xingjian (LR 2), Taichong (LR 3), Ganshu (BL 18) and Sanyinjiao (SP 6), use thumb kneading manipulation on each of them with considerable force at high speed until the area turns hot or the patient has the feelings of soreness, numbness, distension and heaviness in the area; once per day. And it is contraindicated in pregnancy.

2. Spleen Deficiency and Dampness Accumulation Syndrome

(1) Daily life nursing. The ward should be quiet, dry, clean, bright, and full of fresh air. The bedding should be dry and clean and the clothes should be baggy, soft and cotton. Patients should rest in bed more to ensure adequate sleep and may take gentle exercise, such as walking and Taiji.

(2) Diet nursing. The patients may drink ningmeng douya (lemon and bean sprouts) tea and eat foods that invigorate the spleen and drain dampness, such as shanyao (common yam rhizome), and chixiaodou (adzuki bean). Yiyiren (coix seed) porridge is recommended: prepare 30~60 g of yiyiren (coix seed), wash them, add an appropriate amount of rice, and make them into thin porridge; because the property of yiyiren (coix seed) is slightly cold, small amounts of shengjiang (fresh ginger) juice could be added in case of intolerance of cold due to spleen deficiency. Don't eat raw, cold and greasy foods.

(3) Emotion nursing. Due to the prolonged course of the disease, the patients may experience depression. Nurses may use verbal enlightenment therapy and emotional transference and dispositional change therapy, take the initiative to care for them to remove their worries. It is recommended to distract their attention to maintain emotional stability of the patients and prevent damaging the spleen due to overthinking and aggravating the condition.

(4) Medication nursing. Decoction should be taken warm before meals. If the patients have

gastrointestinal discomfort, the decoction can be taken after meals. Explain to the patients the diuretic effect of Chushi Weiling Decoction that there is no need to be nervous about the excessive urine.

(5) Manipulation techniques. ① Umbilical compress therapy: grind into powder tufuling (glabrous greenbrier rhizome) 20 g, aiye (mugwort leaf) 10 g, ganjiang (dried ginger rhizome) 10 g, zhizi (gardenia)10 g, zelan (hirsute shiny bugleweed herb) 10 g, baizhi (angelica root) 10 g, caodoukou (katsumadai) 10 g, and wuzhuyu (medicinal evodia fruit) 10 g; blend the powder with honey into a paste, apply it in the umbilicus, fix it with an adhesive tape and warm it with a hot water bag at a comfortable temperature, one hour each time, and twice per day. After the therapy, wash the umbilicus with warm water. ② Acupressure therapy: select Yinlingquan (SP 9), Zusanli (ST 36), Neiting (ST 44) and Sanyinjiao (SP 6); use thumb kneading manipulation on each of them until the area turns hot or the patient has the feelings of soreness, numbness, distension and heaviness in the area; once per day. And it is contraindicated in pregnancy.

3. Qi Stagnation and Blood Stasis Syndrome

(1) Daily life nursing. The ward should be quiet, warm, and full of gentle light and fresh air. The bedding should be dry and clean and the clothes should be baggy, soft and cotton. Patients should rest in bed more to ensure adequate sleep and may take gentle exercise, such as walking and Taiji.

(2) Diet nursing. The patients may have qi-moving and blood-activating foods, such as shanzha (Chinese hawthorn fruit), white radish, chenpi (dried tangerine peel) and mugua (Chinese quince fruit). Don't eat too-sweet or flatulent foods.

(3) Emotion nursing. Due to the prolonged course of disease, the patients may experience depression. Nurses may use verbal enlightenment therapy, take the initiative to care for them, and share the knowledge of the disease with them to remove their worries. Or use emotional transference and dispositional change therapy, encourage the patients to participate in more social intercourses to move qi and activate blood, and maintain emotional stability.

(4) Medication nursing. Decoction should be taken warm after meals.

(5) Manipulation techniques. ① Ointment application therapy: use Huanglian Ointment; smear the ointment on the skin lesions with cotton swab, once per day, and gently wipe away the ointment the next day with gancao (licorice root) oil. ② Acupressure therapy: Select Ganshu (BL 18), Tianshu (ST 25), Sanyinjiao (SP 6), Xuehai (SP 10) and Ashi (the original lesion spot), use thumb kneading manipulation on each of them until the area turns hot or the patient has the feelings of soreness, numbness, distension and heaviness in the area; once per day. And it is contraindicated in pregnancy. ③ Articular pressure therapy: Select lung (CO14), liver (CO12), shenmen (TF4), endocrine (CO18), subcortical (AT4) and adrenal gland (TG2p); apply specialized pasters on them, press on each of them till the area turns hot and red, 4 ~ 5 times per day, and keep the pasters for 2 ~ 4 days. And it is contraindicated in pregnancy.

Patient Education

Keep the wound surface clean and dry to prevent infection. If there are big blisters, a sterilized syringe can be used to draw fluid from the blisters, keep the outer skin of the blister, and disinfect the wound surface. For those who have infection due to blister rupture, apply Shuanghuanglian Lotion on the skin with gauze strips. It is recommended that patients trim their nails as well as avoid rubbing and scratching skin lesions. When skin lesions affect the eyes, administer eye drops, once every 2~3 hours during the daytime. Ask the patients to blink eyes frequently, and avoid strong light stimulation. Closely observe the disease condition of the eyes and vision change to prevent aganoblepharon and ulcerative keratitis. When skin lesions occur on the scalp, underarms or perineal region, cut the hair of the area. Avoid washing skin lesions with hot water or soap.

Patients with impaired immunity, infants, young children and the elderly should undergo protective quarantine. The patients should live in a single room if possible. For patients who cannot live in a single room, they should keep fresh air in the ward and not live with patients who have compromised immunity.

The patients should live a regular life, and balance work and rest. Be aware of sudden weather change to prevent colds. Keep a normal bowel movement.

The diet should be light, nutritious and digestible. The patients should drink more water, and eat more fresh fruit and vegetables. The patients should refrain from cigarette and alcohol. Too-sweet, sticky, spicy, pungent, and greasy foods should be avoided. Don't eat foods that induce or aggravate disease, such as shengjiang (fresh ginger), dasuan (garlic bulb), chili, rooster meat, beef, mutton and coriander.

The patients should maintain a good mentality, and avoid getting angry or anxious. Nurses should inform patients and their families about the impact of emotional factors on the disease, share the disease-related knowledge and experience of successful treatment, and help the patients build up confidence to effectively cooperate with the doctors during treatment.

第四节 痔 疮

痔疮,泛指因脏腑本虚,或外感风湿,内蕴热毒,导致肛门气血纵横、筋脉交错、结滞不散的一类肛肠病。痔疮包括内痔、外痔、混合痔等。西医的痔可参照本节进行护理。

一、病因病机

痔疮的病因多为外感、过劳、饮食不节、情志内伤、妊娠多产和大便失调。病人外受风湿燥热之邪,津伤便结,瘀血浊气阻于肛门,可发为痔疮。久坐、久立、久行,或房劳过度,暗耗气血津液,中气下陷,经络瘀阻,可发为痔疮。病人过食肥腻炙煿辛辣的食物,积生湿热,下注肛门,可发为痔疮。情志久郁化火,气机失调,内生湿热,下注肛门,可发为痔疮。病人多产或经产用力,气血不畅,肛门血脉瘀滞,或产后血虚津亏,肠燥便秘,排便时临厕久蹲,努责用力,血瘀气陷,均可发为痔疮。病人素体湿热,化燥便结,或久泻伤气,气血不畅,阻于肛门,亦可发为痔疮。

痔疮的病机为脏腑功能失调,气血湿热郁滞于肛门,经络阻隔,血脉瘀滞,冲突为痔。日久气虚,中气下陷,不能摄纳则痔核突出。病位在肛门、直肠,与肺、脾、大肠有关。病性为本虚标实。

二、常见证型

（一）辨证要点

1. 辨虚实 根据出血的颜色、质地,以及舌脉等来辨别。若血色鲜红,如射如滴,苔黄,脉数,多为实证。若血色清淡,面色少华,神疲倦怠,舌淡苔白,脉细弱,则多为虚证。

2. 辨内痔与外痔 根据发病部位和主要症状来辨别。若痔位于肛管齿状线以上,主要症状是便血,多为内痔。若痔位于肛管齿状线以下,主要症状是肛门坠胀、疼痛和异物感,则多为外痔。

（二）证候分型

1. 风伤肠络证

[主要证候] 大便滴血、射血或带血,血色鲜红;大便干结,肛门瘙痒,口干咽燥;舌红,苔黄,脉浮数。

[证候分析] 外感六淫,化热生风,或肝郁化火生风,风热下冲肛门,热伤肠络,血不循经而溢于脉外,或便结擦伤痔核血络,故大便滴血、射血或带血;热灼津液,故血色鲜红,大便干结;风邪致病,故肛门瘙痒;舌红,苔黄,脉浮数,均为风热之象。

[护治原则] 凉血祛风。

[常用方剂] 凉血地黄汤。

2. 湿热下注证

［主要证候］便血色鲜红,量较多,肛门肿物外脱、肿胀、灼热疼痛或有滋水;便干或溏,小便短赤;舌质红,苔黄腻,脉数。

［证候分析］外感湿邪,日久化热,或久食肥甘,内生湿热,湿热下注,灼伤血络,故便血色鲜,量较多;湿热互结,下注大肠,蕴阻肛门,故肛门肿物外脱、肿胀、灼热疼痛或有滋水;舌质红,苔黄腻,脉数,均为湿热之象。

［护治原则］清热燥湿。

［常用方剂］槐花散。

3. 气滞血瘀证

［主要证候］肿物脱出肛外、水肿,内有血栓形成,或有嵌顿,表面紫暗、糜烂、渗液,疼痛剧烈,触痛明显,肛管紧缩;大便秘结,小便不利;舌质紫暗或有瘀斑,脉弦或涩。

［证候分析］气机郁滞日久,气滞血瘀阻于肛门,故肿物脱出肛外、水肿,或有嵌顿,表面紫暗、糜烂、渗液,疼痛剧烈,触痛明显,肛管紧缩;气机不畅,统摄无力,血不循经,故甚则内有血栓形成;舌质紫暗或有瘀斑,脉弦或涩,均为气滞血瘀之象。

［护治原则］活血消肿。

［常用方剂］活血散瘀汤。

4. 脾虚气陷证

［主要证候］肿物脱出肛外,不易复位,肛门坠胀,排便乏力,便血色淡;面色少华,头晕神疲,食少乏力,少气懒言;舌淡胖,苔薄白,脉细弱。

［证候分析］脾气虚弱,中气下陷,固摄无力,故肿物脱出肛外,不易复位,肛门坠胀,排便乏力;脾不统血,气虚无以生血,故便血色淡;脾虚运化失常,故食少;脾虚气血不足,故面色少华,头晕神疲,乏力,少气懒言;舌淡,苔薄白,脉细弱,均为脾虚之象。

［护治原则］益气升提。

［常用方剂］补中益气汤。

三、护理措施

对于痔疮的病人,应观察排便的时段、频次;大便的量、干燥程度;便血的次数、时机;出血的量、色、质;便后有无肿物脱出;脱出物的大小、颜色,表面有无糜烂、分泌物,能否自行回纳、能否用手推回;肛门疼痛或瘙痒的部位、性质、程度和持续时间。若病人发生痔核嵌顿,或者突发血栓外痔,或者长期出血量多,突发面色苍白,脉搏加快,血压下降,头晕心慌,应立即报告医生。

（一）辨证施护

1. 风伤肠络证

（1）生活起居护理 居室凉爽安静,空气新鲜。取侧卧位休息。保持肛周皮肤清洁干燥。避风,防止外感风邪。

（2）饮食护理 多饮水,可饮槐花茶、丝瓜汁。多吃新鲜的水果和蔬菜,如芹菜、西瓜、香蕉。宜食疏风清热的食物,如荷叶、藕节。不宜食辛辣的食物。

(3)情志护理　病人的疾病新起,护士可运用语言开导疗法,耐心为病人解释便血的原因,使病人保持平和的心态,消除恐惧心理。

(4)用药护理　中药汤剂宜武火快煎,饭后温服。服后加盖衣被,使其微微汗出。

(5)操作技术　①熏洗疗法:用芒硝、金银花、连翘,择一煮沸,水温50~70℃时熏蒸肛周,水温降至37~40℃时淋洗、坐浴,每次5分钟,每日2次;若痒甚,可加花椒;女性月经期或妊娠期禁用。②浸洗疗法:排便后用荆防散浸洗肛周;女性月经期或妊娠期禁用。③湿敷疗法:用五倍子汤或苦参汤;以5~6层纱布浸透38~41℃的药液敷于肛周,每次20分钟,每日1次;女性月经期或妊娠期禁用。

2. 湿热下注证

(1)生活起居护理　居室安静凉爽。卧床休息,取侧卧位。避免久坐、久站。保持肛周皮肤清洁干燥。保持大便畅通,排便时不可久蹲或过于用力。便血量较多时应停止排便,尽量减少搬动身体和肛门部位的检查。

(2)饮食护理　多饮水,可饮菊花茶、蒲公英茶、金银花茶。宜食清热利湿的食物,如荸荠、芹菜、槐花、赤小豆、薏苡仁、马齿苋、鱼腥草。食疗方:绿豆冬瓜汤。若出血,可食煮柿饼。不宜食辛辣的食物。

(3)情志护理　病人便血量多,护士可运用移情易性疗法,如读书、看报、听音乐,以转移病人的注意力,使病人保持平和的心态,避免烦躁、恐惧。或运用语言开导疗法,关心体贴病人,为病人讲解本病的常见症状和治疗方法,介绍同类病人的治疗和康复情况,增强病人对于治疗的信心。

(4)用药护理　中药汤剂宜饭后温服或偏凉服。

(5)操作技术　①熏洗疗法:用苦参汤加减;熏洗前排空二便,水温50~70℃时熏蒸,水温降至37~40℃时浸泡、淋洗,每次5分钟,每日2次;若出现皮疹、瘙痒,应立即停止;女性月经期或妊娠期禁用。②涂药法:用九华膏或三黄膏;用棉签蘸药物涂于肛周,每日2次;女性月经期或妊娠期禁用。③刮痧疗法:取大肠俞、腰阳关、天枢、大横,以皮肤出现潮红或起痧为度;女性月经期或妊娠期禁用。④药栓疗法:用肛泰栓或牛黄痔清栓,便后或睡前纳肛;适用于外痔者,女性月经期或妊娠期禁用。

3. 气滞血瘀证

(1)生活起居护理　居室温暖舒适,空气新鲜。卧床休息,取侧卧位,避免久站、久蹲、久坐及负重。保持肛周皮肤清洁干燥。保持大便通畅,养成良好的排便习惯,排便时不可久蹲或过于用力。

(2)饮食护理　可饮玫瑰花茶。宜食理气活血的食物,如山楂、白萝卜、茄子。食疗方:红糖黄花菜、槐花米煲牛脾。不宜食辛辣的食物。

(3)情志护理　护士可运用语言开导疗法,向病人解释烦躁易怒会导致肝气郁滞,加重病情。病人疼痛较甚,可采用音乐疗法、歌吟疗法,帮助病人放松心情。

(4)用药护理　中药汤剂宜饭后温服。

(5)操作技术　①熏洗疗法:取乳香、没药、红花、川芎各20 g;白芷、枳壳、青黛、徐长卿各15 g;合而煮沸,水温50~70℃时熏蒸,水温降至37~40℃时淋洗、坐浴,每次5分钟,每日1次;女性月经期或妊娠期禁用。②灸法:在肛周用艾条温和灸以止痛,灸至病人有温热舒适无灼痛的感觉,每次15~20分钟,每日1次;女性月经期或妊娠期禁用。③穴位按摩法:取足三里、承山,用拇指揉法,按摩至局部发热或有酸麻重胀感,每日 1 次;孕妇禁用。

4. 脾虚气陷证

(1) 生活起居护理　居室温暖干燥。病人应避风,卧床休息,勿久站、久行、剧烈运动。如厕时最好有人陪伴。保持大便通畅,排便时不可久蹲或过于用力。若出现心悸,头晕,气短,应报告医生。若痔核轻微脱出,指导病人用手指涂抹润滑油,将其轻轻纳回,回纳后平卧休息 20 分钟。

(2) 饮食护理　饮食宜温热,少食多餐。宜食健脾利湿的食物,如茯苓、山药、薏苡仁、桑椹、菠菜、鳝鱼。食疗方:白糖炖鱼胶、大枣乌鱼汤。不宜食生冷的食物。

(3) 情志护理　护士可运用语言开导疗法和移情易性疗法,建议病人看喜剧、听相声,保持乐观的情绪,避免悲观、忧愁。

(4) 用药护理　中药汤剂宜饭前温服。

(5) 操作技术　① 灸法:取百会、关元、气海,或肛周,用温和灸,艾条燃着端悬于施灸部位上,距离皮肤 2~3 厘米,灸至病人有温热舒适无灼痛的感觉,皮肤稍有红晕,每日 1 次;孕妇腹部禁用。② 穴位按摩法:取中脘、百会、足三里、脾俞、梁门,用拇指揉法、一指禅推法,按摩至局部发热或有酸麻重胀感,每日 1 次;孕妇禁用。③ 热敷疗法:取小腹部,用水热敷法,以病人感觉温暖舒适为宜,每次 20 分钟,每日 1 次。④ 耳压疗法:取神门、交感、皮质下、直肠、肛门等耳穴,用耳穴压丸贴片贴压,每日按揉 4~5 次,以局部发热泛红为度,留置 2~4 日;孕妇禁用。

(二) 健康教育

养成良好的排便习惯。每日定时排便,可于晨起或早餐后进行,每日 1 次。最好采用坐便。排便时不可阅读、久蹲和过于用力。不可因为害怕便血而拒绝排便。排便疼痛时,可在肛周涂少许润滑剂,以减轻疼痛。保持大便通畅。积极治疗便秘、腹泻、痢疾。若出现便秘,可通过运动和饮食调节,或遵医嘱用药,不可自行长期使用泻药或长期灌肠。

居室安静整洁,空气新鲜。内裤棉质、柔软、宽松。卧床休息,睡眠充足。养成良好的卫生习惯,便后及临睡前用温水坐浴,以保持肛周清洁干燥。根据病人的身体情况,适量运动,以增加肠道蠕动。睡前或晨起时顺时针按摩腹部 20~30 圈,并坚持做提肛运动:取仰卧位、坐位或站立位,吸气时上提肛门,呼气时放松肛门,逐渐延长提肛时间,一个呼吸为 1 遍,每次做 20~30 遍。注意避风。不可过劳,避免久站、久坐、久蹲、负重远行。属久坐、久站工作性质的,应适时变换体位,并加强日常的体育锻炼。避免坐在过热、过冷、潮湿的物体表面。避免肛门局部刺激,厕纸应柔软。

饮食有节,定时定量,荤素搭配。饮食宜清淡、营养、易消化。白天多饮水,晨起时喝 1 杯淡盐水,睡前喝少量蜂蜜水。宜进食杂粮以及高纤维的水果和蔬菜,如芹菜、荠菜。避免暴饮暴食,或者因惧怕便血和疼痛而减少食量。戒烟限酒,不宜食辛辣、煎炸、肥甘、厚味的食物,如大葱、大蒜、辣椒。发作期间忌食发物,如虾、牛肉、羊肉。

保持心情舒畅。病程的反复和症状的变化可使病人烦躁、抑郁,从而加重病情。护士应帮助虚证的病人避免过思伤脾,帮助实证的病人避免暴怒伤肝,了解、关心和鼓励病人,及时予以心理疏导,教病人放松自我和减轻疼痛的方法。建议家属多鼓励和安慰病人,以增强其战胜疾病的信心。

病人应定期复查。可对病人进行电话回访,采取针对性干预。痔疮有保守治疗和手术治疗。保守治疗适用于痔疮早期、老年体弱或兼有其他严重慢性疾病且不适合手术者。手术治疗适用于痔疮中、晚期或经保守治疗无效者。病人康复后,如出现便血、肿物脱出,应及时就医。

Section 4　Hemorrhoids

Hemorrhoids generally refers to a kind of anorectal diseases that is characterized by stagnation of qi and blood in the anus and is caused by deficiency of zang-fu organs, or external contraction of wind-dampness and internal accumulation of heat toxin. It includes internal hemorrhoids, external hemorrhoids and mixed hemorrhoids. This section can be referred to for the nursing of hemorrhoids in Western medicine.

ETIOLOGY AND PATHOGENESIS

The etiology includes external contraction, overstrain, improper diet, internal emotional injury, stool disorder, pregnancy and excessive childbearing. All the following factors might cause hemorrhoids: external contraction of wind, dampness, dryness and heat pathogens brings about fluid damage, dry stool, and obstruction of blood stasis and turbid qi in the anus; long-time sitting, standing and walking or sexual strain consumes qi, blood and body fluids, and leads to sinking of the middle qi and stasis obstruction of the meridians; excessive intake of fatty, greasy, fried, pungent and spicy foodstuffs produces accumulated dampness-heat that pours downward to the anus; long-term emotional depression transforming into fire results in disorder of qi movement and pouring down of internal dampness-heat; excessive childbearing or overexertion in labor induces qi and blood inhibition as well as stasis stagnation of blood vessels in the anus; blood deficiency and fluid depletion after labor and constipation due to intestine dryness that need overexertion and long squatting in defecation trigger blood stasis and qi sinking; constitutional dampness-heat transforms into dryness and causes dry stool; chronic diarrhea consumes qi and causes inhibition of qi and blood in the anus.

The pathogenesis is dysfunction of zang-fu organs and depression of qi, blood, dampness and heat in the anus that blocks meridians and stagnates blood and vessels. Prolonged qi deficiency causes sinking of the middle qi and failure of qi in controlling function, so the hemorrhoid nucleus prolapses. The disease is located in the anus and rectum but related to the lung, spleen and large intestine. And the disease is root deficiency and tip excess in nature.

COMMON SYNDROMES

Key Points in Syndrome Differentiation

1. Differentiation of Deficiency from Excess Syndrome

The differentiation is based on the color and texture of the bleeding, and tongue and pulse manifestations. Spraying or dripping blood of the bright color, yellow tongue coating and rapid pulse indicate excess syndrome. Clear thin blood, lusterless complexion, mental and physical fatigue, pale tongue with white coating and thread weak pulse means deficiency syndrome.

2. Differentiation of Internal from External Hemorrhoids

The differentiation is based on the location of hemorrhoids and main symptoms. What occurs above the dentate line with bloody stool as the main symptom is internal hemorrhoids. What occurs below the dentate line with pain, sagging distension and foreign body sensation of the anus as the main symptoms is external hemorrhoids.

Syndrome Differentiation

1. Wind Injuring Intestine Collaterals Syndrome

[Clinical Manifestations] Blood in stool, dripping or spraying blood in defecation, bright red color, dry stool, pruritus in the anus, dry mouth and throat, red tongue with yellow coating, and float rapid pulse.

[Manifestations Analysis] External contraction of six excesses transforms into heat and generates wind, or liver depression transforms into fire and generates wind. Wind-heat rushes downward into the anus. Heat injures intestine collaterals which makes blood fail to stay in the meridians and flow outside the vessels, or dry stool damages blood collaterals of the hemorrhoid nucleus, resulting in blood in stool, dripping or spraying blood in defecation. Heat scorches body fluids, so the blood is of bright red color and the stool is dry. The disease is caused by wind pathogen, so pruritus in the anus occurs. Red tongue with yellow coating, and float rapid pulse are signs of wind-heat.

[Nursing Principle] Cooling blood and dispelling wind.

[Suggested Formula] Liangxue Dihuang Decoction.

2. Dampness-Heat Pouring Downward Syndrome

[Clinical Manifestations] Large volume of hematochezia in bright red color, prolapse of the intrarectal lump with swelling, distension, burning pain and wet sensation, dry or loose stool, scanty and dark urine, red tongue with yellow slimy coating, and rapid pulse.

[Manifestations Analysis] Long-term external contraction of dampness pathogen transforms into heat or long-term excessive intake of fatty sweet foodstuffs causes internal dampness-heat that pours downward and scorches blood collaterals, causing large volume of hematochezia in bright red color. Dampness binding with heat pours downward into the large intestines and accumulates and obstructs the anus, so prolapse of the intrarectal lump with swelling, distension, burning pain and wet sensation are felt. Red tongue with yellow slimy coating and rapid pulse are signs of dampness-heat.

[Nursing Principle] Clearing heat and drying dampness.

[Suggested Formula] Huaihua Powder.

3. Qi Stagnation and Blood Stasis Syndrome

[Clinical Manifestations] Prolapse of the intrarectal lump with edema, thrombosis or incarceration, dark purple surface, erosion, exudation, severe pain, obvious tenderness, anal canal tightness, constipation, inhibited urination, dark purple tongue or with ecchymosis, and wiry or unsmooth pulse.

[Manifestations Analysis] Long-term qi depression and stagnation causes qi stagnation and blood stasis in the anus, thus leading to symptoms such as prolapse of the intrarectal lump with edema or incarceration, dark purple surface, erosion, exudation, severe pain, obvious tenderness, anal canal tightness. Qi movement inhibition, failure of qi in controlling function, and blood failing to stay in the meridians explains the occurrence of thrombosis. Dark purple tongue or with ecchymosis, and wiry or unsmooth pulse are signs of qi stagnation and blood stasis.

[Nursing Principle] Activating blood and dispersing swelling.

[Suggested Formula] Huoxue Sanyu Decoction.

4. Spleen Deficiency and Qi Sinking Syndrome

[Clinical Manifestations] Prolapse of the intrarectal lump, difficulty in coming back by itself, sagging distension of the anus, lack of strength in defecation, hematochezia with light color, lusterless complexion, dizziness, mental and physical fatigue, reduced appetite, shortness of breath, no desire to speak, pale enlarged tongue with thin white coating, and thready weak pulse.

[Manifestations Analysis] Spleen qi deficiency, sinking of middle qi, and failure of qi in securing and controlling function lead to prolapse of the intrarectal lump, difficulty in coming back by itself, sagging distension of the anus, and lack of strength in defecation. Spleen fails to control blood and qi deficiency cannot generate blood, so hematochezia with light color occurs. Spleen deficiency causes insufficiency of qi and blood, leading to lusterless complexion, dizziness, mental and physical fatigue, shortness of breath and no desire to speak. Pale tongue with thin white coating and thready weak pulse are sings of spleen deficiency.

[Nursing Principle] Replenishing qi to uplift the middle qi.

[Suggested Formula] Buzhong Yiqi Decoction.

NURSING MEASURES

For patients with hemorrhoids, nurses should closely monitor the following factors: the time and frequency of bowel movement; the amount and dryness of the stool; the time and frequency of bleeding; the quantity, color and texture of the blood; the prolapse of intrarectal lump as well as the erosion and excretion on its surface; the possibility of self-retraction or manual-assisted push-back of the prolapse; the location, nature, severity, duration of the anal pain or itch. The doctor should be immediately informed if the patient experiences incarcerated hemorrhoid or sudden thrombosis of external hemorrhoid as well as persistent heavy bleeding, sudden pale complexion, pulse quickening, blood pressure dropping, dizziness and palpitation.

Syndrome-Based Nursing Measures

1. Wind Injuring Intestine Collateral Syndrome

(1) Daily life nursing. The ward should be cool, quiet, and full of fresh air. The patients should

rest in a lateral decubitus position, keep the perianal region clean and dry, and avoid wind to prevent external contraction of pathogenic wind.

(2) Diet nursing. The patients should drink more water, may drink huaihua (pagoda tree flower) tea and luffa juice and eat more fresh fruit and vegetables, such as celery, watermelons, and bananas. They may eat foods that disperse wind and clear heat, such as heye (lotus leaf) and oujie (lotus rhizome node). Pungent and spicy foods should be avoided.

(3) Emotion nursing. Because the disease is newly onset, nurses may use verbal enlightenment therapy to inform the patients about the causes of bloody stool to help them relieve fear and stay in a peaceful state of mind.

(4) Medication nursing. Decoction should be brewed quickly over high heat and taken warm after meals. After taking medicine, they should cover themselves up to get warm and perspire slightly.

(5) Manipulation techniques. ① Fumigating and washing therapy: mangxiao (sodium sulphate), jinyinhua (honeysuckle), and lianqiao (weeping forsythia capsule); decoct one of the three ingredients and fumigate the perineal region with the decoction at a temperature of 50~70℃, and use it for hip bath at a temperature of 37~40℃, five minutes each time, twice per day. For patients with severe itching, add in huajiao (pricklyash peel). And it should be avoided during menstruation or pregnancy. ② Steeping and washing therapy: after defecation, use jingfang (schizonepeta and saposhnikovia) powder to steep and wash the perineal region. And it should be avoided during menstruation or pregnancy. ③ Wet compress therapy: use decoction prepared with wubeizi (gallnut of Chinese sumac) or kushen (light yellow sophora root); soak 5~6 layers of gauze into the decoction at 38~41℃ and apply the gauze to the affected area, 20 minutes each time, once per day. And it should be avoided during menstruation or pregnancy.

2. Dampness-Heat Pouring Downward Syndrome

(1) Daily life nursing. The ward should be quiet and cool. The patients should rest in bed in a lateral decubitus position and avoid prolonged period of sitting or standing. They should keep the perianal region clean and dry, and maintain a normal bowel movement without extended periods of squatting and overexertion in defecation. In case of excessive blood in stool, the patients should stop defecation and minimize movement of the body and get examination of the anal area.

(2) Diet nursing. The patients should drink more water, may drink juhua (chrysanthemum flower) tea, pugongying (dandelion) tea, and jinyinhua (honeysuckle) tea, and eat foods that clear heat and drain dampness, such as biqi (waternut), celery, huaihua (pagoda tree flower), chixiaodou (adzuki bean), yiyiren (coix seed), machixian (purslane) and yuxingcao (heartleaf houttuynia). Food therapy: lüdou donggua (mung bean and Chinese waxgourd) soup. For patients with blood in stool, eat cooked dried persimmon. Pungent and spicy foods should be avoided.

(3) Emotion nursing. Because excessive bleeding often occurs, nurses may apply emotional transference and dispositional change therapy such as reading and listening to music to divert the patients' attention and help them stay in a peaceful state of mind to prevent restlessness and fear. Nurses may also

apply verbal enlightenment therapy to care for the patients and inform them about the common symptoms and treatments as well as other patients' treatments and recovery to boost their confidence in treatment effectiveness.

（4）Medication nursing. Decoction should be taken warm or slightly cool after meals.

（5）Manipulation techniques. ① Fumigating and washing therapy：use modified Kushen Decoction. After emptying both the bladder and bowels, use the decoction for fumigating the anal area when the temperature is 50~70℃ and for washing when the temperature is 37~40℃, five minutes each time, and twice per day. The treatment should be immediately stopped if rash or itching develops. And it should be avoided during menstruation or pregnancy. ② Unction therapy：apply Jiuhua Ointment or Sanhuang Ointment；apply the medicine on the affected area with a cotton swab, twice a day. And it should be avoided during menstruation or pregnancy. ③ Scraping therapy：select Dachangshu（BL 25）, Yaoyangguan（GV 3）, Tianshu（ST 25）, and Daheng（SP 15）；scrape each of the acupoints until it turns red and *sha qi*（rash of measles）occurs. And it should be avoided during menstruation or pregnancy. ④ Medicinal suppository therapy：insert into the anus Gangtai Suppository or Niuhuang Zhiqing Suppository after defecation or before sleep. It is suitable for external hemorrhoid. And it should be avoided during menstruation or pregnancy.

3. Qi Stagnation and Blood Stasis Syndrome

（1）Daily life nursing. The ward should be warm, comfortable, and full of fresh air. The patients should rest in bed with a lateral decubitus position and avoid prolonged period of standing, squatting, sitting or bearing weight. They should keep the perianal region clean and dry, maintain a normal bowel movement, and develop good bowel habits without extended periods of squatting and overexertion in defecation.

（2）Diet nursing. The patients may drink meiguihua（rose flower）tea and eat foods that regulate qi and activate blood, such as shanzha（Chinese hawthorn fruit）, white radish and eggplants. Food therapy：brown sugar and day lily, huaihuami（sophora fruit）stewed with bovine spleen. Pungent and spicy foods should be avoided.

（3）Emotion nursing. Nurses may apply verbal enlightenment therapy to inform patients that irritability and restlessness would lead to liver qi depression that aggravates the condition. For patients with severe pain, music therapy or singing and chanting therapy might help them relax.

（4）Medication nursing. Decoction should be taken warm after meals.

（5）Manipulation techniques. ① Fumigating and washing therapy：ruxiang（frankincense）, moyao （myrrh）, honghua（safflower）and chuanxiong（Sichuan lovage root）20 g respectively, baizhi （angelica root）, zhiqiao（bitter orange）, qingdai（natural indigo）and xuchangqing（paniculate swallowwort root）15 g respectively；decoct the above ingredients and fumigate with the decoction at a temperature of 50~70℃, and wash with it at a temperature of 37~40℃, five minutes each time, once per day. And it should be avoided during menstruation or pregnancy. ② Moxibustion therapy：apply mild moxibustion on the perineal region to relieve pain, until the area turns red and the patient feels warm and comfortable without the sensation of burning pain, 15 ~ 20 minutes each time, once per day. And it should be avoided during menstruation or pregnancy. ③ Acupressure therapy: select Zusanli (ST 36) and Chengshan (BL 57); apply thumb kneading manipulation on each of them till the local area turns hot or feels soreness, numbness and heaviness and distension, once per day. And it is contraindicated in pregnancy.

4. Spleen deficiency and Qi Sinking Syndrome

(1) Daily life nursing. The ward should be warm, dry and away from wind. The patients should rest in bed, be accompanied when using the bathroom, and maintain a normal bowel movement without extended periods of squatting and overexertion in defecation. They should also avoid prolonged period of sitting, standing or strenuous activity. For patients with palpitation, dizziness or shortness of breath, nurses should report the information to the doctor immediately. For patients with slight prolapse of hemorrhoids, nurses should guide them to gently push it back with lubricated fingers and to lie on their back to rest in bed for 20 minutes.

(2) Diet nursing. The diet should be warm. The patients should have small frequent meals and foods that invigorate the spleen and drain dampness, such as fuling (poria), shanyao (common yam rhizome), yiyiren (coix seed), sangshen (mulberry), spinach and eels. Food therapy: sugar stewed with fish gelatin, and dazao wuyu (Chinese date and snakehead fish) soup. Raw and cold foods should be avoided.

(3) Emotion nursing. Nurses may apply verbal enlightenment therapy as well as emotional transference and dispositional change therapy to advise patients to watch comedies or crosstalk show to stay optimistic and keep away from pessimism and sorrow.

(4) Medication nursing. Decoction should be taken warm before meals.

(5) Manipulation techniques. ① Moxibustion therapy: select Baihui (GV 20), Guanyuan (CV 4), Qihai (CV 6) or the perineal region; place the moxa stick 2 ~ 3 centimeters away from the skin to perform mild moxibustion on each of them until the area turns red and the patient feels warm and comfortable without the sensation of burning pain, once per day. And it cannot be applied on the abdomen of pregnant women. ② Acupressure therapy: select Zhongwan (CV 12), Baihui (GV 20), Zusanli (ST 36), Pishu (BL 20), and Liangmen (ST 21); apply thumb kneading and one-finger pushing manipulations on each of them till the local area turns hot or feels soreness, numbness and heaviness and distension, once per day. And it is contraindicated in pregnancy. ③ Hot compress therapy: use warm water to compress the lower abdomen at a comfortable temperature, 20 minutes each time, once per day. ④ Auricular pressure therapy: select shenmen (TF4), sympathetic (AH6a), subcortex (AT4), rectum (HX2), and anus (HX5); apply specialized pasters on the points, press and knead each of them till the area turns hot and red, 4 ~ 5 times per day, and keep the pasters for 2 ~ 4 days. And it is contraindicated in pregnancy..

Patient Education

The patients should develop good habits of defecation, such as following a regular routine of defecation once per day, using toilets instead of squatting, avoiding reading, overexertion, and squatting for extended periods. Don't refuse to defecate because of fear of bleeding and moderate lubrication on the perineal region could relieve pain in defecation. The patients should maintain a normal bowel movement and actively receive treatment for constipation, diarrhea and dysentery. If constipation occurs, it could be regulated with exercise, diet, or drugs prescribed by doctors rather than the extended use of laxatives or enema.

The room should be quiet, tidy, and full of fresh air. The underwear should be cotton, soft and loose. The patients should rest in bed, have sufficient sleep, and develop good sanitary habits, such as having a hip bath before sleep and after defecation, and keeping the perineal region dry and clean. Appropriate activities based on the patients' constitution could improve bowel movement. Before sleep or after getting up in the morning, the patients could massage the abdomen clockwise for 20~30 circles. It is beneficial to practice anus-contraction exercise: sit, stand, or lie on the back, lift the anus during inhalation and relax it during exhalation; the duration of lifting the anus could be gradually lengthened; one inspiration and expiration counts as one act, and one session exercise includes 20~30 such acts; perform one session exercise every day before sleep or after getting up in the morning. The patients should avoid wind, overwork, prolonged period of standing, sitting, squatting and walking with weights. Those who are sedentary and stand for a long time should change their positions regularly and strengthen physical exercise in normal times. They should also refrain from sitting where it is too hot, cold or damp. Avoid anal irritation and the toilet paper should be soft.

The patients should follow a moderate diet by following regular routines and quantities. The diet should include both meat and vegetables and be light, nutritious and digestible. They drink more water in the day, a glass of lightly salted water after getting up in the morning and moderate honey water before sleep, and eat multigrain, fruit and vegetables rich in fiber, such as celery and shepherd's purse. Moreover, they should avoid gluttony or craputence as well as eating less for fear of bloody stool and pain. They should also avoid cigarettes, alcohol as well as pungent, spicy, fried, fatty, sweet, or rich foods, such as scallions, dasuan (garlic bulb) and chili, so do foods that induce or aggravate disease during flare-ups, such as shrimp, beef and mutton.

The patients should stay good-humored. Relapses and changing symptoms might cause irritability, restlessness, depression and deterioration in patients. Nurses should guide patients with deficiency syndrome to avoid excessive contemplation so as not to impair the spleen whereas guide patients with excess syndrome to avoid intense anger so as not to damage the liver. Nurses should get to know the patients, be attentive to them, and provide encouragement, psychological counselling as well as methods of relaxation and pain relief. Families of the patients are advised to encourage and reassure patients to enhance their confidence in overcoming diseases.

The patients should go back to the hospital for regular checks. Nurses could pay a return visit through phone calls and provide individualized interventions. Treatment for hemorrhoids include conservative ones and surgeries. Conservative treatments work best with patients in early phases of hemorrhoids, elderly patients with weak constitution, and patients with serious chronic disease who are unsuitable for surgeries. However, surgeries are most appropriate for patients in the middle or late stages of hemorrhoids and those for whom conservative treatments don't work. Patients should immediately see doctors if they experience some uncomfortable symptoms such as bloody stool or prolapse of intrarectal lumps after recovery.

第三章
妇科病证的中医护理

据《史记·扁鹊仓公列传》记载,在春秋战国时出现了妇产科医生:带下医。在《黄帝内经》中,描述了女性的生殖器官——女子胞,阐释了女性的生殖功能由初发、旺盛到衰竭的过程。在《神农本草经》中,记载了88种妇产科药物。在《金匮要略》中,张仲景论述了月经病、带下病、妊娠病、产后病和妇科杂病的辨证论治。在漫长的时间里,中医妇科学为中华民族的繁衍做出了巨大的贡献。中医妇科学的特色集中在调经、助孕、安胎,以及治疗带下病、调治产后病和养生保健方面。

在中医妇科里,胞宫包含子宫、子管、子核以及胞脉、胞络。胞宫的生理功能与冲脉、任脉、督脉、带脉密切相关。冲脉是全身气血运行的要冲,冲脉的精血充盛是胞宫行经和胎孕的基础。任脉总司精、血、津、液,"任主胞胎",任脉的气机通畅是胞宫行经和胎孕的条件。督脉贯脊属肾,维系元气。带脉横行于腰,状如束带,维持气血循行,约束冲脉、任脉、督脉的生理活动。

中医妇科有独特的月经、带下、妊娠、产育生理。月经与五脏关系密切。心主血,月经以血为本。脾所产生和运化的气血是月经的主要来源。肺可输布精、血、津、液到达子宫。"女子以肝为先天","肝肾同源",肾中精气充盛,则肝血充足。肾主闭藏,肝主疏泄,藏泻相协,形成月经周期。带下是肾精下润之液。受孕的前提是肾气充盛,天癸成熟,冲任二脉功能协调,胞宫藏泻有期,月经正常。妊娠的条件是男女双方生殖之精适时相合。受孕以后,胎元依赖母体的气血持续充养。胎儿形神兼备后就可足月分娩。

妇科疾病的常见病因有六淫邪气、情志内伤、生活失度、病理产物和体质因素。由于经、带、胎、产均以血为用,而寒、热、湿邪最易与血相搏结,所以寒、热、湿邪是妇科疾病的常见病因。七情太过,体内气机受扰,可导致妇科疾病。其中,过怒、过思、过恐最为常见。极端的或者突然改变的生活环境,如房劳多产、饮食不节、劳逸失常、跌仆损伤、迁居异乡,均可导致妇科疾病。由疾病所致的瘀血、痰饮稽留于体内,阻碍气机,也可导致妇科疾病。不同的体质会影响身体对于外界致病因素的易感性和患病以后的证型。

妇科疾病的诊断方法包括望、闻、问、切。在望诊中,常用望形神、面色、毛发、月经、带下和舌象。在闻诊中,常用到听语音高低,以及嗅月经、带下、恶露的气味。在问诊中,要问年龄、月经史、带下史、婚产史、既往史和家族史。若病人有难言之隐,或羞于启齿,应单独问诊,向病人说明病史对于诊断和护理的重要性。女性的脉多沉细而软。在经期、妊娠期和产后,脉象会发生变化。在按诊中,常用按肌肤和按腹部。

妇科疾病的辨证以八纲辨证、脏腑辨证和气血辨证为主。

妇科疾病的常用护理操作技术包括熏洗疗法、药熨疗法、拔罐疗法、灸法、推拿疗法、耳压疗法等。这些技术有祛寒、止痛、止血、止带、清热解毒、杀虫止痒等功效。与内服药物相比,这些操作技术对胃肠道和肝肾的副作用较小。

Chapter 3
Nursing of Gynecological Diseases

As recorded in the section *Biography of Bian Que and Cang Gong* in the book *Records of the Historian*, there were obstetricians and gynecologists called "Daixia doctors" in the Spring and Autumn Period and the Warring States Period. The book *Huangdi's Internal Classic* describes the female reproductive organ (the uterus) and expounds the process of female reproductive function from its initial onset, exuberance to exhaustion. *Shennong's Classic of Materia Medica* recorded 88 kinds of obstetrics and gynecology medicinals. In *Synopsis of the Golden Chamber*, Zhang Zhongjing discussed the syndrome differentiation and treatment of menstrual diseases, leucorrhea diseases, pregnancy diseases, postpartum diseases and miscellaneous gynecological diseases. Over a long period of time, *Gynecology of TCM* has made a great contribution to the reproduction of the Chinese nation. The uniqueness of *Gynecology of TCM* lies in regulating menstruation, assisting pregnancy, calming the fetus, treating leucorrhea and postpartum diseases, and keeping in good health.

In *Gynecology of TCM*, the uterus with appendages includes the uterus, oviduct, ovary, uterine vessels and uterine collateral. The thoroughfare, conception, governor and belt vessels are closely related to the physiological functions of the uterus with appendages. Among them, the thoroughfare vessel is the major pathway of the movement of qi and blood. Its sufficient essence and blood are the foundation of menstruation and pregnancy. The conception governs essence, blood and body fluid. It is the base of pregnancy. The smooth qi movement in the conception vessel is the condition of menstruation and pregnancy. The governor vessel moves along the spine, pertains to the kidney and maintains the original qi. And the belt vessel moves around the waist like a belt, maintains the normal circulation of qi and blood, and restrains the physiological activities of the thoroughfare, conception and governor vessels.

Gynecology of TCM has unique physiology of menstruation, leukorrhea, pregnancy and childbirth. The five zang organs are closely related to menstruation. Specifically speaking, the heart governs blood and menstruation takes the blood as its root. Qi and blood that are produced, transported and transformed by the spleen are the main sources of menstruation. The essence, blood and body fluid all depend on lung qi to distribute them to the uterus. "The liver is the congenital base of life for women" and "the liver and the kidney share the same origin", therefore, sufficient essential qi assures the nourishment of the liver and the fullness of the blood. The kidney governing storage, the liver governing free flow of qi, and their coordinated storing and excreting functions work together to produce the menstruation. Leucorrhea is yin fluid in the body derived from kidney essence that moves downward to moisten the vagina. The premise of female conception is exuberant kidney qi, mature tiangui (reproductive essence), coordinated functions of the thoroughfare and conception vessels, regular storage and excretion of the uterus, and normal menstruation. And the condition of pregnancy is that the reproductive essence of both the male and female combines at the right time. After pregnancy, the fetal original qi depends on the continuous nourishment of mother's qi and blood. When the unity of the fetus' physical form and spirit is well developed, it will be born in full-term.

The common causes of gynecological diseases include six excesses, emotional damage, intemperance in life, pathological products and constitutional factors. Generally speaking, cold, heat and dampness pathogens are the common causes of disease because, on the one hand, the menstruation, leukorrhea, pregnancy and childbirth all depend on the blood, and on the other hand, these three pathogens frequently bind the blood. Excessive emotional damages disturb qi movement in the body that induces gynecological diseases. Among the seven emotions, over-anger, over-thought and over-fear are most frequent ones. Extreme or sudden changes in the living environment (such as sexual overindulgence and multiparity, improper diet, uneven allocation of work, injury due to falling, residence change to a new place, etc.) can lead to gynecological diseases. The blood stasis, phlegm and fluid retention that are produced by diseases stay in the body and hinder qi movement, which in turn causes gynecological diseases. Besides, different constitution will affect the body's susceptibility to external pathogenic factors and the syndrome type of the disease.

The diagnostic methods of gynecological diseases include inspection, listening and smelling, inquiry, and pulse taking and palpation. Inspection method usually includes inspecting the form, spirit, complexion, hair of head and body, menstruation, leucorrhea, and tongue manifestation. Listening and smelling often means listening to voice and smelling the odor of menstruation, leucorrhea and lochia. Inquiry method includes inquiring the age, leucorrhea, menstrual history, marital history, pregnancy and delivery history, past medical history and family medical history. If the patients have some secret information to share or is too shy to talk about the disease, separate inquiry should be made to keep the privacy and it is necessary to let them know the importance of the medical history to diagnosis and care. Generally speaking, the female's pulse is deep, thready and soft, and pulse manifestation varies in menstruation and pregnancy and after childbirth. And palpation usually includes palpating the muscle, skin and abdomen.

Syndrome differentiation methods of gynecological diseases often include eight-principle syndrome differentiation, visceral syndrome differentiation and qi-blood syndrome differentiation.

Common nursing techniques for gynecological diseases include fumigating and washing therapy, medicated ironing therapy, cupping therapy, moxibustion therapy, massage therapy, auricular pressure therapy and so on. The effects of these techniques include: removing cold, relieving pain, stopping bleeding, stopping leukorrhagia, clearing heat and removing toxin, killing worms and relieving itching, etc. Nursing techniques have fewer side effects on the gastrointestinal tract, liver and kidney than oral medicines do.

第一节　月经先期、月经后期、月经先后不定期

月经先期，是指因气虚冲任不固，或因热扰冲任，血海不宁而引起的，以月经周期提前7天以上，连续3个周期以上，经期基本正常为临床特征的月经病。月经后期，是指因肾虚、血虚导致冲任不足，或因血寒、气滞、痰湿导致冲任阻滞，以月经周期延后7天以上，甚或长达3个月至5个月一行，连续3个周期以上，经期正常为临床特征的月经病。月经先后无定期，是指因肝郁、肾虚，导致冲任失调，血海蓄溢失常，以月经周期时或提前时或延后7天以上，交替不定且连续3个周期以上为临床特征的月经病。这三种疾病都是关于月经周期的异常。西医的黄体功能不足、子宫内膜不规则脱落、盆腔炎性疾病、子宫腺肌病、子宫肌瘤，以月经频发、月经稀发、不规律月经为主要表现的，可参照本节进行护理。

一、病因病机

月经先期的病因多为气虚和血热。病人素体脾虚，或饮食不节，或思虑过度，均可因气虚导致冲任不固，发生月经先期。病人为阳盛之体，或过食辛温，或肝郁化火；或病人为阴虚之体，或产多乳众，或久病失血：此二者皆可因血热发生热扰冲任，导致月经先期。

月经后期的病因多为血寒、痰湿、血虚和肾虚。病人平素体寒，或感受寒邪，或过食生冷，或冒雨涉水，均可因血寒导致经血充盈延迟，发生月经后期。病人素来体胖，或脾失健运，水湿内停为痰，均可因痰湿导致胞宫胞脉壅塞，发生月经后期。病人平素气血不足，或久病失血，或堕胎产数伤血，或伤食思虑损脾，均可因血虚导致冲任亏虚，发生月经后期。病人先天肾气不足，或后天肾精亏虚，均可因肾虚导致冲任失养，发生月经后期。

月经先后无定期的病因多为肝郁和肾虚。病人伤于情志，肝失疏泄，可导致胞宫藏泻失常，发生月经先后无定期。病人先天禀赋不足，或房劳多产，均可因肾虚导致肾失封藏，发生月经先后无定期。

月经先期、月经后期、月经先后不定期的病机为冲任气血失调，胞宫藏泻失度。病位在冲任、胞宫，与肾、肝、脾相关。月经先期、月经后期、月经先后不定期的病性多为虚实夹杂和寒热错杂。

二、常见证型

（一）辨证要点

1. 辨虚实　根据病因、体质及伴随症状来辨别。若病人有长期的气血阴阳亏虚，且有近期过劳史，多为虚证。若因肝郁、寒凝、血热而起，有具体的致病邪气，且不伴疲乏、脉无力等虚象，则多为实证。

2. 辨寒热　根据月经的量、色、质，月经周期，病因，体质及伴随症状等来辨别。实热多因素体阳盛或外感热邪，虚热多因素体阴虚或久病伤阴。若月经先期，量多，色深红或紫，质稠，伴口渴面

赤,溲黄便结,舌质红,苔黄,脉滑数,多为阳盛血热。若月经先期,量少,色鲜红,质稠,伴手足心热,潮热盗汗,舌红少苔,脉细数,多为阴虚血热。实寒多因外感寒邪,虚寒多因素体阳虚。若月经后期,量少,色暗或有块,小腹冷痛拒按,多为实寒。若月经后期,量少,色淡质稀,小腹隐痛,喜温喜按,多为虚寒。

3. 辨脏腑　根据月经的量、色、质,月经周期及伴随症状等来辨别。若月经色淡质稀,伴神疲乏力,气短懒言,倦怠嗜卧,纳少便溏,舌淡胖,脉缓弱,多为脾虚。若月经先后不定期,色暗红,有块,伴少腹胀痛,脘闷不舒,脉弦,多为肝郁。若经量或多或少,色暗质稀,伴腰膝酸软,舌淡暗,脉沉细,多为肾虚。

（二）证候分型

1. 脾气虚证

［主要证候］月经周期提前,量或多或少;或经期错后,量少;月经色淡质稀;神疲肢倦,面色萎黄,气短懒言,倦怠嗜卧,小腹空坠,语声低微,脘闷腹胀,纳少便溏;舌质淡胖,边有齿痕,苔薄白,脉缓弱。

［证候分析］脾虚统血无权,冲任不固,故月经周期提前,量或多或少;脾虚气血生化不足,冲任不充,故月经后期且量少;气虚血失温煦,故月经色淡质稀;脾虚中气不足,故神疲肢倦,气短懒言,倦怠嗜卧,小腹空坠,语声低微;脾虚运化失司,故脘闷腹胀,纳少便溏;脾虚气血不足,不能上荣于面,故面色萎黄;舌质淡胖,边有齿痕,苔薄白,脉缓弱均为脾虚之象。

［护治原则］补脾益气,固冲调经。

［常用方剂］补中益气汤。

2. 肾气虚证

［主要证候］月经周期提前,或错后,或先后不定,量或多或少,色淡暗,质清稀;头晕耳鸣,腰膝酸软,小便清长,夜尿频多;面色晦暗或有暗斑;舌淡暗,苔薄白,脉沉细。

［证候分析］肾气不足,冲任不固,故月经提前,量多;肾气虚损,冲任不充,故月经后期,量少;肾虚封藏失司,血海蓄溢失常,故月经前后不定期,量少;肾虚精血不足,故经量少;肾气不足,血失温煦,则经色淡暗,质清稀;肾虚则外府失荣,筋骨不坚,故腰膝酸软;肾虚血海不充,清窍失养,故头晕耳鸣;肾虚气化失司,故小便清长,夜尿频多;肾在色为黑,故面色晦暗或有暗斑;舌淡暗,苔薄白,脉沉细均为肾虚之象。

［护治原则］补肾益气,养血调经。

［常用方剂］固阴煎。

3. 肝气郁结证

［主要证候］月经周期先后不定,经量或多或少,色暗红,有块,经行不畅;胸胁、乳房、少腹胀痛,脘闷不舒,时欲叹息;舌淡红,苔薄白,脉弦。

［证候分析］肝失疏泄,血海蓄溢与胞宫藏泻失常,故月经周期先后不定,经量或多或少;气滞导致血瘀,故经色暗红,有块,经行不畅;肝脉循少腹、布胁肋,肝气郁结,其经脉所过之处气机不利,故胸胁、乳房、少腹胀痛;气郁不达,故脘闷不舒,时欲叹息;舌淡红,苔薄白,脉弦均为肝气郁结之象。

［护治原则］疏肝解郁,理气调经。

［常用方剂］逍遥散。

4. 阳盛血热证

［主要证候］月经周期提前，量多，色深红或紫红，质稠；口渴，喜冷饮，面红唇赤，心烦，溲黄便结；舌质红，苔黄，脉滑数。

［证候分析］热扰冲任，迫血妄行，故月经周期提前，量多；热灼阴血，故经色深红或紫红，质稠；邪热扰心，故心烦；热盛伤津，故口渴，喜冷饮，溲黄便结；面红唇赤，舌质红，苔黄，脉滑数均为实热之象。

［护治原则］清热降火，凉血调经。

［常用方剂］清经散。

5. 阴虚血热证

［主要证候］月经周期提前，量少，色鲜红，质稠；手足心热，口燥咽干，两颧潮红，潮热盗汗，心烦不寐，口舌糜烂；舌质红，苔少，脉细数。

［证候分析］热扰冲任，迫血妄行，则月经周期提前；阴虚血少，冲任不充，故月经量少；热灼阴血，故月经色鲜红，质稠；热盛伤津，故口燥咽干；手足心热，两颧潮红，潮热盗汗，心烦不寐，舌质红，苔少，脉细数均为虚热之象。

［护治原则］养阴清热，凉血调经。

［常用方剂］两地汤。

6. 虚寒证

［主要证候］月经周期延后，量少，色淡，质清稀；小腹冷痛，喜暖喜按，腰酸无力，小便清长，大便溏薄；舌淡，苔白，脉沉迟无力。

［证候分析］阳气不足，脏腑失于温养，气血生化不足，冲任不充，故月经周期延后，量少；阳虚血失温煦，故月经色淡，质清稀；阳虚胞宫失于温养，故小腹冷痛，喜温喜按；阳虚肾气不足，腰府失养，故腰酸无力；阳虚气化不利，故小便清长；舌淡，苔白脉沉迟无力均为虚寒之象。

［护治原则］温经扶阳，养血调经。

［常用方剂］温经汤（《金匮要略》）。

7. 实寒证

［主要证候］月经周期延后，量少，色暗，夹有血块；小腹冷痛拒按，畏寒肢冷；舌暗，苔白，脉沉紧。

［证候分析］感受寒邪，血为寒凝，经血运行不畅，故月经周期延后，量少；寒凝血滞，瘀血内阻，故月经色暗，夹有血块；寒邪阻于胞宫，凝滞气血，不通则痛，故小腹冷痛拒按；寒为阴邪，阳气不能外达，故畏寒肢冷。舌暗，苔白，脉沉紧均为实寒之象。

［护治原则］温经散寒、活血调经。

［常用方剂］温经汤（《妇人大全良方》）。

三、护理措施

对于月经先期、月经后期和月经先后无定期的病人，应观察月经的量、色、质，以及月经周期。对于月经量大的病人，应观察面色，神志和血压，及时发现贫血及休克，如有异常，应立即报告医生。

（一）辨证施护

1. 脾气虚证

（1）生活起居护理 居室温暖安静,干燥舒适,光线充足。卧床休息,注意保暖。若经量过多,更应减少活动。避免过劳,禁止经期冒雨涉水。

（2）饮食护理 宜食益气健脾的食物,如猪瘦肉、茯苓、大枣。食疗方:参芪炖乌鸡。不宜食油腻、生冷、苦寒、酸涩、辛辣的食物。

（3）情志护理 护士可运用语言开导疗法,多与病人沟通,使其保持心情舒畅,避免过思、忧虑。

（4）用药护理 中药汤剂宜饭前温服,少量频服。服药期间,忌食莱菔子、白萝卜,勿用过多滋补之品。

（5）操作技术 ① 灸法:取足三里、气海、关元,用温和灸,艾条燃着端悬于施灸部位上,距离皮肤2~3厘米,灸至病人有温热舒适无灼痛的感觉,皮肤稍有红晕,每日1次;孕妇腹部禁用。② 药熨疗法:取脾俞、胃俞,或中脘、神阙,选择背部或者腹部,用白术、当归、白扁豆、黄芪各20 g,研磨炒热后装入布袋中,制成温度为60~70℃的中药热罨包,药熨20分钟,每日1次;孕妇腹部禁用。

2. 肾气虚证

（1）生活起居护理 居室温暖安静,光线充足。卧床休息。若经量过多,更应减少活动。减少性行为,避免熬夜和过劳,禁止用冷水洗澡和洗头。

（2）饮食护理 宜食益肾固冲的食物,如核桃仁、桑椹、黑芝麻、黑豆、猪肾。食疗方:羊脊汤、蒸乌鸡、银耳鸽蛋羹。不宜食生冷、苦寒、酸涩、辛辣的食物。

（3）情志护理 护士可运用语言开导疗法,鼓励病友相互交流,以避免消沉、沮丧。

（4）用药护理 中药汤剂宜饭前温服。服药期间,忌食莱菔子、白萝卜,勿用过多滋补之品。

（5）操作技术 ① 穴位按摩法:取肾俞、命门、次髎,用拇指揉法、掌平推法,按摩至局部发热或有酸麻重胀感,每日1次;孕妇禁用。② 灸法:取神阙、腰阳关、肾俞,用隔附子饼灸,将附子研磨成粉,与黄酒调成直径2~3厘米、厚0.5~0.8厘米的薄饼,中间以针刺数孔,放置于施灸处,每处5~7壮,每日2次;孕妇禁用。

3. 肝气郁结证

（1）生活起居护理 居室安静舒适,空气新鲜。衣被宜薄。适量锻炼。若经量过多,则减少活动。

（2）饮食护理 可饮佛手茶。宜食疏肝理气的食物,如玫瑰花、金橘、白萝卜、陈皮。食疗方:韭菜炒羊肝。不宜食油腻、酸涩、易产气、温燥助阳的食物。

（3）情志护理 护士可运用顺意疗法,鼓励病人多表达,满足合理要求,减轻心理压力,避免焦虑、抑郁。

（4）用药护理 中药汤剂宜饭后温服。

（5）操作技术 ① 拔罐疗法:取期门、肝俞,留罐10分钟,每周1~2次。② 穴位按摩法:取太冲、行间,反复从太冲向行间慢慢推揉,每次3~5分钟,每日1~2次;孕妇禁用。

4. 阳盛血热证

（1）生活起居护理 居室凉爽湿润,安静舒适,空气新鲜。衣被宜薄。每日清洁外阴。由于月经量多,故应卧床休息;坐卧起立时,动作要缓慢,避免动作过快,以防止发生眩晕跌仆。

(2)饮食护理 饮食宜清淡、易消化。可饮荸荠茅根汁。宜食清热凉血的食物,如藕节、木耳、芹菜、百合。不宜食滋腻、温热动火的食物,如猪蹄、大蒜、辣椒、羊肉。

(3)情志护理 护士可运用语言开导疗法,引导病人正确对待疾病,告诉病人生气会加重症状,心情愉悦则可减轻症状,使病人保持心情舒畅,避免焦虑、暴躁。

(4)用药护理 中药汤剂宜饭后偏凉服或温服。

(5)操作技术 ① 刮痧疗法:取膈俞至胆俞,沿着足太阳膀胱经循行的路线,从上到下采用直线重刮法刮拭,每侧刮拭20~30次,以皮肤出现潮红或起痧为度,两次刮痧之间宜间隔3~6日;女性月经期或妊娠期禁用。② 耳压疗法:选耳尖、卵巢、内分泌等耳穴,用耳穴压丸贴片贴压,每日按揉4~5次,以局部发热泛红为度,留置2~4日;孕妇禁用。

5.阴虚血热证

(1)生活起居护理 居室凉爽湿润,安静舒适。衣被宜薄。卧床休息,禁止熬夜和过劳。

(2)饮食护理 可饮荸荠茅根汁。宜食养阴清热的食物,如猪瘦肉、百合、鳖肉。不宜食辛辣、香燥的食物。

(3)情志护理 护士可运用语言开导疗法,关心体贴病人,减少病人与情绪焦虑人员的接触,营造轻松的氛围,以避免心烦不宁。

(4)用药护理 中药汤剂宜饭前温服或偏凉服。服药期间,忌食莱菔子、白萝卜,勿用过多滋补之品。

(5)操作技术 ① 穴位按摩:取曲池、外关、太溪,用拇指揉法,按摩至局部发热或有酸麻重胀感,每日1次;孕妇禁用。② 耳压疗法:取神门、交感等耳穴,用耳穴压丸贴片贴压,每日按揉4~5次,以局部发热泛红为度,留置2~4日;孕妇禁用。

6.虚寒证

(1)生活起居护理 居室温暖安静,光线充足,避免强风、对流风。衣被宜厚。起居有常,劳逸适度,注意保暖。避免过劳,禁止经期冒雨涉水。

(2)饮食护理 可饮肉桂红茶。宜食温阳养血的食物,如当归、大枣、龙眼肉。食疗方:豆豉生姜炖羊肉。不宜食生冷、苦寒、酸涩的食物。

(3)情志护理 护士可运用语言开导疗法,多与病人沟通,多关心体贴病人,以避免悲观、抑郁。

(4)用药护理 中药汤剂宜饭前温服。

(5)操作技术 ① 灸法:取神阙、关元、肾俞、命门,用隔附子饼灸,将附子研磨成粉,与黄酒调成直径2~3厘米、厚0.5~0.8厘米的薄饼,中间以针刺数孔,放置于施灸处,每处5~7壮,每日2次;孕妇禁用。② 药熨疗法:取肾俞、命门、腰阳关,用菟丝子、青盐各300 g,肉桂末100 g,附子末50 g,炒热后装入布袋中,制成温度为60~70℃的中药热罨包,药熨20分钟,每日1次;孕妇禁用。③ 穴位按摩法:取劳宫、涌泉,用拇指揉法,每晚睡前按摩至局部发热;孕妇禁用。

7.实寒证

(1)生活起居护理 居室温暖安静,光线充足。衣被宜厚。起居有常,劳逸适度,适量锻炼。避免过劳,禁止经期冒雨涉水。

（2）饮食护理 可饮生姜艾叶红糖水。宜食助阳温通的食物，如肉桂、豆豉、羊肉、花椒。不宜食生冷、苦寒、酸涩的食物。

（3）情志护理 护士可运用移情易性疗法，鼓励病人参加娱乐活动，使病人保持心情舒畅。

（4）用药护理 中药汤剂宜饭后热服。

（5）操作技术 ① 足部熏洗疗法：艾叶、干姜、菟丝子、青盐各 30 g，杜仲、当归、川芎、制附子各 20 g，花椒 15 g，肉桂 10 g，水 1 500 mL，合而煮沸，水温 50~70℃时熏蒸，水温降至 37~40℃时浸泡、淋洗，每次 20 分钟，每日 1 次，熏洗后休息 30 分钟方可外出。② 灸法：取关元、八髎、三阴交、足三里，用温和灸，艾条燃着端悬于施灸部位上，距离皮肤 2~3 厘米，灸至病人有温热舒适无灼痛的感觉，皮肤稍有红晕，每日 1 次；孕妇腹部及腰骶部禁用。

（二）健康教育

护士应向病人讲解关于本病的保健知识，耐心回答病人提出的问题，使病人对治疗有信心，积极主动地配合治疗和护理。

经期严禁性行为，不宜浸渍冷水、游泳、盆浴、阴道用药及阴道检查。

饮食宜清淡、营养、易消化。宜食含铁量高、富含维生素 C 和具有补气养血功效的食物，如蛋黄、豆类、动物肝、鸡肉、鱼、大枣、黑芝麻、番茄。戒烟限酒，不宜食生冷、辛辣、香燥、炙煿、难消化的食物。

调经药宜在行经前数日开始服用，一般以 3 个月经周期为一个疗程。服药过程中，注意观察月经经量、经色、经质的改变。

建议月经先后无定期的病人随访，以排除其他妇科疾病。对于月经周期异常且伴腹痛者，应查明病因。

Section 1　Early Menstruation, Delayed Menstruation, and Irregular Menstrual Cycle

Early menstruation is clinically characterized by a menstrual cycle seven or more days earlier than usual for more than three consecutive cycles with basically normal menses duration, which is caused by the insecurity of the thoroughfare and conception vessels due to qi deficiency, or by heat harassing the thoroughfare and conception vessels that causes frenetic movement of the blood. Delayed menstruation is clinically characterized by a menstrual cycle seven or more days later than usual or even only once menstruation in three to five months, continuously for more than three cycles with basically normal menses duration, which is caused by the insufficiency of the thoroughfare and conception vessels due to kidney and blood deficiency, or by the obstruction of the thoroughfare and conception vessels due to blood cold, qi stagnation and phlegm dampness. Irregular menstrual cycle is clinically characterized by a menstrual cycle seven or more days earlier or later than usual alternately and continuously for more than three cycles, which is caused by liver depression, kidney deficiency, and the disharmony of the thoroughfare and conception vessels. All three kinds are related to abnormalities of menstrual cycle. This section can be referred to for the nursing of luteal phase defect, irregular shedding of endometrium, pelvic inflammatory disease, adenomyosis and uterine myoma, fibroid, which are featured by frequent, scarce or abnormal menstruation in Western medicine.

ETIOLOGY AND PATHOGENESIS

The etiology of early menstruation includes qi deficiency and blood heat. First, spleen deficiency constitution, dietary irregularities, and excessive thought all may lead to qi deficiency and the insecurity of the thoroughfare and conception vessels. Thus, early menstruation occurs. Second, yang exuberance constitution, over intake of pungent and warm foods, or liver depression transforming into fire; or yin deficiency constitution, excessive childbearing and lactation, or losing blood due to long illness, all may induce blood heat harassing the thoroughfare and conception vessels that causes early menstruation.

The etiology of delayed menstruation includes blood cold, phlegm dampness, blood deficiency and kidney deficiency. Specifically speaking, cold constitution, invasion of pathogenic cold, overeating raw or cold foods, braving rain or wading in water, all may induce blood cold that causes the delay of the blood and menstruation. Fat constitution, or phlegm due to dysfunction of the spleen in transportation and transformation and internal storage of water and dampness, may cause phlegm dampness that induces the obstruction of the uterus and uterine vessels, and delayed menstruation. Qi and blood deficiency constitution, losing blood due to long illness, blood damage due to abortion or excessive childbearing, spleen damage due to improper diet or excessive thought, may lead to blood deficiency that causes the deficiency of the thoroughfare and conception vessels, and delayed menstruation. Congenital deficiency of kidney qi or acquired deficiency of kidney essence may lead to kidney deficiency that causes the malnourishment of the thoroughfare and conception vessels, and delayed menstruation.

The etiology of irregular menstrual cycle includes liver depression and kidney deficiency. Emotional injury and failure of the liver to govern free flow of qi induce the abnormal storing and excreting function of the uterus, so irregular menstrual cycle occurs. Insufficiency of natural endowment, sexual strain or excessive childbearing induce kidney deficiency that causes the kidney to lose its closing and storing function, thus, irregular menstrual cycle also occurs.

The pathogenesis of early menstruation, delayed menstruation and irregular menstrual cycle is qi-blood disharmony of the thoroughfare and conception vessels, and the abnormal storing and excreting function of the uterus. The disease is located in the thoroughfare and conception vessels as well as uterus, but relates to the kidney, liver and spleen. The disease nature of early menstruation, delayed menstruation and irregular menstrual cycle is mainly deficiency-excess and cold-heat in complexity.

COMMON SYNDROMES

Key Points in Syndrome Differentiation

1. Differentiation of Deficiency from Excess Syndrome

The differentiation is based on disease cause, constitution and accompanied symptoms. Generally speaking, deficiency syndrome is mostly with long-term deficiency of qi, blood, yin and yang, and recent overwork history. Excess syndrome is usually caused by liver depression, cold coagulation and blood heat, which has specific pathogenic factors but without deficiency symptoms such as fatigue and forceless pulse.

2. Differentiation of Cold from Heat Syndrome

The differentiation is based on the amount, color, texture and cycle of the menstruation, disease cause, body constitution and accompanied symptom. Excess heat syndrome mostly shows yang exuberance constitution or external contraction of pathogenic heat whereas deficiency heat syndrome mostly yin deficiency constitution or impairment of yin due to long illness. Yang exuberance and blood heat syndrome may show such symptoms as early menstruation with profuse amount, dark red or purple color and thick texture, accompanied by thirst, red complexion, dark urine, dry stool, red tongue with yellow coating, and slippery rapid pulse. However, yin deficiency and blood heat syndrome may show such symptoms as early menstruation with scanty amount, bright red color and thick texture, accompanied by feverish sensation of the palms and soles, tidal fever, night sweat, red tongue with scanty coating, and thready rapid pulse. On the contrary, excess cold syndrome is mostly caused by external contraction of pathogenic cold while deficiency cold syndrome is mostly with yang deficiency constitution. Symptoms such as delayed menstruation with scanty amount, dark color and blood clots, and unpalpable cold pain in the lower abdomen indicate excess cold syndrome. And symptoms such as delayed menstruation with scanty amount, light color, thin texture, and dull pain in the lower abdomen with preference for warmth and pressure show deficiency cold syndrome.

3. Differentiation of Zang-Fu Organs

The differentiation is mainly based on the amount, color, texture and cycle of the menstruation, and accompanied symptoms. If the menstrual blood is light in color and thin in texture, accompanied by mental and physical fatigue, shortness of breath, no desire to speak, listlessness and sleepiness, reduced appetite and loosing stool, pale enlarged tongue and moderate weak pulse, this case is spleen qi deficiency syndrome. If the menstruation is irregular with dark red color, blood clots, accompanied by lower abdominal distending pain, epigastric oppression and discomfort, and wiry pulse, the case is liver depression syndrome. If the menstrual blood is unstable in amount, dark in color and thin in texture, accompanied by aching lumbus and knees, dark tongue and sunken thready pulse, the case is kidney deficiency syndrome.

Syndrome Differentiation

1. Spleen Qi Deficiency Syndrome

[Clinical Manifestations] Early menstruation with unstable amount or delayed menstruation with scanty amount, light color and thin texture, mental and physical fatigue, sallow complexion, shortness of breath, no desire to speak, listlessness and sleepiness, empty sagging sensation in the lower abdomen, lower voice, epigastric oppression and abdominal distension, reduced appetite and loose stool, pale enlarged tongue with thin white coating and tooth marks on its margins, and moderate weak pulse.

[Manifestations Analysis] Spleen failing to control the blood causes the insecurity of the thoroughfare and conception vessels, causing early menstruation with unstable amount. Spleen qi deficiency leads to deficiency of qi and blood, and insufficiency of the thoroughfare and conception vessels, thus there is delayed menstruation with scanty amount. Qi deficiency fails to warm the blood, so menstruation shows light color and thin texture. Spleen deficiency and insufficiency of middle qi may cause mental and physical fatigue, shortness of breath, no desire to speak, listlessness and sleepiness, empty sagging sensation in the lower abdomen, and lower voice. Failure of the spleen in transportation and transformation may cause epigastric oppression and abdominal distension, reduced appetite and loose stool. Deficient qi and blood can't nourish the face, resulting in sallow complexion. Such symptoms as pale enlarged tongue with thin white coating and tooth marks on its margins, and moderate weak pulse, all are signs of spleen deficiency.

[Nursing Principle] Tonifying the spleen and replenishing qi; securing the thoroughfare vessel and regulating menstruation.

[Suggested Formula] Buzhong Yiqi Decoction.

2. Kidney Qi Deficiency Syndrome

[Clinical Manifestations] Early, delayed or irregular menstrual cycle, with unstable amount, light dark color and thin texture, dizziness and tinnitus, aching lumbus and knees, clear and profuse urine, frequent urination at night, dim complexion or with dark spots, dark tongue with thin white coating, and sunken thready pulse.

〔Manifestations Analysis〕Insufficiency of kidney qi causes the insecurity of the thoroughfare and conception vessels, causing early menstruation. Kidney qi deficiency causes the insufficiency of the thoroughfare and conception vessels, leading to delayed menstruation with scanty menses. Kidney deficiency causes the loss of its closing and storing function, so irregular menstrual cycle occurs with scanty menses. Kidney deficiency causes the insufficiency of essence and blood, resulting in scanty menses. Kidney qi insufficiency fails to warm the blood, causing menses with light dark color and thin texture. Lumbus is the house of the kidney and kidney governs the bones, so kidney deficiency causes the malnourishment of the lumbus and the weakness of sinew and bone, then aching lumbus and weak knees appears. Kidney opens into the ears, so kidney deficiency causes the insufficiency of the blood sea and the malnutrition of clear orifices, then dizziness and tinnitus appear. Kidney deficiency causes the failure of qi transformation, so clear and profuse urine and frequent urination at night occur. Kidney pertains to blackness in color, so there appears dim complexion or with dark spots. Such symptoms as dark tongue with thin white coating, and sunken thready pulse, all are signs of kidney deficiency.

〔Nursing Principle〕Tonifying the kidney and replenishing qi; nourishing blood and regulating menstruation.

〔Suggested Formula〕Guyin Decoction.

3. Liver Qi Depression Syndrome

〔Clinical Manifestations〕Irregular menstrual cycle with unstable amount, dark red color, blood clots, menstrual inhibition, distending pain in chest, hypochondrium, breast and lower abdomen, epigastric oppression and discomfort, frequent sigh, pale red tongue with thin white coating, and wiry pulse.

〔Manifestations Analysis〕Failure of the liver to govern free flow of qi induces the abnormal storing and excreting function of the uterus, so irregular menstrual cycle with unstable menses appears. Qi stagnation causes blood stasis, so menses occurs with dark red color, blood clots, and menstrual inhibition. The liver meridian goes up to the lower abdomen and spreads over the hypochondriac region, so when liver qi is depressed, qi movement in the course of the liver meridian is inhibited, thus, there appears distending pain in chest, hypochondrium, breast and lower abdomen. The depressed qi is not freed timely, so epigastric oppression and discomfort, and frequent sigh are felt. Pale red tongue with thin white coating, and wiry pulse, all are signs of liver qi depression.

〔Nursing Principle〕Soothing the liver and relieving depression; regulating qi and menstruation.

〔Suggested Formula〕Xiaoyao Powder.

4. Yang Exuberance and Blood Heat Syndrome

〔Clinical Manifestations〕Early menstruation with profuse amount, dark red or purple color and thick texture, thirst, preference for cold drink, red complexion and lips, heart vexation, dark urine, dry stool, red tongue with yellow coating, and slippery rapid pulse.

[Manifestations Analysis] Heat harassing the thoroughfare and conception vessels drives the blood to flow frenetically, causing carly menstruation with profuse amount. Heat scorching the blood causes the menses with dark red or purple color and thick texture. Pathogenic heat disturbing the heart induces heart vexation. Heat exuberance consuming body fluids leads to thirst, preference for cold drink, dark urine, and dry stool. Such symptoms as red complexion and lips, red tongue with yellow coating, and slippery rapid pulse, all are signs of excess heat.

[Nursing Principle] Clearing heat and reducing fire; cooling blood and regulating menstruation.

[Suggested Formula] Qingjing Powder.

5. Yin Deficiency and Blood Heat Syndrome

[Clinical Manifestations] Early menstruation with scanty menses, bright red color and thick texture, feverish sensation of the palms and soles, dry mouth and throat, flushed cheeks, tidal fever, night sweat, heart vexation, sleeplessness, ulceration of the mouth and tongue, red tongue with scanty coating, and thready rapid pulse.

[Manifestations Analysis] Heat harassing the thoroughfare and conception vessels drives the blood to flow frenetically, causing early menstruation. Yin deficiency and blood inadequacy causes the insufficiency of the thoroughfare and conception vessels, so the menses is scanty. Heat scorching the blood causes the menses with bright red color and thick texture. Heat exuberance consuming body fluid leads to dry mouth and throat. Such symptoms as feverish sensation of the palms and soles, flushed cheeks, tidal fever, night sweat, heart vexation, sleeplessness, red tongue with scanty coating, and thready rapid pulse, all are signs of deficiency heat.

[Nursing Principle] Nourishing yin and clearing heat; cooling blood and regulating menstruation.

[Suggested Formula] Liangdi Decoction.

6. Deficiency Cold Syndrome

[Clinical Manifestations] Delayed menstruation with scanty amount, light color, thin texture, cold pain in the lower abdomen with preference for warmth and pressure, weak aching lumbus, clear and profuse urine, loose stool, pale tongue with white coating, and sunken slow and forceless pulse.

[Manifestations Analysis] Insufficiency of yang qi fails to warm zang-fu organs, and deficiency of qi and blood causes the insufficiency of the thoroughfare and conception vessels, causing delayed menstruation with scanty menses. Yang deficiency fails to warm the blood, so the menses is with light color and thin texture. Yang deficiency fails to warm and nourish the uterus, therefore leading to cold pain in the lower abdomen with preference for warmth and pressure. Yang deficiency and insufficiency of kidney qi fail to nourish the lumbus, leading to weak aching lumbus. Yang deficiency and inhibited qi transformation result in clear and profuse urine. Pale tongue with white coating, and sunken slow and forceless pulse, all are signs of deficiency cold.

[Nursing Principle] Warming meridian to restore yang; nourishing blood and regulating menstruation.

[Suggested Formula] Wenjing Decoction (in *Synopsis of the Golden Chamber*).

7. Excess Cold Syndrome

[Clinical Manifestations] Delayed menstruation with scanty amount, dark color and blood clots, unpalpable cold pain in the lower abdomen, fear of cold, cold limbs, dark tongue with white coating, and sunken tight pulse.

[Manifestations Analysis] External contraction of pathogenic cold coagulates the blood that causes the unsmooth flow of menses, causing delayed menstruation with scanty amount. Cold coagulation and blood stagnation causes the internal obstruction of blood stasis, leading to menses with dark color and blood clots. Pathogenic cold obstructing the uterus leads to stagnation of qi and blood, therefore, unpalpable cold pain in the lower abdomen is felt because "where there is obstruction, there is pain". Cold belongs to yin pathogen that hinders yang qi to reach the body surface, causing fear of cold and cold limbs. Pale tongue with white coating, and sunken tight pulse are signs of excess cold.

[Nursing Principle] Warming meridian to dissipate cold; activating blood and regulating menstruation.

[Suggested Formula] Wenjing Decoction (in *A Complete Collection of Effective Prescriptions for Women*).

NURSING MEASURES

For patients with early menstruation, delayed menstruation or irregular menstrual cycle, nurses should observe the amount, color, texture and cycle of the menses. Besides, for patients with profuse menses, the complexion, spirit and blood pressure should be observed to timely detect anemia and shock. If something unusual happens, it is advisable to report to the doctor immediately.

Syndrome-Based Nursing Measures

1. Spleen Qi Deficiency Syndrome

(1) Daily life nursing. The ward should be warm, quiet, dry and comfortable, with plenty of light. The patients should keep themselves warm, rest in bed, and reduce activities if the menses is profuse. They should also avoid overstrain, braving rain or wading in water during menstruation.

(2) Diet nursing. The patients may eat foods that replenish qi and invigorate the spleen, such as lean pork, fuling (poria) and dazao (Chinese date). Food therapy: shenqi (ginseng and astragalus root) stewed with black chicken. Don't eat greasy, raw, cold, bitter, sour, astringent, pungent or spicy foods.

(3) Emotion nursing. Nurses may use verbal enlightenment therapy to communicate with the patients to help them stay in a pleasant state of mind and prevent excessive contemplation and anxiety.

(4) Medication nursing. Decoction should be taken warm before meals, multiple times in small portions. Avoid eating white radish and laifuzi (radish seed), and don't take too many tonic products during medication.

(5) Manipulation techniques. ① Moxibustion therapy: select Zusanli (ST 36), Qihai (CV 6), and Guanyuan (CV 4); place the moxa stick 2~3 centimeters away from the skin to perform mild moxibustion on each of them until the area turns red and the patient feels warm and comfortable without the sensation of burning pain, once per day. And it cannot be applied on the abdomen of pregnant women. ② Medicated ironing therapy: select Pishu (BL 20) and Weishu (BL 21), or Zhongwan (CV 12) and Shenque (CV 8); grind into fine powder baizhu (white atractylodes rhizome), danggui (Chinese angelica), baibiandou (white hyacinth bean) and huangqi (astragalus root) 20 g respectively; stir-fry the powder and put it into a cloth bag for medicated ironing at a temperature of 60~70℃; each time apply the bag on the back or the abdomen for 20 minutes, once per day. And it cannot be applied on the abdomen of pregnant women.

2. Kidney Qi Deficiency Syndrome

(1) Daily life nursing. The ward should be warm and quiet, with plenty of light. The patients should rest in bed, and reduce activities if the menses is profuse. They should also reduce the frequency of sexual activities, and avoid overstrain, staying up late, and washing hair and shower with cold water.

(2) Diet nursing. The patients may eat foods that replenish the kidney and secure the thoroughfare vessel, such as hetaoren (walnut), sangshen (mulberry), heizhima (black sesame), heidou (black soybean) and pig kidneys. Food therapy: sheep ridge soup, steamed black chicken, or yin'er gedan (tremella and pigeon egg) thick soup. Don't eat raw, cold, bitter, sour, astringent, pungent, or spicy foods.

(3) Emotion nursing. Nurses may use verbal enlightenment therapy to encourage the patients to communicate with each other to prevent pessimism.

(4) Medication nursing. Decoction should be taken warm before meals. Avoid eating white radish and laifuzi (radish seed), and don't take too many tonic products during medication.

(5) Manipulation techniques. ① Acupressure therapy: select Shenshu (BL 23), Mingmen (GV 4), and Ciliao (BL 32); apply thumb kneading and palm flat pushing manipulation on each of them until the area turns hot the patient has the feelings of soreness, numbness, distension and heaviness in the area, once per day. And it is contraindicated in pregnancy. ② Moxibustion therapy: select Shenque (CV 8), Yaoyangguan (GV 3) and Shenshu (BL 23); apply monkshood-cake-partitioned moxibustion on each of them. The procedure is to mix finely ground fuzi (monkshood) powder with yellow wine to make thin medicated cakes with diameter of 2~3 centimeters and thickness of 0.5~0.8 centimeters, pierce several holes through the cakes with a sharp needle, and place the cakes on the acupoints, five to seven moxa-cones on every acupoint, and twice a day. And it is contraindicated in pregnancy.

3. Liver Qi Depression Syndrome

(1) Daily life nursing. The ward should be quiet, comfortable, and full of fresh air. The coverings should be thin. The patients should keep moderate exercise, and reduce activities if the menses is profuse.

(2) Diet nursing. The patients may drink foshou (finger citron fruit) tea and eat foods that soothe

the liver and regulate qi, such as meiguihua (rose flower), kumquat, white radish, and chenpi (aged tangerine peel). Food therapy: Chinese chives stir-fried with sheep liver. Don't eat greasy, sour, astringent or flatulent foods, or warm-natured, dry-natured or yang-assisting foods.

(3) Emotion nursing. Nurses may use submission therapy to encourage the patients to express their feelings as much as possible, and satisfy their needs to reduce the psychological pressure and prevent anxiety and depression.

(4) Medication nursing. Decoction should be taken warm after meals.

(5) Manipulation techniques. ① Cupping therapy: select Qimen (LR 14) and Ganshu (BL 18); retain the cup on them for ten minutes, once or twice a week. ② Acupressure therapy: select Taichong (LR 3) and Xingjian (LR 2); apply pushing and kneading manipulation from Taichong (LR 3) to Xingjian (LR 2) slowly and repeatedly, 3~5 minutes each time, once to twice every day. And it is contraindicated in pregnancy.

4. Yang Exuberance and Blood Heat Syndrome

(1) Daily life nursing. The ward should be cool, quiet, moist, and full of fresh air. The coverings should be thin. The patients should clean the vulva every day, and rest in bed if the menses is profuse. When sitting or lying up, the action should be slowly to prevent the occurrence of vertigo and fall.

(2) Diet nursing. The diet should be light and digestible. The patients may drink biqi maogen (waternut and woolly grass) juice and eat foods that clear heat and cool blood, such as oujie (lotus rhizome node), muer (wood ear), celery and baihe (lily bulb). Don't eat greasy, warm-natured, or fire-generating foods, such as pig's feet, dasuan (garlic bulb), chili and mutton.

(3) Emotion nursing. Nurses may use verbal enlightenment therapy to make the patients have a right attitude toward the illness. Likewise, they should also inform the patients that anger would aggravate the symptoms whereas happiness would alleviate the symptoms, so the patients should keep a good mood and avoid anxiety and short temper.

(4) Medication nursing. Decoction should be taken slightly cool or warm after meals.

(5) Manipulation techniques. ① Scraping therapy: select the line from Geshu (BL 17) to Danshu (BL 19); use scraping plate to forcefully scrape the line along the bladder meridian of foot-taiyang with the direction from top to bottom, and repeat the manipulation for 20~30 successive times on each side till the area turns red and *sha qi* (rash of measles) occurs. An interval of 3~6 days for rest in between each scraping is preferred and it should be avoided during menstruation or pregnancy. ② Auricular pressure therapy: select ear apex (HX6, 7i), ovary (TF2), and endocrine (CO18); apply specialized pasters on them, press and knead on each of them till the area turns hot and red, 4~5 times per day, and keep the pasters for 2~4 days. And it is contraindicated in pregnancy.

5. Yin Deficiency and Blood Heat Syndrome

(1) Daily life nursing. The ward should be cool, moist, quiet and comfortable. The coverings should be thin. The patients should rest in bed and avoid staying up and overstrain.

(2) Diet nursing. The patients may drink biqi maogen (waternut and woolly grass) juice and eat

foods that clear heat and nourish yin, such as lean pork, baihe (lily bulb) and meat of soft-shelled turtles. Don't eat pungent, spicy, fragrant or dry-natured foods.

(3) Emotion nursing. Nurses may use verbal enlightenment therapy and care much for the patients. And the patients should not contact with anxious person so as to ensure an easy atmosphere and avoid dysphoria.

(4) Medication nursing. Decoction should be taken warm or slightly cool before meals. Avoid ingestion of white radish, laifuzi (radish seed), and excessive tonic products during medication.

(5) Manipulation techniques. ① Acupressure therapy: select Quchi (LI 11), Waiguan (TE 5) and Taixi (KI 3); apply thumb kneading manipulation on each of them until the area turns hot or the patient has the feelings of soreness, numbness, distension and heaviness in the area; once a day. And it is contraindicated in pregnancy. ② Auricular pressure therapy: select shenmen (TF4) and sympathetic (AH6a); apply specialized pasters on them, press and knead on each of them till the area turns hot and red, 4~5 times per day, and keep the pasters for 2~4 days.

6. Deficiency Cold Syndrome

(1) Daily life nursing. The ward should be warm, quiet and full of light, avoiding strong and convective wind. The coverings should be thick. The patients should live a regular life, balance work and rest, and pay attention to keeping warm. They should also avoid overstrain, braving rain or wading in water during menstruation.

(2) Diet nursing. The patients may drink rougui (cinnamon bark) brown sugar tea and eat foods that warm yang and nourish blood, such as danggui (Chinese angelica), dazao (Chinese date), and longyanrou (longan). Food therapy: douchi (fermented soya bean) fresh ginger stewed with mutton. Don't eat raw, cold, bitter, sour, or astringent foods.

(3) Emotion nursing. Nurses may use verbal enlightenment therapy to communicate with and care for the patients as much as possible to prevent the patients from gesting pessimistic and depressed.

(4) Medication nursing. Decoction should be taken warm before meals.

(5) Manipulation techniques. ① Moxibustion therapy: select Shenque (CV 8), Guanyuan (CV 4), Shenshu (BL 23) and Mingmen (GV 4); apply monkshood-cake-partitioned moxibustion on each of them. The procedure is to mix finely ground fuzi (monkshood) powder with yellow wine to make thin medicated cakes with diameter of 2~3 centimeters and thickness of 0.5~0.8 centimeters, pierce several holes through the cakes with a sharp needle, and place the cakes on the acupoints, five to seven moxa-cones on every acupoint, and twice every day. And it is contraindicated in pregnancy. ② Medicated ironing therapy: select Shenshu (BL 23), Mingmen (GV 4) and Yaoyangguan (GV 3); apply the therapy with tusizi (dodder seed) 300 g, qingyan (halite) 300 g, rougui (cinnamon bark) powder 100 g, fuzi (monkshood) powder 50 g, which should be stir-fried and put into a cloth bag for medicated ironing at a temperature of 60~70℃; 20 minutes each time, once per day. And it is contraindicated in pregnancy. ③ Acupressure therapy: select Laogong (PC 8) and Yongquan (KI 1); apply thumb kneading manipulation on each of them before bed every night till the area feels hot. And it is

contraindicated in pregnancy.

7. Excess Cold Syndrome

(1) Daily life nursing. The ward should be warm, quiet and full of light. The coverings should be thick. The patients should live a regular life, balance work and rest, and do moderate exercise. They should also avoid braving rain or wading in water during menstruation.

(2) Diet nursing. The patients may drink shengjiang aiye (fresh ginger and mugwort leaf) brown sugar tea and eat warm and yang-assisting foods, such as rougui (cinnamon bark), douchi (fermented soya bean), mutton and huajiao (pricklyash peel). Don't eat raw, cold, bitter, sour, or astringent foods.

(3) Emotion nursing. Nurses may use emotional transference and dispositional change therapy to encourage the patients to take part in entertainment activities so as to keep a good mood.

(4) Medication nursing. Decoction should be taken hot after meals.

(5) Manipulation techniques. ① Foot fumigating and washing therapy: aiye (mugwort leaf) 30 g, ganjiang (dried ginger rhizome) 30 g, tusizi (dodder seed) 30 g, duzhong (eucommia bark) 20 g, danggui (Chinese angelica) 20 g, chuanxiong (Sichuan lovage root) 20 g, zhifuzi (prepared aconite root) 20 g, huajiao (pricklyash peel) 15 g, rougui (cinnamon bark) 10 g, and water 1 500 mL; decoct the above ingredients for fumigating at a temperature of $50 \sim 70 \, ^{\circ}\text{C}$, and for foot bathing at a temperature of $37 \sim 40 \, ^{\circ}\text{C}$, 20 minutes each time, once per day. After fumigating and washing, the patients need to take a rest for 30 minutes before leaving. ② Moxibustion therapy: select Guanyuan (CV 4), Baliao (BL 31~34), Sanyinjiao (SP 6) and Zusanli (ST 36); place the moxa stick 2~3 centimeters away from the skin to perform mild moxibustion on each of them until the area turns red and the patient feels warm and comfortable without the sensation of burning pain, once per day. And it cannot be applied on the abdomen and lumbosacral region of pregnant women.

Patient Education

The nurses should explain to the patients about the health care knowledge of the disease and answer their problems patiently in order to make them confident and cooperative.

Sexual intercourse is strictly prohibited during menstruation. And it is not appropriate to swim, take tub bath, dip into cold water, and have vaginal medication and examination.

The diet should be light, nutritious and digestible. Eat foods rich in iron and vitamin C, and foods that tonify qi and nourish blood, such as yolk, beans, animal liver, chicken, fish, dazao (Chinses date), heizhima (black sesame) and tomatoes. The patients should refrain from cigarette and alcohol. Raw, cold, pungent, spicy, fragrant, fried, roasted and indigestible foods should be avoided.

Menstruation-regulating medicine should be taken several days before menstruation, generally three cycles as a course of treatment. During medication, pay attention to the changes of menstrual quantity, color and texture.

It is recommended to follow up the patients with irregular menstrual cycle to exclude other gynecological diseases. For abnormal menstrual cycle with abdominal pain, the cause should be identified.

第二节 痛 经

痛经,是指因月经期前后冲任不和,导致气血阻滞,或因精血不足,导致胞脉失养,以经期或经行前后出现周期性小腹疼痛,或痛引腰骶,牵掣大腿内侧,甚则剧痛,汗出,晕厥,伴见面色苍白为临床特征的月经病。西医的痛经分为原发性和继发性两类。原发性痛经者,生殖器无器质性病变。继发性痛经多由盆腔器质性疾病,如盆腔炎性疾病、子宫内膜异位症、子宫腺肌病等引起。这两类痛经均可参照本节进行护理。

一、病因病机

痛经的病因常有虚实两种,以实者居多。其实者多因邪气而起,如气滞、寒凝和湿热阻滞,逢经前、经期气血下注冲任,胞宫气血更加壅滞,不通则痛,发为痛经。气滞血瘀多由天性抑郁或积怒伤肝所致。寒凝血瘀多因冒雨涉水,坐卧湿地,久居寒处而感受外寒,或因过食生冷,寒邪直中所致。湿热瘀阻多因素体湿热或外感湿热之邪所致。其虚者常见于气血两虚和肝肾亏虚,胞宫、冲任失于温煦濡养,经期、经后血海更虚,不荣则痛,发为痛经。气血两虚多由素体脾虚,生化乏源,或失血久病所致。肝肾亏虚多由先天不足,房劳多产和重病久病所致。

痛经的病机分为两大类:冲任、胞宫气血阻滞,“不通则痛”;冲任、胞宫失于濡养,“不荣而痛”。病位在冲任、胞宫,与肝、肾、脾相关。实证多责之于寒、热、湿邪侵袭,虚证多责之于脾肾亏虚。

二、常见证型

(一)辨证要点

1. 辨寒热 根据疼痛的性质和缓解因素来辨别。若疼痛性质为绞痛、冷痛,得热痛减,则多为寒证。若疼痛性质为灼痛,得热痛增,则多为热证。

2. 辨虚实 根据疼痛的发生时间、性质和程度等来辨别。若疼痛发生在经前、月经初期或月经中期,为绞痛、刺痛、灼痛,疼痛剧烈,拒按,则多为实证。若疼痛发生在月经后程或月经结束之后,为隐痛、坠痛,疼痛不剧烈,喜揉喜按,则多为虚证。

3. 辨气滞与血瘀 根据疼痛的性质、部位和持续时间等来辨别。若疼痛位于腹部正中,持续刺痛,块下痛减,胀感较弱,则多为血瘀。若疼痛常窜于两侧少腹,时痛时止,痛无定处,胀甚于痛,则多为气滞。

(二)证候分型

1. 气滞血瘀证

[主要证候]经前或经期小腹胀痛拒按,经行不畅,色紫暗,有血块,块下痛减;经前乳房胀痛;

舌暗红或有瘀点、瘀斑,苔薄白,脉弦。

[证候分析]肝失调达,冲任气血郁滞,故经前或经期小腹胀痛拒按,经行不畅,色紫暗,有血块。血块排出后气血暂通,故块下痛减。肝气郁滞,经脉不利,故经前乳房胀痛;舌暗红或有瘀点、瘀斑,脉弦,均为气滞血瘀之象。

[护治原则]理气活血,化瘀止痛。

[常用方剂]膈下逐瘀汤。

2. 寒凝血瘀证

[主要证候]经前或经期小腹冷痛,得热痛减,色暗,有血块;平素带下量多,质清稀,畏寒肢冷;舌暗或有瘀点、瘀斑,苔白或腻,脉沉紧。

[证候分析]寒邪收引凝滞,与经血抟结,使血行不畅,故经前或经期小腹冷痛;寒凝导致血瘀,故经色暗,有血块;阴寒内盛,气化失司故平素带下量多,质清稀;寒邪伤阳,身体失于温煦,故畏寒肢冷;舌暗或有瘀点、瘀斑,苔白或腻,脉沉紧,均为寒凝血瘀之象。

[护治原则]温经散寒,化瘀止痛。

[常用方剂]少腹逐瘀汤。

3. 湿热瘀阻证

[主要证候]经前或经期小腹疼痛或胀痛拒按,有灼热感,或痛连腰骶,色暗红,质稠,或夹较多黏液;平素带下量多,色黄,质稠,有味,或低热起伏,小便黄赤;舌红,苔黄腻,脉弦数或滑数。

[证候分析]湿热阻滞冲任、胞宫,与血相抟结,气机不通,故小腹疼痛或胀痛拒按,有灼热感;热盛伤津,故经色暗红,质稠,带下量色黄,质稠,小便黄赤;湿为阴邪,气化失司,故月经中或夹较多黏液,平素带下量多;舌红,苔黄腻,脉弦数或滑数,均为湿热瘀阻之象。

[护治原则]清热除湿,化瘀止痛。

[常用方剂]清热调血汤。

4. 气血虚弱证

[主要证候]经期或经后小腹隐隐坠痛,喜按,或小腹阴部空坠,月经量少,色淡,质清稀;面色无华,神疲乏力;舌淡,苔薄白,脉细无力。

[证候分析]气血不足致胞宫、冲任失养,经行之后血海更虚,故经期或经后小腹隐隐坠痛,喜按;气虚不固,故小腹阴部空坠;气虚不充,血虚不荣,故月经量少,色淡,质清稀;气血两虚不能上荣于面,故面色无华;气血两虚,心失所养,脾阳不振,故神疲乏力;舌淡,脉细无力,均为气血虚弱之象。

[护治原则]补气养血,调经止痛。

[常用方剂]八珍汤。

5. 肝肾亏损证

[主要证候]经期或经后小腹绵绵作痛,伴腰骶部酸痛,经量少,色淡暗,质稀;头晕耳鸣,失眠健忘,或伴潮热;舌淡红,苔薄白,脉细弱。

[证候分析]肝肾亏损,精血不足,冲任俱虚,经行之后血海更虚,胞宫、冲任更失于濡养,故经期或经后小腹绵绵作痛,经量少,色淡暗,质稀;腰为肾之府,肾开窍于耳,肾虚故腰骶部酸痛,伴耳鸣;肝肾亏虚,清窍失养,故头晕。脉细弱,为肝肾亏损之象。

[护治原则]补养肝肾,调经止痛。

[常用方剂]调肝汤。

三、护理措施

对于痛经的病人,应询问痛经的发生时间、持续时长;疼痛的部位、性质、程度、缓解因素、加重因素;进行疼痛评定。注意观察月经的量、色、质,有无血块,以及月经周期。对于疼痛剧烈的病人,应观察面色,汗出,血压。若病人出现坐卧不宁,面色苍白,冷汗淋漓,四肢厥冷,甚至血压下降,应立即报告医生。

（一）辨证施护

1. 气滞血瘀证

（1）生活起居护理　居室温暖整洁,空气新鲜,避免油烟和异味刺激。注意腹部和下肢保暖,禁止坐卧潮湿之地。适量锻炼,如散步、打太极拳,以保持大便通畅。

（2）饮食护理　饮食清淡,少食多餐。可饮玫瑰花茶。宜食行滞化瘀的食物,如陈皮、金橘、山楂、佛手。食疗方:茉莉花粥、酒糟蛋。不宜食生冷、肥甘、辛辣的食物。

（3）情志护理　护士可运用顺意疗法,鼓励病人多表达,满足病人的合理要求,以避免焦虑、抑郁。

（4）用药护理　中药汤剂宜武火快煎。饭后温服,少量多次服用。

（5）操作技术　① 穴位按摩法:取气海、太冲、三阴交、内关、次髎,用拇指揉法、掌平推法、一指禅推法,按摩至局部发热或有酸麻重胀感,每日 1 次。② 耳压疗法:取卵巢、内分泌、皮质下、肝等耳穴,用耳穴压丸贴片贴压,每日按揉 4~5 次,以局部发热泛红为度,留置 2~4 日,从经前使用至经行痛止。

2. 寒凝血瘀证

（1）生活起居护理　居室温暖干燥。衣被宜厚。卧床休息,注意腹部和下肢保暖。禁止冒雨涉水,坐卧湿地。

（2）饮食护理　可饮红花酒、山楂肉桂红糖汤。宜食散寒活血的食物,如羊肉、小茴香。食疗方:艾叶生姜煮鸡蛋、桂椒炖猪肚。经前及经期不宜食寒凉、酸涩的食物,如柿子、西瓜、醋、蚌肉、螺蛳。

（3）情志护理　护士可运用语言开导疗法,鼓励家属多陪伴病人,用融洽和睦的氛围温暖病人。

（4）用药护理　中药汤剂宜饭后温服。丸剂可用黄酒或生姜红糖水送服。

（5）操作技术　① 灸法:取神阙、命门、关元、三阴交、肾俞,用隔姜灸,把生姜切成直径 2~3 厘米、厚 0.4~0.6 厘米的薄片,中间以针刺数孔,放置于施灸处,每处 5 壮,每日 2 次。② 敷脐疗法:用吴茱萸、小茴香各 20 g,肉桂 10 g,共研细末备用;从月经将要来临前 3 天开始,取 3 g 药粉与黄酒调成糊状,纳入脐中,用胶布固定后用热水袋加温,每次 2~8 小时;每日 1 次,连用 3 次。③ 热敷疗法:取腹部,用青盐 150 g;炒热装入布袋中,制成温度为 60~70℃的布包,热敷 20 分钟,每日 1 次。

3. 湿热瘀阻证

（1）生活起居护理　居室凉爽舒适,空气新鲜。衣被宜薄。避免剧烈运动,禁止冒雨涉水,坐卧湿地。

（2）饮食护理　宜食清热除湿的食物,如薏苡仁、苦瓜、赤小豆、丝瓜叶。食疗方:田螺塞肉。忌饮酒过度,不宜食辛辣、油腻、热性的食物,如辣椒、韭菜、羊肉。

（3）情志护理　护士可运用移情易性疗法,营造轻松的氛围。可请病人聆听舒缓的音乐,以保持情绪稳定,避免烦躁、焦虑。

（4）用药护理　中药汤剂宜饭后温服或偏凉服。

（5）操作技术　① 耳压疗法:取卵巢、内分泌、皮质下等耳穴,用耳穴压丸贴片贴压,每日按揉4~5次,以局部发热泛红为度,留置2~4日,从经前使用至经行痛止。② 穴位按摩:取次髎、阴陵泉,用拇指揉法,按摩至局部发热或有酸麻重胀感,每日1次。

4. 气血虚弱证

（1）生活起居护理　居室温暖安静。衣被宜厚。卧床休息,注意腹部和下肢保暖,睡眠充足。适量运动,如散步、打太极拳。避免过劳,禁止坐卧潮湿之地。

（2）饮食护理　宜食益气补血的食物,如乌贼、龙眼肉、山药。食疗方:当归生姜羊肉汤、乌鸡良姜汤。糯米阿胶粥:阿胶30 g,糯米50 g,将阿胶捣碎炒黄研磨备用,将糯米加水500 mL煮粥,待粥熟后加阿胶末搅匀服食,每日2次。不宜食过甜、滋腻、生冷、辛辣的食物。

（3）情志护理　护士可运用语言开导疗法,多关心鼓励病人,以避免抑郁、消沉。

（4）用药护理　中药汤剂宜文火久煎,饭前温服。勿过用滋补之品。

（5）操作技术　① 灸法:取命门、肾俞、关元、足三里、脾俞,用温和灸,艾条燃着端悬于施灸部位上,距离皮肤2~3厘米,灸至病人有温热舒适无灼痛的感觉,皮肤稍有红晕,每日1次,从经前使用至经行痛止。② 穴位按摩法:取脾俞、胃俞、足三里,用拇指揉法,按摩至局部发热或有酸麻重胀感,每日1次。

5. 肝肾亏损证

（1）生活起居护理　居室温暖安静。卧床休息,注意腹部和下肢保暖,睡眠充足。适量运动,如散步、打太极拳。平时应节制性行为,避免过劳,禁止淋雨涉水,坐卧湿地。

（2）饮食护理　可饮枸杞子茶、桑椹茶。宜食益肾养肝的食物,如黑芝麻、紫米、猪肾、猪肝、核桃仁。食疗方:枸杞炖兔肉。不宜食生冷、辛辣的食物。

（3）情志护理　护士可运用语言开导疗法,经常巡视病房,多关心鼓励病人,使病人保持心情愉悦,避免紧张、恐惧。

（4）用药护理　中药汤剂宜文火久煎,饭前温服。

（5）操作技术　① 灸法:取肾俞、肝俞、太溪、复溜、归来,用温和灸,艾条燃着端悬于施灸部位上,距离皮肤2~3厘米,灸至病人有温热舒适无灼痛的感觉,皮肤稍有红晕,每日1次,从经前使用至经行痛止。② 推拿疗法:取背部督脉以及肾俞、命门,用擦法,按摩至局部透热。

（二）健康教育

从月经将要开始前的3~5天起,避免剧烈运动和重体力劳动。保持外阴清洁,每日用温开水清洗。保持大便通畅。月经未尽时,忌性行为、盆浴、游泳、涉水。

从月经将要开始前的3~5天起,饮食以清淡、易消化为主,可食补血活血的食物,如大枣、苹果,不宜吃太咸、过甜的食物。月经期间应少食多餐,多吃温性的以及高纤维的食物,如红薯。忌烟酒、浓茶、咖啡,不宜食生冷、酸性的食物。

保持乐观豁达,平和舒畅的心情。对于原发性痛经,消除紧张的心理能在一定程度上缓解痛经。护士应向病人宣教关于预防痛经的知识,解答病人的疑问。

规律用药,遵医嘱从疼痛发生前的3~5天开始,用至痛止。坚持周期性治疗,连续治疗3个月经周期以上。

在痛经的症状缓解后,应明确病因。必要时到医院进行妇科检查。

Section 2   Dysmenorrhea

Dysmenorrhea refers to the menstrual disease characterized by periodic lower abdominal pain that may radiate to the lumbosacral area and inner thigh, or even by severe pain, sweating, fainting, and pale complexion, before, after or during menstruation. It is mainly caused by the disharmony of the thoroughfare and conception vessels and the stagnation of qi and blood before or after menstruation, or by insufficiency of essence and blood, and the malnourishment of the uterine vessels. Dysmenorrhea in Western medicine can be divided into primary and secondary dysmenorrhea. Primary dysmenorrhea is without pelvic organic lesions. And secondary dysmenorrhea is often caused by pelvic organic lesions, such as pelvic inflammation disease, endometriosis, adenomyosis, etc. This section can be referred to for the nursing of these two types of dysmenorrhea in Western medicine.

ETIOLOGY AND PATHOGENESIS

The etiology includes deficiency and excess, with the latter mostly seen. The excess cause mainly refers to pathogenic factors, such as qi stagnation, cold coagulation and dampness-heat obstruction, which further congest and stagnate the movement of qi and blood in the uterus and the thoroughfare and conception vessels before or during menstruation. Among the pathogenic factors, qi stagnation and blood stasis is mostly due to one's emotional depression in nature or accumulated anger injuring the liver; cold coagulation and blood stasis are mainly caused by the contraction of external cold (due to such factors as wading in rain, sitting and lying in damp places, and living in cold places for a long time), or by cold pathogen directly attacking the body (due to overeating raw and cold foods); dampness-heat and stasis obstruction is frequently caused by dampness-heat constitution or external contraction of pathogenic dampness-heat. And the deficiency cause is often seen in qi and blood deficiency syndrome, and liver and kidney deficiency syndrome. In these cases, the uterus and the thoroughfare and conception vessels lose its due warmth and nourishment. And the blood sea becomes more insufficient during or after menstruation, so painful menstruation happens. Among them, qi and blood deficiency syndrome is mostly caused by spleen deficiency constitution that lacks the source of generation and transformation, or by loss of blood and chronic diseases; liver and kidney deficiency syndrome is usually caused by congenital inadequacy, sexual strain, fertility, and serious or chronic diseases.

The pathogenesis is divided into two categories: one is the obstruction of qi and blood in the uterus and the thoroughfare and conception vessels, and the other is the malnourishment of the uterus and the thoroughfare and conception vessels. Obviously, the disease is located in the uterus and the thoroughfare and conception vessels but relates to the liver, spleen and kidney. Excess syndromes of dysmenorrhea are often caused by cold, heat and dampness pathogens whereas deficiency syndromes often result from spleen and kidney deficiency.

COMMON SYNDROMES

Key Points in Syndrome Differentiation

1. Differentiation of Cold from Heat Syndrome

The differentiation is based on the nature of the pain and alleviating factors. Colic pain, cold pain, and pain alleviated with warmth pertain to cold syndrome. And burning pain and pain worsened with warmth belong to heat syndrome.

2. Differentiation of Deficiency from Excess Syndrome

The differentiation is based on the onset time, nature and severity of the pain. Colic pain, stabbing pain, burning pain, severe pain, unpalpable pain, or pain that takes place before, at the beginning of, or during menstruation belong to excess syndrome. And dull pain, sagging pain, mild pain, preference for kneading and pressure, or pain that appears after or at the end of menstruation pertain to deficiency syndrome.

3. Differentiation of Qi Stagnation from Blood Stasis

The differentiation is based on the nature, location and duration of the pain. Continuous stabbing pain, pain located in the middle of the abdomen, pain alleviated after the release of blood clots, or severer pain with milder distension mostly indicates blood stasis. And intermittent pain, migrant pain, pain often scurrying on both sides of the lower abdomen, or severer distension with milder pain mostly suggests qi stagnation.

Syndrome Differentiation

1. Qi Stagnation and Blood Stasis Syndrome

[Clinical Manifestations] Unpalpable distending pain in lower abdomen before or during menstruation, unsmooth menstruation with dark purple color and blood clots, pain alleviated after the release of blood clots, breast distending pain before menstruation, dark red tongue with thin white coating, or with stasis speckle and macule, and wiry pulse.

[Manifestations Analysis] Liver fails to act freely, and qi and blood stagnate in the thoroughfare and conception vessels, causing unpalpable distending pain in lower abdomen before or during menstruation, and unsmooth menstruation with dark purple color and blood clots. The removal of the clots temporarily normalizes the movement of qi and blood, so the pain is alleviated. Liver qi is depressed and meridian vessel is inhibited, therefore, breast distending pain before menstruation occurs. And dark red tongue, or with stasis speckle and macule, and wiry pulse, all are signs of qi stagnation and blood stasis.

[Nursing Principle] Regulating qi and activating blood; resolving stasis and relieving pain.

[Suggested Formula] Gexia Zhuyu Decoction.

2. Cold Coagulation and Blood Stasis Syndrome

[Clinical Manifestations] Cold pain in lower abdomen before or during menstruation, pain alleviated with warmth, menstruation with dark color and blood clots, profuse leucorrhea with clear thin texture in normal times, fear of cold, cold limbs, dark tongue with white or slimy coating, or with stasis speckle and macule, and sunken tight pulse.

[Manifestations Analysis] Cold pathogen with contraction and coagulation attribute binds with the blood, which inhibits the smooth movement of blood, causing cold pain in lower abdomen before or during menstruation. Cold coagulation causes blood stasis, leading to menstruation with dark color and blood clots. Inner exuberance of yin cold causes the failure of qi transformation, therefore, there is profuse leucorrhea with clear thin texture in normal times. Cold pathogen damages yang that makes the body lose the warmth of yang qi, so fear of cold and cold limbs is felt. Dark tongue with white or slimy coating, or with stasis speckle and macule, and sunken tight pulse, all are signs of cold coagulation and blood stasis.

[Nursing Principle] Warming meridian and dissipating cold; resolving stasis and relieving pain.

[Suggested Formula] Shaofu Zhuyu Decoction.

3. Dampness-Heat and Stasis Obstruction Syndrome

[Clinical Manifestations] Pain or unpalpable distending pain in lower abdomen before or during menstruation, burning heat sensation, or pain radiating to the lumbosacral area, menstruation with dark red color and thick texture, or accompanying with more mucus, profuse leucorrhea with yellow color and thick texture as well as odor smell in normal times, or fluctuated low fever, dark urine, red tongue with yellow slimy coating, and wiry rapid pulse or slippery rapid pulse.

[Manifestations Analysis] Dampness-heat that obstructs the thoroughfare and conception vessels and the uterus binds with the blood, which causes the blockage of qi movement, leading to pain or unpalpable distending pain in lower abdomen and burning heat sensation. Heat exuberance damages body fluid, causing such symptoms as dark urine, menstruation with dark red color and thick texture, profuse leucorrhea with yellow color and thick texture as well as odor smell. Dampness of yin pathogen attribute causes the failure of qi transformation, therefore, there are such symptoms as menstruation accompanying with more mucus, and profuse leucorrhea in normal times. And red tongue with yellow slimy coating, and wiry rapid pulse or slippery rapid pulse, all are signs of dampness-heat and stasis obstruction.

[Nursing Principle] Clearing heat and removing dampness; resolving stasis and relieving pain.

[Suggested Formula] Qingre Tiaoxue Decoction.

4. Qi and Blood Deficiency Syndrome

[Clinical Manifestations] Dull sagging pain in lower abdomen during or after menstruation, preference for pressure, or empty sagging sensation in lower abdomen and vulva area, scanty menstruation with light color and clear thin texture, lusterless complexion, mental and physical fatigue, pale tongue with thin white coating, and thready weak pulse.

[Manifestations Analysis] Qi and blood deficiency causes the malnourishment of the uterus and the thoroughfare and conception vessels. And the blood sea becomes more insufficient after menstruation, causing such symptoms as dull sagging pain in lower abdomen during or after menstruation and preference for pressure. Qi deficiency with its poor secure function leads to empty sagging sensation in lower abdomen and vulva area. Qi deficiency fails to fill the blood vessels and blood deficiency can't nourish the body, resulting in scanty menstruation with light color and clear thin texture. Dual deficiency of qi and blood fails to nourish the face, causing lusterless complexion. Dual deficiency of qi and blood fails to nourish the heart and devitalizes spleen yang, so mental and physical fatigue is felt. And pale tongue and thready weak pulse are signs of qi and blood deficiency.

[Nursing Principle] Tonifying qi and nourishing blood; regulating menstruation and relieving pain.

[Suggested Formula] Bazhen Decoction.

5. Liver and Kidney Deficiency Syndrome

[Clinical Manifestations] Incessant pain in lower abdomen after or during menstruation, accompanying with aching pain in lumbosacral area, scanty menstruation with light dark color and thin texture, dizziness, tinnitus, insomnia, forgetfulness, or accompanying with tidal fever, light red tongue with thin white coating, and thready weak pulse.

[Manifestations Analysis] Liver and kidney deficiency causes the insufficiency of essence and blood, and the deficiency of the thoroughfare and conception vessels. And the blood sea becomes more insufficient after menstruation, causing such symptoms as incessant pain in lower abdomen after or during menstruation, and scanty menstruation with light dark color and thin texture. Lumbus is the house of the kidney and the kidney opens into the ears, so kidney deficiency causes aching pain in lumbosacral area and tinnitus. Liver and kidney deficiency fails to nourish the clear orifices, so dizziness is felt. And thread weaky pulse is the sign of liver and kidney deficiency.

[Nursing Principle] Tonifying and nourishing the liver and kidney; regulating menstruation and relieving pain.

[Suggested Formula] Tiaogan Decoction.

NURSING MEASURES

For patients with dysmenorrhea, nurses should check the onset, duration, location, nature, intensity and cause of relief or aggravation of the pain, and perform pain evaluation. They should also observe the amount, color, texture, clot and other accompanying symptoms of the menses. For patients experiencing severe pain, their complexion, perspiration, and blood pressure should be checked. If the patient exhibits white complexion, fidgetiness, dripping cold sweat, reversal cold of the limbs, or even a drop in blood pressure, it is advisable to timely report to the doctor.

Syndrome-Based Nursing Measures

1. Qi Stagnation and Blood Stasis Syndrome

(1) Daily life nursing. The ward should be warm, tidy, and full of fresh air. The patients should keep abdomen and the lower limbs warm, and do moderate exercise such as walking or Taiji to maintain a normal bowel movement. They should avoid fumes, odor irritation, and damp places when sitting or lying down.

(2) Diet nursing. The diet should be light. The patients should have small frequent meals, and may drink meiguihua (rose flower) tea and eat foods that remove food stagnation and resolve stasis, such as chenpi (aged tangerine peel), kumquat, shanzha (Chinese hawthorn fruit) and foshou (finger citron fruit). Food therapy: jasmine flower porridge and jiuzao (distillers' grains) boiled with eggs. Raw, cold, fatty, sweet, pungent and spicy foods should be avoided.

(3) Emotion nursing. Nurses may use submission therapy to encourage the patients to express their feelings as much as possible, and satisfy their needs to prevent anxiety and depression.

(4) Medication nursing. Decoction should be brewed fast with strong fire and taken warm, multiple times in small portions.

(5) Manipulation techniques. ① Acupressure therapy: select Qihai (CV 6), Taichong (LR 3), Sanyinjiao (SP 6), Neiguan (PC 6), and Ciliao (BL 32); apply thumb kneading, palm flat pushing and one-finger pushing manipulations on each of them until the area turns hot or the patient has the feelings of soreness, numbness, distension and heaviness in the area; once per day. ② Auricular pressure therapy: select ovary (TF2), endocrine (CO18), subcortex (AT4), and liver (CO12); apply specialized pasters on the points, press on each of them till the area turns hot and red, 4~5 times per day, and keep the pasters for 2~4 days. Use this therapy before the menses and end it till the pain recedes during the menses.

2. Cold Coagulation and Blood Stasis Syndrome

(1) Daily life nursing. The ward should be warm and dry. The coverings should be thick. The patients should have enough rest and keep the abdomen and lower limbs warm. They should avoid braving rain or wading in water, and damp places when sitting or lying down.

(2) Diet nursing. The patients may drink honghua (safflower) wine, shanzha rougui hongtang (Chinese hawthorn fruit, cinnamon bark and brown sugar) soup, and eat foods that dissipate cold and activate blood, such as mutton and xiaohuixiang (fennel). Food therapy: aiye (mugwort leaf) ginger boiled with egg, and guijiao (cinnamon bark and white pepper) stewed with pig stomach. Cold, sour and astringent foods should be avoided before and during menstruation, such as persimmons, watermelons, vinegar, mussel and river snails.

(3) Emotion nursing. Nurses may use verbal enlightenment therapy to encourage family members to accompany patients and warm them in a harmonious atmosphere.

(4) Medication nursing. Decoction should be taken warm after meals. Pills could be taken with yellow wine or brown-sugared shengjiang (fresh ginger) water.

（5）Manipulation techniques. ① Moxibustion therapy: select Shenque（CV 8）, Mingmen（GV 4）, Guanyuan（CV 4）, Sanyinjiao（SP 6）, and Shenshu（BL 23）; apply ginger-partitioned moxibustion on each of them. The procedure is to slice shengjiang（fresh ginger）into thin pieces with diameter of 2~3 centimeters and thickness of 0.4~0.6 centimeters, pierce several holes through the ginger slice with a sharp needle, and place the ginger slices on the acupoints, five moxa-cones on every acupoint until the area turns red, and twice every day. ② Umbilical compress therapy: grind into powder wuzhuyu（medicinal evodia fruit）20 g, xiaohuixiang（fennel）20 g, and rougui（cinnamon bark）10 g; blend 3 g of the powder with yellow wine to make a paste, apply the paste on the navel three days before menses, fix it with an adhesive tape, and warm it with hot water bag, 2~8 hours each time, once per day, and three consecutive use. ③ Hot compress therapy: put 150 g of heated qingyan（halite）into a cloth bag to compress the abdomen at a temperature of 60~70℃, 20 minutes each time, once per day.

3. Dampness-Heat and Stasis Obstruction Syndrome

（1）Daily life nursing. The ward should be cool, comfortable and full of fresh air. The coverings should be thin. The patients should avoid strenuous activity, braving rain or wading in water, and damp places when sitting or lying down.

（2）Diet nursing. The patients may eat foods that clear heat and remove dampness, such as yiyiren（coix seed）, balsam pear, chixiaodou（adzuki bean）and luffa leaf. Food therapy: meat-stuffed field snail. Pungent, spicy, greasy and hot-natured foods should be avoided, such as chili, Chinese chives and mutton. Avoid excessive drinking.

（3）Emotion nursing. Nurses may use emotional transference and dispositional change therapy to create a relaxing atmosphere and invite the patients to listen to soothing music so as to keep them calm and prevent agitation and anxiety.

（4）Medication nursing. Decoction should be taken warm or slightly cool after meals.

（5）Manipulation techniques. ① Auricular pressure therapy: select ovary（TF2）, endocrine（CO18）, and subcortex（AT4）; apply specialized pasters on them, press and knead on each of them till the area turns hot and red, 4~5 times per day, and keep the pasters for 2~4 days. Use this therapy before the menses and end it till the pain recedes during the menses. ② Acupressure therapy: select Ciliao（BL 32）and Yinlingquan（SP 9）; apply thumb kneading manipulation on each of them until the area turns hot or the patient has the feelings of soreness, numbness, distension and heaviness in the area; once per day.

4. Qi and Blood Deficiency Syndrome

（1）Daily life nursing. The ward should be warm and quiet. The coverings should be thick. The patients should keep abdomen and the lower limbs warm, and have sufficient sleep and do moderate exercise, such as walking and Taiji. They should avoid overstrain, and damp places when sitting or lying down.

（2）Diet nursing. The patients may eat foods that replenish qi and nourish blood, such as cuttlefish, longyanrou（longan）and shanyao（common yam rhizome）. Food therapy: danggui shengjiang yangrou（Chinese angelica, fresh ginger and muton）soup; wuji liangjiang（black chicken and galangal）soup;

nuomi ejiao (glutinous rice and donkey-hide gelatin) porridge: pound ejiao (donkey-hide gelatin) 30 g into powder and stir-fry it yellow for late use, boil 50 g of glutinous rice with 500 mL of water till it is well cooked, then blend the powder into the porridge, twice a day. Sweet, greasy, raw, cold, pungent and spicy foods should be avoided.

(3) Emotion nursing. Nurses may use verbal enlightenment therapy to care for and encourage the patients as much as possible to prevent distress and depression.

(4) Medication nursing. Decoction should be brewed slowly over low heat and taken warm before meals. Don't take too many tonic products during medication.

(5) Manipulation techniques. ① Moxibustion therapy: select Mingmen (GV 4), Shenshu (BL 23), Guanyuan (CV 4), Zusanli (ST 36), and Pishu (BL 20); place the moxa stick 2~3 centimeters away from the skin to perform mild moxibustion on each of them until the area turns red and feels warm and comfortable without the sensation of burning pain, once per day. Use this therapy before the menses and end it till the pain recedes during the menses. ② Acupressure therapy: select Pishu (BL 20), Weishu (BL 21) and Zusanli (ST 36); apply thumb kneading manipulation on each of them until the area turns hot or the patient has the feelings of soreness, numbness, distension and heaviness in the area; once per day.

5. Liver and Kidney Deficiency Syndrome

(1) Daily life nursing. The ward should be warm and quiet. The patients should rest in bed, keep abdomen and the lower limbs warm, have sufficient sleep and do moderate exercise, such as walking or Taiji. They should avoid overstrain, sexual indulgence, braving rain or wading in water, and damp places when sitting or lying down.

(2) Diet nursing. The patients may drink gouqizi (Chinese wolfberry fruit) tea and sangshen (mulberry) tea, and eat foods that replenish the kidney and nourish the liver, such as heizhima (black sesame), purple rice, pig kidneys, pig liver, and hetaoren (walnut). Food therapy: gouqi (Chinese wolfberry fruit) stewed with rabbit meat. Raw, cold, pungent and spicy foods should be avoided.

(3) Emotion nursing. Nurses should often make rounds of the wards and may use verbal enlightenment therapy to care for and encourage the patients as much as possible to help them maintain good moods and prevent nervousness and fear.

(4) Medication nursing. Decoction should be brewed slowly over low heat and taken warm before meals.

(5) Manipulation techniques. ① Moxibustion therapy: select Shenshu (BL 23), Ganshu (BL 18), Taixi (KI 3), Fuliu (KI 7), and Guilai (ST 29); place the moxa stick 2~3 centimeters away from the skin to perform mild moxibustion on each of them until the area turns red and the patient feels warm and comfortable without the sensation of burning pain, once per day. Use this therapy before the menses and end it till the pain recedes during the menses. ② Tuina therapy: select the governor vessel on the back, Shenshu (BL 23) and Mingmen (GV 4); apply rubbing manipulation on each of them until the area feels warm.

Patient Education

The patients should maintain perineal hygiene by rinsing with warm water every day and keep a normal bowel movement. On the other hand, they should avoid strenuous exercise and heavy labor from 3~5 days before the menses through to the end. Moreover, sex, swimming, wading in water, and tub bath should be avoided during menses.

From 3~5 days before the menses on, the diet should be light and digestible rather than too-salty or too-sweet, and foods that tonify blood and activate blood are preferred, such as dazao (Chinese date) and apple. During menstruation, the patients should have small frequent meals and foods of warm nature or rich in fiber, such as sweet potatoes, and refrain from cigarette, alcohol, and raw cold and sour foods.

Stay optimistic, open-minded, peaceful and good-humored. For primary dysmenorrhea, releasing tension can help relieve it to a certain extent. Nurses should instruct patients about the prevention of dysmenorrhea and answer their questions.

Take medicine regularly. Generally, follow the doctor's advice to take medicine from 3~5 days before the pain occurs, until it is relieved. Adhere to periodic treatment for more than three continuous menstrual cycles.

After the symptoms of dysmenorrhea are relieved, the causes should be clarified. And patients may visit hospital for gynecological examination if necessary.

第三节 胎 动 不 安

胎动不安,是指因冲任气血不和,导致胎元不固,或因跌仆举重,导致胎气损伤,以妊娠期间自觉胎动,或有轻微腰酸、腹痛,或伴见下腹坠胀,少量阴道出血为临床特征的胎孕病。西医的早期先兆流产可参照本节进行护理。

一、病因病机

胎动不安的病因分为胎元与母体两方面。在胎元方面,病因多为胎元先天精气薄弱,胎不成实,或母体孕后为外邪、毒物所伤,胎元不健。在母体方面,病因多为肾虚、气血不足、血热和血瘀。母体先天肾虚,或久病伤肾,或房劳多产,均可因肾虚导致冲任不固,胎失所养,胎动不安。母体素体气血不足,或过劳伤及气血,或饮食不节伤脾,或孕后恶阻伤脾,或久病重病伤及气血,均可因气不载胎,血不养胎,导致胎元不固,胎动不安。母体素体阳盛、阴虚,或孕后过食辛热,或外感热邪,或五志化火,均可因热扰冲任,损伤胎元,导致胎动不安。母体素有症瘕,或孕后跌仆创伤,均可因瘀阻胞宫导致胎元不固,胎动不安。

胎动不安的病机是冲任损伤,胎元不固。病位在胞宫。胎动不安的病性多为虚证,或为虚实夹杂之证。

二、常见证型

（一）辨证要点

1. 辨肾虚和气血虚弱　根据阴道出血的量、色、质,以及伴随症状等来辨别。若妊娠期间阴道出血,量少,色淡暗,伴腰酸,头晕耳鸣,夜尿频多,脉沉细滑,则多为肾虚。若妊娠期间阴道出血,量少,色淡质稀,伴小腹坠痛,神疲肢倦,面色无华,心悸气短,舌质淡,苔薄白,脉细滑,则多为气血虚弱。

2. 辨血热与血瘀　根据阴道出血的量、色、质,伴随症状,以及有无外伤史来辨别。若妊娠期间阴道出血,色鲜红,伴小便短黄,大便秘结,舌红苔黄,脉数,则多为血热。若妊娠期间阴道少量出血,色暗红,有妊娠期外伤史或宿有症瘕,脉滑无力,则多为血瘀。

（二）证候分型

1. 肾虚证

［主要证候］妊娠期,阴道少量出血,色淡暗,质薄;腰膝酸软,下腹坠痛,伴头晕耳鸣,小便频数,夜尿频多,面色晦暗或有暗斑,或曾屡有堕胎;舌淡暗,苔薄白,脉沉细滑。

［证候分析］肾为冲任之本,肾虚则冲任失固,故妊娠期阴道少量出血;肾虚血失阳化,故血色

淡暗,质薄;胎元欲坠,故下腹坠痛;腰为肾之府,肾虚外府失荣,故腰酸;肾虚髓海不充,脑失所养,故头晕耳鸣;肾虚膀胱失约,故小便频数,夜尿频多;肾虚难于系胎,故曾屡有堕胎;舌淡暗,脉沉细滑,均为肾虚之象。

[护治原则]补肾益气安胎。

[常用方剂]寿胎丸。

2. 气血虚弱证

[主要证候]妊娠期,阴道少量出血,色淡红,质稀薄;小腹坠痛隐隐,喜按,神疲肢倦,伴面色无华或萎黄,头晕眼花,心悸气短,唇甲色淡;舌质淡,苔薄白,脉细滑。

[证候分析]气虚胎失所载,血虚胎失所养,胎元不固,故妊娠期阴道少量流血,色淡红,质稀薄;气虚升举无力,血虚胞脉失养,故小腹坠痛隐隐,喜按;神疲肢倦,面色无华或萎黄,头晕眼花,心悸气短,唇甲色淡,舌质淡,苔薄白,脉细滑,均为气血虚弱之象。

[护治原则]益气养血安胎。

[常用方剂]胎元饮。

3. 血热证

[主要证候]妊娠期,阴道出血,色鲜红,量或多或少;腰酸痛或小腹下坠,口干咽燥,伴心烦少寐,手足心热,小便短黄,大便秘结;舌质红,苔黄,脉滑数或滑细数。

[证候分析]热扰冲任,冲任不固,迫血妄行,血海不宁,故妊娠期阴道出血,腰酸痛或小腹下坠;血为热灼,故血色鲜红;热扰心神,故心烦少寐;热伤津液,故口干咽燥,小便短黄,大便秘结;手足心热,舌质红,苔黄,脉滑数或滑细数,均为血热之象。

[护治原则]滋肾凉血安胎。

[常用方剂]寿胎丸合保阴煎。

4. 血瘀证

[主要证候]妊娠期,阴道少量出血,色暗红;有妊娠期外伤史或宿有症瘕,腰酸痛,伴小腹刺痛;舌质正常,脉滑无力。

[证候分析]妊娠期外伤或宿有症瘕结于胞宫,均可致气血失和,瘀阻胞宫胞脉,损伤冲任,出现阴道出血,腰酸痛,小腹刺痛;脉无力,为血瘀之象。

[护治原则]益肾祛瘀安胎。

[常用方剂]寿胎丸合加味圣愈汤。

三、护理措施

对胎动不安的病人,应严密观察阴道出血的量、色、质;腰酸和小腹坠胀的程度;腹痛的性质和程度;结合孕产史和外伤史进行综合评估。若阴道出血量超过月经量,且伴腹痛,腰酸,尿频,甚至出现面色苍白,冷汗淋漓,神情淡漠等危急症状,考虑为保胎失败,应立即报告医生。

(一)辨证施护

1. 肾虚证

(1)生活起居护理　居室温暖安静,明亮整洁。卧床休息,注意腰腹部保暖。腰后垫软枕以缓解腰痛。病人体虚,应随天气变化及时增减衣物,避开强风和对流风。改变体位时动作宜慢,如厕及外出时需有人陪护,以免发生跌仆损伤。避免过劳,禁止负重及大幅度的动作,如腰部后伸、用力咳嗽等。

(2)饮食护理　可饮枸杞子茶、桑椹茶。宜食补肾益气的食物,如芡实、鲤鱼、鸡肝、猪肾、猪骨髓、鳖肉、核桃仁。食疗方:莲子黑豆糯米粥。如有呕吐,可食砂仁鲫鱼汤。不宜食过咸、生冷的食物。

(3)情志护理　护士可运用移情易性疗法,如听音乐、读书,以使病人保持情绪稳定。对于有堕胎史的病人,告知病人七情过极可导致胎动不安,应避免焦虑、恐惧;发动家属配合治疗,帮助病人建立信心。

(4)用药护理　中药汤剂宜文火久煎,饭前温服。服药后静卧少动。

(5)操作技术　① 灸法:遵医嘱取隐白,用温和灸,艾条燃着端悬于施灸部位上,距离皮肤 2~3 厘米,灸至病人有温热舒适无灼痛的感觉,皮肤稍有红晕,每日 1 次。② 足浴疗法:菟丝子、桑寄生、黄芪各 50 g,杜仲、青盐各 30 g;煎煮后待水温降至 37~42℃时洗按足部,每次 20 分钟,每日 1 次;血压过低者慎用。

2. 气血虚弱证

(1)生活起居护理　居室温暖安静,明亮整洁。卧床休息,可取左侧卧位,以避免压迫下腔动、静脉。注意腰腹部保暖,随天气变化及时增减衣物,避开强风和对流风。睡眠充足,少说话,少会客,避免过劳。动作幅度不宜太大,尽量避免下蹲和弯腰,以防止发生跌仆损伤。

(2)饮食护理　饮食有节,避免过饥、过饱。宜食益气养血的食物,如乌贼、龙眼肉、莲子、山药。食疗方:阿胶鸡子黄汤。不宜食生冷、寒凉、滋腻的食物。

(3)情志护理　护士可运用移情易性疗法,让病人听音乐、读书,以避免过思伤脾。或运用语言开导疗法,向病人及家属做好解释工作,发动家属配合治疗,帮助病人建立信心。

(4)用药护理　中药汤剂宜文火久煎,饭前温服,服药后静卧少动。若服药时恶心欲呕,可于服药前在舌根滴几滴生姜汁。

(5)操作技术　① 灸法:遵医嘱取足三里,用温和灸,艾条燃着端悬于施灸部位上,距离皮肤 2~3 厘米,灸至病人有温热舒适无灼痛的感觉,皮肤稍有红晕,每日 1 次。② 敷贴疗法:遵医嘱取至阴、神阙,用杜仲、补骨脂等研磨成粉调糊敷贴。

3. 血热证

(1)生活起居护理　居室安静凉爽,空气新鲜。衣被宜薄。卧床休息。保持外阴清洁,每日用温水清洗外阴。

(2)饮食护理　可饮荸荠豆浆、荷叶红糖水、木耳芝麻茶。宜食清热凉血的食物,如冬瓜、豆腐、鳖肉、鸭肉。若大便干结,可食蜂蜜、玉米、红薯、香蕉。戒烟限酒,不宜食煎炸、辛热动火的食物,如牛肉、羊肉、狗肉、生姜、韭菜、香菜。

(3)情志护理　护士可运用移情易性疗法,以避免激动、焦虑。

(4)用药护理　中药宜温服或偏凉服,服药后静卧少动。

(5)操作技术　敷贴疗法。遵医嘱取天枢,用桑寄生 15 g,炒黄芩、川续断、菟丝子各 9 g,打粉后与蜂蜜调成糊状敷贴,每次 4 小时,每日 1 次。

4. 血瘀证

（1）生活起居护理　居室安静温暖。卧床休息，睡眠充足，可取左侧卧位。注意腰腹部保暖，避开强风和对流风。改变体位时动作宜慢，如厕及外出时需有人陪护。禁止负重及大幅度的动作。

（2）饮食护理　宜食益气和血的食物，如阿胶（遵医嘱食用）。食疗方：苎麻根鸡蛋汤（遵医嘱食用）。不宜食酸涩收敛、壅阻气机的食物。

（3）情志护理　护士可运用语言开导疗法，向病人讲解情绪舒畅的益处，指导病人掌握控制情绪的方法，如听轻音乐，以保持心态平和。

（4）用药护理　中药汤剂宜饭后温服，服药后静卧少动。严禁自行使用活血化瘀的膏药或者活血通络、舒筋行气的药物。

（二）健康教育

胎动不安者需绝对卧床。待阴道流血停止 3~5 天后，方可下床适量活动。活动时穿平底软鞋。若治疗后血止胎安，仍需再观察 2 周。观察期间宜在家静养，少去人多拥挤的公共场所。避免过劳，禁止登高、负重，以免跌仆闪挫。但也不可过于安逸，如久坐、久卧，以防止气血停滞，胎失所养。

生活规律，睡眠充足，防寒保暖。衣裤宽松、柔软，不可紧身、束腰。保持外阴清洁，每日用温水清洗外阴，勤换消毒卫生垫及内裤。若大便干结，切忌用力排便和按摩腰腹部。禁止盆浴和性行为。

饮食宜清淡、营养、易消化。饮食有节，不可过饱。饮食多样化，不可偏嗜。多补充肉、鱼、蛋、奶、动物肝。多吃高纤维的水果和蔬菜，以保持大便通畅。注意饮食卫生，避免因腹泻诱发胎动不安。戒烟限酒，不宜食辛辣、温燥、滑利、动血、生冷、肥甘的食物，如桃仁、山楂、螃蟹。

调畅情志。解除心理压力，避免恐惧、焦虑的情志刺激。

禁止病人自行使用峻下、滑利、破气、苦寒、活血化瘀、舒筋行气或有毒的药物。避免接触放射性物质和重金属，如汞、铅、砷等。若大便干结，禁止使用泻下药。

如果保胎失败，应安慰病人，并告知病人要加强锻炼，保证身体和心理健康。夫妇双方应做有关检查，找出病因，休息半年至 1 年后才可怀孕。再次怀孕后应立即保胎，服保胎药时间和绝对卧床时间均应超过既往堕胎孕周。定期产前检查，避免不必要的妇科检查及阴道冲洗。若必须检查，动作应轻柔。

Section 3 Threatened Abortion

Threatened abortion is clinically characterized by abnormal fetal movement, mild aching lumbus, abdominal pain, lower abdominal sagging distention or mild virginal bleeding during pregnancy, which is caused by disharmony of qi and blood in the thoroughfare and conception vessels, insecurity of fetal original qi, or damage to fetal qi due to injury or weightlifting. This section can be referred to for the nursing of early threatened abortion in Western medicine.

ETIOLOGY AND PATHOGENESIS

The causes of threatened abortion lie in two aspects: the fetal original qi and the maternal body. From the aspect of fetal original qi, the etiology is congenital weakness of the fetal original qi, the abnormal growth of fetus, or the unhealthy state of fetal original qi due to damage to the maternal body by external pathogens and toxins. From the aspect of maternal body, the etiology is kidney deficiency, insufficient qi and blood, blood heat and blood stasis. Maternal congenital kidney deficiency, kidney damage due to long-term illness, or sexual strain and prolificacy can lead to kidney deficiency that causes insecurity of the thoroughfare and conception vessels, loss of nourishment for the fetus, and even threatened abortion. Insufficient qi and blood in the maternal body, qi-blood damage due to overwork, spleen damage due to improper diet or morning sickness in pregnancy, or qi-blood damage due to chronic and serious illness, all can lead to the failure of qi and blood to nourish the fetus that induces insecurity of fetal original qi and threatened abortion. The maternal body's yang exuberance and yin deficiency, excessive eating of acrid or hot food after pregnancy, external contraction of pathogenic heat, or five emotions transforming into fire, all can lead to heat harassing the thoroughfare and conception vessels and damage to the fetus that causes threatened abortion. The abdominal mass in the maternal body, or falling and trauma after pregnancy, can result in blood stasis obstructing the uterus that causes insecurity of fetal original qi and threatened abortion.

The pathogenesis is the damage to the thoroughfare and conception vessels and the insecurity of fetal original qi. The disease is located in the uterus. And the nature of disease is mostly deficiency syndrome, or deficiency-excess in complexity.

COMMON SYNDROMES

Key Points in Syndrome Differentiation

1. Differentiation of Kidney Deficiency from Qi-Blood Deficiency

The differentiation is based on the amount, color and texture of vaginal bleeding, and accompanied symptoms. Kidney deficiency is marked by mild vaginal bleeding during pregnancy, light dark color, aching lumbus, dizziness, tinnitus, frequent urination at night, and sunken, thready and slippery pulse. Deficiency of qi and blood is marked by mild vaginal bleeding during pregnancy, light color, thin texture, lower abdominal sagging pain, mental and physical fatigue, pale complexion, palpitation, shortness of breath, pale tongue with thin white coating, and thready slippery pulse.

2. Differentiation of Blood Heat from Blood Stasis

The differentiation is based on the amount, color and texture of vaginal bleeding, accompanied symptoms and history of trauma. Blood heat is marked by vaginal bleeding during pregnancy, bright red color, scanty dark urine, constipation, red tongue with yellow coating, and slippery rapid pulse. Blood stasis is marked by mild vaginal bleeding during pregnancy, dark red color, trauma during pregnancy, abdominal mass, and slippery weak pulse.

Syndrome Differentiation

1. Kidney Deficiency Syndrome

［Clinical Manifestations］ Mild vaginal bleeding during pregnancy, light dark color, thin texture, aching lumbus and knees, lower abdominal sagging pain, dizziness, tinnitus, frequent urination (especially at night), dim complexion or dark macule, induced abortion histories, light dark tongue with thin white coating, and sunken, thready and slippery pulse.

［Manifestations Analysis］ Kidney is the basis of the thoroughfare and conception vessels. Kidney deficiency leads to insecurity of the thoroughfare and conception vessels that causes mild vaginal bleeding during pregnancy. The kidney yang fails to warm the blood, so the blood is light dark and thin. The fetal original qi is insecure and tends to fall, therefore, the lower abdominal sagging pain occurs. The lumbus is the house of the kidney and kidney deficiency leads to malnourish of the lumbus, therefore, aching lumbus is felt. Kidney deficiency with unfilled sea of marrow fails to nourish the brain, so dizziness and tinnitus occur. Kidney deficiency fails to constrain the bladder, leading to frequent urination, especially at night. Kidney deficiency leads to insecurity of fetus and causes frequent abortions. Light dark tongue and sunken, thready and slippery pulse are signs of kidney deficiency.

［Nursing Principle］ Tonifying the kidney, replenishing qi and calming fetus.

［Suggested Formula］ Shoutai Pills.

2. Qi and Blood Deficiency Syndrome

［Clinical Manifestations］ Mild vaginal bleeding during pregnancy, light red color, thin texture, lower abdominal sagging dull pain, preference for pressure, mental and physical fatigue, lusterless or sallow complexion, dizziness, palpitations, shortness of breath, pale lips and nails, pale tongue with thin white coating, and thready slippery pulse.

［Manifestations Analysis］ Qi and blood deficiency fails to secure and nourish the fetal original qi, so mild vaginal bleeding occurs during pregnancy, with light red color and thin texture. Qi deficiency fails to lift the fetus and blood deficiency fails to nourish the uterine vessels, so lower abdominal sagging dull pain and preference for pressure occur. Mental and physical fatigue, lusterless or sallow complexion, dizziness, palpitations, shortness of breath, pale lips and nails, pale tongue with thin white coating, and thready slippery pulse, all are signs of deficiency of qi and blood.

［Nursing Principle］ Replenishing qi, nourishing blood and calming fetus.

［Suggested Formula］ Taiyuan Drink.

3. Blood Heat Syndrome

［Clinical Manifestations］ Vaginal bleeding during pregnancy, bright red color, unstable amount, aching painful lumbus or sagging lower abdomen, dry mouth and throat, vexation with reduced sleep, heat in two soles and palms, scanty dark urine, constipation, red tongue with yellow coating, and slippery rapid pulse, or slippery, thready and rapid one.

［Manifestations Analysis］ Heat harassing the thoroughfare and conception vessels, and insecurity of the thoroughfare and conception vessels, cause the frenetic movement of the blood, leading to vaginal bleeding during pregnancy, aching painful lumbus or sagging lower abdomen. The blood is scorched by heat, so the color is bright red. Heat harasses the mind, so vexation with reduced sleep is felt. Heat damages body fluids, resulting in a dry mouth and throat, scanty dark urine, and constipation. Heat in two soles and palms, red tongue with yellow coating, and slippery rapid pulse, or slippery, thready and rapid pulse, all are signs of blood heat.

［Nursing Principle］ Nourishing the kidney, cooling blood and calming fetus.

［Suggested Formula］ Shoutai Pills and Baoyin Decoction.

4. Blood Stasis Syndrome

［Clinical Manifestations］ Mild vaginal bleeding during pregnancy, dark red color, trauma or abdominal mass during pregnancy, aching painful lumbus, stabbing pain in lower abdomen, normal tongue, and slippery weak pulse.

［Manifestations Analysis］ Trauma or abdominal mass during pregnancy causes the disharmony of qi and blood, the obstruction of blood stasis in the uterus and uterine vessels, and the damage to the thoroughfare and conception vessels, therefore, there present such symptoms as vaginal bleeding, aching painful lumbus, and stabbing pain in lower abdomen. And weak pulse is the sign of blood stasis.

［Nursing Principle］ Replenishing the kidney, dispelling stasis and calming fetus.

［Suggested Formula］ Shoutai Pills and Jiawei Shengyu Decoction.

NURSING MEASURES

For patients with threatened abortion, nurses should closely monitor the amount, color and texture of vaginal bleeding; the severity of aching lumbus and sagging distension of lower abdomen; and the nature and severity of bellyache. Histories of pregnancy, delivery and trauma should also be considered so as to make comprehensive evaluations. If vaginal bleeding exceeds that of menses and is accompanied by bellyache, aching lumbus, frequent urination, or even such critical symptoms as pale complexion, dripping cold sweat and indifferent look, the patient is likely to have a miscarriage and the doctor should be informed immediately.

Syndrome-Based Nursing Measures

1. Kidney Deficiency Syndrome

(1) Daily life nursing. The ward should be warm, quiet, bright and tidy. The patients should rest in bed and keep the waist and abdomen warm. Pillows could be placed behind the waist to ease the pain. The patients with weak constitution should adjust their clothing to match the change of weather and avoid gusty winds and draughts. Slow motion is preferable when changing body gestures. The patients should be accompanied when using the bathroom or going outside to prevent traumatic impairment. They should avoid overstrain, extra burden and dramatic movements such as lumbar backward extension and coughing forcefully.

(2) Diet nursing. The patients may drink Gouqizi (Chinese wolfberry fruit) tea and sangshen (mulberry) tea, and eat foods that tonify the kidney and replenish qi, such as qianshi (euryale seed), carp, chicken liver, pig kidneys, pig bone marrow, meat of soft-shelled turtles, and hetaoren (walnut). Food therapy: lianzi heidou nuomi (lotus seed, black soybean and glutinous rice) porridge. For vomiting patients, sharen jiyu (villous amomum fruit and crucian) soup is desirable. Patients should refrain from overly salty, raw or cold foods.

(3) Emotion nursing. Nurses may use emotional transference and dispositional change therapy such as listening to music and reading books to keep the patients calm. For patients with history of abortion, they should be informed that extremity of seven emotions may cause threatened abortion whereas their families should be encouraged to cooperate with the treatment and help patients build up confidence.

(4) Medication nursing. Decoction should be brewed slowly over low heat and taken warm before meals. After taking medicine, they should lie still and avoid movement.

(5) Manipulation techniques. ① Moxibustion therapy: follow the doctor's advice to select Yinbai (SP 1); place the moxa stick 2~3 centimeters away from the skin and apply mild moxibustion on the acupoint until the area turns red and the patient feels warm and comfortable without the sensation of burning pain, once per day. ② Foot bath therapy: decoct tusizi (dodder seed) 50 g, sangjisheng (Chinese taxillus) 50 g, huangqi (astragalus root) 50 g, duzhong (eucommia bark) 30 g, and qingyan (halite) 30 g; wash feet with the decoction and massage at a temperature of 37~42°C, 20 minutes each

time, once per day. And it should be used with caution for patients with hypotension.

2. Qi and Blood Deficiency Syndrome

(1) Daily life nursing. The ward should be warm, quiet, bright and tidy. The patients should rest in bed and lie in a left lateral recumbent position so as not to press the inferior vena cava and artery. They should keep the waist and abdomen warm, adjust clothes to match the change of weather and avoid gusty winds and draughts. They should also have sufficient sleep and minimize talking and receiving visitors. Moreover, they should avoid overstrain, and dramatic movements such as squatting and stooping to prevent traumatic impairment.

(2) Diet nursing. The patients should follow a moderate diet without being too hungry or too full, and eat foods that replenish qi and nourish blood, such as cuttlefish, longyanrou (longan), lianzi (lotus seed) and shanyao (common yam rhizome). Food therapy: ejiao jizihuang (donkey-hide gelatin and egg yolk) soup. Raw, cold or greasy foods should be avoided.

(3) Emotion nursing. Nurses may use emotional transference and dispositional change therapy such as listening to music and reading books to guide the patients to prevent spleen damage due to excessive contemplation. Nurses may also use verbal enlightenment therapy to explain disease condition to the patients and family members whereas their families should be encouraged to cooperate with the treatment and help patients build up confidence.

(4) Medication nursing. Decoction should be brewed slowly over low heat and taken warm before meals. After taking medicine, the patients should lie still and avoid movement. A few drops of shengjiagnzhi (fresh ginger juice) could prevent nausea and vomiting resulting from taking medicine.

(5) Manipulation techniques. ① Moxibustion therapy: follow the doctor's advice to select Zusanli (ST 36); place the moxa stick 2~3 centimeters away from the skin and apply mild moxibustion on the acupoint until the area turns red and the patient feels warm and comfortable without the sensation of burning pain, once per day. ② Paste application therapy: follow the doctor's advice to select Zhiyin (BL 67) and Shenque (CV 8); grind into powder duzhong (eucommia bark) and buguzhi (psoralea fruit) to make pastes and apply them to the acupoints.

3. Blood Heat Syndrome

(1) Daily life nursing. The ward should be quiet, cool, and full of fresh air. The coverings should be thin. The patients should rest in bed, and maintain genital hygiene by washing vulva with warm water.

(2) Diet nursing. The patients may drink biqi (waternut) soybean milk, heye hongtang (lotus leaf and brown sugar) water, and muer zhima (wood ear and sesame) tea. They may eat foods that clear heat and cool blood, such as Chinese waxgourd, bean curd, meat of soft-shelled turtles and duck meat. For patients with dry stool, honey, corn, sweet potatoes or banana could help. The patients should also refrain from cigarette and alcohol as well as fried, pungent and hot foods that engender fire, such as beef, mutton, dog meat, shengjiang (fresh ginger), Chinese chives and coriander.

(3) Emotion nursing. Nurses may use emotional transference and dispositional change therapy to avoid excitement and anxiety.

（4）Medication nursing. Decoction should be taken warm or slightly cool. After taking the medicine, the patients should lie still and avoid movement.

（5）Manipulation techniques. Follow the doctor's advice to select Tianshu（ST 25）, use sangjisheng（Chinese taxillus）15 g, chaohuangqin（stir-fried scutellaria root）9 g, chuanxuduan（Himalayan teasel root）9 g, and tusizi（dodder seed）9 g; grind the above medicinals into powder and blend it with honey to make pastes, then apply them on the acupoint, four hours each time, once per day.

4. Blood Stasis Syndrome

（1）Daily life nursing. The ward should be warm and quiet. The patients should rest in bed to ensure sufficient sleep and lie in a left recumbent position. They should keep the waist and abdomen warm and avoid gusty winds and draughts. Slow motion is preferable when changing body gestures. The patients should be accompanied when using the bathroom or going outside to prevent traumatic impairment. Moreover, they should avoid overstrain and dramatic movements.

（2）Diet nursing. The patients may eat foods that replenish qi and harmonize blood, such as ejiao（donkey-hide gelatin）（follow the doctor's advice）. Food therapy: zhumagen jidan（ramie root and chicken egg）soup（follow the doctor's advice）. Sour and astringent foods or those that obstruct qi movement should be avoided.

（3）Emotion nursing. Nurses may use verbal enlightenment therapy to instruct the patients on the benefits of being good-humored and on how to control their emotions, such as listening to soft music.

（4）Medication nursing. Decoction should be taken warm after meals. After taking the medicine, the patients should lie still and avoid movement. It is forbidden to use blood-activating and stasis-resolving plasters and medicinals that activate blood, dredge collaterals, soothe sinews and move qi.

Patient Education

Patients with threatened abortion should be kept at absolute rest in the bed. Movement off the bed wearing soft shoes with flat sole could be attempted only three to five days after vaginal bleeding stops. The patients should be monitored for another two weeks after the bleeding stops and the fetus is calmed. After the fetus is calmed, it is advisable to rest at home or work moderately, not to visit crowded public places. Overwork, extra burden and scaling heights should be avoided to prevent traumatic impairment. Sedentary behaviors such as prolonged periods of sitting or resting in bed should be avoided to prevent the stagnation of qi and blood and the fetal malnourishment.

The patients should follow a regular daily routine, have sufficient sleep, and keep warm. Clothing should loose-fitting and soft rather than tight or belted. They should also maintain genital hygiene by washing vulva with warm water every day and changing sanitary towel and underwear regularly. For those with dry stool, avoid defecation with much exertion and massage of waist and abdomen regions. Tub bath and sexual intercourse are also prohibited.

The diet should be light, nutritious, diversified and digestible, with moderate food intake and without flavor predilection. Meat, fish, eggs, milk and animal livers should be supplemented. Fresh fruit and vegetables rich in fiber should also be added to ensure smooth defecation. Food hygiene should be maintained to prevent threatened abortion caused by diarrhea. The patients should refrain from cigarette and alcohol as well as the following kinds of foods: pungent, spicy, raw, cold, fatty, sweet and lubricant foods, or warm-natured, dry-natured, and blood-activating foods, such as taoren (peach kernel), shanzha (Chinese hawthorn fruit) and crabs.

The patients should regulate their moods. Stress, fear or anxiety should be alleviated.

Some special drugs should be prohibited, including poisonous, lubricant, purgative, drastically purgative, qi-breaking, bitter-cold, blood-activating and stasis-resolving, and sinew-soothing and qi-moving ones. So are radioactive substances and heavy metals, such as mercury, lead and arsenic. Purgatives are prohibited when the patient has constipation.

For patients suffering from miscarriages, nurses should console and encourage them to be more physically active and to strive for physical and psychological well-being. Both of the couple should have physical check-ups to identify the causes of abortion. Only after an interval of half a year to one year might they attempt the next pregnancy. Efforts to prevent miscarriages should ensue immediately after detection of pregnancy. The durations of medication and absolute rest in bed for preventing miscarriages should exceed those of the previous abortion. When the patients have regular antenatal examinations, necessary examinations should be performed gently and unnecessary gynecologic exams and vaginal rinsing should be avoided.

第四节　产后恶露不绝

产后恶露不绝,是指因气虚、血热、血瘀,导致冲任损伤,气血运行失常,或因感染邪毒而引起的,以产后血性恶露淋漓不尽,持续10天以上为临床特征的产后病。恶露是指妇女产后由阴道排出的随子宫蜕膜脱落的含有血液、坏死蜕膜等的组织。正常的恶露有血腥味,但无臭味,持续4~6周,总量约250~500 mL。西医的子宫复旧不全,以及人工流产和药物流产后阴道流血、淋漓不净可参照本节进行护理。

一、病因病机

产后恶露不绝的病因多为气虚、血热和血瘀。病人体质虚弱,或孕中摄生不慎,或产时伤血耗气,或产后劳倦伤脾致中气下陷,均可因气虚而致冲任不固,产后恶露不绝。病人为阳盛之人,或产时感受邪毒而致热,或产后过食甘热,或情志不遂致五志化火;或病人为阴虚之体,产时耗伤津血,亏耗营阴而致虚火妄动:此二者均可因血热而扰动冲任,迫血妄行,导致产后恶露不绝。病人产后因感受寒邪而致血瘀,或因情志不畅导致血瘀,或素有症瘕瘀阻冲任,均可因脉道瘀阻,血不归经而致产后恶露不绝。

产后恶露不绝的病机是胞宫藏泻失度,冲任不固,气血运行失常。病位在冲任。虚证多为气虚冲任不固,血失统摄。实证多为热扰冲任,迫血下行;或瘀血内阻,血不归经。

二、常见证型

(一)辨证要点

辨气虚、血热、血瘀　根据恶露的量、色、质、气味等来辨别。若恶露量多,色淡红,质清稀,无臭味,则多为气虚。若恶露量多,色红或深红,质稠,气秽臭,则多为血热。若恶露量时多时少,色紫暗,有血块,则多为血瘀。

(二)证候分型

1. 气虚证

[主要证候]产后恶露逾期不止,量多或淋漓不止,色淡红,质清稀,无臭味;小腹空坠,神疲乏力,气短懒言,面色苍白;舌质淡,苔薄白,脉缓弱。

[证候分析]气虚不能摄血,故恶露逾期不止,量多;气虚血少,见恶露色淡质稀,面色不容而苍白;中气虚弱,脾阳不升,致小腹空坠,神疲倦怠,气短懒言;舌质淡,苔薄白,脉缓弱,均为气血两亏之象。

[护治原则]补气摄血固冲。

［常用方剂］补中益气汤。

2. 血热证

［主要证候］产后恶露逾期不止,量多,色红或深红,质稠,或色如败酱,气秽臭;面色红赤,唇色深红,口咽干燥,或伴有腹痛,便秘,或可兼五心烦热;舌质红,苔黄燥或少苔,脉滑数或细数。

［证候分析］热扰冲任,迫血妄行,故恶露逾期不止,量多;热邪灼伤津液,故恶露色深红,质稠,伴面色红赤,口燥咽干,或伴便秘,五心烦热;血热相互抟结成瘀,日久化腐,故恶露色如败酱而臭秽,或伴腹痛;舌质红,苔黄燥或少苔,脉数,均为热盛伤阴之象。

［护治原则］实热证,清热固冲止血;虚热证,养阴清热,固冲止血。

［常用方剂］实热证,保阴煎;虚热证,两地汤合二至丸。

3. 血瘀证

［主要证候］产后恶露逾期不止,量时多时少,色紫暗,有血块;小腹疼痛拒按,块下痛减,胸腹胀痛;舌紫暗,边尖有瘀斑瘀点,脉弦涩。

［证候分析］瘀阻胞宫,血不归经,致恶露延期不止。瘀血阻滞气血运行,故恶露量时多时少,色紫暗,有血块,腹痛拒按;块下则气血暂通,故腹痛得到缓解;舌紫暗,边尖有瘀斑瘀点,脉弦涩,均为瘀血之象。

［护治原则］活血化瘀止血。

［常用方剂］生化汤。

三、护理措施

对于产后恶露不绝的病人,应观察恶露的量、色、质,以及有无臭味和血块。询问病人有无腹部压痛。若病人恶露过多,色红,有血块,伴头晕心慌,面色苍白,腹痛明显,考虑为胞衣残留,应及时向医生报告。

（一）辨证施护

1. 气虚证

（1）生活起居护理　居室温暖。注意保暖,及时更换湿衣,以避免受凉。卧床休息,睡眠充足。劳逸适度,适量活动,避免久坐、久站、久走。护士应将病人经常使用的物品放置于其伸手可及处,并把障碍物从病人经常走动的区域移开。

（2）饮食护理　饮食有节,少食多餐,不可大补、过饱。宜食益气健脾的食物,如猪瘦肉、海参、龙眼肉、大枣、山药、乌鸡蛋。食疗方:白参莲子汤。不宜食清热的食物。

（3）情志护理　护士可运用语言开导疗法,经常关心鼓励病人,以避免悲观、紧张。

（4）用药护理　中药汤剂宜文火久煎,饭前温服。

（5）操作技术　① 药熨疗法:取气海,用白术、黄芪,研磨炒热后装入布袋中,制成温度为60~70℃的中药热罨包,药熨20分钟,每日1次。② 灸法:取脾俞、天枢、气海、关元、足三里,用温和灸,艾条燃着端悬于施灸部位上,距离皮肤2~3厘米,灸至病人有温热舒适无灼痛的感觉,皮肤稍有红晕,每日1次。③ 腹带法:腹带法可预防由气虚导致的产后恶露不绝;在腹壁上放4~5层棉花,用软布围缚,以通过加压帮助子宫复旧,维持腹部温暖从而防止感寒损气,防止腹壁肌肉松弛和内脏下垂。

2. 血热证

(1) 生活起居护理　居室凉爽湿润,空气新鲜。衣被宜薄。若出血量多,应减少活动。

(2) 饮食护理　增加饮水量,可饮雪梨汁。宜食性凉清热的食物,如苦瓜、芹菜、白木耳。食疗方:赤小豆荸荠羹。不宜过食补益的食物,如大枣、龙眼肉。

(3) 情志护理　护士可运用语言开导疗法,向病人介绍产后的调养知识,指导病人调节情绪,以避免激动、焦虑。

(4) 用药护理　中药宜饭后偏凉服。

(5) 操作技术　① 刮痧疗法:取膈俞至胆俞,从上到下采用直线重刮法刮拭,每侧刮拭 20~30 次,以皮肤出现潮红或起痧为度;两次刮痧之间宜间隔3~6日。② 拔罐疗法:取血海、膈俞,留罐10分钟,隔日1次。③ 穴位按摩法:取合谷、大椎、外关、三阴交,用拇指揉法,按摩至局部发热或有酸麻重胀感,每日1次。

3. 血瘀证

(1) 生活起居护理　居室温暖。衣被宜厚。注意保暖,避免受凉。可取半仰卧位,以促进恶露排出。适量活动,以促进气血运行。

(2) 饮食护理　可饮红糖水、黄酒。宜食活血化瘀的食物。食疗方:山楂木耳汤。不宜食生冷的食物。

(3) 情志护理　护士可运用顺意疗法和移情易性疗法,营造无刺激的环境,鼓励病人表达内心感受,以防止因情志不畅导致肝气郁滞而加重血瘀。

(4) 用药护理　中药汤剂宜饭后温服。

(5) 操作技术　① 灸法:取归来、血海、三阴交,用温和灸,艾条燃着端悬于施灸部位上,距离皮肤2~3厘米,灸至病人有温热舒适无灼痛的感觉,皮肤稍有红晕,每日1次。② 药熨疗法:取子宫、归来,用桃仁、红花,炒热装入布袋中,制成温度为60~70℃的中药热罨包,药熨20分钟,每日1次。③ 乳房按摩:用热毛巾(温度以皮肤能耐受为宜)敷乳房10分钟,病人双手拇指和其余4指自然分开,由下向上承托乳房,用指腹由四周向乳头方向轻轻按摩乳房,然后用双手提拉乳头,每次15~20分钟,每日3~4次。

(二) 健康教育

居室空气新鲜,避免强风和对流风。病人因产后虚弱,容易感受外邪,应增强正气,注意保暖,慎避外邪,以防止感冒。保持外阴清洁干燥,每日用温水清洗,勤换消毒卫生垫和内裤。加强二便后的伤口护理,每日用1∶1000高锰酸钾溶液清洗1~2次。当血量不多、病情平稳时,鼓励病人下床走动,逐渐增大活动量,以加强气血运行,促进子宫收缩。活动间歇要充分休息,勿过劳。忌盆浴及性行为。

加强营养,多吃高热量、高蛋白的食物。宜食富含维生素 E 的食物,如葵花籽、核桃仁。戒烟限酒,不宜食寒凉、辛辣的食物,如辣椒、大蒜。

心情愉悦,避免激动,以防止五志化火。

坚持母乳喂养,以促进子宫收缩和恶露排出。

Section 4   Postpartum Lochiorrhea

Postpartum lochiorrhea is characterized by incessant bloody lochia for over ten days after delivery, which is caused by the infection due to virulent factors or by the damage of the thoroughfare and conception vessels as well as the abnormal movement of qi and blood due to qi deficiency, blood heat or blood stasis. Lochia refers to the tissue containing blood and necrotic decidua that is discharged from the vagina after delivery and along with the decidua of the uterus. Normal lochia with the total amount about 250~500 mL and duration of 4~6 weeks has the smell of blood but without foul odor. This section can be referred to for the nursing of incessant vaginal bleeding in subinvolution of uterus, induced abortion, and medical abortion in Western medicine.

ETIOLOGY AND PATHOGENESIS

The etiology includes qi deficiency, blood heat and blood stasis. First, the patient's weak constitution, improper regimen during pregnancy, qi consumption following blood loss in delivery, or the sinking of middle qi after delivery resulted from the spleen damage due to overstrain, all may lead to qi deficiency and the insecurity of the thoroughfare and conception vessels. Thus, incessant postpartum lochiorrhea occurs. Second, the patient's yang exuberance constitution, fever due to infection in delivery, over intake of too-sweet and hot foods after delivery, or five emotions transforming into fire, all may induce excess heat. And the patient's yin deficiency constitution or blood and fluid damages in delivery that further consumes nutrient yin results in the frenetic stirring of deficiency fire. Blood heat in these two cases harasses the thoroughfare and conception vessels and causes frenetic movement of the blood. Thus, incessant postpartum lochiorrhea occurs. Third, the invasion of pathogenic cold after delivery, the internal damage due to the seven emotions, or the abdominal masses obstructing the thoroughfare and conception vessels all may trigger blood stasis, which obstructs the blood vessels and makes the new blood failing to stay in the meridians. Thus, incessant postpartum lochiorrhea occurs.

The pathogenesis is the abnormal storing and excreting function of the uterus, which leads to the insecurity of the thoroughfare and conception vessels and the abnormal movement of qi and blood. The location of disease is in the thoroughfare and conception vessels. Deficiency syndrome is mostly due to qi deficiency that makes insecurity of the thoroughfare and conception vessels as well as failure of qi to control blood. However, excess syndrome is mainly caused by heat harassing the thoroughfare and conception vessels, which forces the blood to flow downward, or by internal obstruction of blood stasis that makes blood fail to stay in the meridians.

COMMON SYNDROMES

Key Points in Syndrome Differentiation

Differentiation of Qi Deficiency, Blood Heat from Blood Stasis

The differentiation is mainly based on the amount, color, texture, and odour of lochia. Qi deficiency syndrome is marked by profuse amount, light red color, clear thin texture, and without foul odor; blood heat syndrome by profuse amount, red or crimson color, thick sticky texture, or with foul odor; and blood stasis syndrome by unstable amount, dark purple color, and often with blood clots.

Syndrome Differentiation

1. Qi Deficiency Syndrome

〔Clinical Manifestations〕Postpartum incessant or profuse lochiorrhea with prolonged duration, light red color, clear thin texture, and without foul odor, empty sagging sensation in the lower abdomen, fatigue, lack of strength, shortness of breath, no desire to speak, bright white complexion, pale tongue with thin white coating, and moderate weak pulse.

〔Manifestations Analysis〕Qi fails to control blood, causing incessant or profuse lochiorrhea with prolonged duration. Qi deficiency with insufficient blood explains light red color, clear thin texture and bright white complexion. Weak middle qi with the failure of clear yang to ascend, so the patients feel empty sagging sensation in the lower abdomen, fatigue, lack of strength, shortness of breath, and no desire to speak. Pale tongue with thin white coating and moderate weak pulse are all manifestations of depletion of qi and blood.

〔Nursing Principle〕Tonifying qi, controlling blood, and securing the thoroughfare vessel.

〔Suggested Formula〕Buzhong Yiqi Decoction.

2. Blood Heat Syndrome

〔Clinical Manifestations〕Postpartum profuse lochiorrhea with prolonged duration, red or crimson color, thick texture, or sauce-colored texture with foul odor, red complexion and lips, dry throat and mouth, or with abdominal pain and constipation, or with vexing heat in the chest, palms and soles, red tongue with dry yellow coating or with scanty coating, slippery rapid pulse or thready rapid one.

〔Manifestations Analysis〕Heat harasses the thoroughfare and conception vessels and causes frenetic movement of the blood. Therefore, there is incessant profuse lochiorrhea with prolonged duration. Heat scorching fluid causes crimson color, thick texture, red complexion and lips, dry throat and mouth, or accompanied with constipation or vexing heat in the chest, palms and soles. Blood binding with heat produces blood stasis that transforms putridity and inhibits the movement of qi and blood, leading to sauce-colored lochiorrhea with foul odor or accompanied with abdominal pain. Rapid pulse and red tongue with dry yellow coating or with scanty coating are all manifestations of exuberant heat damaging yin.

〔Nursing Principle〕For excess heat syndrome: clearing heat, securing the thoroughfare vessel, and stopping bleeding. For deficiency heat syndrome: nourishing yin and clearing heat; securing the thoroughfare vessel and stopping bleeding.

[Suggested Formula] For excess heat syndrome: Baoyin Decoction. For deficiency heat syndrome: Liangdi Decoction and Erzhi Pills.

3. Blood Stasis Syndrome

[Clinical Manifestations] Postpartum lochiorrhea with prolonged duration, unstable amount, dark purple color, blood clots, unpalpable pain in the lower abdominal, alleviation of pain after removal of the clot, distending pain in the chest and abdomen, dark purple tongue with ecchymoses and spots on the tip and margins of the tongue, and wiry unsmooth pulse.

[Manifestations Analysis] Blood stasis obstructing the uterus makes the new blood failing to stay in the meridians, so the lochia has a prolonged duration. Blood stasis obstructing the movement of qi and blood brings about the lochia with unstable amount, dark purple color, blood clots, and unpalpable pain in the lower abdominal. The removal of the clot temporarily normalizes the movement of qi and blood, so the pain is alleviated. Dark purple tongue with ecchymoses and spots on the tip and margins of the tongue and wiry unsmooth pulse are all manifestations of blood stasis.

[Nursing Principle] Activating blood, resolving stasis, and stopping bleeding.

[Suggested Formula] Shenghua Decoction.

NURSING MEASURES

For patients with postpartum lochiorrhea, nurses should observe the amount, color, texture, odor and clot of the lochia, and the presence or absence the tenderness in the abdomen. Then the nursing measures are applied according to the general rules and different circumstances. If the patient has excessive red and clotted lochia, vertigo, palpitation, white complexion and severe abdominal pain, in this case, it is advisable to timely report to the doctor because it may be retention of the placenta.

Syndrome-Based Nursing Measures

1. Qi Deficiency Syndrome

(1) Daily life nursing. The ward should be warm. The patients should keep themselves warm and change the wet clothes timely to prevent getting cold. They should rest in bed to get enough sleep, take moderate activities, and avoid sitting, standing and walking for a long time. Nurses should assist the patients in daily life, place frequently-used items within their reach and move obstacles away from the area where the patients often walk.

(2) Diet nursing. The patients should follow a moderate diet and have small frequent meals, without over-tonics and over-eating. They may eat foods that replenish qi and invigorate the spleen, such as lean meat, sea cucumber, longyanrou (longan), dazao (Chinese date), shanyao (common yam rhizome) and eggs of black chicken. Food therapy: baishen lianzi (white ginseng and lotus seed) soup. Moreover, the patients should avoid heat-clearing foods.

（3）Emotion nursing. Nurses may use verbal enlightenment therapy to care for and encourage the patients as much as possible to prevent pessimism and nervousness.

（4）Medication nursing. Decoction should be brewed slowly over low heat and taken warm before meals.

（5）Manipulation techniques. ① Medicated ironing therapy: select Qihai（CV 6）to apply the therapy with baizhu（white atractylodes rhizome）and huangqi（astragalus root）, which should be finely ground, stir-fried and put into a cloth bag for medicated ironing at a temperature of $60 \sim 70℃$, 20 minutes each time, once per day. ② Moxibustion therapy: select Pishu（BL 20）, Tianshu（ST 25）, Qihai（CV 6）, Guanyuan（CV 4）and Zusanli（ST 36）; place the moxa stick $2 \sim 3$ centimeters away from the skin to perform mild moxibustion on each of them until the area turns red and the patient feels warm and comfortable without the sensation of burning pain, once per day. ③ Abdominal belt therapy: this therapy can prevent postpartum lochiorrhea caused by qi deficiency. The method is to put $4 \sim 5$ layers of cotton on the abdominal wall and bind them with a soft cloth. The therapy helps the recovery of the uterus by a little pressure from the external, keeps the abdomen warm to prevent qi consumption due to cold contraction, and prevent abdominal wall muscle flabby and internal organ prolapses.

2. Blood Heat Syndrome

（1）Daily life nursing. The ward should be cool, moist and full of fresh air. The coverings should be thin. For patients with profuse bleeding, reduce activities as much as possible.

（2）Diet nursing. The patients should increase the water intake, may drink snow pear juice, and eat cool-natured foods that clear heat, such as balsam pear, celery and muer（wood ear）. Food therapy: chixiaodou biqi（adzuki bean and waternut）thick soup. They should avoid intake of too many tonics, such as dazao（Chinese date）and longyanrou（longan）.

（3）Emotion nursing. Nurses may use verbal enlightenment therapy to introduce postpartum recuperation knowledge to patients and guide them to regulate their moods so as to prevent excitement and anxiety.

（4）Medication nursing. Decoction should be taken cool after meals.

（5）Manipulation techniques. ① Scraping therapy: select the line from Geshu（BL 17）to Danshu（BL 19）; use a scraping plate to forcefully scrape the straight line with the direction from top to bottom, and repeat the manipulation for $20 \sim 30$ consecutive times on each side till the area turns red and *sha qi*（rash of measles）occurs. An interval of $3 \sim 6$ days for rest in between scraping is preferred. ② Cupping therapy: select Xuehai（SP 10）and Geshu（BL 17）; retain the cup on them for ten minutes, once every other day. ③ Acupressure therapy: select Hegu（LI 4）, Dazhui（GV 14）, Waiguan（TE 5）, and Sanyinjiao（SP 6）; apply thumb kneading manipulation on each of them until the area turns hot or the patient has the feelings of soreness, numbness, distension and heaviness in the area; once per day.

3. Blood Stasis Syndrome

（1）Daily life nursing. The ward should be warm. The coverings should be thick. The patients should keep themselves warm to prevent getting cold, and may take a semi-supine position to facilitate lochia excretion and take moderate exercise to promote the movement of qi and blood.

(2) Diet nursing. The patients may drink brown sugar water or yellow wine, and eat foods that activate blood and resolve stasis. Food therapy: shanzha muer (Chinese hawthorn fruit and wood ear) soup. And don't eat raw or cold foods.

(3) Emotion nursing. Nurses may use submission therapy as well as emotional transference and dispositional change therapy to create an easy environment and encourage the patients to express feelings to prevent liver qi depression and blood stasis due to inhibited emotion.

(4) Medication nursing. Decoction should be taken warm after meals.

(5) Manipulation techniques. ① Moxibustion therapy: select Guilai (ST 29), Xuehai (SP 10) and Sanyinjiao (SP 6); place the moxa stick 2 ~ 3 centimeters away from the skin to perform mild moxibustion on each of them until the area turns red and the patient feels warm and comfortable without the sensation of burning pain, once per day. ② Medicated ironing therapy: select Zigong (EX – CA1) and Guilai (ST 29) with the use of taoren (peach kernel) and honghua (safflower), which should be stir-fried and put into a cloth bag for medicated ironing at a temperature of 60 ~ 70℃, 20 minutes each time, once per day. ③ Breast massage: apply a hot towel (the temperature should be suitable for skin tolerance) to the breasts for ten minutes; the patient's thumbs and other four fingers of both hands naturally separate to support the breasts from the bottom up, gently massage the breasts with finger pulps from all sides to the nipple direction, and then lift the nipples with both hands, 15 ~ 20 minutes each time, 3 ~ 4 times a day.

Patient Education

The room should be full of fresh air without strong winds and countercurrents. The patients are vulnerable to external pathogenic qi due to constitution weakness after delivery, therefore, it's necessary for them to reinforce healthy qi to resist pathogenic factors. And they should also keep warm to prevent colds; keep vulvae hygiene and dry, washing it with warm water every day and frequently changing disinfected sanitary pads and underwear; pay attention to wound care after defecation and urination, cleaning the wound with 1 : 1 000 potassium permanganate solution once or twice a day. When the blood volume is not much and the condition allows, encourage the patients to get up to walk and gradually increase the amount of activity in order to promote the movement of qi and blood as well as the uterine contraction, however, adequate rest is needed to avoid exhaustion. Moreover, tub bath and sexual intercourse are prohibited.

Eat more foods with high calories and high protein, or rich in Vitamin E, such as sunflower seed and hetaoren (walnut). The patients should refrain from cigarette and alcohol. Cold, pungent and spicy foods should be avoided, such as chili and dasuan (garlic bulb).

The patients should keep a good mood and avoid mood fluctuations to prevent five emotions transforming into fire.

Breastfeeding is advisable because it can promote uterine contractions and lochia discharge.

第四章
儿科病证的中医护理

据《史记·扁鹊仓公列传》记载,在春秋战国时期已有儿科医生:小儿医。《黄帝内经》论述了小儿的生长发育。隋朝,巢元方在《诸病源候论》中介绍了小儿病证255候。唐朝,孙思邈著《备急千金要方》,详细论述了多种儿科疾病的理、法、方、药。北宋,"儿科之圣"钱乙著《小儿药证直诀》,创立小儿辨证。金元时期,"金元四大家"均有关于儿科的论述。清朝,陈复正著《幼幼集成》,记载了新生儿疾病的防治和诊法。公元16至17世纪,我国应用"人痘接种"预防天花,该技术广泛传播到了世界各国。数千年来,中医儿科学在小儿喂养、保健、预防和医疗等方面,为中华民族的繁衍昌盛做出了不可磨灭的贡献。

小儿成长可划分为胎儿期、新生儿期、婴儿期、幼儿期、学龄前期、学龄期和青春期。临床常用的小儿体格指标有:体重、身高(长)、头围、囟门、胸围、牙齿等。

小儿疾病的病因,在外多为六淫和疫疠之邪,在内多为乳食不节、饮食不节。除此之外,还有先天因素、意外伤害和药品所伤。情志致病在小儿疾病中相对较少,其中惊恐较为常见。

小儿与成人相比,在生理方面有诸多不同。小儿脏腑娇嫩,尤其以肺、脾、肾三脏为甚,故有小儿"肺常不足""脾常不足""肾常虚"之说。小儿形气未充,"稚阴稚阳"。"稚阴"表现为精、血、津液,以及脏腑、筋骨、脑髓、肌肤等有形之质皆未充实与完善。"稚阳"指脏腑功能幼稚不足或处于不稳定的状态。小儿生机蓬勃,发育迅速。凡孩子在3岁以下,为"纯阳"之体。

小儿因为生理特点与成人不同,所以拥有独特的病理特点。小儿发病容易,传变迅速,容易发生肺、脾、肾疾病和时行疾病。发病后,"易虚易实,易寒易热",但因其脏气清灵,故易趋康复。

儿科疾病的诊断方法包括望、闻、问、切,尤其重视望诊。在望诊中,常用望神色、形态、苗窍、斑疹、二便和指纹。望指纹可归纳为"浮沉分表里,红紫辨寒热,淡滞定虚实,三关测轻重"。在闻诊中,常用听小儿啼哭、呼吸、咳嗽、说话,以及嗅口中气味,嗅大小便、痰液、汗液和呕吐物的气味。问诊则常通过询问患儿家长来完成。要注意询问小儿的年龄和个人史。小儿的脉软而较数,在安静或入睡时较易诊得。在按诊中,常用按颅囟、颈腋、四肢、皮肤、胸腹,以观察冷、热、软、硬,以及是否有症瘕痞块。

在儿科疾病的内治法中,治疗要及时、正确、谨慎,中病即止。服药时,每日煎出药的药量为:新生儿30~50 mL,婴儿60~100 mL,幼儿150~200 mL,学龄儿童200~300 mL,分3~5次服用。喂药时鼓励小儿自愿服药,不可强行灌服。凡大辛、大热、大苦、大寒、有毒、重镇、攻伐、峻下、壅补的药物,要谨慎使用。

　　小儿肌肤柔弱,脏气清灵,外治疗法尤为有效,它不仅规避了小儿害怕打针、服药困难的问题,还避免了口服给药对于胃肠道的刺激。常用的外治疗法有:熏洗疗法、敷贴疗法、药熨疗法、雾化吸入疗法等。除此之外,还有小儿推拿疗法、小儿捏脊疗法、挑治疗法、灸法、拔罐疗法、耳压疗法等。

Chapter 4
Nursing of Pediatric Diseases

As recorded in the section *Biography of Bian Que and Cang Gong* of the book *Records of the Historian*, there were pediatricians called "Xiaoer doctors" in the Spring and Autumn Period and the Warring States Period. In *Huangdi's Internal Classic*, the growth and development of children are recorded. In the Sui Dynasty, Dr. Chao Yuanfang introduced 255 kinds of pediatric diseases in *Treatise on the Pathogenesis and Manifestations of All Diseases*. In the Tang Dynasty, Dr. Sun Simiao wrote *Essential Prescriptions Worth a Thousand Gold for Emergencies*, in which the theories, principles, formulas, and medicinals in curing pediatric diseases have been detailedly discussed. In the Northern Song Dynasty, Dr. Qian Yi, "the saint of pediatric medicine", has established syndrome differentiation for children in his book, *Key to Therapeutics of Children's Diseases*. During the Jin and Yuan dynasties, the four great physicians all have made contributions to the development of pediatric medicine. In the Qing Dynasty, Dr. Chen Fuzheng recorded the prevention and treatment of pediatric diseases for neonates in his book of *Compendium of Pediatrics*. Between 16 to 17 century A.D., human smallpox vaccination technology invented in China were broadly shared in many countries around the world. For thousands of years, the Pediatrics of TCM has made great contribution to the prosperity of Chinese nation in the fields of feeding, health care, prevention and medical treatment of children.

The development of children can be classified into different periods, including fetal period, neonatal period, infant period, toddler period, preschool period, school-age period and adolescent period. The physical indexes often used in clinical practice are weight, height (length), head circumference, fontanelle, chest circumference, and teeth.

The external causes of pediatric diseases are mostly six excesses and epidemic pestilence, and the internal causes are mostly improper milk feeding or diet. Apart from those, there are congenital factors, accidental injuries and drug injuries. Emotional diseases are relatively rare in pediatric diseases, among which, fright is the most common one.

The physiology of children is sufficiently distinct from that of adults. Children has tender zang-fu organs, especially the lung, spleen and kidney, so there are theories that "lung is often insufficient" "spleen is often insufficient", and "kidney is often vacuous" for children. Children have the underdeveloped physique and qi with immature yin and yang. Immature yin is manifested in the insufficiency and incompleteness of essence, blood, body fluids, zang-fu organs, tendons and bones, marrow and skin. Immature yang is manifested in the deficiency or unstable state of visceral functions. However, children also enjoy a full vigor and rapid development. For children under three years old, they have pure-yang constitution.

Due to the unique physiology, children have distinctive pathology. Pediatric diseases are characterized by easy onset, quick transmission, and susceptible to lung, spleen and kidney diseases and seasonal pestilence. After onset, the nature of disease is always shifting within deficiency, excess, cold, or heat. Nevertheless, thanks to the keen visceral qi, the prognosis is good and the duration is short most of the time.

The diagnostic methods in pediatric diseases are inspection, smelling and listening, inquiry, pulse taking and palpation. Among them, the method of inspection is the most important one. In inspection, spirit, complexion, physique, posture, signal orifices, macula, papule, urine, stool, and finger venules should be examined. The inspection of finger venules can be concluded as, "differentiate the exterior or interior syndrome by the floating or sinking venules; the cold or heat syndrome by the red or purple color; the deficiency or excess syndrome by light or stagnant venules; and differentiate the severity of the disease by the length of three passes". In smelling and listening, children's crying sound, breathing, cough, and voice should be listened to, and their smell in the mouth, urine, stool, phlegm, sweat and vomitus should be smelt. Inquiry method is usually done by asking children's parents about their disease condition, especially the age and personal history. Children's pulse are normally soft and slightly rapid, which can be easily taken when in quietness or sleep. In palpation, the cranial fontanelle, neck, armpit, four limbs, skin, chest or abdomen should be palpated to observe the cold, heat, softness or hardness, and the presence of lumps or masses under the skin.

In the internal treatment of pediatric diseases, the treatment should be timely, correct and cautious. Treatment should be immediately stopped once the disease is cured. The daily dosage of decoction is 30~ 50 mL for neonates, 60~100 mL for infants, 150~200 mL for toddlers, and 200~300 mL for school-age children, taken 3~5 times per day. Children should be encouraged to take the medicine willingly without forced feeding. The medicinals that are highly pungent, highly hot, highly bitter, highly cold, toxic, heavily sedative, offensive-attacking, drastic purgative, stagnant tonifying should be used with caution.

Because the children have tender and soft skin and muscles with keen visceral qi, external therapies are quite effective for them. External therapies circumvent the feared injection and medicine among children, and avoid the gastrointestinal tract irritation from oral administration. The commonly used external therapies are fumigating and washing therapy, paste application therapy, medicated ironing therapy, and spray inhalation therapy. Moreover, there are also infantile tuina therapy, infantile spine pinching therapy, fibrous tissue-pricking therapy, moxibustion therapy, cupping therapy and auricular pressure therapy.

第一节 肺炎喘嗽

肺炎喘嗽,是指因外感时邪,或温热疫毒犯肺,导致痰阻气道,肺气郁闭,甚或邪陷心肝而引起的,以发热,咳嗽,气喘,鼻翕,痰壅,甚则高热不已,迅即神昏,谵语,惊厥,抽搐为临床特征的小儿肺系病。西医的小儿肺炎可参照本节进行护理。

一、病因病机

肺炎喘嗽的病因分为外因和内因。外因多为外感风邪。内因多为小儿脏腑娇嫩,卫外不固,或痰湿内伏,火热内蕴。小儿外感风邪,风为百病之长,夹寒热之邪侵犯肺卫,肺失宣降,发为肺炎喘嗽。若邪在肺卫不解,化热入里,炼液成痰,痰热互结,闭阻肺络,肺气郁闭,则发为痰热闭肺。本病后期,若邪热伤肺,肺阴耗伤,余邪留恋,则见阴虚肺热;若素体虚弱,或久咳伤肺,肺病及脾,则见肺脾气虚。若正气不足,邪毒内陷,可出现心阳虚衰或邪陷厥阴等严重变证。

肺炎喘嗽的病机为肺气郁闭。病位主要在肺,常累及脾,亦可内窜心、肝。

二、常见证型

(一)辨证要点

1. 辨常证与变证　根据神志情况,发热程度,持续时间,以及是否累及他脏来辨别。若主要表现为发热,咳嗽,气喘,多为常证中的轻证。若壮热不退,喘憋,鼻翼翕动,则多为常证中的重证。若出现神萎淡漠,面色苍白,唇指紫绀,四肢不温,或谵语狂躁,口噤项强,四肢抽搐,则多为变证。

2. 辨风寒与风热　根据恶寒与发热的程度,痰的颜色和质地,是否有汗、口渴来辨别。若恶寒重,发热轻,痰白质稀,无汗,口不渴,多为风寒。若发热重,恶寒轻,痰稠色黄,有汗,咽红疼痛,口渴欲饮,则多为风热。

3. 辨痰热与毒热　根据津液是否亏少,以及伴随症状来辨别。若气急鼻翕,喉间痰鸣,泛吐痰涎,苔黄腻,多为痰热。若喘憋,涕泪俱无,鼻孔干燥,苔黄燥,多为毒热。

(二)证候分型

1. 常证

(1)风寒闭肺证

[主要证候]恶寒发热,头身痛,无汗,鼻塞流清涕,喷嚏,咳嗽,气喘鼻翕,痰稀白易咯,可见泡沫样痰或闻喉间痰鸣;咽不红,口不渴,面色淡白,纳呆,小便清;舌淡红,苔薄白,脉浮紧,指纹浮红。

[证候分析]风寒之邪外袭犯肺,肺失肃降,其气上逆,故咳嗽,气喘鼻翕;卫阳为寒邪所遏,阳气不能敷布周身,故恶寒发热,无汗;肺为水之上源,肺气闭塞,水液输化无权,凝而为痰,故痰稀白

易咯,可见泡沫样痰或闻喉间痰鸣;舌淡红,苔薄白,脉浮紧,指纹浮红,均为风寒之象。

［护治原则］辛温宣肺,化痰降逆。

［常用方剂］华盖散。

（2）风热闭肺证

［主要证候］发热恶风,头痛有汗,鼻塞流清涕或黄涕,咳嗽,气喘,咯黄痰,或闻喉间痰嘶,鼻翼翕动;声高息涌,胸膈满闷,咽红肿,口渴欲饮,纳呆,便秘,小便黄少,面色红赤,烦躁不安;舌质红,苔薄黄,脉浮数,指纹浮紫。

［证候分析］风热闭肺,肺气失宣,气逆不顺,故咳嗽,气喘,鼻翼翕动;热灼肺津,炼液成痰,故咯黄痰,或闻喉间痰嘶;肺热蒸腾,故发热,咽红肿;舌质红,苔薄黄,脉浮数,指纹浮紫,均为风热之象。

［护治原则］辛凉宣肺,降逆化痰。

［常用方剂］银翘散合麻杏石甘汤。

（3）痰热闭肺证

［主要证候］发热,有汗,咳嗽,咯痰黄稠或喉间痰鸣,气急喘促,鼻翼翕动,声高息涌,呼吸困难,胸高胁满,张口抬肩;口唇紫绀,咽红肿,面色红,口渴欲饮,纳呆,便秘,小便黄少,烦躁不安;舌质红,苔黄腻,脉滑数,指纹紫滞。

［证候分析］痰热胶结,闭阻于肺,肺气失宣,故咳嗽,咯痰黄稠或喉间痰鸣,气急喘促,鼻翼翕动,呼吸困难;肺热壅盛,故发热,烦躁不安;气为血之帅,肺气郁闭,气滞血瘀,故口唇紫绀;舌质红,苔黄腻,脉滑数,指纹紫滞,均为痰热之象。

［护治原则］清热涤痰,开肺定喘。

［常用方剂］五虎汤合葶苈大枣泻肺汤。

（4）毒热闭肺证

［主要证候］壮热不退,咳嗽剧烈,痰黄稠难咯或痰中带血,气急喘促,喘憋,呼吸困难,鼻翼翕动,胸高胁满,胸膈满闷,张口抬肩;鼻孔干燥,面色红赤,口唇紫绀,涕泪俱无,烦躁不宁或嗜睡,甚至神昏谵语,呛奶,恶心呕吐,口渴引饮,便秘,小便黄少;舌红少津,苔黄腻或黄燥,脉洪数,指纹紫滞。

［证候分析］肺热炽盛,宣肃失司,故壮热不退,咳嗽剧烈;毒热内闭肺气,气道不利,故气急喘促,喘憋,呼吸困难;毒热耗液伤津,故鼻孔干燥,涕泪俱无,口渴引饮,便秘,小便黄少;舌红少津,苔黄腻或黄燥,脉洪数,指纹紫滞,均为毒热内盛之象。

［护治原则］清热解毒,泻肺开闭。

［常用方剂］黄连解毒汤合麻杏石甘汤。

（5）肺脾气虚证

［主要证候］久咳,咳痰无力,痰稀白易咯,气短,喘促乏力,动则喘甚;低热起伏,面白少华,神疲乏力,形体消瘦,自汗,纳差,口不渴,便溏,病程迁延,反复感冒;舌质淡红,舌体胖嫩,苔薄白,脉无力或细弱,指纹淡。

［证候分析］肺虚气无所主,故久咳、咳痰无力,气短,喘促乏力,动则喘甚;肺气不足,卫外失固,故自汗;脾虚运化不利,痰涎内生,故痰稀白易咯;脾虚运化失司,气血生化乏源,故面白少华,神

疲乏力,形体消瘦,纳差;脾气不足,运化失职,清浊不分,故便溏;舌质淡红,舌体胖嫩,苔薄白,脉无力或细弱,指纹淡,均为肺脾气虚之象。

[护治原则]补肺健脾,益气化痰。

[常用方剂]人参五味子汤。

（6）阴虚肺热证

[主要证候]咳喘持久,时有低热,手足心热,干咳,痰量少或无痰,咯痰带血;面色潮红,口干,口渴欲饮,神疲倦怠,夜卧不安,形体消瘦,盗汗,便秘,小便黄少,病程迁延;舌红少津,苔少或花剥,脉细数,指纹淡紫。

[证候分析]久热久咳,耗伤肺阴,加之余热留恋不去,故时有低热,手足心热,面色潮红,口干,口渴欲饮;津液亏少,肺失濡养,故干咳,痰量少或无痰;虚火上炎,阳加于阴,逼蒸外泄,故盗汗;舌红少津,苔少或花剥,脉细数,指纹淡紫,均为阴虚肺热之象。

[护治原则]养阴清肺,润肺止咳。

[常用方剂]沙参麦冬汤。

2. 变证

（1）心阳虚衰证

[主要证候]面色苍白,唇指紫绀,呼吸浅促、困难,四肢不温,多汗,胁下痞块,心悸动数,虚烦不安,神萎淡漠,小便减少;舌质淡紫,脉疾数、细弱欲绝,指纹紫滞。

[证候分析]肺为邪闭,气机不利,心血运行不畅,心阳不能敷布全身,故面色苍白,四肢不温;阳气虚衰,气不行血,故唇指紫绀,胁下痞块,舌质淡紫;心主藏神,心阳虚衰,故虚烦不安,神萎淡漠;肺病及肾,金不生水,肾不纳气,故呼吸浅促、困难;心主血脉,心阳虚衰,运血无力,故脉疾数、细弱欲绝。

[护治原则]温补心阳,救逆固脱。

[常用方剂]参附龙牡救逆汤。

（2）邪陷厥阴证

[主要证候]壮热不退,口唇紫绀,气促,喉间痰鸣,烦躁不安,谵语狂躁,神识昏迷,口噤项强,角弓反张,四肢抽搐;舌质红绛,脉细数,指纹紫。

[证候分析]毒热炽盛,内陷手厥阴心包经,故壮热不退,烦躁不安,谵语狂躁,神识昏迷;毒热内陷足厥阴肝经,引动肝风,故口噤项强,角弓反张,四肢抽搐;肺闭不宣,有垂绝之势,故气促,喉间痰鸣;舌质绛红,脉细数,指纹紫,均为毒热炽盛,邪陷厥阴,病势垂危之象。

[护治原则]清心开窍,平肝熄风。

[常用方剂]羚角钩藤汤合牛黄清心丸。

三、护理措施

对于肺炎喘嗽的患儿,应观察基础生命体征以及咳嗽、气急、鼻翕、面色、尿量、紫绀的情况。加强对重症患儿的巡视,密切观察神志和呼吸情况,记录出入量、体温、脉搏、呼吸、血压、血氧饱和度。若患儿出现面白肢冷,口唇发绀,呼吸困难,神昏抽搐,考虑为变证,应立即报告医生,并配合抢救。

（一）辨证施护

1. 风寒闭肺证

（1）生活起居护理 居室温暖舒适，阳光充足，空气新鲜。衣被宽大轻暖。卧床休息，睡眠充足。保持呼吸道通畅，经常变换体位，进行有效的咳嗽、咳痰，护士可协助翻身、拍背，必要时进行中药雾化吸入或使用吸痰器。可用温水擦浴，操作时注意避风，禁用冷敷法。

（2）饮食护理 可饮姜豉饴糖饮，也可浓煎紫苏叶取汁，兑生姜汁频服。宜食祛风散寒的食物。

（3）情志护理 本病起病急，症状明显，患儿常因发热、咳嗽、气急而哭闹不安，护士应向年长儿及家长讲解疾病的知识，取得患儿及家长的配合。

（4）用药护理 中药汤剂宜武火快煎，饭后热服。若咳嗽频繁，可少量频服。服药后进食热饮，如热米汤，加盖衣被，使其微微汗出。避免大汗、吹风。

（5）操作技术 ① 小儿推拿疗法：揉天突，搓摩胁肋，推揉膻中，运内八卦，揉肺俞，清肺经，推三关，揉外劳宫。② 灌肠疗法：对于服药困难的患儿，可选用疏风散寒，化痰平喘的中药煎汤，进行保留灌肠。③ 敷贴疗法：取肺俞，用白芥子粉、面粉各 20 g，加水调成糊状敷贴，每次 10 分钟，以皮肤潮红为宜，避免起泡，每日 1 次，连用 3 日。

2. 风热闭肺证

（1）生活起居护理 居室凉爽湿润。衣被宜薄。卧床休息，睡眠充足。保持呼吸道通畅。若痰多且稠，可遵医嘱进行中药雾化吸入或使用吸痰器。若体温偏高，可用温水擦浴或用温水足浴，操作时注意避风。慎用物理降温。

（2）饮食护理 多饮水，可饮桑菊杏仁茶、雪梨冰糖饮，或饮温热的藕汁、荸荠汁。宜食辛凉化痰的食物，如薄荷、金银花。若咳嗽痰多，可饮鲜竹沥。不宜食过甜的食物和饮料。

（3）情志护理 护士应加强巡视，对患儿关护体贴，以稳定患儿的情绪。护理时，态度和蔼，根据患儿的喜好转移其注意力，以使其配合治疗，减少因治疗或因环境改变而引起的恐惧和哭闹。

（4）用药护理 中药汤剂宜武火快煎，饭后温服。若咳嗽频繁或呕吐，可少量频服。服药后进食热饮，如热米汤，加盖衣被，使其微微汗出。避免大汗、吹风。

（5）操作技术 ① 小儿推拿疗法：揉天突，揉丰隆，搓摩胁肋，揉定喘，推揉膻中，运内八卦，揉肺俞，揉内劳宫，推小横纹，清肺经，清天河水。② 灌肠疗法：对于服药困难的患儿，可选用疏风清热，化痰平喘的中药随证加减后保留灌肠。③ 敷贴疗法：取肺俞，用薄荷、麻黄、白芥子等，研磨成粉后与生姜汁调成糊状敷贴，每次 10 分钟，以皮肤潮红为宜，避免起泡，每日 1 次，连用 3 日。

3. 痰热闭肺证

（1）生活起居护理 病室凉爽湿润，安静舒适。衣被宜薄。卧床休息，年长儿取半仰卧位，婴幼儿取 20°～30° 的低斜坡卧位，经常变换体位，睡眠充足。注意口腔清洁，保持呼吸道通畅。若高热，应观察体温的变化，每 4 小时测 1 次体温，可用温水擦浴降温。若汗多，应及时擦干，并换掉湿衣被，避免汗出当风。若痰多，帮助其排痰，采用拍背法或体位引流法。若痰多且稠，可遵医嘱进行中药雾化吸入或使用吸痰器。

（2）饮食护理 多饮水，可饮丝瓜花蜂蜜饮、热白萝卜汁。宜食清热化痰的食物，如雪梨、荸荠、冬瓜、鱼腥草。若高热，予清淡、易消化的流食。若咳嗽痰多，可饮鲜竹沥。不宜食过甜的食物和饮料。

（3）情志护理　小儿存在恐医心理,护士应有高度的责任心,对待患儿和蔼可亲,鼓励其更好地配合治疗和护理。

（4）用药护理　中药汤剂宜饭后温服,少量频服。

（5）操作技术　① 小儿推拿疗法:开天门,推坎宫,揉太阳,揉耳后高骨,清天河水,揉足三里,推涌泉穴;或在背部用中指、示指的指腹在脊柱自上而下直推 50~100 下,每次 40~60 分钟;每日 2 次。② 雾化吸入疗法:用甘草、金银花、鱼腥草各 20 g,桑叶、知母各 15 g,杏仁、前胡、白前各 10 g,桔梗 6 g,煎煮后雾化吸入,每次 10 分钟,每日 3 次;适用于痰多黄稠,口唇紫绀的患儿。③ 敷贴疗法:取两肩胛间或肺部听诊湿啰音密集处,用大黄、芒硝与大蒜各 20 g,捣泥后用纱布包裹,敷贴厚度 3~5 毫米,敷前先在皮肤上涂润滑油以减轻刺激;1~2 岁的患儿每次 15 分钟,3~5 岁每次 20 分钟,5 岁以上每次 25 分钟,以皮肤潮红为度,避免起泡,每日 1 次;敷药结束后,用温水擦净。

4. 毒热闭肺证

（1）生活起居护理　居室凉爽安静。衣被宜薄。卧床休息,年长儿取半仰卧位,婴幼儿取 20°~30° 的低斜坡位,经常变换体位,睡眠充足。密切观察患儿,指导患儿家长了解高热惊厥的早期表现:若患儿出现烦躁或表情呆滞,四肢有微小抽动,应立即报告医生和护士。

（2）饮食护理　多饮水,可饮热白萝卜汁。宜食清热化痰的食物,如雪梨、荸荠、冬瓜、马齿苋。若咳嗽痰多,可饮鲜竹沥。若高热,予清淡、易消化的流食。不宜食过甜的食物和饮料。

（3）情志护理　护士可运用语言开导疗法,向家长说明小儿的生理特点和疾病转归,安慰和鼓励患儿,以使其保持情绪稳定。

（4）用药护理　中药汤剂宜饭后温服,少量频服。

（5）操作技术　① 刺血疗法:取耳尖,皮肤消毒后揉按局部使其充血,用三棱针的 3 毫米针尖,快速刺入并出针,放出 1.0 mL 以下的血液,用无菌干棉球擦拭或按压,双耳各操作 1 次;或取十宣、八风、大椎,放出 1.0 mL 以下的血液或黏液;适用于高热的患儿。② 电离子导入疗法:取肺俞、定喘、膻中,选择清热解毒,泻肺开闭的中药,浓煎备用;每次取药液 50~100 mL,用药物离子透入仪导入,每次 15 分钟,每日 1 次;婴儿禁用。③ 敷贴疗法:取肺俞或肺部听诊啰音处,用红花、当归、川芎、赤芍、透骨草各 30 g,肉桂、丁香、川乌、草乌、乳香、没药各 15 g,黄芩、黄连、大黄各 10 g;研磨成粉与芝麻油调成糊状敷贴,用胶布固定,每次 2 小时,每日 1 次;用于肺部湿啰音明显者。

5. 肺脾气虚证

（1）生活起居护理　居室温暖安静,阳光充足。衣被宽大轻暖。卧床休息,年长儿取半仰卧位,婴幼儿取 20°~30° 的低斜坡位,经常变换体位,睡眠充足。待症状好转后,逐渐增加运动量。注意避风,不可过劳。

（2）饮食护理　饮食宜清淡、营养、易消化。进食肉、鱼、蛋、奶,以增强体质。宜食补气健脾的食物,如芡实、莲子、薏苡仁。食疗方:百合猪肺汤,山药杏仁粥。

（3）情志护理　小儿情志单纯,护士应帮助其树立战胜疾病的信心。

（4）用药护理　中药汤剂宜久煎,饭前温服。若咳嗽频繁或呕吐,可少量频服。

（5）操作技术　① 小儿推拿疗法:补脾经,补肺经,运内八卦,推揉膻中,揉脾俞,揉天突,揉定喘,揉肺俞,按揉足三里。② 敷贴疗法:取肺俞,用党参、炒白术、白芥子,研磨成粉后与生姜汁调成糊状敷贴,每次 10 分钟,以皮肤潮红为宜,避免起泡,每日 1 次,连用 3 日。③ 捏脊疗法:提捏背部的督脉和足太阳膀胱经,每次 3~5 分钟,每日 1 次,以增强体质。④灸法:取百会、气海、关元,用隔姜灸,把生姜切成直径 2~3 厘米,厚 0.3 厘米的薄片,中间以针刺数孔,放置于施灸处,每处 1~3 壮,灸至皮肤稍有红晕;或取神阙,用隔盐灸。⑤药熨疗法:取腹部,用连须葱白 30 g,生姜 15 g;药物捣烂炒热装入布袋中,制成温度为 60~70℃的中药热罨包,每次药熨 30 分钟,每日 2 次。⑥敷脐疗法:取神阙,将白胡椒、吴茱萸、五倍子、苍术、公丁香按 1∶2∶4∶2∶1 的比例配伍,打成粉后与生姜汁调成药饼,用无菌敷料封于神阙,每晚睡前敷脐至次晨约 10 小时。

6. 阴虚肺热证

(1)生活起居护理　居室凉爽安静。卧床休息,年长儿取半仰卧位,婴幼儿取 20°~30°的低斜坡位,经常变换体位,睡眠充足。若盗汗,应及时擦干,并换掉湿衣被。待症状好转后,逐渐增加运动量。注意避风,不可过劳。

(2)饮食护理　饮食宜清淡、营养、易消化。可用百合、杏仁、糯稻根煎水频服。进食肉、鱼、蛋、奶,以增强体质。宜食养阴清热的食物,如泥鳅、藕、酸枣仁。食疗方:银耳雪梨膏。不宜食煎炸、烘烤的食物。

(3)情志护理　在疾病的恢复期,护士应了解患儿和家长的思想状况,运用语言开导疗法,鼓励其坚持治疗。

(4)用药护理　中药汤剂宜久煎,饭前温服。

(5)操作技术　①小儿推拿疗法:补脾经,清肺经,清天河水,揉二马,揉按足三里,推涌泉,揉肺俞,揉脾俞。②敷贴疗法:取肺俞,用北沙参、炒白术、白芥子,研磨成粉后与生姜汁调成糊状敷贴,每次 10 分钟,以皮肤潮红为宜,避免起泡,每日 1 次,连用 3 日。③拔罐疗法:取肺俞、肺部听诊啰音明显处或肩胛骨下方,留罐 5~10 分钟,每日 1 次;适用于 3 岁以上,湿啰音久不消退者。④敷脐疗法:取神阙,用五倍子,研磨成粉后与醋调成糊状,每日睡前敷于脐中,第二天清晨清洗干净,连用 3 次;适用于盗汗的患儿。

7. 心阳虚衰证

(1)生活起居护理　居室温暖安静。衣被宽大轻暖。卧床休息,年长儿取半仰卧位,婴幼儿取 20°~30°的低斜坡位,经常变换体位,睡眠充足。若多汗,应及时擦干,并换掉湿衣被。严格监控心率,记录出入量。吸氧,氧气应湿化、温化。给氧前清除鼻痂、鼻涕及口腔积物,以保证呼吸道通畅。

(2)饮食护理　严格控制水、盐的摄入量。轻者予少盐饮食,重者无盐饮食。昏迷时,宜静脉补液。清醒后,可进食清淡的流食或半流食。使用利尿剂者,用药期间应补充富含钾的食物,如香蕉、柑橘、绿叶蔬菜。

(3)情志护理　患儿病情危重,家长存在不同程度的恐惧和焦虑。护士可运用语言开导疗法,说明病情的发展情况,安慰和鼓励家长,以使其保持情绪稳定。

(4)用药护理　中药汤剂宜急煎、浓煎,频频热服。对于昏迷的患儿,可用鼻饲法给药。尽量减少静脉输液量,输液速度宜慢。使用利尿剂者,应尽量在早晨及上午给药,以避免夜尿过多影响患儿休息。

(5)操作技术　①灸法:取百会、气海、关元、神阙,用隔姜灸,把生姜切成直径 2~3 厘米,厚 0.3 厘米的薄片,中间以针刺数孔,放置于施灸处,每处 1~3 壮,每日 2 次。②耳压疗法:取肺、气管、交感、神门等耳穴,用耳穴压丸贴片贴压,每日按揉 4~5 次,以局部发热泛红为度,留置 2~4 日。

8. 邪陷厥阴证

（1）生活起居护理　居室凉爽安静。卧床休息,年长儿取半仰卧位,婴幼儿取 20°~30°的低斜坡位,经常变换体位。记录出入量,监测血氧饱和度。观察体温变化,体温高于 39℃时应立即采用物理降温,如冷敷前额、温水擦浴,警惕高热惊厥的发生。若发生抽搐,患儿宜平卧,头后垫以柔软的物品,头偏向一侧,保持呼吸道通畅,解开衣领,松解衣物,不可强行按压,以免肢体受伤。

（2）饮食护理　昏迷时,宜静脉补液。清醒后,予清淡的流食或半流食。

（3）情志护理　患儿病情危重,家长存在不同程度的恐惧和焦虑。护士可运用语言开导疗法,说明病情发展情况,安慰和鼓励家长。多关心、安慰和抚触患儿,以减少恐惧感。

（4）用药护理　中药汤剂宜急煎、浓煎,温服。对于昏迷的患儿,可用鼻饲法给药。

（5）操作技术　①穴位按摩法:取水沟、涌泉、十宣、四缝,用力挤掐,直至患儿苏醒;取肩井、委中、承山,用拿法,直至抽搐停止;适用于高热惊厥的患儿。②敷贴疗法:取前胸剑突部,用三黄散(大黄、黄连、黄芩各 10 g,共研细末)与热酒调匀敷贴,每次 2 小时,重症者换药再敷;适用于高热喘促的患儿。③药栓疗法:蜂蜜浓煎,搓成小栓形,塞肛;适用于大便秘结的患儿。

（二）健康教育

经常变换体位,婴幼儿可常抱起,年长儿可取坐位或半仰卧位。指导年长患儿进行有效的咳嗽,协助以拍背。若痰黏难排,可使用吸痰器,负压不宜过大,动作要轻快,以免损伤口腔黏膜。

饮食宜清淡、营养、易消化。多吃高纤维的水果和蔬菜,以保持大便通畅。对于婴儿,鼓励继续母乳喂养。若气急、鼻翕严重,可暂停哺乳,待症状缓解后再继续进食。不宜食辛辣、生冷、油腻、肥甘、质地干燥的食物,如辣椒、冷饮、肥肉、饼干。哺乳期间,乳母也应注意饮食禁忌。

遵医嘱用药。中药宜浓煎,温服,少量多次,徐徐喂服。切勿暴躁急进或捏鼻灌服,致使患儿躁动气急,甚至呛咳,引起窒息。

积极开展体育锻炼,以增强体质。寒冷季节或天气骤变时注意保暖。冬春季节时,应经常到户外,于无风处晒太阳。上呼吸道疾病流行期间,尽量不去公共场所。注意个人卫生,勤洗手,远离烟雾刺激。若发生感冒、咳嗽,应及时治疗,以避免发展为肺炎喘嗽。

Section 1 Pneumonia with Dyspnea and Cough

Pneumonia with dyspnea and cough refers to a lung disease in children characterized by fever, cough, dyspnea, flaring nostrils, phlegm congestion, or even high fever with immediate coma, delirious speech, fright reversal and convulsion. It is caused by external contraction of seasonal pathogen or invasion of warm febrile epidemic toxin to the lung that causes blockage of phlegm in the air passage, depression of lung qi, or even invasion of pathogen in the heart and the liver. This section can be referred to for the nursing of infantile pneumonia in Western medicine.

ETIOLOGY AND PATHOGENESIS

The etiology includes exogenous and endogenous causes. The former mainly refers to external contraction of wind pathogen while the latter is mainly due to children's delicacy of zang-fu organs and insecurity of the defensive exterior, or internal accumulation of phlegm-dampness or fire-heat. Pathogenic wind is the leading cause of all diseases. When children contract external wind pathogen, the wind intermingles with cold and heat to invade the lung-defense, which induces failure of lung qi to disperse and descend, so pneumonia with dyspnea and cough occurs. If the pathogen in the lung-defense is not resolved, it would transform into heat and further enter the interior to scorch body fluids into phlegm. Phlegm binding with heat blocks lung collaterals and depresses lung qi, so phlegm-heat blocks the lung. In the late period, pathogenic heat damages the lung and consumes lung yin, so there may be yin deficiency and lung heat. Constitutional weakness, lung damage due to prolonged cough, or involvement of lung disorder in the spleen would lead to qi deficiency of the lung and spleen. Deficiency of healthy qi and inward invasion of pathogenic toxin would bring about deteriorated syndromes such as deficiency and debilitation of heart-yang or pathogenic invasion to jueyin meridian.

The pathogenesis is the blockage of lung qi. And the disease is located in the lung and often involves the spleen, or inward in the heart and liver.

COMMON SYNDROMES

Key Points in Syndrome Differentiation

1. Differentiation of Common from Deteriorated Syndrome

The differentiation is based on mental condition, degree and duration of fever, and whether spreading to other zang-organs. The main manifestations such as fever, cough and dyspnea are judged as minor ones of common syndrome; the manifestations such as persistent high fever, dyspnea with stifling oppression, and flaring nostrils are judged as serious ones of common syndrome. The manifestations such as dispiritedness and indifference, pale complexion, cyanotic lips and fingers nails, cold four limbs, or delirious speech and mania, clenched jaw and neck rigidity, and convulsion of the limbs are judged as deteriorated syndrome.

2. Differentiation of Wind-Cold from Wind-Heat Syndrome

The differentiation is based on the degree of aversion to cold and fever, color and texture of phlegm, and presence or absence of sweating and thirst. Serious aversion to cold, light fever, white thin phlegm, no sweating and no thirst are manifestations of wind-cold; serious fever, light aversion to cold, thick yellow phlegm, sweating, sore throat and thirst are manifestations of wind-heat.

3. Differentiation of Phlegm-Heat from Toxin-Heat

The differentiation is based on the consumption of body fluids and accompanied symptoms. Rapid breathing and flaring nostrils, wheezing sound in the throat, saliva and yellow sticky tongue coating are judged as phlegm-heat; dyspnea with stifling oppression, no snivel and tear, dry nose, and yellow dry tongue coating are judged as toxin-heat.

Syndrome Differentiation

1. Common Syndromes

(1) Wind-Cold Blocking the Lung Syndrome

[Clinical Manifestations] Aversion to cold, fever, headache, generalized pain, no sweating, nasal congestion, thin nasal discharge, sneezing, cough, dyspnea, flaring nostrils, white thin phlegm with easy expectoration, phlegm with bubbles or wheezing sound in the throat, no swollen throat, no thirst, pale complexion, torpid intake, clear urine, light red tongue with white thin coating, floating tight pulse, and floating-red finger venules.

[Manifestations Analysis] External pathogenic wind-cold invading the lung leads to the failure of the lung to descend and counterflow ascending of lung qi, so cough and dyspnea with flaring nostrils occur. Defensive yang being constrained by pathogenic cold makes yang qi fail to protect the body, so there are aversion to cold, fever and no sweating. The lung is upper source of water, it fails to dredge and regulate water passage when lung qi is blocked, thus, water condenses into phlegm, causing white and thin phlegm with easy expectoration, bubbles in the phlegm or wheezing sound in the throat. Light red tongue with white thin coating, floating tight pulse and floating-red finger venules are all the manifestations of wind-cold.

[Nursing Principle] Ventilating the lung with pungent-warm; resolving phlegm and descending adverse qi.

[Suggested Formula] Huagai Powder.

(2) Wind-Heat Blocking the Lung Syndrome

[Clinical Manifestations] Fever, aversion to wind, headache, sweat, nasal congestion with clear or yellow snivel, cough, dyspnea, expectoration of yellow phlegm or wheezing sound in the throat, flaring nostrils, high voice and rough breathing, fullness and oppression in the chest and diaphragm, swollen throat, thirst with desire to drink, torpid intake, constipation and dark scanty urine, red complexion, dysphoria, red tongue with yellow thin coating, floating rapid pulse and floating-purple finger venules.

[Manifestations Analysis] Wind-heat blocking the lung leads to failure of the lung to disperse and descend and lung qi counterflow, causing cough, and dyspnea with flaring nostrils. Heat scorches lung fluids into phlegm, resulting in yellow phlegm or wheezing sound in the throat. Steaming of lung heat leads to fever and swollen throat. Red tongue with yellow thin coating, floating rapid pulse, and floating-purple finger venules are the manifestations of wind-heat.

[Nursing Principle] Ventilating the lung with pungent-cool; descending adverse qi and resolving phlegm.

[Suggested Formula] Yinqiao Powder and Maxing Shigan Decoction.

(3) Phlegm-Heat Blocking the Lung Syndrome

[Clinical Manifestations] Fever, sweat, cough with yellow thick phlegm or wheezing sound in the throat, rapid breathing, dyspnea with flaring nostrils, high voice, rough breathing, difficult breathing, raised and full chest, gaping mouth and raised shoulders, cyanotic lips, swollen throat, red complexion, thirst with desire to drink, torpid intake, constipation, dark scanty urine, dysphoria, red tongue with yellow slimy coating, slippery rapid pulse and purple stagnant finger venules.

[Manifestations Analysis] Phlegm and heat jelling together blocks the lung and causes failure of the lung to disperse and descend, leading to cough with thick yellow phlegm or wheezing sound in the throat, rapid breathing, dyspnea with flaring nostrils and difficulty breathing. Exuberance of lung heat leads to fever and dysphoria. Qi is being commander of blood, so qi stagnation and blood stasis occurs when lung qi is depressed. This is the reason for cyanotic lips. Red tongue with yellow slimy coating, slippery rapid pulse and purple stagnant finger venules are manifestations of phlegm heat.

[Nursing Principle] Clearing heat and removing phlegm; ventilating the lung and relieving dyspnea.

[Suggested Formula] Wuhu Decoction and Tingli Dazao Xiefei Decoction.

(4) Toxin-Heat Blocking the Lung Syndrome

[Clinical Manifestations] Persistent high fever, severe cough, yellow thick phlegm with blood or difficult expectoration, rapid breathing, dyspnea with stifling oppression, difficult breathing, flaring nostrils, raised and full chest, fullness and oppression in the chest and diaphragm, gaping mouth and raised shoulders, dry nostrils, red complexion, cyanotic lips, no tear or snivel, dysphoria or somnolence, even coma and delirious speech, chocking when drinking milk, nausea and vomiting, thirst with desire to drink, constipation, dark scanty urine, red tongue with scanty fluids, yellow slimy coating or dry yellow coating, surging rapid pulse and purple stagnant finger venules.

[Manifestations Analysis] Exuberance of lung heat leads to failure of the lung to disperse and descend, causing persistent high fever and severe cough. Toxic heat blocking lung qi causes inhibition of air passage, leading to rapid breathing, dyspnea with stifling oppression, and difficult breathing. Toxic heat consuming body fluids is responsible for dry nostrils, no snivel or tear, thirst with desire to drink, constipation, and dark scanty urine. Red tongue with scanty fluids, yellow slimy coating or dry yellow coating, surging rapid pulse with purple stagnant finger venules are manifestations of internal exuberance of toxic heat.

［Nursing Principle］Clearing heat and removing toxin; purging the lung and opening blockage.

［Suggested Formula］Huanglian Jiedu Decoction and Maxing Shigan Decoction.

（5）Lung-Spleen Qi Deficiency Syndrome

［Clinical Manifestations］Prolonged cough, weak expectoration, white thin phlegm, shortness of breath, hasty panting that aggravates with exertion, fluctuating low fever, pale complexion, mental and physical fatigue, emaciation, spontaneous sweating, poor appetite, no thirst, loose stool, prolonged course of disease with recurrent cold, tender enlarged tongue with light red color and white thin coating, feeble pulse or weak thready pulse with pale finger venules.

［Manifestations Analysis］The lung fails to govern qi due to its deficiency, causing prolonged cough, weak expectoration, shortness of breath, and hasty panting that aggravates with exertion. Insufficiency of lung qi brings about insecurity of the defensive exterior, so spontaneous sweating occurs. Dysfunction of the spleen in transportation and transformation generates internal dampness and saliva, so phlegm is white, thin and easily expectorated. Deficient spleen cannot provide enough source for the generation of qi and blood, resulting in pale complexion, mental and physical fatigue, emaciation, and poor appetite. Spleen deficiency also fails to ascend the clear and descend the turbid, so loose stool occurs. Light red tender enlarged tongue with light red color and white thin coating, feeble pulse or weak thready pulse with pale finger venules, all are signs of qi deficiency of the lung and spleen.

［Nursing Principle］Tonifying the lung and invigorating the spleen; replenishing qi and resolving phlegm.

［Suggested Formula］Renshen Wuweizi Decoction.

（6）Yin Deficiency and Lung Heat Syndrome

［Clinical Manifestations］Prolonged cough, intermittent low fever, feverish sensation in palms and soles, dry cough with little or no phlegm, expectoration with blood, flushed face, thirst with desire to drink, mental and physical fatigue, unquiet sleep, emaciation, night sweat, constipation, dark scanty urine, prolonged course of disease, red tongue with scanty fluids, little coating or peeling coating, thin rapid pulse, and light red finger venules.

［Manifestations Analysis］Prolonged fever and cough consume lung yin, leading to yin deficiency with yang hyperactivity and lingering fever, causing intermittent low fever, feverish sensation in palms and soles, flushed face, and thirst with desire to drink. Insufficient fluids fail to nourish and moisten the lung, so there is dry cough with little or no phlegm. Insufficiency of lung yin causes deficiency fire to flame upward, so night sweat is induced. Red tongue with scanty fluids, little coating or peeling coating, thin rapid pulse, and light red finger venules all are manifestations of yin deficiency and lung heat.

［Nursing Principle］Nourishing yin and clearing the lung; moistening the lung and relieving cough.

［Suggested Formula］Shashen Maidong Decoction.

2. Deteriorated Syndrome

（1）Heart Yang Debilitation Syndrome

［Clinical Manifestations］Pale complexion, cyanotic lips and fingers, hasty breathing, dyspnea, lack of warmth in the limbs, profuse sweating, lump glomus below the costal region, rapid palpitation, vacuity vexation, restlessness, dispiritedness and indifference, reduced urine, light purple tongue with swift rapid pulse and faint pulse verging on expiry and purple stagnant finger venules.

［Manifestations Analysis］Pathogenic factors blocking the lung causes disturbance of qi movement, inhibited movement of heart blood, and failure of heart yang to spread to the whole body, causing pale complexion and lack warmth of the limbs. Debilitation of yang qi fails to promote the circulation of blood, resulting in cyanotic lips and fingers, lump glomus below the costal region, and light purple tongue. The heart governs spirit, and debilitation of heart yang is the reason for vacuity vexation, restlessness, dispiritedness and indifference. Disease of the lung affecting the kidney brings about failure of metal to generate water and failure of the kidney to receive qi, so the patients feel hasty breathing and dyspnea. The heart governs blood and vessels, so debilitation of heart yang cannot forcefully propel the movement of blood, hence there are swift rapid pulse and faint pulse verging on expiry.

［Nursing Principle］Warming and tonifying heart yang; restoring yang to stop collapse.

［Suggested Formula］Shenfu Longmu Jiuni Decoction.

（2）Pathogen Invading Jueyin Meridian Syndrome

［Clinical Manifestations］Persistent high fever, cyanotic lips, hasty breathing, wheezing sound in the throat, dysphoria, delirious speech, manic agitation, coma, clenched jaw, neck rigidity, arched-back rigidity, convulsion of the limbs, crimson tongue with thready rapid pulse and purple finger venules.

［Manifestations Analysis］Exuberant heat toxin invades pericardium meridian of hand-jueyin, causing persistent high fever, dysphoria, delirious speech, manic agitation and coma. Heat toxin invades liver meridian of foot-jueyin and stirs liver wind, so exhibit clenched jaw, neck rigidity, arched-back rigidity, and convulsion of the limbs. Lung qi is blocked with the tendency of exhaustion and danger, so the patients have hasty breathing and wheezing sound in the throat. Crimson tongue with thready rapid pulse and purple finger venules are manifestations of exuberant heat toxin invading jueyin meridian, which is a dangerous condition.

［Nursing Principle］Clearing heart and opening orifice; pacifying the liver and extinguishing wind.

［Suggested Formula］Lingjiao Gouteng Decoction and Niuhuang Qingxin Pills.

NURSING MEASURES

For patients with pneumonia with dyspnea and cough, nurses should observe the basic vital signs and cough, hasty breathing, flaring nostrils, complexion, urine volume and cyanosis. For critically ill children, intensified inspection should be performed and their mental and respiratory conditions should be observed closely. Nurses should also record their intake and output, body temperature, pulse, respiration, blood pressure and blood oxygen saturation, etc. If there is deteriorated syndrome with the symptoms of pale complexion, cold limbs, cyanotic lips, difficult breathing, coma and convulsion, nurses should report to the doctor and help give emergency treatment.

Syndrome-Based Nursing Measures

1. Wind-Cold Blocking the Lung Syndrome

（1）Daily life nursing. The ward should be warm, comfortable, sunny and full of fresh air. The children should rest in bed with light, loose and warm clothes and quilts, ensure adequate sleep, and keep the respiratory tract unobstructed and change positions frequently to ensure effective cough and expectoration. Nurses may assist with turning-over and back-patting, give herbal spray inhalation or sputum aspiration if necessary. Sponge bath with warm water could be applied for the patients rather than cold compress method. And the children should keep away from wind when they have sponge bath.

（2）Diet nursing. Jiangchi yitang（fresh ginger, prepared soybean and malt sugar）tea is recommended. Zisuye（perilla leaf）can be decocted dense for frequent drinking with addition of shengjiang（fresh ginger）juice. The patients may eat foods with function of expelling wind and dissipating cold.

（3）Emotion nursing. Due to the sudden attack of the disease with apparent symptoms, the children may often be agitated with fever, cough and hasty breathing. Nurses should inform the elder children and parents the knowledge about the disease to get their cooperation.

（4）Medication nursing. Decoction should be brewed quickly with strong fire and taken warm after meals, one dose per day. For the cases with frequent cough, decoction could be taken multiple times in small portions. After taking decoction, the children could have hot drinks such as hot rice juice and wear more clothes to induce slight sweating. Profuse sweating and wind should both be avoided.

（5）Manipulation techniques. ① Infantile tuina therapy: kneading Tiantu（CV 22）, twisting and rubbing Xielei（hypochondrium）, pushing and kneading Danzhong（CV 17）, circularly pushing Neibagua, kneading Feishu（BL 13）, clearing Feijing（lung meridian）, pushing Sanguan（triple pass）, and kneading Wailaogong（EX‐UE8）. ② Enema therapy: for those who have difficulty in drinking decoction, Chinese medicinals of dispersing wind, dissipating cold, resolving phlegm and relieving dyspnea can be decocted for retention enema. ③ Paste application therapy: prepare baijiezi（white mustard seed）powder and flour 20 g respectively; blend them with water to make pastes and apply them on Feishu（BL 13）till the area turns red without blister, ten minutes each time, once per day, and continuous application for three days.

2. Wind-Heat Blocking the Lung Syndrome

（1）Daily life nursing. The ward should be cool and moist. The children should rest in bed with thin clothes and quilts, ensure adequate sleep, and keep the respiratory tract unobstructed. If there is much thick and sticky phlegm, give herbal spray inhalation or sputum aspiration. If the body temperature is high, sponge bath or foot bath with warm water could be applied for the patients rather than physical cooling method. And the children should keep away from wind when they have sponge bath or foot bath.

（2）Diet nursing. The children should drink more water and may drink sangju xingren（mulberry leaf, chrysanthemum flower and apricot kernel）tea, snow pear crystal sugar juice, warm lotus root juice, or warm biqi（waternut）juice. They may eat pungent and cool foods with function of releasing exterior and resolving phlegm such as bohe（field mint）and jinyinhua（honeysuckle flower）. If there is cough with profuse phlegm, zhuli（bamboo sap）can be taken. They should not take too-sweet foods or drinks.

（3）Emotion nursing. Nurses should pay great attention to and care for the children to stabilize their moods. Nurses should be kind and divert children's attention considering their preference so as to make them cooperate with the treatment and reduce the fear or crying caused by the change of environment or treatment.

（4）Medication nursing. Decoction should be brewed quickly with strong fire and taken warm after meals. If there is frequent cough or vomiting, decoction could be taken multiple times in small portions. After taking decoction, the children could have hot drinks such as hot rice juice and wear more clothes to induce slight sweating. Profuse sweating and wind should both be avoided.

（5）Manipulation techniques. ① Infantile tuina therapy: kneading Tiantu（CV 22）, kneading Fenglong（ST 40）, kneading Dingchuan（EX - B1）, twisting and rubbing Xielei（hypochondrium）, pushing and kneading Danzhong（CV 17）, circularly pushing Neibagua, kneading Feishu（BL 13）, kneading Neilaogong（inner part of palm）, pushing Xiaohengwen（small transverse crease）, clearing Feijing（lung meridian）and clearing Tianheshui（heaven river water）. ② Enema therapy: for those who have difficulty in drinking decoction, Chinese medicinals of dispersing wind, clearing heat, resolving phlegm and relieving dyspnea can be decocted for retention enema. ③ Paste application therapy: grind into powder bohe（field mint）, mahuang（ephedra）, and baijiezi（white mustard seed）; blend the powder with shengjiang（fresh ginger）juice to make pastes, and apply them on Feishu（BL 13）till the area turns red without blister, ten minutes each time, once per day, and continuous application for three days.

3. Phlegm-Heat Blocking the Lung Syndrome

（1）Daily life nursing. The ward should be cool, moist, quiet and comfortable. The children should rest in bed with thin clothes and quilts, ensure adequate sleep and change positions frequently. The older children can take a semi-supine position and infants a low slope position of 20° ~ 30° height. They should also pay attention to oral hygiene and keep the respiratory tract unobstructed. In case of high fever, nurses should observe the change of body temperature and take the temperature every four hours, and sponge bath with warm water could be applied for them. If there is much sweating, it is necessary to promptly wipe out sweat and change the wet clothes and quilts to avoid exposure after sweating. If there is much phlegm, nurses should help to expel phlegm by patting the back or using postural drainage method. If there is much thick phlegm, follow the doctor's advice to give herbal spray inhalation or sputum aspiration.

(2) Diet nursing. The children should drink more water and may take hot white radish juice, or luffa flower juice with honey, and cat foods with function of clearing heat and resolving phlegm such as snow pear, biqi (waternut), Chinese waxgourd, and yuxingcao (heartleaf houttuynia). If there is high fever, light digestible liquid foods are preferred. If there is cough with profuse phlegm, zhuli (bamboo sap) can be taken. The children should not take too-sweet foods or drinks.

(3) Emotion nursing. Children are afraid of treatment, so nurses should be highly responsible kind to them and encourage them to better cooperate with treatment and care.

(4) Medication nursing. Decoction should be taken warm after meals, multiple times in small portions.

(5) Manipulation techniques. ① Infantile tuina therapy: opening Tianmen (heaven gate), pushing Kangong, kneading Taiyang (EX－HN5), kneading Erhougaogu (prominent bone behind the ears), clearing Tianheshui (heaven river water), kneading Zusanli (ST 36), and pushing Yongquan (KI 1); or straightly pushing the spine from top to bottom with the bellies of middle and index fingers 50~100 times, about 40~60 minutes each time; twice per day. ② Spray inhalation therapy: gancao (licorice root), jinyinhua (honeysuckle flower) and yuxingcao (heartleaf houttuynia) 20 g respectively, sangye (mulberry leaf) and zhimu (common anemarrhena rhizome) 15 g respectively, xingren (apricot kernel), qianhu (hogfennel root) and baiqian (cynanchum root and rhizome) 10 g respectively, and jiegeng (platycodon root) 6 g; decoct the above medicinals and instruct the patient to inhale the decoction steam into respiratory tract, ten minutes each time, three times per day. It is suitable for children with profuse thick yellow phlegm and lip cyanosis. ③ Paste application therapy: pound into mud dahuang (rhubarb root and rhizome), mangxiao (sodium sulphate) and dasuan (garlic bulb) 20 g respectively; use gauze to wrap the mud with a thickness of 3~5 millimeters, and apply it between the two shoulder blades or moist-rale-concentrated place in lung auscultation till the area turns red without blister; for children aged 1~2 year(s) old, 15 minutes each time, for those aged 3~5 years old, 20 minutes each time, and for those aged above five years old, 25 minutes each time, once per day; apply lubricating oil on the skin before paste application to reduce irritation, and clean the skin with warm water after the paste is removed.

4. Toxin-Heat Blocking the Lung Syndrome

(1) Daily life nursing. The ward should be cool and quiet. The children should rest in bed with thin clothes and quilts, ensure adequate sleep and change positions frequently. The older children may take a semi-supine position and infants a low slope position of 20°~30° height. Nurses should observe the children closely and instruct the parents about the early manifestations of febrile convulsions: if the children appear irritable or have dull expression and slight twitching of the limbs, immediately report to the doctors and nurses.

(2) Diet nursing. The children should drink more water and may take hot white radish juice and eat foods with function of clearing heat and resolving phlegm such as snow pear, biqi (waternut), Chinese

waxgourd and machixian (purslane). If there is cough with profuse phlegm, zhuli (bamboo sap) can be taken. If there is high fever, light digestible liquid foods are preferred. The children should not take too-sweet foods or drinks.

(3) Emotion nursing. Nurses may inform the parents about their children's physiological characteristics and disease development as well as use verbal enlightenment therapy to comfort and encourage the children to help them maintain emotional stability.

(4) Medication nursing. Decoction should be taken warm after meals, multiple times in small portions.

(5) Manipulation techniques. ① Blood-letting therapy: select the Erjian (EX - HN6); after the skin is disinfected, rub the local area to make it hyperemic, use a three-edged needle to quickly pierce the skin at a depth of 3 millimeters, remove the needle to release blood less than 1.0 mL, wipe or press the pierced point with a sterile dry cotton ball, once for each ear. Or select Shixuan (EX - UE11), Bafeng (EX - LE10) and Dazhui (GV 14) to perform the pricking with the same method above to release blood or mucus less than 1.0 mL; it is suitable for children with high fever. ② Electrical iontophoresis therapy: select Feishu (BL 13), Dingchuan (EX - B1) and Danzhong (CV 17); first decoct the medicinals for late use that clear heat, remove toxin, purge the lung and remove blockage; take 50~100 mL of the decoction each time, and use medicinal iontophoresis apparatus to conduct the medicinal ions of the decoction into the accupoints; 15 minutes each time, once per day. And it should be avoided for children aged below one year old. ③ Paste application therapy: grind into powder honghua (safflower), danggui (Chinese angelica), chuanxiong (Sichuan lovage root), chishao (red peony root) and tougucao (impatientis stem) 30 g respectively, rougui (cinnamon bark), dingxiang (clove flower), chuanwu (prepared monkshood mother root), caowu (prepared kusnezoff monkshood root), ruxiang (frankincense) and moyao (myrrh) 15 g respectively, huangqin (scutellaria root), huanglian (coptis rhizome) and dahuang (rhubarb root and rhizome) 10 g respectively; blend the powder with sesame oil to make pastes, apply them on Feishu (BL 13) or moist-rale-concentrated place in lung auscultation, and fix them with adhesive plaster, two hours each time, once per day; it is suitable for patients with obvious moist-rale in the lung.

5. Lung-Spleen Qi Deficiency Syndrome

(1) Daily life nursing. The ward should be warm, quiet and sunny. The children should rest in bed with loose, light and warm clothes and quilts, ensure adequate sleep and change positions frequently. The older children may take a semi-supine position and infants a low slope position of 20°~30° height. After the symptoms get improved, the children should gradually increase the amount of exercise but pay attention to avoiding wind and overwork.

(2) Diet nursing. The diet should be light, nutritious and digestible. The children may take milk, egg, lean meat and fish to enhance body constitution, and eat foods with function of tonifying qi and invigorating the spleen such as qianshi (euryale seed), lianzi (lotus seed) and yiyiren (coix seed). Food therapy: baihe zhufei (lily bulb and pig lung) soup, and shanyao xingren (common yam rhizome

and apricot kernel) porridge.

(3) Emotion nursing. Children are very simple and naive, and nurses should help them build up confidence in overcoming the disease.

(4) Medication nursing. Decoction should be brewed for long time and taken warm before meals. If there is frequent cough or vomiting, decoction could be taken multiple times in small portions.

(5) Manipulation techniques. ① Infantile tuina therapy: tonifying Pijing (spleen meridian), tonifying Feijing (lung meridian), circularly pushing Neibagua, pushing and kneading Danzhong (CV 17), kneading Pishu (BL 20), kneading Tiantu (CV 22), kneading Dingchuan (EX-B1), kneading Feishu (BL 13), and pressing and kneading Zusanli (ST 36). ② Paste application therapy: grind into powder dangshen (codonopsis root), chaobaizhu (stir-fried white atractylodes rhizome) and baijiezi (white mustard seed); blend the powder with shengjiang (fresh ginger) juice to make pastes and apply them on Feishu (BL 13) till the area turns red without blister, ten minutes each time, once per day, and continuous application for three days. ③ Spine pinching therapy: lift and pinch the governor vessel and bladder meridian of foot-taiyang to enhance body constitution, once per day, 3~5 minutes each time. ④ Moxibustion therapy: perform ginger-partitioned moxibustion on Baihui (GV 20), Qihai (CV 6) and Guanyuan (CV 4). The procedure is to slice shengjiang (fresh ginger) into thin pieces with diameter of 2~3 centimeters and thickness of 0.3 centimeters, pierce several holes through the ginger slice with a sharp needle, and place the ginger slices on the acupoints, 1~3 moxa-cone(s) on every acupoint until the area turns red. Or apply salt-partitioned moxibustion on Shenque (CV 8). ⑤ Medicated ironing therapy: pound 30 g of congbai (scallion white) with root and 15 g of shengjiang (fresh ginger) into mud; stir-fry the mud hot and put it into a cloth bag for medicated ironing at a temperature of 60~70℃; 30 minutes each time, twice per day. ⑥ Umbilical compress therapy: grind into powder baihujiao (white pepper), wuzhuyu (medicinal evodia fruit), wubeizi (gallnut of Chinese sumac), cangzhu (atractylodes rhizome), and dingxiang (clove flower) in a ratio of 1 : 2 : 4 : 2 : 1; blend the powder with shengjiang (fresh ginger) juice to make a medicated cake; place the cake on Shenque (CV 8) and seal it with sterile dressing; every night about ten hours from before going to bed to the next morning.

6. Yin Deficiency and Lung Heat Syndrome

(1) Daily life nursing. The ward should be cool and quiet. The children should rest in bed, ensure adequate sleep and change positions frequently. The older children may take a semi-supine position and infants a low slope position of 20°~30° height. If there is night sweat, it is necessary to promptly wipe out sweat and change the wet clothes and quilts. After the symptoms get improved, the children should gradually increase the amount of exercise but pay attention to avoid wind and overwork.

(2) Diet nursing. The diet should be light, nutritious and digestible. The children may drink frequently the decoction of baihe (lily bulb), xingren (apricot kernel), and nuodaogen (glutinous rice root), take milk, egg, lean meat and fish to enhance body constitution, and eat foods with function of nourishing yin and clearing heat such as loach, lotus root and suanzaoren (spiny date seed). Food

therapy: yin'er xueli (tremella and snow pear) extract. And they should avoid eating fried and baked foods.

(3) Emotion nursing. During the recovery period of the disease, nurses should know well the state of mind of both the children and parents, and may employ verbal enlightenment therapy to encourage them to stay in treatment.

(4) Medication nursing. Decoction should be brewed for long time and taken warm before meals.

(5) Manipulation techniques. ① Infantile tuina therapy: tonifying Pijing (spleen meridian), clearing Feijing (lung meridian), clearing Tianheshui (heaven river water), kneading Erma, pressing and kneading Zusanli (ST 36), pushing Yongquan (KI 1), kneading Feishu (BL 13), and kneading Pishu (BL 20). ② Paste application therapy: grind into powder beishashen (straight ladybell root), chaobaizhu (stir-fried white atractylodes rhizome) and baijiezi (white mustard seed); blend the powder with shengjiang (fresh ginger) juice to make pastes, and apply them on Feishu (BL 13) till the area turns red without blister, about ten minutes each time, once per day, and continuous application for three days. ③ Cupping therapy: select Feishu (BL 13), moist-rale-concentrated place in lung auscultation, or the area below the scapula for cupping, 5~10 minutes each time, once per day; it is suitable for children over three years old with persistent moist rale. ④ Umbilical compress therapy: grind wubeizi (gallnut of Chinese sumac) into powder; blend the powder with vinegar to make a paste, and place it on Shenque (CV 8); every night from before going to bed to the next morning, once per day, and three consecutive times; it is suitable for children with night sweat.

7. Heart Yang Debilitation Syndrome

(1) Daily life nursing. The ward should be warm and quiet. The children should rest in bed with loose, light and warm clothes and quilts, ensure adequate sleep and change positions frequently. The older children may take a semi-supine position and infants a low slope position of $20° \sim 30°$ height. If there is night sweat, it is necessary to promptly wipe out sweat and change the wet clothes and quilts. Nurses should strictly monitor heart rate and record intake and output. Nurses can apply moistened and warmed oxygen inhalation. Before oxygen inhalation, nurses should remove the children's nasal crust, nasal mucus, and clean oral cavity to ensure a clear airway.

(2) Diet nursing. Strictly control water and salt intake. Mild cases can be given a low-salt diet, and severe cases a salt-free diet. In the case of coma, intravenous infusion is recommended. After regaining consciousness, light liquid foods or semi-liquid foods are preferred. For those using diuretics, potassium-rich foods such as bananas, oranges, and green leafy vegetables should be supplemented during medication.

(3) Emotion nursing. When critical illness occurs, the parents have varying degrees of fear and anxiety. Nurses should inform the parents knowledge about disease development as well as use verbal enlightenment therapy to comfort and encourage the parents to maintain emotional stability.

(4) Medication nursing. Decoction should be quickly brewed dense and taken warm frequently. In comatose children, decoction can be administered by nasal feeding. Minimize the amount of intravenous

infusion with slow input speed. If diuretics are used, administration should be offered in the early morning or as much as possible to avoid excessive nighttime urination that affects sleep.

（5）Manipulation techniques. ① Moxibustion therapy: select Baihui (GV20), Qihai (CV 6), Guanyuan (CV 4) and Shenque (CV 8); perform ginger-partitioned moxibustion on each of them. The procedure is to slice shengjiang (fresh ginger) into thin pieces with diameter of 2~3 centimeters and thickness of 0.3 centimeters, pierce several holes through the ginger slice with a sharp needle, and place the ginger slices on the acupoints, 1~3 moxa-cone(s) on every acupoint until the area turns red, and twice every day. ② Auricular pressure therapy: select lung (CO14), trachea (CO16), sympathetic (AH6a) and shenmen (TF4); apply specialized pasters on them, press on each of them till the area turns hot and red, 4~5 times per day, and keep the pasters for 2~4 days.

8. Pathogen Invading Jueyin Meridian Syndrome

（1）Daily life nursing. The ward should be cool and quiet. The children should rest in bed and change positions frequently. The older children may take a semi-supine position and infants a low slope position of 20°~30° height. Nurses should strictly record intake and output, and monitor blood oxygen saturation. Nurses should also observe the change of body temperature, and immediately use physical cooling, such as cold compress on forehead or sponge bath with warm water, when the body temperature is higher than 39℃ in case of convulsions due to high fever. If convulsions occur, the following measures should be adopted for emergency: lie in a supine position, place a soft object under the head to tilt the head to one side in order to keep the respiratory tract open, unfasten the collar and loosen the clothing. And don't press patients forcibly to prevent limb injury.

（2）Diet nursing. In the case of coma, intravenous infusion is recommended. After regaining consciousness, light liquid foods or semi-liquid foods are preferred.

（3）Emotion nursing. When critical illness occurs, the parents have varying degrees of fear and anxiety. Nurses should inform the parents knowledge about disease development as well as use verbal enlightenment therapy to comfort and encourage the parents. Nurses should also care for, comfort and gently touch the children as much as possible to reduce their fear.

（4）Medication nursing. Decoction should be quickly brewed dense and taken warm. In comatose children, decoction can be administered by nasal feeding.

（5）Manipulation techniques. ① Acupressure therapy: select Shuigou (GV 26), Yongquan (KI 1), Shixuan (EX－UE11) and Sifeng (EX－UE10), and forcefully squeeze and nip these acupoints until the children regain consciousness; select Jianjing (GB 21), Weizhong (BL 40) and Chengshan (BL 57), and grasp these acupoints until the convulsion stops; it is suitable for children with high fever and convulsion. ② Paste application therapy: grind into powder dahuang (rhubarb root and rhizome), huanglian (coptis rhizome) and huangqin (scutellaria root) 10 g respectively; blend the powder with hot liquor to make a paste; apply it on the anterior thoracic xiphoid process for about two hours, and renew the paste for severe cases; it is suitable for dyspnea children with high fever. ③ Medicinal suppository therapy: decoct the honey dense and rub it into a small suppository to plug the anus; it is suitable for children with constipation.

Patient Education

Sick children should often change positions. Infants may be held frequently while older children may take a semi-supine position. Nurses should instruct older children how to cough effectively, and assist in resonant sputum discharge by patting the back. If sputum is sticky and difficult to discharge, apply sputum aspiration, but the action should be gentle and fast and the negative pressure should not be too large so as not to damage the oral mucosa.

The diet should be light, nutritious and digestible. More vegetables and fruit rich in fiber should be supplemented to maintain smooth stool. For infants, breastfeeding is preferred. If rapid breathing and flaring nostrils are serious, breastfeeding can be suspended. The mother may continue to breastfeed after the symptoms are relieved. Sick children should avoid pungent, spicy, raw, cold, fatty, too-sweet and dry-natured foods such as chili, cold drinks, fatty meats and cookies. During breastfeeding, the lactating mother should pay the same attention to dietary contraindications.

Doctor's instructions should be followed for medication. Decoction should be quickly brewed dense, taken warm and slowly, multiple times in small portions. Avoid irritable feeding or forced intake with the nose pinched because it may cause agitation, rapid breathing, chocking cough or even suffocation of the children.

The children should actively carry out physical exercise to enhance physical fitness, and keep warm during the cold season or when the weather changes suddenly, go outdoors frequently during winter and spring to bask in the sun in a windless place. It is better for children not to go to public places during an upper respiratory disease epidemic and pay attention to personal hygiene, such as washing hands regularly, and staying away from smoke. If there is cold or cough, prompt treatment should be carried out to prevent it from developing into pneumonia with dyspnea and cough.

第二节 积 滞

积滞，是指因喂养不当，导致乳食内积，或因饮食失节，导致食滞脾胃，以小儿脘腹胀满、疼痛，伴见呕吐、嗳腐、吐酸、腹泻或便秘，久则睡眠不安，磨牙，龋齿，吮指嗜异为临床特征的小儿脾系病。西医的小儿消化功能紊乱、功能性消化不良可参照本节进行护理。

一、病因病机

积滞的病因包括先天禀赋不足、乳食失节、病后失调和用药不当。哺乳过频过急过量，添加辅食过多过快，或饥饱无度，过食肥甘厚腻、生冷坚硬，或久泻久痢后调养失宜，或过用苦寒攻伐之药，均可导致脾胃受损，运化失宜，宿食内停，积而不化，形成积滞。若先天禀赋不足，后天失于调养，则更容易形成积滞。

积滞的病机为乳食停聚中焦，积而不化，气滞不行。病位在脾胃。

二、常见证型

（一）辨证要点

1. 辨虚实 根据体质、病程长短、症状剧烈程度和指纹来辨别。若平素体健，新病，症状剧烈，表现为哭闹不宁，腹胀拒按，大便秘结，舌红苔黄，指纹紫滞，多为实证。若先天禀赋不足，久病，症状不剧烈，表现为神疲肢倦，形体消瘦，腹满喜按，大便溏薄，舌淡苔白，指纹淡滞，多为虚实夹杂。

2. 辨寒热 根据体质、饮食偏好、伴随症状和舌象来辨别。若素体阳盛，喜食肥甘厚味，脘腹胀满，得热胀甚，得凉稍缓，心烦易怒，大便臭秽秘结，腹部灼热，舌红苔黄，多为热证。若素体阳虚，贪食生冷，或过用寒凉药物，脘腹胀满，遇冷胀甚，喜温喜按，面黄唇淡，大便稀溏，舌淡苔白，多为寒证。

（二）证候分型

1. 乳食内积证

[主要证候] 乳食不思或少思，脘腹胀满，疼痛拒按，呕吐食物、乳片；夜寐不安，哭闹不宁，大便酸臭或秘结；舌淡红，苔白厚腻，脉弦滑，指纹紫滞。

[证候分析] 乳食内积中焦，气机郁滞，运化失司，故乳食不思或少思，脘腹胀满，疼痛拒按；气机郁滞，胃气不降反升，故呕吐食物、乳片；食滞不化，腐秽内结，故大便酸臭或秘结；苔白厚腻，脉弦滑，指纹紫滞，均为食积之象。

[护治原则] 消乳化食，导滞和中。

[常用方剂] 乳积者，消乳丸；食积者，保和丸。

2. 食积化热证

［主要证候］不思乳食,口干,脘腹胀满,腹部灼热;午后发热,心烦易怒,夜寐不安,小便黄,大便臭秽或秘结;舌红,苔黄腻,脉滑数,指纹紫。

［证候分析］小儿素体阳盛,或食积日久,郁而化热,灼伤津液,故口干,腹部灼热,午后发热,小便黄,大便臭秽;热扰心神,故心烦易怒,夜寐不安;食积于内,气机壅塞,大肠传导失司,故大便秘结;舌红,苔黄腻,脉滑数,指纹紫,均为食积化热之象。

［护治原则］清热导滞,消积和中。

［常用方剂］枳实导滞丸。

3. 脾虚夹积证

［主要证候］不思乳食,食则饱胀,呕吐酸馊;腹满喜按,喜俯卧,夜寐不安,面色萎黄,形体消瘦,神疲肢倦,大便稀糊或溏,夹食物残渣;唇舌色淡,苔白腻,脉细滑,指纹淡滞。

［证候分析］脾胃虚弱,运化失司,故不思乳食,食则饱胀;脾胃虚弱,故腹满喜按,喜俯卧;胃气不和,故夜寐不安;中焦气机不利,胃气上逆,故呕吐酸馊;脾虚食少,气血生化乏源,故面色萎黄,形体消瘦,神疲肢倦;食滞不化,故大便稀糊或溏,夹食物残渣;舌淡苔白腻,脉细滑,指纹淡滞,均为脾虚夹积之象。

［护治原则］健脾助运,消积化滞。

［常用方剂］健脾丸。

三、护理措施

对于积滞的患儿,应观察呕吐的次数、时间;呕吐物的量、性状;排便的次数;大便的量、性状;腹胀的部位;腹痛的部位、性质、程度。注意观察神色、口唇、舌象、指纹。进行腹部按诊,询问患儿的食欲、食量、喂养方式、饮食行为和体重的变化情况。

（一）辨证施护

1. 乳食内积证

（1）生活起居护理　居室安静温暖,干燥舒适,空气新鲜,阳光充足。多休息,睡眠充足,适当增加户外运动。

（2）饮食护理　宜食消食化积的食物,如炒山楂、炒神曲、炒麦芽。食疗方:莱菔鸡胗粥。可遵医嘱予鸡内金粉:3 岁以下的幼儿,每次 0.3 g;3～5 岁,每次 0.6 g。若呕吐剧烈,应暂停进食,待病情好转后,逐渐恢复正常饮食。

（3）情志护理　保持情绪愉快。在进餐时,不可批评或突然惊吓患儿,避免因情志不舒,肝郁乘脾而加重积滞。

（4）用药护理　中药汤剂宜浓煎,饭后分次热服。丸剂宜用温水溶化后喂服。

（5）操作技术　① 小儿推拿疗法:清天河水,清补脾,平肝;或清胃经,揉板门,运内八卦,推四横纹,按揉中脘、足三里,推下七节骨,分腹阴阳。② 拔罐疗法合敷脐疗法:取神阙、命门,留罐 5～10 分钟;再取神阙,用焦神曲、焦麦芽、焦山楂各 15 g,炒莱菔子 6 g,鸡内金、广木香、川厚朴各 5 g,研磨后取 15 g 药粉和 1 g 淀粉拌匀,与白开水调成糊状,做成药饼,烘热后敷贴在肚脐中;每日 1 次。

③ 膏摩疗法:取中脘、胃俞、脾俞,以消积膏为介质进行推拿;消积膏:青皮、麸炒枳壳、厚朴、砂仁、芒硝、焦三仙、生姜各 10 g,研成细小粉末,在 75% 的医用酒精中浸泡 24 小时,加入适量凡士林,用小火加热,当颜色开始变成微黄时停止加热,过滤药渣,冷却备用。④ 挑治疗法:取四缝;皮肤消毒后揉按局部使其充血,用三棱针的 2 毫米针尖,避开血管,挑破皮肤,挤出 1.0 mL 以下的黏液,用无菌干棉球擦拭或按压。⑤ 耳压疗法:取胃、大肠、神门、脾,用耳穴压丸贴片贴压,每日按揉 4~5 次,以局部发热泛红为度,留置 2~4 日。

2. 食积化热证

(1)生活起居护理　居室安静舒适,空气新鲜,阳光充足。多休息,睡眠充足。适量锻炼,以保持大便通畅。

(2)饮食护理　可饮温白萝卜汁。宜食清热消积的食物,如刺梨、荸荠。若便秘,可饮蜂蜜水。

(3)情志护理　护士可运用移情易性疗法,如看电视、赏花,使患儿保持心情愉快,避免烦躁、焦虑。

(4)用药护理　中药汤剂宜浓煎,饭后分次温服。丸剂宜用温水溶化后喂服。

(5)操作技术　① 小儿推拿疗法:清天河水,清大肠,揉曲池,清胃经,揉板门,运内八卦,推四横纹,按揉中脘、足三里,推下七节骨,分腹阴阳。② 敷贴疗法:取内关,用白术、桃仁、苦杏仁、栀子各 50 g,枳实、砂仁各 10 g,樟脑、冰片适量;研磨后取药粉 2~3 g,与蛋清调成糊状外敷。③ 拔罐疗法:取中脘、脾俞、胃俞,留罐 5~10 分钟,隔日 1 次。④ 敷脐疗法:取神阙,用神曲、麦芽、山楂各 30 g,芒硝 20 g,槟榔、大黄各 10 g,研磨成粉后与芝麻油调成糊状敷贴,每次 2~4 小时;隔日 1 次。

3. 脾虚夹积证

(1)生活起居护理　居室安静舒适,温暖干燥,空气新鲜,阳光充足。衣被宽大轻暖,避免受凉。多休息,睡眠充足。适量运动,不可过劳。保持肛周清洁干燥。若大便次数多,大便稀糊或溏,指导家长在患儿便后用温水清洗肛周,用软毛巾轻轻擦干。

(2)饮食护理　饮食宜清淡、温热、软烂。可饮山楂谷芽饮。宜食健脾消积的食物,如芡实、薏苡仁、陈皮。食疗方:小米山药粥、焦米粥。若发生呕吐,可在舌根滴少许生姜汁。

(3)情志护理　护士可向患儿家长宣教喂养知识,鼓励患儿参加娱乐活动,保持乐观、放松的情绪,愉快进食。对年长儿要讲解饮食营养的重要性。

(4)用药护理　中药汤剂宜温服,少量频服。

(5)操作技术　① 小儿推拿疗法:补脾,平肝,揉一窝风;或补脾经,运内八卦,摩中脘,清补大肠,揉按足三里。② 捏脊疗法:用双手拇指和食指将脊柱处的皮肤捏起,自长强向上捏至大椎,并在肾俞、脾俞各重提 1 下,最后压肾俞 3 下,每次 3~5 遍,每日 1 次。③ 敷贴疗法:取神阙、脾俞、肾俞、涌泉,用肉桂 60 g,丁香、苍术、焦三仙各 30 g,枳壳、玄明粉 10 g,研磨成粉后与芝麻油调成糊状敷贴,每次 1 小时,每日 1 次。④ 敷脐疗法:取神阙,用槟榔 4 g,高良姜 2 g,研磨成粉后与芝麻油调匀敷贴,每次 2~4 小时,每日 1 次;适用于腹胀者。⑤ 热敷疗法:取腹部,用 60~70℃ 的热水袋热敷;或用酒糟 100 g,入锅炒热,分 2 次装袋,交替置于腹部热敷;每次 2~3 小时,每日 1 次;适用于腹部胀痛者。

(二)健康教育

起居有常,睡眠充足。适量运动,以保持大便通畅。注意保暖,不去寒冷、潮湿的地方,谨防受凉。

　　饮食宜清淡、营养、易消化,定时定量,少食多餐。根据患儿的年龄选取细、软、烂的食物。注意饮食卫生。不偏食、挑食、过饥、过饱,忌妄加滋补,不宜食生冷、肥甘、辛辣、煎炸的食物。

　　保持情绪愉快。积滞容易使患儿抑郁、焦虑,应注意观察患儿的情绪变化,及时进行心理疏导。对于食量下降的患儿,应积极寻找原因,不要强迫进食,以免引起逆反心理。乳母的心情也应舒畅。

　　对于呕吐的患儿,应暂停进食,待胃肠功能恢复后,再少量进食。可予生姜汁数滴,滴于舌根,或揉按内关以止呕。注意口腔护理,及时清理呕吐物,每日用淡盐水或银芩汤漱口2~3次。

　　积极向家长宣教喂养知识。小儿对营养物质的需求很大,但其脏腑功能尚未发育完善,加之饮食尚不能自节,所以哺乳应有规律,人工喂养要定时定量。婴幼儿的饮食应是清淡、营养、易消化的流食或半流食。按时添加辅食,3月龄加菜汁、果汁,4~6月龄加菜泥、果泥、肉汤、米汤、稀粥,每次1种;若小儿大便正常,再给第2种,逐渐加量加稠。

Section 2　Food Accumulation

Food accumulation is a gastrointestinal disorder caused by improper feeding and internal accumulation of milk or food, or improper diet and food retention in the spleen and stomach. It is featured by abdominal and epigastric distension, fullness and pain, accompanied with vomiting, sour belching, acid regurgitation, diarrhea or constipation. If it lasts long, it may also go with restlessness in sleeping, teeth grinding, finger sucking and parorexia. This section can be referred to for the nursing of digestive disorders and functional dyspepsia in children in Western medicine.

ETIOLOGY AND PATHOGENESIS

The etiology includes poor constitution, inappropriate diet of milk or foods, inadequate care after an illness, and inappropriate medication. Specifically speaking, all the following factors may damage the spleen and stomach, and cause impaired transportation and transformation as well as food retention and accumulation. They include but are not limited to frequent, urgent or excessive breastfeeding, excessive or too early addition of complementary foods, excessive hunger or satiety, over-ingestion of sweet, rich, greasy, raw, cold or hard foods, inadequate care after chronic diarrhea or dysentery, overdose of bitter-cold medicines, etc. Infants with insufficient congenital endowment or inadequate acquired care are easier to suffer from food accumulation.

The pathogenesis is retention and accumulation of milk or foods in the middle energizer. And the location of disease is in the spleen and stomach.

COMMON SYNDROMES

Key Points in Syndrome Differentiation

1. Differentiation of Deficiency from Excess Syndrome

The differentiation is based on body constitution, course of disease, severity of symptoms, and finger venules. Excess syndrome may present robust constitution in normal times, new disease, severe symptoms, such as persistent crying, unpalpable abdominal distension, constipation, red tongue with yellow coating, and purple stagnant finger venules. However, deficiency-excess in complexity syndrome may show insufficient congenital endowment, prolonged illness, mild symptoms, such as mental and physical fatigue, emaciation, abdominal fullness with preference for pressure, loose stool, pale tongue with white coating, and light stagnant finger venules.

2. Differentiation of Cold from Heat Syndrome

The differentiation is based on the constitution, dietary preference, accompanying symptoms, and tongue and pulse manifestations. Yang exuberance constitution, predilection for sweet, rich and greasy foods, abdominal and epigastric distension and fullness that aggravates with heat and alleviates with cool, heart vexation and irritability, constipation with foul smell, abdominal burning sensation, red tongue with yellow coating, all belong to heat syndrome. Yang deficiency constitution, predilection for raw or cold foods, overdose of bitter-cold medicines, abdominal and epigastric distension and fullness that aggravates with cold and alleviates with heat, preference for warmth and pressure, yellow complexion and pale lips, loose stool, pale tongue with white coating, all indicate cold syndrome.

Syndrome Differentiation

1. Syndrome of Internal Accumulation of Milk or Foods

［Clinical Manifestations］Poor or reduced appetite, abdominal and epigastric distension and fullness, unpalpable pain, vomitus of milk or foods, restless sleep, persistent crying, stool of sour and foul odor or constipation, light red tongue with white dirty and slimy coating, wiry slippery pulse, and purple stagnant finger venules.

［Manifestations Analysis］Internal accumulation of milk or foods causes depression and stagnation of qi movement and dysfunction of transportation and transformation, causing poor or reduced appetite, abdominal and epigastric distension and fullness, and unpalpable pain. Depression and stagnation of qi movement and adverse rising of stomach qi are responsible for vomitus of milk or foods. Internal retention of food and staleness in the middle energizer explains stool of sour and foul odor or constipation. White dirty and slimy tongue coating, wiry slippery pulse, and purple stagnant finger venules are signs of food accumulation.

［Nursing Principle］Promoting digestion, removing food stagnation and harmonizing the middle.

［Suggested Formula］Xiaoru Pills for milk accumulation, and Baohe Pills for food accumulation.

2. Syndrome of Food Accumulation Transforming into Heat

［Clinical Manifestations］Poor appetite, dry mouth, abdominal and epigastric distension and fullness, abdominal burning sensation, afternoon fever, heart vexation and irritability, restless sleep, dark urine, stool of foul odor or constipation, red tongue with yellow slimy coating, slippery rapid pulse, and purple finger venules.

［Manifestations Analysis］Yang exuberance constitution, or long-time depression of food accumulation that transforms into heat and scorches body fluids, resulting in dry mouth, abdominal burning sensation, afternoon fever, dark urine, and stool of foul odor. Heat harasses heart spirit, so heart vexation and irritability, and restless sleep are felt. Internal accumulation of foods and congestion of qi movement make the large intestine fail to govern conveyance, therefore, constipation happens. Red tongue with yellow slimy coating, slippery rapid pulse, and purple finger venules signify food accumulation transforming into heat.

［Nursing Principle］Clearing heat and removing food stagnation; resolving accumulation and harmonizing the middle.

［Suggested Formula］Zhishi Daozhi Pills.

3. Syndrome of Spleen Deficiency with Food Accumulation

［Clinical Manifestations］Poor appetite, immediate abdominal fullness after intake of milk or foods, vomitus of sour smell, abdominal fullness with preference for pressure, fond of prone position, restless sleep, sallow complexion, emaciation, mental and physical fatigue, thin-paste-like or loose stool with food residue, pale tongue and lips, white slimy coating, thready slippery pulse, and light stagnant finger venules.

［Manifestations Analysis］Spleen and stomach deficiency causes dysfunction of transportation and transformation, so the patients have poor appetite, immediate abdominal fullness after intake of milk or foods and abdominal fullness with preference for pressure, and is fond of prone position. Stomach disharmony leads to restless sleep. Inhibition of qi movement in the middle energizer and adverse rising of stomach qi is the reason for vomitus of sour smell. Spleen deficiency with reduced appetite cannot ensure the enough origin of qi and blood, leading to symptoms such as sallow complexion, emaciation, and mental and physical fatigue. Food accumulation is not transported and transformed timely, so there appears thin-paste-like or loose stool with food residue. Pale tongue with white slimy coating, thready slippery pulse, and light stagnant finger venules manifest spleen deficiency with food accumulation.

［Nursing Principle］Invigorating the spleen and assisting food transportation; resolving accumulation and removing food stagnation.

［Suggested Formula］Jianpi Pills.

NURSING MEASURES

For patients with food accumulation, nurses should observe the frequency and time of vomiting; the quantity, shape and properties of vomitus; the frequency of defecation; the quantity, shape and properties of the stool; the place of abdominal distension and pain; the nature and degree of pain; the changes in spirit, complexion, lips, tongue manifestation and finger venules. The abdomen must be carefully palpated. Moreover, nurses should enquire about the children's appetite, food intake, feeding mode, dining behavior and body weight changes.

Syndrome-Based Nursing Measures

1. Syndrome of Internal Accumulation of Milk or Foods

（1）Daily life nursing. The ward should be quiet, warm, dry, comfortable and full of fresh air, with sufficient sunshine. The sick children should have proper rest and sufficient sleep and moderately increase outdoor activity.

（2）Diet nursing. The children may eat foods that promote digestion and resolve accumulation, such as chaoshanzha（stir-fried Chinese hawthorn fruit）, chaoshenqu（stir-fried medicated leaven）and chaomaiya（stir-fried germinated barley）. Food therapy: laifu jizhen（radish seed and chicken gizzard） porridge. Patients could take ji'neijin (chicken gizzard lining) powder as prescribed: for infants under three years old, 0.3 g every time; for infants of 3 ~ 5 years old, 0.6 g every time. If the vomiting is severe, the patients should stop eating. When the condition improves, the diet should be normalized gradually.

(3) Emotion nursing. The afflicted children should stay in a cheerful state of mind. During mealtime, scolding or fright should be avoided to prevent emotional disorder as well as liver depression overwhelming the spleen that result in aggravation of food accumulation.

(4) Medication nursing. Decoction should be brewed thick and taken warm after meals. Pills should melt with warm water before taken.

(5) Manipulation techniques. ① Infantile tuina therapy: clearing Tianheshui (heaven river water), clearing and tonifying Pijing (spleen meridian), pacifying Ganjing (liver meridian); or clearing Weijing (stomach meridian), kneading Banmen (major thenar), circularly pushing Neibagua, pushing Sihengwen (four transverse ceases), pressing and kneading Zhongwan (CV 12) and Zusanli (ST 36), pushing Qijiegu (seven lumbrosacral vertebrae) from top to bottom, separately pushing abdominal yin and yang. ② Cupping therapy plus umbilical compress therapy: first, select Shenque (CV 8) and Mingmen (GV 4) for cupping therapy and retain the cup on them for 5 ~ 10 minutes; second, grind into powder the following ingredients, blend 15 g of the powder with boiled water and 1 g of starch to make a paste, heat the paste and apply it on the navel, once every day. The ingredients are jiaoshenqu (scorch-fried medicated leaven) 15 g, jiaomaiya (scorch-fried germinated barley) 15 g, jiaoshanzha (scorch-fried Chinese hawthorn fruit) 15 g, chaolaifuzi (stir-fried radish seed) 6 g, ji'neijin (chicken gizzard lining) 5 g, guangmuxiang (saussurae root) 5 g, and houpo (magnolia bark) 5 g. ③ Therapy of massage with ointment: select Zhongwan (CV 12), Weishu (BL 21) and Pishu (BL 20); apply massage manipulation with the medium of Xiaoji Ointment. The ingredients of Xiaoji Ointment are qingpi (green tangerine peel), chaozhiqiao (bitter orange stir-fried with bran), houpo (magnolia bark), sharen (villous amomum fruit), mangxiao (sodium sulphate), jiaoshenqu (scorch-fried medicated leaven), jiaomaiya (scorch-fried germinated barley), jiaoshanzha (scorch-fried Chinese hawthorn fruit), and shengjiang (fresh ginger) respectively 10 g. Grind the above ingredients into fine powder, soak it in 75% medical alcohol for 24 hours, add in appropriate amount of vaseline, heat it with low fire, and stop heating when it begins to turn yellowish, then filter the residue and cool it for later use. ④ Fibrous tissue-pricking therapy: select Sifeng (EX - UE10); after the skin is disinfected, rub the local area to make it hyperemic. Use a three-edged needle to quickly pierce the skin away from blood vessels at a depth of 2 millimeters, remove the needle and squeeze the skin to release mucus less than 1.0 mL. Wipe or press the pierced point with a sterile dry cotton ball. ⑤ Auricular pressure therapy: select stomach (CO4), large intestine (CO7), shenmen (TF4), and spleen (CO13); apply specialized pasters on them, press on each of them till the area turns hot and red, 4 ~ 5 times per day, and keep the pasters for 2 ~ 4 days.

2. Syndrome of Food Accumulation Transforming into Heat

(1) Daily life nursing. The ward should be quiet, comfortable and full of fresh air, with sufficient sunshine. The afflicted children should have proper rest and sufficient sleep. And they should do adequate exercise to maintain a normal bowel movement.

(2) Diet nursing. The children may drink warm white radish juice and eat foods that clear heat and resolve accumulation, such as cili (rosa roxburghii) and biqi (waternut). For patients with constipation, honey water could relieve the symptom.

(3) Emotion nursing. Nurses may use emotional transference and dispositional change therapy, such as watching TV, enjoying flowers, to keep the afflicted children stay in a cheerful state of mind and avoid dysphoria and anxiety.

(4) Medication nursing. Decoction should be brewed thick and taken warm after meals. Pills should melt with warm water before taken.

(5) Manipulation techniques. ① Infantile tuina therapy: clearing Tianheshui (heaven river water), clearing Dachang (large intestine), kneading Quchi (LI 11), Weijing (stomach meridian), kneading Banmen (major thenar), circularly pushing Neibagua, pushing Sihengwen (four transverse ceases), pressing and kneading Zhongwan (CV 12) and Zusanli (ST 36), pushing Qijiegu (seven lumbrosacral vertebrae) from top to bottom, separately pushing abdominal yin and yang. ② Paste application therapy: grind into powder baizhu (white atractylodes rhizome), taoren (peach kernel), kuxingren (bitter apricot kernel) and zhizi (gardenia) 50 g respectively, zhishi (immature bitter orange) and sharen (villous amomum fruit) 10 g respectively, and appropriate amounts of zhangnao (camphor) and bingpian (borneol); whisk 2~3 g of the powder with egg white to make pastes, and apply the pastes on the acupoints. ③ Cupping therapy: select Zhongwan (CV 12), Pishu (BL 20) and Weishu (BL 21); retain the cup on them for 10~15 minutes, once every other day. ④ Umbilical compress therapy: select Shenque (CV 8); prepare the following medicinals: shenqu (medicated leaven), maiya (germinated barley), and shanzha (Chinese hawthorn fruit) 30 g respectively, binglang (betel nut) and dahuang (rhubarb root and rhizome) 10 g respectively, and mangxiao (sodium sulphate) 20 g; grind into powder the above medicinals, whisk it with sesame oil to make a paste, and apply the paste on the acupoint, 2~4 hours each time, once every other day.

3. Syndrome of Speen Deficiency with Food Accumulation

(1) Daily life nursing. The ward should be quiet, warm, dry, comfortable, and full of fresh air, with sufficient sunshine. The afflicted children should wear loose, light and warm clothes. They should have proper rest, sufficient sleep and moderate exercise. They should also be protected from catching cold or getting overstrained. The perianal region should be kept dry and clean. Nurses should inform the parents of the patients to wash their perianal region with warm water and wipe it dry with soft towels if the patients defecate frequently with pasty or loose stool.

(2) Diet nursing. The diet should be light, warm, tender and thoroughly cooked. The children may drink shanzha guya (Chinese hawthorn fruit and grain sprout) decoction and eat foods that invigorate the

spleen and resolve accumulation, such as qianshi (euryale seed), yiyiren (coix seed), and chenpi (aged tangerine peel). Food therapy: xiaomi shanyao (millet and common yam rhizome) porridge and scorch-fried-rice porridge. Children with vomiting could have a few drops of shengjiang (fresh ginger) juice on the root of the tongue.

(3) Emotion nursing. Nurses should inform the parents of the patients about proper feeding, encourage the children to engage in recreational activities, stay optimistic and relaxed, and enjoy dining. For elder children, the importance of food nutrition should be explained.

(4) Medication nursing. Decoction should be taken warm, multiple times in small portions.

(5) Manipulation techniques. ① Infantile tuina therapy: tonifying Pijing (spleen meridian), pacifying Ganjing (liver meridian), kneading Yiwofeng (a cave of wind); or tonifying Pijing (spleen meridian), circularly pushing Neibagua, circularly rubbing Zhongwan (CV 12), clearing and tonifying Dachang (large intestine), pressing and kneading Zusanli (ST 36). ② Spine pinching therapy: use thumbs and forefingers to pinch the skin along the spine, from Changqiang (GV 1) upward to Dazhui (GV 14); during the process, forcefully pinch Shenshu (BL 23) and Pishu (BL 20) once respectively; finally press Shenshu (BL 23) three times. Perform three to five successive sessions of pinching every day. ③ Paste application therapy: select Shenque (CV 8), Pishu (BL 20), Shenshu (BL 23), and Yongquan (KI 1); grind into powder rougui (cinnamon bark) 60 g, dingxiang (clove flower), cangzhu (atractylodes rhizome) and jiaosanxian (scorch-fried Chinese hawthorn fruit, germinated barley and medicated leaven) 30 g respectively, zhiqiao (bitter orange) and xuanmingfen (exsiccated sodium sulphate) 10 g respectively; whisk the powder with sesame oil to make pastes, and apply the pastes on the acupoints, one hour each time, once every day. ④ Umbilical compress therapy: select Shenque (CV 8); grind into powder binglang (betel nut) 4 g and gaoliangjiang (galangal) 2 g; whisk it with sesame oil into a paste, then apply it on the navel; 2 ~ 4 hours each time, once per day; it is effective for patients with abdominal distension. ⑤ Hot compress therapy: put the hot-water bag on the abdomen for hot compress at a temperature of 60 ~ 70℃; or stir-fry hot 100 g of distillers' grains, divide it into two equal portions and put them in bags, then apply them on the abdomen alternately; 2 ~ 3 hours each time, once per day. This therapy is suitable for patients with abdominal distending pain.

Patient Education

The patients should follow a regular daily routine and ensure adequate sleep. The patients should also take part in moderate physical activities to maintain a normal bowel movement. Besides, the children should keep warm and avoid damp cold places to prevent catching cold.

The diet should be light, nutritious and digestible. The patients should follow a regular dietary schedule and amount as well as have small frequent meals. Fine, tender or thoroughly cooked foods are offered according to the children's age. Great attention should be paid to food hygiene and safety. The children should not be too hungry, too full, or faddy about food. Extra tonics should be avoided, so are foods that are raw, cold, too-sweet, greasy, rich, pungent, spicy and fried.

The patients should stay in a pleasant state of mind. Children with food accumulation are prone to depression and anxiety. Nurses should pay attention to mood changes in the patients and provide timely psychological counseling. For children with decreased food intake, causes should be pinpointed and force-feeding should be avoided to trigger rebellion. Nursing mothers should also keep a pleasant state of mind.

For patients with vomiting, feeding should temporarily stop until gastrointestinal functions are restored. Only then could the children consume small portions of food. Children could have a few drops of shengjiang (fresh ginger) juice on the root of the tongue or Neiguan (PC 6) kneaded to stop vomiting. Children should be monitored to maintain oral hygiene, have their vomitus cleaned, use lightly salted water or Yinqin Decoction to rinse the mouth two to three times every day.

Nurses should actively inform the patients' parents of the proper feeding. Children have a great demand for nutrients but without fully developed visceral functions or self-restraint in diet. Therefore, mothers should follow a regular schedule of breastfeeding, and a regular timetable and food amount should also be followed for artificial feeding. Infants should have light, nutritious, digestible liquid or semi-liquid diet. Moreover, supplementary food should be added on time. For instance, vegetable juice and fruit juice could be added for three-month-olds; vegetable puree, fruit puree, broth, rice soup, and thin porridge could be added one kind at a time for babies four to six months old; on this basis if the stool is normal, another kind of supplementary food could be added, with gradually increasing amount and thickness.

第三节　水　　痘

水痘,是指因外感时邪风毒,内蕴湿热,发于肤表而引起的,以发热,咳嗽,皮肤分批出现皮疹,斑丘疹、疱疹、结痂同时并见为临床特征,多见于小儿的出疹性温疫病。西医的水痘可参照本节进行护理。

一、病因病机

水痘的病因多为外感时邪病毒、内蕴湿热。时行邪毒由口鼻而入,蕴郁于肺胃(脾),与内湿相搏,外透于肌表,发为水痘。邪毒尚轻,病在肺卫,肺失宣发,卫表不和,故发热,咳嗽,流涕。邪毒入里,郁于肺脾,肺失通调,脾失健运,水湿内停,正气抗邪外出,时邪夹湿透于肌表,则疱疹稀疏,疹色红润,疱浆清亮,全身症状较轻。若小儿素体虚弱,加之感邪较重,邪毒炽盛,内传气营,气营内燔,发于肌表,则见水痘分布稠密,疹色紫暗,疱浆混浊,全身症状较重。若正气极衰,邪毒内陷,则会出现昏迷,抽搐等邪陷心肝之证,或高热、咳嗽、气喘、鼻翕、口唇青紫等邪毒闭肺之证。

水痘的病机为水痘时毒郁于肺胃(脾),与内湿相搏,外泄肌肤。病位在肺、脾,少数重病患儿可累及心、肝。

二、常见证型

(一) 辨证要点

辨轻重　根据水痘的数量、大小、颜色、疱浆、根脚和全身症状来辨别。若轻度发热,痘疹形小稀疏,颜色红润,疱浆清亮,根脚红晕不明显,无其他兼症,多为轻证。若壮热不解,痘疹形大稠密,颜色紫暗,疱浆混浊,根脚红晕明显,或有兼证,多为重证。

(二) 证候分型

1. 常证

(1) 邪伤肺卫证

[主要证候] 全身性皮疹,向心性分布,躯干为多,点粒稀疏,疱疹形小,疹色红润,根盘红晕不显,疱浆清亮,此起彼伏,瘙痒感;伴发热,多为低热,恶风或恶寒,头痛,鼻塞,流涕,喷嚏,咳嗽,纳差;舌质红,苔薄白或薄黄,脉浮数,指纹浮紫。

[证候分析] 邪郁肺卫,肺失宣发,卫表不和,故发热,恶风或恶寒,鼻塞,流涕,喷嚏,咳嗽;邪毒入里,郁于肺脾,肺失通调,脾失健运,水湿内停,正气抗邪外出,时邪夹湿透于肌表,故疱疹布露;邪轻病浅,尚在卫分,故点粒稀疏,疱疹形小,疹色红润,根盘红晕不显,疱浆清亮;舌质红,苔薄白或薄黄,脉浮数,指纹浮紫,均为邪伤肺卫之象。

［护治原则］疏风清热,利湿解毒。

［常用方剂］银翘散合六一散。

（2）邪炽气营证

［主要证候］全身性皮疹分布范围较广,疹点密布,根盘红晕较明显,疱疹形大,疹色红赤或紫暗,疱浆混浊,出血性皮疹,口腔、睑结膜、会阴部可见疱疹;壮热,烦躁,口渴欲饮,面赤唇红,目赤,口舌生疮,牙龈肿痛,纳差,大便干结,小便短赤;舌质红绛,苔黄糙而干或苔黄腻,脉滑数,指纹紫滞。

［证候分析］邪炽气分,气分热盛,故壮热,烦躁,口渴欲饮,面赤唇红;毒传营分,营分热炽,与内湿相搏外透肌表,故疹点密布,根盘红晕较明显,疱疹形大,疹色红赤或紫暗,疱浆混浊;邪热上熏于面,故面赤唇红,目赤,口舌生疮,牙龈肿痛;热盛津伤,故大便干结,小便短赤;舌质红绛,苔黄糙而干或苔黄腻,脉滑数,指纹紫滞,均为邪炽气营之象。

［护治原则］清气凉营,解毒化湿。

［常用方剂］清瘟败毒饮。

2. 变证

（1）邪陷心肝证

［主要证候］发热,常壮热持续,头痛,呕吐,甚或喷射性呕吐,烦躁不安或狂躁,神识不清,谵语,嗜睡,或昏愦不语,口噤,项强,四肢抽搐,角弓反张;痘疹密布,无规律分布,疹色紫暗,疱浆混浊,根盘较硬;舌质红绛,苔黄燥或黄厚,脉弦数,指纹紫滞。

［证候分析］小儿正气极衰,邪毒内陷心肝,故发热,常壮热持续,头痛,呕吐,甚或喷射性呕吐,烦躁不安或狂躁,神识不清,谵语,嗜睡,或昏愦不语;小儿肝常有余,邪毒炽盛化火,引发肝风内动,故口噤,项强,四肢抽搐,角弓反张;痘疹密布,无规律分布,疹色紫暗,疱浆混浊,根盘较硬,舌质红绛,苔黄燥或黄厚,脉弦数,指纹紫滞,均为热毒内盛之象。

［护治原则］镇惊熄风,清热解毒。

［常用方剂］清瘟败毒饮合羚角钩藤汤。

（2）邪毒闭肺证

［主要证候］发热,常高热不退,咳嗽频作,喉间痰鸣,气急喘促,鼻翕,胸高胁满,张口抬肩,口唇紫绀;痘疹密布,无规律分布,疹色紫暗,疱浆混浊,根盘较硬;舌质红或红绛,苔黄或黄腻,脉滑数或洪数,指纹紫滞。

［证候分析］邪毒内闭,肺气失宣,故咳嗽频作,气急喘促,鼻翕,胸高胁满,张口抬肩;热毒内陷,炼津成痰,故发热,常高热不退,喉间痰鸣;邪毒与内湿相搏外透肌表,故痘疹密布,无规律分布,疹色紫暗,疱浆混浊,根盘较硬;舌质红或红绛,苔黄或黄腻,脉滑数或洪数,指纹紫滞,均为邪毒内闭,湿热熏蒸之象。

［护治原则］清热解毒,开肺定喘。

［常用方剂］麻杏石甘汤合黄连解毒汤。

三、护理措施

对于水痘的患儿,应观察疱疹的出现时间、部位、色泽、形态、疏密程度,以及疱液是否清亮。对于持续高热的患儿,应密切观察神志、体温、呼吸。若体温持续在 39.5℃ 以上,并出现神昏、烦躁、气急、鼻翼翕动、呼吸困难,甚至惊厥,考虑为变证,应立即报告医生。

（一）辨证施护

1. 邪伤肺卫证

（1）生活起居护理　居室凉爽安静,空气新鲜。被褥松软轻薄,衣服宽大、棉质、松软。卧床休息,睡眠充足。保持身体微汗,以利透疹,及时换掉汗湿的衣被。若体温低于 38.5℃,则不必进行降温处理。注意避风。

（2）饮食护理　以流食或半流食为宜,如白萝卜泥。多饮水,可频频喂服黄花菜马齿苋饮、菊花茶、荸荠汁、甘蔗汁;或用金银花 15 g,生甘草 5 g,煎水代茶饮。宜食疏风清热的食物,如薄荷、薏苡仁、绿豆芽。遵医嘱使用食疗方:牛蒡粥。

（3）情志护理　对于皮肤瘙痒的患儿,护士应安慰患儿,耐心解释不搔抓皮肤的重要性。若患儿因皮肤瘙痒而吵闹不休,可运用讲故事、听音乐、看动画等移情易性疗法,转移其注意力。

（4）用药护理　中药汤剂不宜久煎,应饭后温服。服后加盖衣被,使其微微汗出。

（5）操作技术　① 沐浴疗法:用蒲公英、黄柏、千里光、野菊花、生地、玄参、苦参、白矾,煎煮后兑水浸洗皮损处,药液温度 38~40℃,每次 20 分钟左右,每日 1~2 次,适用于痘疹初起无皮肤破溃者;或用苦参、芒硝各 30 g,浮萍 15 g,煎水外洗,每日 2 次,适用于皮疹稠密,瘙痒明显者。② 敷贴疗法:用青黛粉、滑石粉,与芝麻油调成糊状,敷于患处,厚度以完全覆盖疱疹为宜;适用于水痘中后期,斑丘疹已演变成疱疹,且无疱疹破溃及皮肤感染者。③ 涂药法:用炉甘石洗剂涂擦;适用于皮肤瘙痒剧烈处。④ 小儿推拿疗法:开天门,推坎宫,运太阳,揉耳后高骨,掐揉二扇门,清天河水,退六腑,清肺经,清、补脾经,水底捞明月,分手阴阳,掐十宣,拿风池。

2. 邪炽气营证

（1）生活起居护理　居室凉爽安静,空气新鲜。被褥松软轻薄,衣服宽大、棉质、松软。卧床休息,睡眠充足。若体温高于 39.5℃,可予温水擦浴,不可使用冷敷法。注意口腔清洁,进食前后用金银花甘草水含漱,以防发生口腔溃疡。

（2）饮食护理　以流食或半流食为宜。多饮水,可饮西瓜汁、鲜芦根茶。宜食清热利湿的食物,如荸荠、绿豆。食疗方:荸荠酒酿、薏苡仁粥。若大便干结,可食蜂蜜水、香蕉。

（3）情志护理　护士应耐心细致,多与患儿沟通,鼓励患儿及家长积极配合治疗,帮助患儿及家长正确认识水痘,说明只要积极治疗,痘疹不会留下瘢痕。

（4）用药护理　中药汤剂宜饭后温服。中病即止,以免损伤脾胃。

（5）操作技术　① 涂药法:若眼结膜溃疡,用生理盐水清洗,涂金霉素眼膏;若口腔溃疡,用生理盐水清洗,用冰硼散涂在创面上,每日 3~4 次。② 沐浴疗法:用蒲公英、黄芩、益母草、苦参各 20 g,黄连、黄柏各 10 g,每日 1 剂,煎水,每日外洗 2 次。③ 敷贴疗法:用煅石膏、滑石各 50 g,青黛 30 g,黄柏 15 g,冰片、黄连各 10 g;研磨成粉后与芝麻油调匀,搽于患处;适用于水痘疱浆浑浊或疱疹破溃者。

3. 邪陷心肝证

（1）生活起居护理　病室安静凉爽,光线昏暗,空气新鲜。衣被宜薄。卧床休息。注意观察体温变化,若患儿的体温高于 39.5℃,可予温水擦浴。警惕高热惊厥的发生。若发生抽搐,平卧,头后垫以柔软的物品,头偏向一侧,保持呼吸道通畅,解开衣领,松解衣物,不可强行按压,以免肢体受伤。

(2) 饮食护理　宜鼻饲清热开窍的流食,如马齿苋。可用鲜芦根 60 g,菊花 10 g,水煎鼻饲。

(3) 情志护理　护士应注意患儿家长的情绪,及时安慰和鼓励患儿家长,保持其情绪稳定,避免恐惧、焦虑。

(4) 用药护理　中药汤剂宜微温鼻饲。中药丸剂宜用温水溶化后鼻饲。

(5) 操作技术　① 敷贴疗法:用青黛散,与芝麻油调匀;或用煅石膏、滑石各 50 g,青黛 30 g,黄柏 15 g,冰片、黄连各 10 g,研磨成粉后与芝麻油调匀;敷贴于皮疹处,每日 1~2 次;适用于疱疹破溃化脓者。② 吹药疗法:用锡类散、冰硼散或珠黄散,吹向口内破溃处,每日 2~3 次;适用于口腔黏膜的水疱破溃处。③ 刺血疗法:取大椎、天柱、曲池或合谷,皮肤消毒后揉按局部使其充血,用三棱针的 3 毫米针尖,快速刺入并出针,放出 1.0 mL 以下的血液,用无菌干棉球擦拭或按压;适用于高热的患儿。④ 点穴疗法:掐人中,按合谷、太冲;适用于高热惊厥时。

4. 邪毒闭肺证

(1) 生活起居护理　病室安静凉爽,光线昏暗,空气新鲜。衣被宜薄。若患儿的体温高于 39.5℃,可予温水擦浴。

(2) 饮食护理　宜鼻饲清热化痰的流食,如杏仁、鱼腥草、枇杷、雪梨。可用荸荠、竹叶心、鲜芦根各 30~60 g,水煎鼻饲。

(3) 情志护理　患儿发病时,患儿及家长均存在不同程度的恐惧和焦虑。患儿容易在采取隔离措施后情绪低落,孤独感增强,护理人员可运用情志相胜疗法、移情易性疗法,安慰和鼓励患儿,使其保持情绪稳定。

(4) 用药护理　中药汤剂宜微温鼻饲。中药丸剂宜用温水溶化后鼻饲。

(5) 操作技术　① 刺血疗法:取少商或耳尖,皮肤消毒后揉按局部使其充血,用三棱针的 3 毫米针尖,快速刺入并出针,放出 1.0 mL 以下的血液,用无菌干棉球擦拭或按压;适用于高热的患儿。② 小儿推拿疗法:开天门,推坎宫,清肺经,清天河水,揉曲池、大椎、合谷;适用于高热的患儿。③ 湿敷疗法:用黄连膏、如意金黄散调敷于疱疹局部;适用于皮疹破溃、感染者。

(二) 健康教育

居室空气新鲜,避免强风、对流风。患儿发热及出疹期间,应卧床休息,避免劳累。保持皮肤清洁干燥。勤换内衣,内衣要柔软。若水痘较重,暂时不要洗澡或擦洗。修剪患儿的指甲,避免抓破皮肤引起感染,婴幼儿的手部可用纱布包裹。

饮食宜清淡、营养、易消化,少食多餐。多饮水,多吃新鲜的水果和蔬菜。对于体质虚弱的患儿,当病情好转以后,应加强营养,增强体质。忌食生姜、辣椒,不宜食燥热、油腻的食物。

向患儿家长宣教水痘的传播途径及预防、消毒、隔离和护理方法。对婴幼儿要耐心哄抱,细心照顾生活起居。向年长患儿介绍医院环境及医护人员,讲解疾病的发展过程及治疗措施。夜间加强巡视,留地灯,避免患儿因黑暗而感到恐惧。

水痘的皮疹特点为:皮肤分批出现皮疹,斑丘疹、疱疹、结痂同时并见,每批历时 1~6 天;皮疹呈向心性分布,首发于躯干,后发展至脸、肩、四肢。待全部结痂后,可轻轻用温水擦洗。当痂盖脱落不完全时,应等待其自行脱落,不可强行撕扯。必要时,可用无菌剪刀剪掉痂盖,涂上石蜡油。

水痘的传染源为水痘患儿,经飞沫和直接接触传播。水痘从出疹前1天到疱疹全部结痂期间,均有很强的传染性,所以发病后应采取呼吸道隔离。在接触患儿时,必须衣帽整齐,戴口罩。护理后,护士必须进行手部消毒。要经常对被水痘患儿污染的被服、用具进行消毒。室内应每日进行空气消毒、物表及物品消毒。

Section 3　Chickenpox

Chickenpox is an epidemic eruptive disease clinically characterized by fever, cough, skin rashes in batches, and coexistence of maculopapules, herpes and scabs. It is more common in children and caused by external contraction of seasonal pathogenic wind-toxin and internal accumulation of dampness-heat that occur on the skin surface. This section can be referred to for the nursing of chickenpox in Western medicine.

ETIOLOGY AND PATHOGENESIS

The etiology includes external contraction of seasonal epidemic toxin and internal accumulation of dampness-heat. The seasonal epidemic toxin that enters the body from the mouth and nose accumulates in the lung and stomach (spleen), contends with internal dampness, and outthrusts to the muscles and skin, then chickenpox occurs. Pathogenic toxin still in defense aspect with mild disease condition causes failure of the lung to disperse and descend as well as disharmony of defensive exterior, thus fever, cough and running nose occur. Internal entrance of pathogenic toxin and its accumulation in the lung and spleen leads to failure of the lung to dredge and regulate water passage as well as failure of the spleen to transport and transform, which causes internal stoppage of water and dampness. The healthy qi drives out pathogenic qi, and epidemic pathogen with dampness outthrusts to the muscles and skin, thus sparse rashes and herpes with ruddy color and lucid blister liquid occur, and systemic symptoms are relatively mild. Infantile constitutional weakness and severe contraction of intense epidemic toxin that enters qi and nutrient aspects causes blazing of both qi and nutrient aspects and outthrusts to muscles and skin, then dense chickenpox with dark purple color and turbid blister liquid occur, and systemic symptoms are severe. Extreme weakness of infants' healthy qi and inward sinking of pathogenic toxin may cause deteriorated syndromes such as syndrome of pathogen invading the heart and liver with symptoms such as coma, convulsion, or syndrome of pathogenic toxin blocking the lung with symptoms such as high fever, cough, panting, flapping of nasal wings and cyanotic mouth and lips.

The pathogenesis is contraction of seasonal epidemic toxin (varicella virus) that accumulates in the lung and stomach (spleen), contends with internal dampness and outthrusts to the muscles and skin. The location of diseases is in the lung and spleen but for some critical cases it may involve the heart and liver.

COMMON SYNDROMES

Key Points in Syndrome Differentiation

Differentiation of Severity of the Disease

The differentiation is based on the quantity, size, color, base, blister liquid, and systemic symptoms of chickenpox. Mild syndrome shows mild fever, small sparse rashes and herpes with ruddy color, lucid blister liquid, inapparent areolae around the base and without other concurrent symptoms. However, severe syndrome displays high fever without abatement, big dense rashes and herpes with dark purple color, turbid blister liquid, apparent areolae around the base and with other concurrent symptoms.

Syndrome Differentiation

1. Common Syndromes

(1) Syndrome of Pathogen Invading the Lung-Defense

[Clinical Manifestations] Spare generalized and centripetally-distributed skin rashes, with more rashes on the trunk, small herpes with ruddy color, inapparent areolae around the base, lucid blister liquid, itching skin, accompanied by fever (mostly low fever), aversion to wind or cold, headache, nasal congestion, running nose, sneezing, cough, poor appetite, red tongue with thin white coating or thin yellow coating, floating rapid pulse, and floating purple finger venules.

[Manifestations Analysis] Pathogen depression in lung-defense leads to failure of the lung to disperse and descend as well as disharmony of defensive exterior, thus there are fever, aversion to wind or cold, nasal congestion, running nose, sneezing and cough. Internal entrance of pathogenic toxin and its accumulation in the lung and spleen leads to failure of the lung to dredge and regulate water passage as well as failure of the spleen to transport and transform, which causes internal stoppage of water and dampness. The healthy qi drives out pathogenic qi, and epidemic pathogen with dampness outthrusts to the muscles and skin, thus herpes occurs. Pathogens still in defense aspect with mild disease condition is responsible for spare skin rashes, small herpes with ruddy color, inapparent areolae around the base, and lucid blister liquid. Red tongue with thin white coating or thin yellow coating, floating rapid pulse, and floating purple finger venules, all are signs of pathogen invading the lung-defense.

[Nursing Principle] Dispersing wind and clearing heat; draining dampness and removing toxin.

[Suggested Formula] Yinqiao Powder and Liuyi Powder.

(2) Syndrome of Pathogen Blazing Qi- and Nutrient Aspects

[Clinical Manifestations] Dense, generalized and widely-distributed skin rashes, big herpes with red or dark purple color, apparent areolae around the base, turbid blister liquid, hemorrhagic skin rashes, visible herpes on the oral mucosa, palpebral conjunctiva and vulva, high fever, irritability, thirst with desire to drink, red complexion, lips and eyes, orolingual ulcer, gingival pain and swelling, poor appetite, dry stool, short dark urine, deep red tongue with rough yellow and dry coating or slimy yellow coating, slippery rapid pulse, and stagnant purple finger venules.

[Manifestations Analysis] Pathogen blazing qi aspect causes exuberant heat in the qi aspect, causing high fever, irritability, thirst with desire to drink, and red complexion and lips. Pathogenic toxin transmitting to the nutrient aspect triggers exuberance heat in the nutrient aspect. The exuberance heat contends with internal dampness and outthrusts to muscles and skin, resulting in dense skin rashes, big herpes with red or dark purple color, apparent areolae around the base, and turbid blister liquid. Pathogenic heat upward fumigating face induces red complexion, lips and eyes, orolingual ulcer, and gingival pain and swelling. Exuberant heat damaging fluids explains dry stool and short dark urine. Deep red tongue with rough yellow and dry coating or slimy yellow coating, slippery rapid pulse, and stagnant purple finger venules, all are signs of pathogen blazing qi and nutrient aspects.

[Nursing Principle] Clearing qi and cooling nutrient; removing toxin and draining dampness.

[Suggested Formula] Qingwen Baidu Drink.

2. Deteriorated Syndrome

(1) Syndrome of Pathogen Invading Heart and Liver

[Clinical Manifestations] Fever (usually persistent high fever), headache, vomiting, even projectile vomiting, restlessness or manic agitation, coma, delirious speech, lethargy, or coma with inability to speak, lock jaw, stiffness of the neck, convulsion of the limbs, arched back rigidity, dense skin rashes with irregular distribution, dark purple color, turbid blister liquid and hard base, deep red tongue with yellow dry coating or thick yellow coating, wiry rapid pulse and stagnant purple finger venules.

[Manifestations Analysis] Extreme weakness of infants' healthy qi and pathogenic toxin invading the heart and liver causes fever (usually persistent high fever), headache, vomiting, even projectile vomiting, restlessness or manic agitation, coma, delirious speech, lethargy, or coma with inability to speak. The liver being often in superabundance for infants and intense pathogenic toxin transforming into fire triggers internal stirring of liver wind, then there are lock jaw, stiffness of the neck, convulsion of the limbs, and arched back rigidity. Dense skin rashes with irregular distribution, dark purple color, turbid blister liquid, hard base, deep red tongue with yellow dry coating or thick yellow coating, wiry rapid pulse and stagnant purple finger venules, all are signs of internal exuberance of heat toxin.

[Nursing Principle] Calming fright and extinguishing wind; clearing heat and removing toxin.

[Suggested Formula] Qingwen Baidu Drink and Lingjiao Gouteng Decoction.

(2) Syndrome of Pathogenic Toxin Blocking Lung

[Clinical Manifestations] Fever (usually persistent high fever), frequent cough, phlegm rale in the throat, rapid breathing, hasty panting, flapping of nasal wings, raised chest and hypochondriac fullness, breathing with raised shoulders and opened mouth, cyanotic mouth and lips, dense skin rashes with irregular distribution, dark purple color, turbid blister liquid and hard base, red or deep red tongue with yellow coating or slimy yellow coating, slippery rapid pulse or surging rapid pulse, and stagnant purple finger venules.

[Manifestations Analysis] Internal blockage of pathogenic toxin induces failure of lung qi to disperse and descend, causing frequent cough, rapid breathing, hasty panting, flapping of nasal wings, raised chest and hypochondriac fullness, and breathing with raised shoulders and opened mouth. Inward sinking of pathogenic toxin condenses fluids to phlegm, leading to fever (usually persistent high fever), and phlegm rale in the throat. Pathogenic toxin contends with internal dampness and outthrusts to muscles and skin, showing dense skin rashes with irregular distribution, dark purple color, turbid blister liquid, and hard base. Red or deep red tongue with yellow coating or slimy yellow coating, slippery rapid pulse or surging rapid pulse, and stagnant purple finger venules, all are signs of internal blockage of pathogenic toxin as well as steaming and fumigating of dampness-heat.

[Nursing Principle] Clearing heat and removing toxin; ventilating the lung and arresting panting.

[Suggested Formula] Maxing Shigan Decoction and Huanglian Jiedu Decoction.

NURSING MEASURES

For patients with chickenpox, nurses should observe the occurrence time, location, color, shape and density of blister, and lucidity of blister liquid. Besides, for children with persistent high fever, their spirit, body temperature and respiration should be observed closely. If the body temperature is over 39.5℃ with coma, restlessness, rapid breathing, flapping of nasal wings, dyspnea, even convulsions, the condition can be considered as deteriorated syndrome. It is advisable to report to the doctor immediately.

Syndrome-Based Nursing Measures

1. Syndrome of Pathogen Invading the Lung-Defense

(1) Daily life nursing. The ward should be cool, quiet, and full of fresh air. The bedding should be loose, soft, light and thin and the clothes should be baggy, soft and cotton. The patients should rest in bed, have adequate sleep, keep the body perspiring slightly to promote eruption of skin rashes, and change the sweaty clothes and quilts in time. If the body temperature is below 38.5℃, there is no need to cool down. But the patients should take shelter from the wind.

(2) Diet nursing. Liquid or semi-liquid diet is appropriate, such as white radish puree. Patients should drink more water and may drink huanghuacai machixian (day lily and purslane) decoction, juhua (chrysanthemum flower) tea, water chestnut juice, sugarcane juice, or herbal tea made with jinyinhua (honeysuckle flower) 15 g and shenggancao (raw licorice root) 5 g. They may eat foods that disperse wind and clear heat, such as bohe (flied mint), yiyiren (coix seed), and mung bean sprouts. Follow the doctor's advice to take food therapy: niubang (great burdock achene) porridge.

(3) Emotion nursing. For children with itching, the nurses should comfort them and patiently explain the importance of not scratching the skin. When children are noisy due to itching, emotional transference and dispositional change therapy such as telling stories, listening to music and watching animations could be used to divert their attention.

(4) Medication nursing. Decoction should not be brewed for long time, and should be taken warm

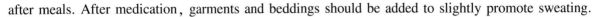

after meals. After medication, garments and beddings should be added to slightly promote sweating.

（5）Manipulation techniques. ① Medicated bath therapy: prepare pugongying（dandelion）, huangbai（amur cork-tree bark）, qianliguang（climbing groundsel）, yejuhua（wild chrysanthemum flower）, shengdi（rehmannia root）, xuanshen（figwort root）, kushen（light yellow sophora root）, and baifan（alum）; first decoct the above medicinals, then add water into the decoction to steep and wash the skin lesions at a temperature of 38 ~ 40℃, 20 minutes each time, once or twice per day. It is appropriate for the initial stage of chickenpox without skin ruptures. Or prepare kushen（light yellow sophora root）and mangxiao（sodium sulphate）30 g respectively, and fuping（duckweed）15 g; decoct the above medicinals to wash the skin lesions, twice per day. It is suitable for patients with plenty of skin rashes and severe itching. ② Paste application therapy: whisk Qingdai Powder and Huashi Powder with sesame oil to make a paste and apply it on the affected area. The paste should be thick enough to cover the herpes completely. It is appropriate for the middle or late stage of chickenpox where maculopapules have evolved into herpes but without skin ruptures and infection. ③ Unction therapy: use calamine lotion for external application, which is appropriate for the patients with severe itching. ④ Infantile tuina therapy: opening Tianmen（heaven gate）, pushing Kangong, circularly pushing Taiyang（EX－HN5）, kneading Erhougaogu（prominent bone behind the ears）, nipping and kneading Ershanmen（double gate）, clearing Tianheshui（heaven river water）, pushing Liufu（six fu-organs）, clearing Feijing（lung meridian）, clearing and tonifying Pijing（spleen meridian）, performing manipulation of Shui Di Lao Yue（scooping the moon from the bottom of water）, separately pushing Dahengwen（major transverse crease）that is also known as separate yin and yang, nipping Shixuan（EX－UE11）, and grasping Fengchi（GB 20）.

2. Syndrome of Pathogen Blazing Qi- and Nutrient Aspects

（1）Daily life nursing. The ward should be cool, quiet, and full of fresh air. The bedding should be loose, soft, light and thin, and the clothes should be baggy, soft and cotton. The patients should rest in bed, have adequate sleep, keep oral hygiene, and gargle the mouth with jinyinhua gancao（honeysuckle flower and licorice root）liquid before and after meals to prevent oral ulcers. If the body temperature is above 39.5℃, sponge bath with warm water can be used rather than cold compress.

（2）Diet nursing. Liquid or semi-liquid diet is appropriate. Patients should drink more water, and may drink watermelon juice and xianlugen（fresh reed rhizome）tea and eat foods that clear heat and drain dampness, such as biqi（waternut）, lüdou（mung bean）, and yiyiren（coix seed）. Food therapy: biqi jiuniang（waternut stewing fermented glutinous rice）, yiren（coix seed）porridge. Patients with dry stool can take honey water and bananas.

（3）Emotion nursing. Nurses should communicate with children patiently and carefully, and encourage them and their parents to cooperate with the treatment actively. Nurses should also inform children and their parents the knowledge about chickenpox and that skin rashes and herpes will not leave scars after incrustation with active treatment.

（4）Medication nursing. Decoction should be taken warm after meals. Discontinue medication immediately after recovery so as not to damage the spleen and stomach.

（5）Manipulation techniques. ① Unction therapy: eye conjunctival ulcer can be cleaned with physiological saline and apply aureomycin eye ointment; oral ulcer can be cleaned with physiological saline and coat the wound with Bingpeng Powder, 3 ~ 4 times per day. ② Medicated bath therapy: prepare pugongying (dandelion), huangqin (scutellaria root) 20 g, yimucao (motherwort) 20 g, kushen (light yellow sophora root) 20 g, huanglian (coptis rhizome) 10 g, and huangbai (amur cork-tree bark) 15 g; decoct the above medicinals for external use, one dose per day, twice per day. ③ Paste application therapy: grind into powder qingdai (natural indigo) 30 g, duanshigao (dried gypsum) 50 g, huashi (talcum) 50 g, huangbai (amur cork-tree bark) 15 g, binpian (borneol) 10 g and huanglian (coptis rhizome) 10 g; whisk the powder with sesame oil to coat the affected area. It is appropriate for patients with turbid blister liquid or herpes ruptures.

3. Syndrome of Pathogen Invading Heart and Liver

（1）Daily life nursing. The ward should be cool, quiet, dark, and full of fresh air. The coverings should be thin. The patients should rest in bed as much as possible. If the body temperature is above 39.5℃, sponge bath with warm water can be used. Nurses should be alert to the occurrence of high fever and convulsion. If convulsions occur, the following measures should be adopted for emergency: lie in a supine position, place a soft object under the head to tilt the head to one side in order to keep the respiratory tract open, unfasten the collar, loosen the clothing. And don't press patients forcibly to prevent limb injury.

（2）Diet nursing. Patients should be nasal fed with liquid foods that clear heat and open orifices, such as machixian (purslane). Juhua lugen decoction may be used for nasal feeding: lugen (reed rhizome) 60 g and juhua (chrysanthemum flower) 10 g.

（3）Emotion nursing. Nurses should pay attention to the emotions of children's parents, comfort and encourage them in time to maintain their emotional stability and prevent fear and anxiety.

（4）Medication nursing. Decoction should be nasal fed when it is warm. Chinese medicine pills should be melted with warm water for nasal feeding.

（5）Manipulation techniques. ① Paste application therapy: whisk Qingdai Powder with sesame oil for external use; or grind into powder duanshigao (dried gypsum) 50 g, huashi (talcum) 50 g, qingdai (natural indigo) 30 g, huangbai (amur cork-tree bark) 15 g, binpian (borneol) 10 g and huanglian (coptis rhizome) 10 g; whisk the powder with sesame oil to coat the affected area, once to twice per day. It is appropriate for the cases with festered herpes. ② Insufflation therapy: insufflate Xilei Powder, Bingpeng Powder or Zhuhuang Powder to the ulcers of the mouth, 2 ~ 3 times per day. It is appropriate for the cases with oral mucosa ruptures. ③ Blood-letting therapy: select Dazhui (GV 14), Tianzhu (BL 10), Quchi (LI 11) or Hegu (LI 4); after the skin is disinfected, rub the local area to make it hyperemic, use a three-edged needle to quickly pierce the skin at a depth of 3 millimeters, remove the needle to release blood less than 1.0 mL, and wipe or press the pierced point with a sterile dry cotton ball. It is appropriate for patients with high fever. ④ Acupressure therapy: nip Renzhong (GV 26), and press Hegu (LI 4) and Taichong (LR 3). It is appropriate for patients with high fever and convulsion.

4. Syndrome of Pathogenic Toxin Blocking Lung

(1) Daily life nursing. The ward should be cool, quiet, dark, and full of fresh air. The coverings should be thin. If the body temperature is above 39.5℃, sponge bath with warm water can be used.

(2) Diet nursing. Patients should be nasal fed with liquid foods that clear heat and resolve phlegm, such as xingren (apricot kernel), yuxingcao (heartleaf houttuynia), loquats and snow pears. Decoction for nasal feeding: biqi (waternut), zhuyexin (lophatherum), and xianlugen (fresh reed rhizome), 30~60 g respectively.

(3) Emotion nursing. When children are sick, they and their parents have varying degrees of fear and anxiety. Children are easy to be depressed and lonely after quarantine. Therefore, nurses may use emotional inter-resistance therapy as well as emotional transference and dispositional change therapy to comfort and encourage them in time to maintain their emotional stability.

(4) Medication nursing. Decoction should be nasal fed when it is warm. Chinese medicine pills should be melted with warm water for nasal feeding.

(5) Manipulation techniques. ① Blood-letting therapy: select Shaoshang (LU 11) or Erjian (EX − HN6); after the skin is disinfected, rub the local area to make it hyperemic, use a three-edged needle to quickly pierce the skin at a depth of 3 millimeter, remove the needle to release blood less than 1.0 mL, and wipe or press the pierced point with a sterile dry cotton ball. It is appropriate for patients with high fever. ② Infantile tuina therapy: opening Tianmen (heaven gate), pushing Kangong, clearing Feijing (lung meridian), clearing Tianheshui (heaven river water), kneading Quchi (LI 11), Dazhui (GV 14) and Hegu (LI 4). It is appropriate for patients with high fever. ③ Wet compress therapy: whisk Huanglian Oinmemt with Ruyi Jinhuang Powder to compress the localized herpes. It is appropriate for patients with infection and rash ruptures.

Patient Education

The room should be full of fresh air without strong or convective wind. During fever and rash eruption, patients should rest in bed as much as possible and avoid exhaustion. The patients should keep skin clean and dry. Underwear should be soft and changed frequently. For patients with severe chickenpox, bathing or sponge bathing should temporarily be prohibited. Patients' nails should be trimmed to avoid scratching the skin and causing infection. And infants' hands can be wrapped with gauze.

Foods should be light, nutritious and digestible. The patients should drink more water and eat more fresh fruit and vegetables as well as multiple small meals. For those with weak constitution, nutrition should be supplemented to improve physical fitness after conditions are improved. Don't eat shengjiang (fresh ginger), hujiao (pepper fruit), and greasy foods or those generating dryness-heat.

Nurses should inform children's parents about the transmission, prevention, disinfection, quarantine and nursing measures of chickenpox. For infants, it is suggested to cuddle and care for them patiently and carefully. For elder children, it is necessary to introduce the hospital environment and medical staffs to them and explain the disease development and treatment measures. At night, pay much attention to make rounds of the wards and leave the floor lighted to allay children's fear of darkness.

Characteristics of skin rashes of chickenpox are: skin rashes occur in batches and maculopapules, herpes and scabs coexist simultaneously; each batch may last one to six days; the rashes distribute centripetally and appear first on the trunk, then on the face, shoulders and limbs. The scars can be washed gently with warm water only after all the herpes are incrusted. When scabs fall off incompletely, patients should wait for them to naturally fall off rather than tear them off forcibly. If necessary, nurses may use sterile scissors to cut them off, and then apply paraffin oil.

The infection source of chickenpox is children with chickenpox and its infection routes are droplets and direct contact. From one day before rash eruption to the time when all the herpes incrust, chickenpox is highly infectious. Therefore, respiratory tract quarantine should be taken immediately after the onset. Nurses should wear a face mask and dress neatly when dealing with children. After care, nurses must disinfect their hands. The bedding and clothing contaminated by children with chickenpox should be sterilized constantly. And the air, objects and their surfaces in the ward should be disinfected every day.

第四节 手 足 口 病

手足口病,是指因手足口病疫毒从口鼻而入,与内蕴湿热搏击,蕴郁于肺脾,外发于肌表而引起的,以口腔颊黏膜出现疱疹或溃疡,手足出现皮疹或水疱,可伴见发热、流涕、咽痛,甚则出现邪毒内陷、邪毒犯心变证为临床特征的小儿温疫病。西医的手足口病可参照本节进行护理。

一、病因病机

手足口病的病因是感受手足口病时邪。小儿肺脏娇嫩,腠理疏松,不耐邪扰;脾常不足,易受损伤。若小儿素有湿热内蕴,或因调护失宜,饮食不节,加之夏秋季节湿热之气偏盛,同气相求,则水湿内生。手足口病疫毒由口鼻而入,内犯于肺,下侵于脾,邪毒蕴郁,气化失司,内停水湿与时行邪毒相搏,蕴蒸于外,则发生本病。若小儿素体虚弱,邪毒炽盛,可出现邪闭心肺,气虚阳脱之危重变证。

手足口病的病机为时邪蕴郁肺脾,外透肌表。病位主要在肺、脾,严重者可累及心、肝。

二、常见证型

(一)辨证要点

辨轻重 根据病程长短、疱疹特点、伴随症状来辨别。若病程短,疱疹局限于手足掌心及口腔,分布稀疏,疹色红润,根盘红晕不明显,疱液清亮,全身症状轻微,多为轻证。若病程长,疱疹累及四肢及臀部,分布稠密,或成簇出现,疹色紫暗,根盘红晕明显,疱液混浊,全身症状较重,多为重证。体弱而邪毒炽盛者,正不胜邪,极易发生嗜睡易惊,肢体抽搐,或喘憋紫绀,神昏厥冷,大汗淋漓,脉微欲绝等邪陷厥阴或气虚阳脱的变证。

(二)证候分型

1. 湿热蕴毒,郁结脾肺证

[主要证候]手、足、口、臀部等部位出现斑丘疹、丘疹、疱疹;疱疹分布稠密,疹色紫暗,根盘红晕显著,疱液浑浊,疱疹疼痛瘙痒,伴有发热或无发热,倦怠,流涎,咽痛,纳差,便秘;甚者可出现大疱、手指脱甲;舌质红绛,苔黄腻,脉数,指纹紫。

[证候分析]邪犯肺脾,通调运化失常,水湿内停与时邪相搏,外发肌肤,故见手、足、口、臀部等部位出现斑丘疹、丘疹、疱疹;热邪犯肺,肺气失宣,故伴有发热或无发热,咽痛;邪热壅盛,灼伤津液,故肠燥便秘;阴血不足,肝失所养,故甚者出现手指脱甲;邪入于脾,故流涎,纳差;舌质红绛,苔黄腻,脉数,指纹紫,均为湿热蕴毒,郁结脾肺之象。

[护治原则]清热解毒,化湿透邪。

　　[常用方剂] 甘露消毒丹。

　　2. 毒热内壅, 肝热惊风证

　　[主要证候] 高热, 易惊, 肌肉眴动, 瘛疭, 或抽搐, 或肢体痿软无力, 呕吐, 嗜睡, 甚则昏蒙、昏迷; 疱疹稠密, 疱浆浑浊紫暗, 疱疹可形小, 甚则无疹; 舌暗红或红绛, 苔黄腻或黄燥, 脉弦细数, 指纹紫滞。

　　[证候分析] 湿热毒盛, 化火内陷, 浸及厥阴, 肝风内动, 故易惊, 肌肉眴动, 瘛疭, 或抽搐; 毒热内扰心神, 故嗜睡, 甚则昏蒙、昏迷; 舌暗红或红绛, 苔黄腻或黄燥, 脉弦细数, 指纹紫滞, 均为毒热内壅, 肝热惊风之象。

　　[护治原则] 解毒清热, 熄风定惊。

　　[常用方剂] 清瘟败毒饮合羚角钩藤汤。

　　3. 邪闭心肺, 气虚阳脱证

　　[主要证候] 壮热, 喘促, 神昏, 手足厥冷, 大汗淋漓, 面色苍白, 口唇紫绀; 疱疹稠密, 疱浆浑浊, 疱疹可波及四肢、臀部、肛周, 或可见疱疹稀疏; 舌质紫暗, 脉细数或沉迟, 或脉微欲绝, 指纹沉紫。

　　[证候分析] 邪热闭肺, 肺气失宣, 故壮热, 喘促; 邪毒内陷心包, 气血运行不利, 故口唇紫绀; 心阳暴脱, 神随气散, 故神昏; 阳脱不运, 不能向四肢透达, 故手足厥冷, 面色苍白; 阳脱无力推动血行, 脉道失充, 故脉微欲绝; 阳气衰亡不能固表, 故大汗淋漓; 舌质紫暗, 脉细数或沉迟, 指纹紫暗, 均为邪闭心肺, 气虚阳脱之象。

　　[护治原则] 固脱开窍, 清热解毒。

　　[常用方剂] 参附汤、生脉散合安宫牛黄丸。

　　4. 气阴不足, 络脉不畅证

　　[主要证候] 乏力, 纳差, 或伴肢体痿软, 或肢体麻木; 舌淡红, 苔薄腻, 脉细, 指纹色淡或青紫。

　　[证候分析] 邪毒伤及肝脾, 邪去正虚, 脾气不足, 运化失司, 气血生化乏源, 故乏力, 纳差; 肝血亏耗, 筋失所养, 络脉不畅, 故肢体痿软, 或肢体麻木; 舌淡红, 苔薄腻, 脉细, 指纹色淡或青紫, 均为气阴不足, 络脉不畅之象。

　　[护治原则] 益气通络, 养阴健脾。

　　[常用方剂] 生脉散合七味白术散。

三、护理措施

　　对于手足口病的患儿, 应观察皮疹的部位、形态、色泽和疏密程度, 以及疱液是否清亮。对于重型的患儿, 应每1~2小时观察1次, 重点观察体温, 脉搏, 心率, 心律, 呼吸, 血压, 精神状态, 末梢循环状况和神经系统症状, 注意皮疹, 口腔溃疡, 饮食等一般情况。随时了解病情的变化, 尤其注意有无神经源性肺水肿、心肺功能衰竭或脑功能衰竭等病情突变。若有异常, 应立即报告医生, 并配合抢救。

　　(一) 辨证施护

　　1. 湿热蕴毒, 郁结脾肺证

　　(1) 生活起居护理　居室凉爽安静, 空气新鲜。患儿需隔离, 卧床休息, 慎避风寒。做好口腔和皮肤护理,保持皮肤清洁干燥,防止疱疹破溃感染,勤剪指甲以防抓伤皮肤。进食前后用生理盐水或金银花甘草液漱口。密切观察体温变化,若体温超过 38.5℃,可物理降温,比如用温水擦浴。

(2)饮食护理　饮食为流食或半流食。多饮水,可饮薄荷茶、淡竹叶茶。宜食清热利湿的食物,如薏苡仁、白扁豆。若患儿为 3~5 岁且素有内热,可用山楂 10 g,菊花 6 g,甘草 3 g,以沸水 200 mL 浸泡后,加冰糖适量频饮。不宜食肥腻的食物。

(3)情志护理　保持患儿情绪稳定。部分患儿在病后 2~4 周会出现脱甲,可能会引起患儿的恐惧、焦虑,护士可运用语言开导疗法,解释新甲会于 1~2 月内长出。

(4)用药护理　中药汤剂宜饭后温服,每日 1 剂,水煎 100~150 mL,分 3~4 次或少量多次服用。若服药困难,可将中药煎剂浓缩取汁 50~100 mL 后灌肠,每日 1 剂。若呕吐,可用少量生姜汁,滴于舌根止呕。

(5)操作技术　① 涂药法:用青黛散、双料喉风散或冰硼散,与蜂蜜调匀后外涂,每日 2~3 次;适用于口咽部疱疹。② 含漱疗法:用薄荷 15 g,黄芩、黄连、黄柏、五倍子、淡竹叶各 10 g,煎水 100 mL,漱口;适用于口腔部疱疹、溃疡。③ 敷贴疗法:用金黄散或青黛散,与芝麻油调成糊状后,敷于手足疱疹患处,每日 2 次;适用于疱疹较多者。④ 灌肠疗法:薏苡仁 20 g,败酱草 12 g,青蒿 10 g,藿香 9 g,黄芩 6 g,栀子 5 g;煎汤后进行保留灌肠。

2. 毒热内壅,肝热惊风证

(1)生活起居护理　居室凉爽安静,空气新鲜。患儿需隔离,发热时绝对卧床,退热后可在室内轻微活动,慎避风寒。保持呼吸道通畅,予以吸氧。做好口腔和皮肤护理,保持皮肤清洁干燥,防止疱疹破溃感染,勤剪指甲以防抓伤皮肤。进食前后用生理盐水或金银花甘草液漱口。密切观察体温变化,若体温超过 38.5℃,可物理降温,如用温水擦浴。注意观察生命体征,若患儿出现头痛、烦躁不安,或出现嗜睡、惊厥、呼吸微弱,应立即报告医生,并配合抢救。

(2)饮食护理　多饮水。宜食清淡、易消化的流食。若进食差或不能进食,可采用鼻饲。不宜食肥甘、油腻、生冷、硬固、辛辣的食物。

(3)情志护理　保持患儿情绪稳定。由于疱疹疼痛难忍,实验室检查项目较多,患儿经常哭闹不止,护士应耐心和蔼,运用移情易性疗法,转移其注意力,或运用鼓励表扬的方法,帮助患儿克服疼痛,积极配合治疗和护理。

(4)用药护理　中药汤剂可口服,每日 1 剂,水煎 100~150 mL,分 3~4 次服用;或灌肠,每日 1 剂,煎煮取汁 50~100 mL。

(5)操作技术　① 涂药法:用金黄散、青黛散或紫金锭,与芝麻油调匀,敷于手足疱疹处,每日 3 次。② 灌肠疗法:用酒大黄、生石膏、生薏苡仁、钩藤、天麻、桂枝,进行保留灌肠。③ 浸洗疗法:用金银花、板蓝根、蒲公英、车前草、浮萍各 15 g,黄柏 10 g,水煎,浸洗手足疱疹处;适用于症状较重的患儿。④ 敷贴疗法:用煅石膏 30 g,黄柏、蛤壳各 15 g,白芷 10 g,研磨成粉后与芝麻油调匀,外敷手足疱疹处;适用于疱疹多而痛痒剧烈的患儿。

3. 邪闭心肺,气虚阳脱证

(1)生活起居护理　居室安静舒适,空气新鲜。患儿需隔离,绝对卧床,头肩抬高 15°~30°,保持中立位。留置胃管、导尿管。保持呼吸道通畅,予以吸氧。做好口腔和皮肤护理,保持皮肤清洁干燥,防止疱疹破溃感染,勤剪指甲以防抓伤皮肤。

（2）饮食护理　发作时禁食。缓解后,可通过鼻饲予营养支持。

（3）情志护理　患儿急性发作时,护士应沉着冷静,多关心和安慰病人及家属。

（4）用药护理　中药汤剂可口服,每日1剂,水煎100~150 mL,分3~4次服用;或灌肠,煎煮取汁50~100 mL,每日1剂。若高热神昏,中药丸剂宜用温水溶化后鼻饲。

（5）操作技术　① 熏洗疗法:用野菊花、蒲公英、紫花地丁、土茯苓各30 g,水杨梅20 g;煎煮后水温50℃时熏蒸皮损处,水温降至37~40℃时浸泡、淋洗皮损,每次20分钟,每日1次。② 耳压疗法:取肺、脾、心、神门等耳穴,用耳穴压丸贴片贴压,每日按揉4~5次,以局部发热泛红为度,留置2~4日。

4. 气阴不足,络脉不畅证

（1）生活起居护理　居室安静舒适,空气新鲜。衣被宽大轻暖。患儿需隔离,绝对卧床。做好口腔和皮肤护理,保持皮肤清洁干燥。不可过劳。

（2）饮食护理　宜进食清淡、营养、易消化、刺激性较小的流食或半流食,如蛋羹、菜粥、米汤。宜食益气养阴的食物,如茯苓、葛根,研磨成粉后与木瓜汁调成糊状,煮熟后喂食。不宜食肥甘、油腻、生冷、辛辣、过咸的食物。

（3）情志护理　患儿重病初愈,护士可运用语言开导疗法,多鼓励和夸奖患儿。对于合并瘫痪的患儿,运用移情易性疗法,转移患儿的注意力,避免悲观、焦虑。

（4）用药护理　中药汤剂每日1剂,水煎100~150 mL,分3~4次服用。

（5）操作技术　① 捏脊疗法:提捏背部的督脉和足太阳膀胱经,每次3~5分钟,每日1次。② 穴位按摩法:取足三里、血海、太溪、合谷、百会,用拇指揉法,按摩至局部发热或有酸麻重胀感,每日1次;适用于手足口病合并弛缓型瘫痪者,进入恢复期后应尽早开展。

（二）健康教育

预防手足口病,关键在于保持良好的个人卫生习惯。饭前、便后、外出返回后都要洗手。衣物置于阳光下暴晒,小儿常接触的物品应使用中效或高效消毒剂定期消毒。本病流行期间,避免到人群聚集、空气流通性差、潮湿闷热的公共场所。

可选用芳香辟秽,清热解毒的中药,如藿香、佩兰、艾叶,配制成香囊随身佩戴。加强体育锻炼,睡眠充足,防止过度疲劳。饮食应清淡、营养、易消化,不喝生水。

避免健康小儿与患儿密切接触。避免接触被病毒污染的毛巾、手绢、牙杯、玩具、食具、奶具、床上用品、内衣。对患儿进行呼吸道隔离和消化道隔离。对患儿的呕吐物、排泄物、用具等进行严格消毒。患儿的衣服和被褥应清洁、柔软,以减少皮肤刺激。对于臀部有皮损的患儿,应及时清理大小便,保持局部清洁干燥。

Section 4　Hand-Foot-Mouth Disease

Hand-foot-mouth disease（HFMD）is an infantile epidemic disease clinically characterized by herpes or ulcer on the oral buccal mucosa, rash or blister on the hands and feet, possibly accompanied by fever, runny nose, sore throat, or even occurrence of deteriorated syndromes such as inward invasion of pathogenic toxin and pathogenic toxin invading the heart. It is caused by the epidemic toxin of HFMD, which enters the body from the nose and mouth, contends with the internal dampness-heat, accumulates in the lung and spleen, and finally manifests in the fleshy exterior. This section can be referred to for the nursing of HFMD in Western medicine.

ETIOLOGY AND PATHOGENESIS

The etiology is invasion of seasonal epidemic toxin. Infants' delicate lung and insecure striae and interstice make them susceptible to the invasion of pathogens. And their spleen is often in deficiency, so the spleen is vulnerable to injury. If the infants have interior accumulation of dampness-heat and improper nursing and diet, interior water-dampness will be generated because the exuberance of dampness-heat in summer and fall likes to be together with the pathogens of the same kind. The epidemic toxin of HFMD enters the body through the nose and mouth, then it invades inward the lung and downward the spleen, leading to internal accumulation of pathogenic toxin, failure of qi transformation as well as internal stoppage of water-dampness. The water-dampness contends with seasonal epidemic toxin and finally manifests in the fleshy exterior. If the infants are weak and the epidemic toxin is exuberance, critical deteriorated syndromes may occur, such as pathogen blocking the heart and lung, qi deficiency and yang collapse.

The pathogenesis is seasonal epidemic toxin accumulation in the lung and spleen that manifests in the fleshy exterior. The location of disease is mainly in the lung and spleen while the serious cases may involve the heart and liver.

COMMON SYNDROMES

Key Points in Syndrome Differentiation

Differentiation of Severity of the Disease

The differentiation is based on the course of disease, characteristics of herpes, and accompanying symptoms. The mild cases show a short course of disease, localized and sparsely-distributed herpes on the hands, palms and mouth, with ruddy color, inapparent areolae around the base, lucid blister liquid and mild generalized symptoms. However, severe cases have a long course of disease, herpes on the limbs and buttocks with dense or clustered distribution, dark purple color, apparent areolae around the base, turbid blister liquid and severe generalized symptoms. The patients who are weak and overwhelmed by exuberant epidemic toxin are prone to suffering from deteriorated syndromes such as syndrome of pathogen invading jueyin or syndrome of qi deficiency with yang collapse, with symptoms of drowsiness, susceptibility to fright, limb convulsions, or dyspnea, suffocation, cyanosis, coma, reversal cold, profuse dripping sweating and faint pulse verging on expiry.

Syndrome Differentiation

1. Syndrome of Dampness-Heat Toxin Accumulation in the Spleen and Lung

[Clinical Manifestations] Maculopapules, papules and herpes on the hands, feet, mouth and buttocks; herpes with dense distribution, dark purple color, apparent areolae around the base, turbid lister liquid and aching itching sensation, accompanied with fever or no fever, fatigue, salivation, sore throat, poor appetite, constipation, or even large blisters and fingernail shedding, crimson tongue with yellow and slimy coating, rapid pulse, and purple finger venules.

[Manifestations Analysis] Pathogens invading the lung and spleen causes failure of the lung to dredge and regulate water passage as well as dysfunction of the spleen in transportation and transformation, which induces internal stoppage of water and dampness. The water and dampness contend with seasonal epidemic pathogens and outthrust to the muscles and skin, causing maculopapules, papules and herpes on the hands, feet, mouth and buttocks. Pathogenic heat invading the lung makes lung qi fail to disperse and descend, so there are fever or no fever, and sore throat. Exuberance of pathogenic heat scorches fluids, so intestinal dryness and constipation occur. Yin blood insufficiency cannot nourish the liver, so exhibits fingernail shedding. Pathogens attacking the spleen is responsible for salivation and poor appetite. Crimson tongue with yellow and slimy coating, rapid pulse, and purple finger venules, all are signs of dampness-heat toxin accumulation in the spleen and lung.

[Nursing Principle] Clearing heat and removing toxin; resolving dampness and expelling pathogen.

[Suggested Formula] Ganlu Xiaodu Pellets.

2. Syndrome of Liver Heat Convulsion due to Internal Congestion of Toxic Heat

[Clinical Manifestations] High fever, susceptibility to fright, muscular twitching, clonic convulsion, or spasm, or weakness and flaccidity of limbs, vomiting, somnolence, even coma; herpes with dense distribution, turbid and dark purple color blister liquid, or small herpes, or even no herpes; dark red or deep red tongue with yellow slimy or dry yellow coating, wiry thready, rapid pulse and purple stagnant finger venules.

[Manifestations Analysis] Exuberance of toxic dampness-heat transforms into fire, inward enters jueyin meridian and causes internal stirring of liver wind, causing susceptibility to fright, muscular twitching, clonic convulsion, or spasm. Toxic heat harasses heart spirit, leading to somnolence or even coma. Dark red or deep red tongue with yellow slimy or dry yellow coating, wiry thready, rapid pulse and purple stagnant finger venules, all are manifestations of liver heat convulsion due to internal congestion of toxic heat.

[Nursing Principle] Removing toxin and clearing heat; extinguishing wind and arresting convulsion.

[Suggested Formula] Qingwen Baidu Drink and Lingjiao Gouteng Decoction.

3. Syndrome of Qi Deficiency and Yang Collapse due to Pathogens Blocking the Heart and Lung

[Clinical Manifestations] High fever, panting, coma, reversal cold of four limbs, profuse sweating, pale complexion, cyanotic lips; herpes on the limbs, buttocks and perianal area with dense distribution and turbid blister liquid, or sparsely-distributed herpes; dark purple tongue with thready rapid pulse, or sunken slow pulse, or paint pulse verging on expiry, and sunken and purple finger venules.

[Manifestations Analysis] Pathogenic heat blocking the lung makes failure of lung qi to disperse and descend, so high fever and panting occur. Pathogenic toxin sinking inward in the pericardium triggers inhibited movement of qi and blood, so the lips are cyanotic. Sudden collapse of heart yang causes loss of spirit following qi depletion, so the patients are in coma. Yang qi cannot reach four extremities due to yang collapse, so exhibit reversal cold of four limbs and pale complexion. Yang collapse fails to propel the movement of blood and fill the vessels with blood, so paint pulse verging on expiry is felt. Yang qi cannot secure the exterior due to yang exhaustion, so there appears profuse sweating. And dark purple tongue with thready rapid pulse, or sunken slow pulse, or paint pulse verging on expiry, and sunken and purple finger venules, all are signs of qi deficiency and yang collapse due to pathogens blocking the heart and lung.

[Nursing Principle] Stopping collapse and opening orifices; clearing heat and removing toxin.

[Suggested Formula] Shenfu Decoction, Shengmai Powder and Angong Niuhuang Pills.

4. Syndrome of Qi-Yin Deficiency and Collateral Inhibition

[Clinical Manifestations] Fatigue, poor appetite, possible numbness or flaccidity of limbs, pale red tongue with thin slimy coating, thready pulse, and pale or cyanotic finger venules.

[Manifestations Analysis] Pathogenic toxin damages the liver and spleen, causing healthy qi deficiency after the elimination of pathogens as well as deficiency of spleen qi. It causes dysfunction of spleen qi in transportation and transformation, and insufficient source of qi and blood, hence fatigue and poor appetite occur. Liver blood depletion brings about malnourishment of the sinews and collateral inhibition, so the patients feel numbness or flaccidity of limbs. Pale red tongue with thin slimy coating, thready pulse, and pale or cyanotic finger venules, all are manifestations of qi-yin deficiency and collateral inhibition.

[Nursing Principle] Replenishing qi and dredging collateral; nourishing yin and invigorating the spleen.

[Suggested Formula] Shengmai Powder and Qiwei Baidu Powder.

NURSING MEASURES

For patients with hand-foot-and-mouth disease, nurses should observe the location, morphology, color and density of skin rashes as well as the lucidity of blister liquid. For severe patients, in every 1~2 hour(s), nurses should closely monitor some basic aspects, such as the temperature, pulse, the rate and rhythm of heart, respiration, blood pressure, mentality, peripheral circulation and symptoms of nervous system, and pay attention to the rashes, mouth ulcer and diet. Changes in the condition such as neurogenic pulmonary edema, cardiopulmonary or cerebral failure should be heeded. Nurses should report every anomaly to the doctor and help give emergency treatment.

Syndrome-Based Nursing Measures

1. Syndrome of Dampness-Heat Toxin Accumulation in the Spleen and Lung

(1) Daily life nursing. The ward should be cool, quiet, and full of fresh air. The sick children should be isolated, rest in bed, keep away from wind and cold, maintain oral and skin hygiene, keep the skin dry and clean, avoid diabrosis and infection of herpes, and have nails trimmed frequently to prevent the skin from getting scratched. They should gargle the mouth with normal saline or jinyinhua gancao (honeysuckle flower and licorice root) liquid before and after meals. Nurses should also closely monitor the changes in temperature. Physical cooling, such as sponge bath with warm water, could be applied for patients with a body temperature above 38.5℃.

(2) Diet nursing. Liquid or semi-liquid diet are preferred. The patients should drink more water, and may drink bohe (field mint) tea or danzhuye (lophatherum herb) tea and eat foods that clear heat and drain dampness, such as yiyiren (coix seed) and biandou (hyacinth bean). For patients 3~5 years old with persistent internal heat, they could frequently drink the following herbal tea: soak shanzha (Chinese hawthorn fruit) 10 g, juhua (chrysanthemum flower) 6 g, and gancao (licorice root) 3 g in 200 mL of boiling water with moderate amounts of rock candies. They should avoid fatty and greasy foods.

(3) Emotion nursing. Nurses should help maintain emotional stability in patients. Some patients' nails might become detached in 2~4 weeks, which could induce fear and anxiety. For those patients, nurses may use verbal enlightenment therapy to tell them that new nails would grow in 1~2 month(s).

(4) Medication nursing. Decoction should be taken warm after meals. A dosage of 100~150 mL per day, taken 3~4 times or small doses taken multiple times per day. For patients with difficulty taking medicine, use 50~100 mL of concentrated decoction for enema therapy, one dose per day. Patients with vomiting could have a few drops of shengjiang (fresh ginger) juice on the root of the tongue to relieve the sickness.

(5) Manipulation techniques. ① Unction therapy: blend Qingdai Powder, Shuangliao Houfeng Powder or Bingpeng Powder with honey and then apply to the affected area 2~3 times per day. This is effective for herpes in the mouth and pharynx. ② Mouth gargling therapy: bohe (field mint) 15 g,

huangqin （scutellaria root）, huanglian （coptis rhizome）, huangbai （amur cork-tree bark）, wubeizi （gallnut of Chinese sumac）, and danzhuye （lophatherum herb） 10 g respectively; brew them to get 100 mL of liquid for mouth gargling; this is effective for herpes and ulcer in the mouth. ③ Paste application therapy: blend Jinhuang Powder or Qingdai Powder with sesame oil and then apply to the herpes on hands and feet, twice per day; this is appropriate for patients with multiple herpes. ④ Enema therapy: decoct yiyiren （coix seed） 20 g, baijiangcao （patrinia） 12 g, qinghao （sweet wormwood） 10 g, huoxiang （agastache） 9 g, huangqin （scutellaria root） 6 g, and zhizi （gardenia） 5 g; and use the decoction for retention enema.

2. Syndrome of Liver Heat Convulsion due to Internal Congestion of Toxic Heat

（1） Daily life nursing. The ward should be cool, quiet, and full of fresh air. The sick children should be isolated, have absolute rest in bed in the presence of a fever, and may do moderate activities after the fever is abated. They should keep away from wind and cold, maintain oral and skin hygiene, keep the skin dry and clean, avoid diabrosis and infection of herpes, and have nails trimmed frequently to prevent the skin from getting scratched. Patients should gargle the mouth with normal saline or jinyinhua gancao （honeysuckle flower and licorice root） liquid before and after meals. Nurses should keep the patients' respiratory tract obstructed, give them oxygen inhalation, and closely monitor the changes in temperature. Physical cooling, such as sponge bath with warm water, could be applied for patients with a body temperature above 38.5℃. Nurses should also watch closely the vital signs, report to the doctor immediately and assist in emergency treatment if the patient experiences headache, irritability, restlessness, or drowsiness, convulsion or shallow breathing.

（2） Diet nursing. Patients should drink more water and take liquid diet that are light and digestible. For patients with difficulty taking food, nasal feeding can be used instead. They should avoid fatty, sweet, greasy, raw, cold, hard, solid, pungent and spicy foods.

（3） Emotion nursing. Nurses should help maintain emotional stability in patients. Some patients might cry incessantly because of the unbearable pain from herpes and the numerous medical examinations. For those sick children, nurses should be kind and patient, and may use emotional transference and dispositional change therapy to divert their attention or encourage and praise them to help them withstand the pain and comply with treatment and nursing.

（4） Medication nursing. A dosage of 100~150 mL brewed decoction per day, taken 3~4 times per day; or, 50~100 mL of concentrated decoction for enema therapy, one dose per day.

（5） Manipulation techniques. ① Unction therapy: blend Jinhuang Powder, Qingdai Powder or Zijin Troche with sesame oil and then apply to herpes on hands and feet, three times per day. ② Enema therapy: decoct dahuang （rhubarb root and rhizome） prepared with yellow wine, unprepared shigao （gypsum）, unprepared yiyiren （coix seed）, gouteng （gambir plant）, tianma （tall gastrodis tuber）, and guizhi （cinnamon twig）; and use the decoction for retention enema, once per day. ③ Steeping and washing therapy: Jinyinhua （honeysuckle flower） 15 g, banlan'gen （isatis root） 15 g, pugongying （dandelion） 15 g, cheqiancao （plantain） 15 g, fuping （duckweed） 15 g, huangbai （amur cork-tree bark) 10 g; decoct the medicinals and wash the herpes on the hands and feet with the decoction; this is effective for patients with severe symptoms. ④ Paste application therapy: grind into powder duanshigao (dried gypsum) 30 g, huangbai (amur cork-tree bark) 15 g, geqiao (clam shell) 15 g, and baizhi (angelica root) 15 g; blend the powder with sesame oil, and apply the mixture to herpes on hands and feet; this is appropriate for patients with numerous herpes and severe itch.

3. Syndrome of Qi Deficiency and Yang Collapse due to Pathogens Blocking the Heart and Lung

(1) Daily life nursing. The ward should be quiet, comfortable and full of fresh air. The sick children should be isolated, have absolute rest in bed with head and shoulder raised $15° \sim 30°$ upward, and stay in a neutral position. Nurses should keep patients' gastric tube and urinary catheter in place, keep their respiratory tract obstructed, and give them oxygen inhalation. The sick children should maintain oral and skin hygiene, keep the skin dry and clean, avoid diabrosis and infection of the herpes, and have nails trimmed frequently to prevent the skin from getting scratched.

(2) Diet nursing. Food intake is forbidden during the acute onset of the disease. After the symptoms are relieved, nutrition could be provided through nasal feeding.

(3) Emotion nursing. Nurses should stay calm and composed as well as provide care and comfort to the patients and their family during acute episodes of the disease.

(4) Medication nursing. A dosage of $100 \sim 150$ mL brewed decoction per day, taken $3 \sim 4$ times per day; or $50 \sim 100$ mL of concentrated decoction for enema therapy, one dose per day. Patients with high fever and unconsciousness could use a nasal feeding tube to take the melted pills in warm water.

(5) Manipulation techniques. ① Fumigating and washing therapy: yejuhua (wild chrysanthemum flower), pugongying (dandelion), zihuadiding (tokyo violet) and tufuling (glabrous greenbrier rhizome) 30 g respectively, and shuiyangmei (throat root) 20 g; decoct the above ingredients for fumigating the skin lesion at a temperature of $50℃$, and for steeping and washing at a temperature of $37 \sim 40℃$, 20 minutes each time, once per day. ② Auricular pressure therapy: select lung (CO14), spleen (CO13), heart (CO15), and shenmen (TF4); apply specialized pasters on the points, press on each of them till the area turns hot and red, $4 \sim 5$ times per day, and keep the pasters for $2 \sim 4$ days.

4. Syndrome of Qi-Yin Deficiency and Collateral Inhibition

(1) Daily life nursing. The ward should be quiet, comfortable and full of fresh air. The sick children should be isolated, have absolute rest in bed, and wear loose, light and warm clothes. They should also maintain oral and skin hygiene, keep the skin dry and clean as well as avoiding overstrain.

(2) Diet nursing. The sick children may have liquid or semi-liquid diet that are light, nutritious, digestible and minimally irritating, such as egg custard, porridge with vegetables, and rice soup. They may eat foods that replenish qi and nourish yin, such as fuling (poria) and gegen (kudzuvine root), both of which could be finely ground and blended with juice of mugua (Chinese quince fruit) to make paste, and cooked to feed the children. They should avoid foods that are fatty, sweet, greasy, raw, cold, pungent, spicy or salty.

（3）Emotion nursing. Nurses may use verbal enlightenment therapy to encourage and praise the patients who just recover from severe illness. For patients with paralysis, nurses may use emotional transference and dispositional change therapy to divert their attention and prevent them from getting pessimistic and anxious.

（4）Medication nursing. A dosage of 100~150 mL decoction per day, taken 3~4 times per day.

（5）Manipulation techniques. ① Spine pinching therapy: lift and pinch the governor vessel and bladder meridian of foot-taiyang on the back for 3~5 minutes to promote recovery, once per day. ② Acupressure therapy: select Zusanli（ST 36）, Xuehai（SP 10）, Taixi（KI 3）, Hegu（LI 4）, and Baihui（GV 20）; perform thumb kneading manipulation on each of them until the area turns hot or the patient has the feelings of soreness, numbness, distension and heaviness in the area, once per day; this is effective for hand-foot-mouth patients with flaccid paralysis and should best be given early in the recovery phase.

Patient Education

The key to preventing hand-foot-mouth disease is maintaining good personal hygiene. Hands should be washed before meals, after using the bathroom, or returning from outdoors. Clothes should be exposed to strong sunlight. Items that patients are frequently exposed to should be sterilized regularly with moderately or highly effective disinfectants. During the pandemic of the disease, the patients should avoid going to public places that are crowded, poorly ventilated or humid.

Patients may wear sachets made with herbal medicine that clears heat and removes toxin as well as dispels filth with aromatic herbs, such as huoxiang（agastache）, peilan（eupatorium）, and aiye（mugwort leaf）. Patients should also be more physically active, have adequate sleep and avoid overstrain and unboiled water. Besides, the diet should be light, nutritious and digestible.

Healthy children should not contact patients with hand-foot-mouth disease or their virus-contaminated items such as towels, handkerchiefs, tooth glasses, toys, table wares, milk containers, bedding and underwear. Sick children should be put in strict respiratory tract quarantine and digestive tract quarantine. Their vomitus, excrea and utensils should be thoroughly sterilized. Their clothes and bedding should be clean, soft and minimally irritating. For patients with herpes on the bottom, urine and feces should be cleaned in time to keep the area dry and clean.

参 考 文 献

1. 孙秋华. 中医护理学［M］. 4 版. 北京：人民卫生出版社,2017.

2. 徐桂华,张先庚. 中医临床护理学［M］. 2 版. 北京：人民卫生出版社,2007.

3. 孙秋华. 中医临床护理学［M］. 3 版. 北京：中国中医药出版社,2016.

4. 胡慧. 中医临床护理学［M］. 北京：人民卫生出版社,2016.

5. 中医病证分类与代码：GB/T 15657—2021［S］. 北京：中国标准出版社,2021.

6. 中医临床诊疗术语：GB/T 16751—1997［S］. 北京：中国标准出版社,1997.

7. 国家中医药管理局医政司. 33 个病种中医护理方案［M］. 北京：中国中医药出版社,2014.

8. 国家中医药管理局医政司. 19 个病种中医护理方案［M］. 北京：中国中医药出版社,2015.

9. 刘秀英. 中医护理技术［M］. 北京：人民卫生出版社,2005.

10. 杨英豪,潘晓彦. 中医临证施护［M］. 北京：中国中医药出版社,2019.

11. 贺永清. 中医辨证护理学［M］. 西安：陕西科学技术出版社,1986.

12. 王莉. 实用中医护理方案手册［M］. 武汉：华中科技大学出版社,2020.

13. 张廷模. 临床中药学［M］. 北京：中国中医药出版社,2004.

14. 施洪飞,方泓. 中医食疗学［M］. 北京：中国中医药出版社,2016.

15. 广州中医药大学《中医饮食调补学》编委会. 中医饮食调补学［M］. 广州：广东科技出版社,
2002.

16. 夏翔,施杞. 中国食疗大全［M］. 3 版. 上海：上海科学技术出版社,2011.

17. 周文泉. 中国药膳辨证治疗学［M］. 北京：人民卫生出版社,2002.

18. 陈佩仪. 中医护理学基础［M］. 2 版. 北京：人民卫生出版社,2017.

19. 丁晓群. 江西省护理技术操作规程［M］. 南昌：江西科学技术出版社,2020.

20. 金宏柱,李照国. 推拿学［M］. 2 版. 北京：人民卫生出版社,2007.

21. 针灸技术操作规范：GB/T 21709—2008［S］. 北京：中国中医药出版社,2008.

22. 中华中医药学会. 中医治未病技术操作规范（一）：T/CACM 1075—1076—2018［S］. 北京：中国
中医药出版社,2019.

23. 戴新娟. 中医护理健康教育［M］. 长沙：湖南科学技术出版社,2003.

24. 刘玉珍. 中医标准护理计划·内科分册［M］. 长沙：湖南科学技术出版社,2003.

25. 张伯礼,吴勉华. 中医内科学［M］. 4 版. 北京：中国中医药出版社,2017.

26. 王永炎. 中医内科学[M]. 2版. 北京：人民卫生出版社,2011.

27. 余小萍,方祝元. 中医内科学[M]. 3版. 上海：上海科学技术出版社,2018.

28. 张伯礼. 中医内科学[M]. 北京：中国中医药出版社,2019.

29. 韦绪性,杨德全. 中医内科学[M]. 北京：中国中医药出版社,2015.

30. 张伯礼,薛博瑜. 中医内科学[M]. 2版. 北京：人民卫生出版社,2012.

31. 葛均波,徐永健,王辰. 内科学[M]. 9版. 北京：人民卫生出版社,2018.

32. 中华中医药学会. 中医外科常见病诊疗指南[M]. 北京：中国中医药出版社,2012.

33. 中华中医药学会. 中医外科临床诊疗指南[M]. 北京：中国中医药出版社,2020.

34. 朱仁康. 中医外科学[M]. 北京：人民卫生出版社,1987.

35. 艾儒棣. 中医外科学[M]. 成都：四川科学技术出版社,1991.

36. 谭新华,陆德铭. 中医外科学[M]. 北京：人民卫生出版社,1999.

37. 巫和蓉,张素秋. 中医标准护理计划·外科分册[M]. 长沙：湖南科学技术出版社,2003.

38. 陈红风. 中医外科学[M]. 4版. 北京：中国中医药出版社,2016.

39. 何清湖,秦国政. 中医外科学[M]. 3版. 北京：人民卫生出版社,2016.

40. 陈孝平,汪建平,赵继宗. 外科学[M]. 9版. 北京：人民卫生出版社,2018.

41. 张学军,郑捷. 皮肤性病学[M]. 9版. 北京：人民卫生出版社,2018.

42. 中华中医药学会. 中医妇科常见病诊疗指南[M]. 北京：中国中医药出版社,2012.

43. 中华中医药学会. 中医妇科临床诊疗指南[M]. 北京：中国中医药出版社,2019.

44. 林金萍,王庆国. 中医标准护理计划·妇产科、儿科分册[M]. 长沙：湖南科学技术出版社,2003.

45. 马宝璋,杜惠兰. 中医妇科学[M]. 3版. 上海：上海科学技术出版社,2018.

46. 罗颂平,刘雁峰. 中医妇科学[M]. 3版. 北京：人民卫生出版社,2016.

47. 罗颂平,孙卓君. 中医妇科学[M]. 北京：科学出版社,2007.

48. 谈勇. 中医妇科学[M]. 北京：人民卫生出版社,2007.

49. 谢幸,孔北华,段涛. 妇产科学[M]. 9版. 北京：人民卫生出版社,2018.

50. 中华中医药学会. 中医儿科常见病诊疗指南[M]. 北京：中国中医药出版社,2012.

51. 中华中医药学会. 中医儿科临床诊疗指南[M]. 北京：中国中医药出版社,2020.

52. 马融. 中医儿科学[M]. 4版. 北京：中国中医药出版社,2016.

53. 孟陆亮. 中医儿科学[M]. 2版. 北京：中国中医药出版社,2018.

54. 姜之炎,赵霞. 中医儿科学[M]. 2版. 上海：上海科学技术出版社,2020.

55. 马融. 中医儿科学[M]. 2版. 北京：人民卫生出版社,2012.

56. 王卫平,孙锟,常立文. 儿科学[M]. 9版. 北京：人民卫生出版社,2018.

57. 李振吉. 中医基本名词术语中英对照国际标准[M]. 北京：人民卫生出版社,2008.

58. 李照国. 中医基本名词术语英译国际标准化研究——理论研究、实践总结、方法探索[M]. 上海：上海科学技术出版社,2008.

59. 李照国. 汉英双解中医临床标准术语辞典[M]. 上海：上海科学技术出版社,2017.

60. 李照国. 中医英语翻译教程[M]. 上海：上海三联书店,2019.

61. 李照国. 简明汉英中医词典［M］. 上海：上海科学技术出版社,2002.

62. 谢竹藩. 中医药常用名词术语英译［M］. 北京：中国中医药出版社,2005.

63. 金魁和. 汉英医学大词典［M］. 2 版. 北京：人民卫生出版社,2004.

64. Li Zhenji, He Xingdong, Wang Kui. International Standard Chinese-English Basic Nomenclature of Chinese Medicine［M］. Beijing：People's Medical Publishing House, 2008.

65. Word Health Organization (Western Pacific Region). WHO International Standard Terminologies on Traditional Medicine in the Western Pacific Region［M］. Beijing：Pecking University Medical Press, 2009.

66. Huang Longxiang, Gang Weijuan. WHO Standard Acupuncture Point Locations in the Western Pacific Region［M］. Beijing：People's Medical Publishing House, 2010.

67. Nigel Wiseman. Dictionary of Chinese Medicine［M］. 2nd ed. Changsha：Hunan Science & Technology Press, 2006.

68. Wu Changguo, Zhu Zhongbao. Basic Theory of Traditional Chinese Medicine［M］. Shanghai：Shanghai Pujiang Education Press, 2002.

69. Sun Guangren, Douglas Darwin Eisenstark, Zhang Qingrong. Fundamentals of Chinese Medicine (International Standard Library of Chinese Medicine)［M］. Beijing：People's Medical Publishing House, 2008.

70. Chen Jiaxu, Jane Frances Wilson. Diagnostics in Chinese Medicine (International Standard Library of Chinese Medicine)［M］. Beijing：People's Medical Publishing House, 2011.

71. Peng Bo, Xie Jianqun. Traditional Chinese Internal Medicine［M］. 2nd ed. Beijing：People's Medical Publishing House, 2000.

72. Zhai Yachun, Huang Guoqi. Surgery of Traditional Chinese Medicine［M］. Shanghai：Publishing House of Shanghai University of Traditional Chinese Medicine, 2002.

73. Tan Yong, Li Zhaoguo, Cheng Peili. Gynecology of Traditional Chinese Medicine［M］. Shanghai：Shanghai Pujiang Education Press, 2002.

74. Wang Shouchuan. Pediatrics in Chinese Medicine［M］. Beijing：People's Medical Publishing House, 2011.

75. Jin Hongzhu, Li Zhaoguo. Science of Tuina［M］. 2nd ed. Beijing：People's Medical Publishing House, 2012.

76. Ge Meifei, Shan Baozhi, Guo Xiaolin. Three-Character-Scripture School Pediatric Massage［M］. Beijing：China Press of Traditional Chinese Medicine, 2016.